生物医用高分子
在皮肤疾病诊疗和健康中的应用
（双语版）

主　　编　朱锦涛　陶　娟

副 主 编　张连斌

编　　者　（按姓氏笔画排序）

邓仁华　华中科技大学化学与化工学院

朱今巾　华中科技大学同济医学院附属协和医院

朱锦涛　华中科技大学化学与化工学院

刘奕静　华中科技大学化学与化工学院

刘倩倩　华中科技大学化学与化工学院

安湘杰　华中科技大学同济医学院附属协和医院

许江平　华中科技大学化学与化工学院

李　延　华中科技大学同济医学院附属协和医院

李　军　华中科技大学同济医学院附属武汉中心医院

李钰策　华中科技大学化学与化工学院

杨　井　华中科技大学同济医学院附属协和医院

杨　柳　华中科技大学同济医学院附属协和医院

张连斌　华中科技大学化学与化工学院

陈森斌　华中科技大学化学与化工学院

周诺娅　华中科技大学同济医学院附属协和医院

索慧男　华中科技大学同济医学院附属协和医院

陶　娟　华中科技大学同济医学院附属协和医院

董励耘　华中科技大学同济医学院附属协和医院

蒋　皓　华中科技大学化学与化工学院

谢　君　武汉大学中南医院

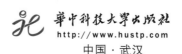

华中科技大学出版社

http://www.hustp.com

中国·武汉

内 容 简 介

　　本教材共分为十一章,每一章均用中、英双语进行介绍。内容包括皮肤结构与功能,皮肤健康与代表性皮肤疾病,生物医用高分子简介,皮肤防护、清洁与消毒,皮肤影像学诊断技术,高分子纳米药物载体及其在皮肤疾病治疗中的应用,生物医用高分子在黑素瘤免疫治疗中的应用,透皮给药技术,生物医用高分子在皮肤美容中的应用,可穿戴电子皮肤器件,生物医用高分子在皮肤伤口修复中的应用。

　　本教材可供高等院校高分子科学、材料化学、化学生物学、生物医学、临床医学相关专业的研究生(含留学生)使用,也可作为选修课教材供高年级本科生(含留学生)使用,亦可作为相关专业青年教师和科研人员的自学参考书。

图书在版编目(CIP)数据

　　生物医用高分子在皮肤疾病诊疗和健康中的应用:双语版:英、汉/朱锦涛,陶娟主编.—武汉:华中科技大学出版社,2021.12
　　ISBN 978-7-5680-7695-1

　　Ⅰ.①生… Ⅱ.①朱… ②陶… Ⅲ.①生物材料-医用高分子材料-应用-皮肤病-诊疗-英、汉 Ⅳ.①R751

中国版本图书馆 CIP 数据核字(2021)第 262625 号

生物医用高分子在皮肤疾病诊疗和健康中的应用(双语版)	朱锦涛　陶　娟　主编

Shengwu Yiyong Gaofenzi zai Pifu Jibing Zhenliao he Jiankang zhong de Yingyong(Shuangyu Ban)

策划编辑:余　雯
责任编辑:丁　平　曾奇峰
封面设计:原色设计
责任校对:李　琴
责任监印:周治超
出版发行:华中科技大学出版社(中国·武汉)　　电话:(027)81321913
　　　　　武汉市东湖新技术开发区华工科技园　　邮编:430223
录　　排:华中科技大学惠友文印中心
印　　刷:湖北恒泰印务有限公司
开　　本:787mm×1092mm　1/16
印　　张:31.5
字　　数:800 千字
版　　次:2021 年 12 月第 1 版第 1 次印刷
定　　价:149.00 元

主/编/简/介

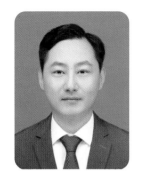

朱锦涛　教授，博士生导师。现任华中科技大学化学与化工学院院长、材料成形与模具技术国家重点实验室副主任、能量转换与存储材料化学教育部重点实验室常务副主任、中国化学会理事、中国化学会高分子学科委员会委员。国家杰出青年科学基金获得者、国家"万人计划"科技创新领军人才、科技部中青年科技创新领军人才、英国皇家化学学会会士、中国化学会青年化学奖获得者。主要从事聚合物有序结构材料的构筑及其光电存储性能、生物医用与防护材料及其在组织修复与治疗领域应用的研究。在 *Nat Commun*、*JACS*、*Angew Chem Int Ed*、*Adv Mater*，*Biomaterials*、*Macromolecules* 等期刊上发表论文230余篇，参与编写中英文专著3部，授权国家发明专利30余项。

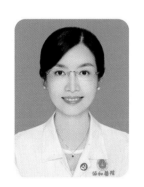

陶　娟　教授，主任医师，博士生导师，长江学者特岗教授。华中科技大学同济医学院附属协和医院皮肤性病科主任，皮肤疾病诊疗与健康湖北省工程研究中心主任。目前担任中国医师协会皮肤科医师分会副会长、中华医学会皮肤性病学分会委员、中国女医师协会皮肤病专家委员会副主任委员、全国卫生产业企业管理协会护肤技术发展分会副会长、湖北省医学会皮肤科学分会候任主任委员等。主要从事重症皮肤疾病免疫机制和临床转化研究，获国之名医、全国优秀科技工作者等荣誉称号，获宝钢优秀教师奖、湖北省科学技术进步奖一等奖等奖项。参编9部教材或担任副主编。担任 *JAAD* 杂志中文版的副主编、*BJD* 杂志的 Editorial Consultants。

前言

Qianyan

　　交叉是学科发展重要的原动力。许多新理论、新发明的产生,都是建立在学科交叉的基础上的;增强学科交叉融合的意识,积极探索学科交叉融合的有效途径,是学科发展的重要手段之一。生物医学的发展、新的诊疗手段的出现,都离不开相关学科的快速发展与提升。生物医用高分子在临床医学(特别是皮肤疾病诊疗和健康)的发展过程中发挥着越来越重要的作用,引起了研究者广泛的兴趣。在华中科技大学创新研究院的支持下,我们开设了交叉学科研究生高水平课程,并在教学实践基础上编写了研究生教材《生物医用高分子在皮肤疾病诊疗和健康中的应用(双语版)》。

　　本教材编写人员包括临床经验丰富的一线医生和多年来从事功能高分子、生物医用高分子材料研究的教学科研人员,凝结了编写人员多年来在科研创新、交叉融合与教学探索中的体会与心得。本教材以临床问题为导向,结合高分子材料科学的发展,系统地介绍了生物医用高分子材料在皮肤疾病的诊断、治疗和皮肤美容等方面的应用。本教材以解决临床工作中面临的实际问题为出发点,介绍了生物医用高分子材料的设计与制备原则、生物医用高分子在解决这些问题中发挥的关键作用,不断打通材料科学与临床医学间的学科壁垒、架起基础研究与临床应用的桥梁,有望在培养学科交叉复合型高级人才方面发挥积极作用。同时,本教材具有如下特点:①以临床问题为主线安排各章结构,应用性强;②双语编写,有助于学生了解国际前沿,适用于相关专业的留学生和研究生学习;③设有思考题和扩展阅读,有助于学生开阔思维、拓宽知识面;④设有挑战与展望,增加了学习的挑战性。本教材的适用对象以高等院校高分子科学、材料科学、化学生物学、生物医学、临床医学相关专业的研究生(含留学生)为主,有助于培养学生思考和解决临床问题的能力,深化对生物医用高分子材料的理解,同时也可作为选修课教材供高年级本科生(含留学生)使用。此外,本教材亦可作为相关专业的青年教师和科研人员的自学参考书。

　　本教材由李军、陶娟编写第一章,杨柳、安湘杰、索慧男、杨井、董励耘编写第二章,陈森斌、朱锦涛编写第三章,周诺娅、陶娟编写第四章,蒋皓编写第五章,邓仁华、刘奕静、李钰策编写第六章,刘倩倩、谢君、刘奕静编写第七章,朱今巾编写第八章,李延编写第九章,许江平编写第十章,张连斌编写第十一章。本教材由朱锦涛、陶娟任主编,张连斌任副主编。

　　本教材在编写过程中得到了华中科技大学出版社的大力支持,在此表示衷心的感谢。本教材覆盖的知识面广,编者的经验和水平有限,书中难免有缺漏和不当之处,恳请广大专家和读者提出批评和建议。

编　者

目录

■■ Mulu

第一章
皮肤结构与功能

第一节　皮肤的结构

皮肤覆于体表,与人体所处的外界环境直接接触,是人体的第一道防线,具有十分重要的功能。皮肤结构通常被分为三层:表皮、真皮和皮下组织。表皮和真皮之间由基底膜带相连接。皮肤中除各种皮肤附属器(如毛发、皮脂腺、汗腺和甲等)外,还含有丰富的血管、淋巴管、神经和肌肉。皮肤是人体最大的器官,总重量约占体重的 16%,成人皮肤总面积约为 1.5 m^2,新生儿皮肤总面积约为 0.21 m^2。皮肤厚度存在个体、年龄和部位的差异,通常为 $0.5\sim4.0$ mm。眼睑、外阴、乳房处的皮肤较薄,厚度为 $0.8\sim1.4$ mm;掌跖部位皮肤较厚,可达 $3\sim4$ mm。皮肤颜色因种族、年龄、性别、营养状况及部位不同而有所差异。

一、表皮

表皮为复层鳞状上皮,主要由角质形成细胞、黑素细胞、朗格汉斯细胞和梅克尔细胞等构成。

(一)角质形成细胞

角质形成细胞是表皮的主要细胞,起源于外胚层,具有产生角蛋白的功能。角蛋白是角质形成细胞的主要结构蛋白之一,可作为细胞骨架维持细胞结构并参与表皮分化、角化等生理病理过程。根据角质形成细胞的分化阶段和特点可以将表皮分为 5 层,由深至浅分别为基底层、棘层、颗粒层、透明层和角质层(图 1-1)。

(1) 基底层:位于表皮底层,由一层圆柱状基底细胞所组成,通常排列整齐,如栅栏状;其长轴与表皮和真皮之间的交界线垂直。基底细胞胞质具有深嗜碱性,胞核呈卵圆形,核仁明显,核分裂现象较常见,胞核上方可见黑素颗粒聚集或呈帽状排列。通常,基底细胞之间以及与其上方的棘细胞之间通过细胞间桥相连接。基底细胞的底部借半桥粒附着于表皮下基底膜带,此带在 HE 染色时不易辨认,只有用特殊染色剂(如过碘酸-希夫(PAS))染色时方能显示。基底细胞表达角蛋白 K5/K14。

基底细胞经分裂、逐渐分化成熟为角质层细胞,并最终从皮肤表面脱落,这是一个受到精密调控的过程。正常情况下,约 30% 的基底细胞处于核分裂期,新生的角质形成细胞有序上

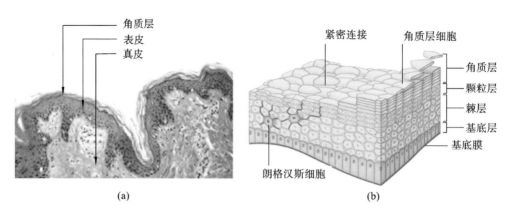

图 1-1　皮肤结构示意图

(a)皮肤 HE 染色；(b)表皮结构示意图

Figure 1-1　Illustration showing the skin structure

(a)HE staining of the skin；(b) Illustration showing the structure of the epidermis

移，由基底层移行至颗粒层约需 14 天，再移行至角质层表面并脱落又需要 14 天(共 28 天)，这一过程被称为表皮通过时间或更替时间。

(2) 棘层：位于基底层上方，此层由 4～8 层多角形细胞构成。越接近表层，细胞形态越扁平。每个细胞有很多胞质突，称为棘突，因此这层细胞也被称为棘细胞。正常皮肤的棘突在高倍镜下看不清楚，但当存在细胞间水肿时，棘突则清晰可见。电镜下可见胞质内有许多张力细丝聚集成束，并附着于桥粒上；棘层上部细胞胞质中散在分布有直径为 100～300 nm 的包膜颗粒，称为角质小体或 Odland 小体。棘细胞表达角蛋白 K1/K10。

(3) 颗粒层：位于棘层上方，通常由 1～3 层扁平或菱形细胞组成，细胞长轴与皮面平行。胞质内充满粗大、深嗜碱性的透明角质颗粒。正常皮肤颗粒层的厚度与角质层的厚度成正比，在角质层薄的部位，颗粒层仅 1～3 层；而在角质层厚的部位(如掌跖)，颗粒层则较厚，可多达 10 层。此层细胞中细胞核和细胞器溶解，胞质中可见大量形态不规则的透明角质颗粒沉积于张力细丝束之间。

(4) 透明层：位于颗粒层和角质层之间，仅见于掌跖等表皮较厚的部位，特别是在足跟部位皮肤组织切片中，此层最明显。此层由 2～3 层较扁平细胞构成。细胞界限不清，易被伊红染色，光学显微镜下胞质呈均质状并有强折光性。

(5) 角质层：位于表皮最上层，由 5～20 层已经死亡的扁平细胞构成，在掌跖部位可厚达 40～50 层。细胞正常结构消失，染色呈嗜酸性；胞质中充满由张力细丝与均质状物质结合而形成的角蛋白。角质层上部细胞间桥粒消失或形成残体，故易于脱落。由于角质层外层不断脱落，因此其厚度难以确定。在福尔马林固定的标本中，角质层内因有较大的细胞内外间隙，往往呈网状。

(二) 黑素细胞

黑素细胞起源于外胚层的神经嵴，位于表皮基底层和毛囊，约占基底细胞总数的 10%。黑素细胞数量随不同身体部位和年龄而异，且在紫外线反复照射后可增多。不同种族人群黑素细胞数量和分布无明显差异，肤色的差异主要是由于其产生的黑素的量和分布的不同。HE 染色切片中，黑素细胞有一小而浓染的核和透明的胞质，故又名透明细胞。但在常规切片中并非所有见到的透明细胞都是黑素细胞,因为基底细胞偶尔也可出现人工性的皱缩,这种皱缩的基底细胞与黑素细胞很难区分。黑素细胞具有生成黑素的功能,因此其多巴反应呈阳性。同时,由于其含有黑素,故银染色呈阳性。黑素可通过黑素细胞的树突状突起输送到基底细胞内。透射电镜下观察可见,黑素细胞胞质内可见特征性黑素小体,黑素小体是含酪氨酸酶的细胞器,是合成黑素的场所。1 个黑素细胞可通过其树枝状突起向周围 10～36 个角质形成细胞提供黑素,称为表皮黑素单元。黑素能遮挡和反射紫外线,保护真皮和深部组织(图 1-2)。

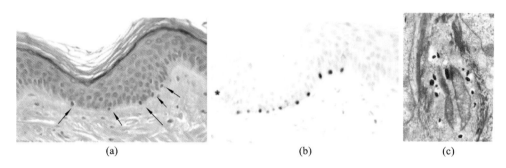

(a)　　　　　　　　(b)　　　　　　　　(c)

图 1-2　黑素细胞的形态、分布与透射电镜图

(a)HE 染色(箭头所示为黑素细胞);(b)免疫组化染色;(c)黑素细胞透射电镜照片

Figure 1-2　The morphology, distribution and transmission electron microscope image of melanocytes

(a)HE staining(arrows:melanocytes);(b)Immunohistochemistry staining;(c)Transmission electron microscope

(三)朗格汉斯细胞

朗格汉斯细胞(Langerhans cell)是起源于骨髓单核-巨噬细胞的免疫活性细胞,分布于基底层以上的表皮和毛囊上皮中,占表皮细胞总数的 3%～5%。朗格汉斯细胞的密度因部位不同而异,一般面颈部较多而掌跖部较少。若用氯化金浸染,朗格汉斯细胞可呈树突状细胞形态,但其多巴反应呈阴性,而 ATP 酶反应呈阳性。光学显微镜下,这类细胞呈多角形,胞质透明,胞核较小并呈分叶状,线粒体、高尔基体和内质网丰富,并有溶酶体。电子显微镜下,其胞质内有独特的伯贝克颗粒,可与黑素细胞区分(图 1-3)。目前,伯贝克颗粒被认为是由朗格汉斯细胞吞噬外来抗原时包膜内陷形成的,其是一种消化细胞外物质的吞噬体或抗原储存形式。表皮定居朗格汉斯细胞可识别、摄取、加工并呈递抗原给 T 细胞,在抗肿瘤免疫应答中发挥重要作用。朗格汉斯细胞具有多种表面标志,包括 IgG 和 IgE 的 FcR、C3b 受体、MHCⅡ类分子(如 HLA-DR、DP、DQ)及 CD4、CD45、S-100 等抗原。朗格汉斯细胞表面的特异性标志为CD1a 和 Langerin(CD207)(见扩展阅读 1)。

(四)梅克尔细胞

梅克尔细胞是位于表皮基底层内的触觉感受细胞,多见于掌跖、口腔与生殖器黏膜、甲床及毛囊漏斗部;细胞有短指状突起,借助桥粒与周围的角质形成细胞连接,常固定于基底膜,不随角质形成细胞向上迁移。梅克尔细胞在光学显微镜下难以辨认。在哺乳动物有毛皮肤中,梅克尔细胞聚集成盘状,形态较特殊,称为毛盘或梅克尔盘。在银染色切片中,每个梅克尔细胞基底部紧贴一个半月板样的神经末梢,形成梅克尔盘,并有一根感觉神经纤维在梅克尔盘处终止。梅克尔细胞在感觉敏锐部位(如指尖和鼻尖)密度较大,这些部位的神经纤维在临近表皮时失去髓鞘,扁盘状的轴突末端与梅克尔细胞基底面形成突触样结构,构成梅克尔细胞-轴突复合体,可能具有非神经末梢介导的感觉作用。

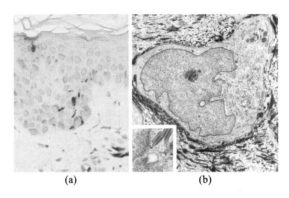

(a)   (b)

图 1-3　朗格汉斯细胞的形态、分布与透射电镜图

(a)免疫组化染色,红色为朗格汉斯细胞;(b)朗格汉斯细胞的透射电镜照片,左下角小图为伯贝克颗粒

Figure 1-3　The morphology, distribution and transmission electron microscope image of Langerhans cells

(a)Immunohistochemistry staining(red ones:Langerhans cells);(b)Transmission electron microscope(lower left: Birbeck granule)

（五）角质形成细胞间及其与真皮间的连接

（1）桥粒:表皮角质形成细胞之间主要通过桥粒连接,其他连接方式还有黏附连接、空隙连接和紧密连接。桥粒是角质形成细胞间连接的主要结构,由相邻细胞的局部胞膜发生卵圆形致密增厚而形成。电镜下桥粒呈盘状,为成对的纽扣样结构,直径为 $0.2 \sim 0.5 \mu m$,厚度为 $30 \sim 60 nm$,其中央有 $20 \sim 30 nm$ 宽的电子透明间隙,内含低密度张力细丝;间隙中央电子密度较高的致密层称中央层;中央层的中间还可见一条更深染的间线,为高度嗜锇层。构成桥粒的相邻细胞膜内侧各有一增厚的盘状附着板,长 $0.2 \sim 0.3 \mu m$,厚度约为 $30 nm$。许多直径约为 $10 nm$ 的张力细丝呈袢状附于附着板上,又折回到胞质内。另外,尚有较细的跨膜细丝起于附着板内部,延伸至细胞间隙,与中央层的细丝交错相连(图 1-4)。构成桥粒的蛋白质主要包括以下两种:①跨膜蛋白,主要由桥粒芯糖蛋白和桥粒芯胶蛋白构成,它们形成桥粒的电子透明细胞间隙和细胞间接触层;②胞质内的桥粒斑是盘状附着板的组成部分,主要由桥粒斑蛋

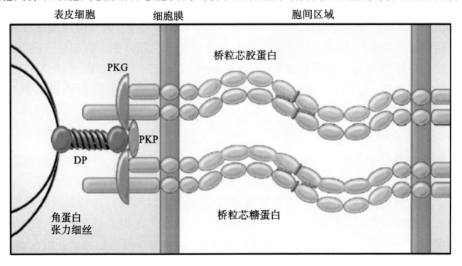

图 1-4　桥粒结构示意图

Figure 1-4　Illustration showing the structure of desmosome

白和桥粒斑珠蛋白构成。桥粒本身有很强的抗牵张力,而相邻细胞间由张力细丝构成的连续结构网进一步加固了细胞间的紧密连接。桥粒结构的破坏可导致角质形成细胞相互分离,形成表皮内水疱,导致大疱性皮肤病的发生,如天疱疮。

(2)半桥粒:基底细胞与下方基底膜带之间的主要连接结构,由基底层角质形成细胞真皮侧胞膜的不规则突起与基底膜带相互嵌合形成的类似于半个桥粒的结构,但其构成蛋白与桥粒有很大不同。在电子显微镜观察下,半桥粒内侧部分为高密度附着斑,基底细胞的角蛋白张力细丝附着于其上;胞膜外侧部分为亚基底致密斑。两侧致密斑与中央胞膜构成夹心饼样结构。致密斑中含大疱性类天疱疮抗原 1 或 2(BPAG1 或 BPAG2)、整合素等蛋白质(图1-5)。

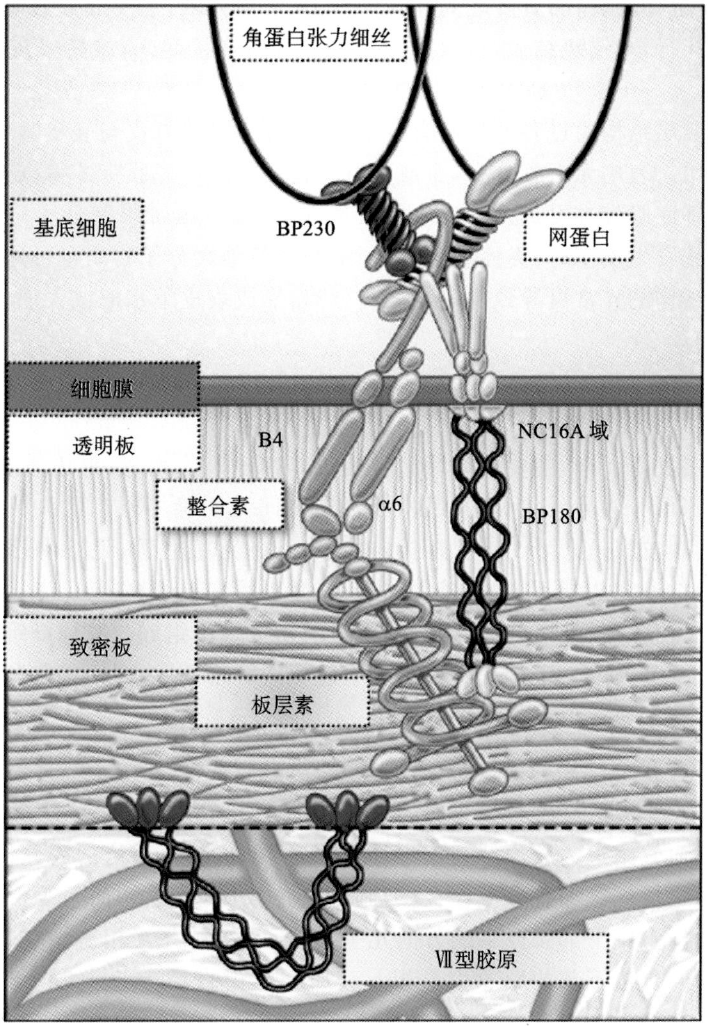

图 1-5 半桥粒结构示意图

Figure 1-5 Illustration showing the structure of hemidesmosome

(3)基底膜带:位于真皮与表皮之间。光学显微镜下,PAS 染色(过碘酸-希夫反应)可将基底膜带染成一条 $0.5\sim1.0~\mu m$ 的紫红色均质带,银浸染法可染成黑色。皮肤附属器与真皮之间、血管周围也存在基底膜。电子显微镜下基底膜带由胞膜层、透明层、致密层和致密下层四层结构组成。

①胞膜层:主要由基底层角质形成细胞真皮侧的胞质膜所构成(厚度约 8 nm),半桥粒横跨其间,半桥粒细胞侧借助附着斑与胞质内张力细丝相连接;另一侧借助多种跨膜蛋白(如BPAG2、整合素 $\alpha_6\beta_4$ 等)与透明层黏附,在基底膜带中形成"铆钉"样连接。

②透明层:位于半桥粒及基底细胞底部细胞膜之下(厚度为 35~40 nm),因电子密度低而显得透明。主要成分为板层素及其异构体组成的细胞外基质和锚丝,锚丝可穿过透明层达致密层,具有连接和固定作用。

③致密层:带状结构(厚度为 35~45 nm),主要成分为Ⅳ型胶原和少量板层素。Ⅳ型胶原分子间交联形成高度稳定的连续三维网格,是基底膜带的重要支撑结构。

④致密下层:也称网板,与真皮之间互相移行,无明显界限,主要成分为Ⅶ型胶原。致密下层中有锚原纤维穿行,与锚斑结合,将致密层和下方真皮连接起来,维持表皮与下方结缔组织之间的连接。

基底膜带的四层结构通过各种机制有机结合在一起,除使真皮与表皮紧密连接外,还具有渗透和屏障等作用。表皮无血管分布,血液中营养物质通过基底膜带才得以进入表皮,而表皮的代谢产物通过基底膜带方可进入真皮。一般情况下,基底膜带限制分子量大于 40000 的大分子通过。但当其发生损伤时,炎症细胞、肿瘤细胞及其他大分子物质也可通过基底膜带进入表皮。基底膜带结构的异常可导致真皮与表皮分离,形成表皮下水疱或大疱,代表性疾病为类天疱疮(见扩展阅读2)。

二、真皮

真皮由中胚层发育而来,主要由结缔组织构成,含有神经、血管、淋巴管、肌肉和皮肤附属器。真皮由浅至深可分为乳头层和网状层,但两层之间无明确界限。乳头层为凸向表皮底部的乳头状隆起,与表皮突呈犬牙交错状相接,内含丰富的毛细血管、毛细淋巴管和感觉神经末梢。网状层较厚,位于乳头层下方,有较大的血管、淋巴管和神经穿行。

真皮结缔组织由胶原纤维、弹性纤维、基质以及众多细胞组成。胶原纤维和弹性纤维互相交织在一起,分散于基质内。正常真皮中的细胞包括成纤维细胞、组织细胞和肥大细胞等。胶原纤维、弹性纤维和基质都由成纤维细胞产生。

(一)胶原纤维

真皮结缔组织中,胶原纤维最为丰富,HE 染色呈浅红色,其直径为 2~15 μm。真皮乳头层、表皮附属器和血管附近的胶原纤维细小且无一定取向,其他部位的胶原纤维均结合成束。在胶原束中,有少量成纤维细胞分散存在,细胞核染色较深,其纵切面呈菱形。真皮中的胶原束由上至下逐渐增粗,中下部胶原束的方向几乎与皮面平行,并互相交织在一起;在同一水平面向各个方向延伸,真皮下部的胶原束最粗。胶原纤维由直径为 70~140 nm 的胶原原纤维聚合而成,主要成分为Ⅰ型胶原,也有少量Ⅲ型胶原。胶原纤维伸展性较差,但很坚韧,对平行拉力抵抗力很强。

(二)网状纤维

网状纤维(直径仅为 0.2~1.0 μm)并非独立的纤维成分,而是幼稚、纤细的未成熟胶原纤维,HE 染色难以显示,但因其具有嗜银性,可用硝酸银溶液浸染而呈黑色,故又称嗜银纤维。在胚胎时期,网状纤维最早出现。网状纤维主要分布在乳头层及皮肤附属器、血管周围。在创伤愈合、成纤维细胞增生活跃或有新胶原形成的病变中，网状纤维大量增生。

（三）弹性纤维

弹性纤维直径为 $1\sim3~\mu m$，HE 染色不易辨认，醛品红染色呈紫色。染色后可见弹性纤维缠绕在胶原束之间，呈波浪状，相互交织成网。弹性纤维在真皮下最粗，其排列方向与胶原束相同，与表皮平行。正常真皮内弹性纤维数量较少（占 $2\%\sim4\%$）。弹性纤维具有较强的弹性。

（四）基质

基质是一种无定形物质，主要成分为蛋白多糖、糖蛋白和葡萄糖胺聚糖，存在于纤维和纤维束间隙及细胞间，在正常皮肤中含量甚少。蛋白多糖和葡萄糖胺聚糖复合物具有很强的吸水性，在调节结合水、真皮可塑性方面发挥重要作用。基质参与细胞成分和纤维成分的连接，影响细胞的增殖分化、组织修复和结构重建。

（五）细胞

真皮中的常驻细胞主要包括成纤维细胞、巨噬细胞和肥大细胞，它们主要分布于真皮乳头层、乳头层下的血管周围和胶原纤维束之间。真皮中还含有少量真皮树突状细胞和淋巴细胞等。①成纤维细胞来源于中胚层，能合成、降解纤维和基质等成分，在真皮网络构建和表皮与真皮的联系中发挥重要作用。②巨噬细胞来源于骨髓造血干细胞，其分化为循环中的单核细胞并移行至真皮分化为巨噬细胞，有吞噬、抗原呈递、杀伤病原微生物和肿瘤细胞等作用。③肥大细胞能合成、释放炎症介质，如组胺、肝素、胰蛋白酶等，参与 I 型超敏反应。真皮树突状细胞是真皮中的专职性抗原呈递细胞，能高效地识别并呈递抗原，合成及分泌细胞因子，并迁移至局部引流淋巴结激活 T 细胞诱发免疫应答。

三、皮下组织

皮下组织又称皮下脂肪组织，位于真皮下方；其下与肌膜等组织相连，由疏松结缔组织及脂肪小叶组成。结缔组织包裹脂肪小叶，形成小叶间隔。皮下组织中含有血管、淋巴管、神经、小汗腺和顶泌汗腺等。其厚度随部位、性别及营养状况而异，在臀部和腹部较厚，在鼻部和胸骨部较薄。皮下组织具有提供皮肤弹力、参与脂肪和糖代谢、储存能量及内分泌等功能。

四、皮肤附属器

皮肤附属器包括毛发、毛囊、皮脂腺、汗腺和甲等，均由外胚层分化而来。

（一）毛发和毛囊

毛发由同心圆状排列的角质形成细胞角化而成。掌跖、指（趾）屈面及其末节伸面、唇、乳头、龟头、包皮内侧、小阴唇、大阴唇内侧、阴蒂等部位皮肤无毛，称为无毛皮肤；其他部位均有长短、直径及颜色不同的毛，称为有毛皮肤。通常毛发可分为硬毛与毳毛两种。硬毛粗硬，具有髓质，颜色较深。硬毛又可分为两种：①长毛，如头发、胡须、腋毛与阴毛等；②短毛，如眉毛、睫毛、鼻毛与耳毛等，通常较长毛短。毳毛细软，无髓质，颜色较淡，主要见于面部、四肢和躯干。毛发位于体表可见的部分为毛干，位于皮肤以内的部分为毛根。毛根末端膨大呈葱头状，称为毛球。纵切面上毛干由内向外可分为髓质、皮质和毛小皮。髓质是毛发的中心部分，由 $2\sim3$ 层立方形细胞构成，细胞质染色较淡；在毛发末端通常无髓质。皮质是毛发的主要组成部分,由数层梭形上皮细胞构成;毛小皮为一层薄而透明的角质形成细胞,彼此重叠如屋瓦状(图 1-6)。

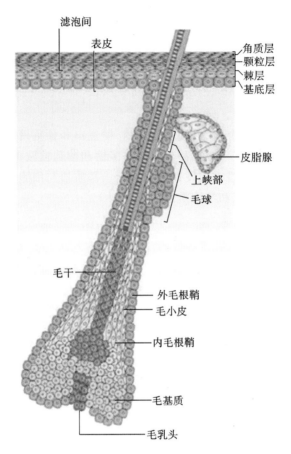

图 1-6　毛发和毛囊结构示意图

Figure 1-6　Illustration showing the structure of hair and hair follicle

毛囊位于真皮和皮下组织中,是毛发生长所必需的结构,由上皮细胞和结缔组织构成。皮脂腺开口于毛囊,自皮脂腺开口以上的部分称为毛囊漏斗部;皮脂腺开口以下至立毛肌附着处之间的部分称为毛囊峡部。毛囊由内、外毛根鞘及结缔组织鞘组成,内、外毛根鞘的细胞均起源于表皮,而结缔组织鞘则起源于真皮。

毛发的生长周期可分为生长期、退行期和休止期(图 1-7),分别约为 3 年、3 周和 3 个月。各部位毛发并非同时生长和脱落,全部毛发中约 80% 处于生长期;正常人每天可脱落 70～100 根头发,同时也有等量的头发再生。毛发性状与遗传、健康状况、激素水平(性激素、甲状腺激素和糖皮质激素等)、药物和气候等多种因素相关。

(二) 皮脂腺

皮脂腺产生皮脂,属于泡状腺体,由腺泡和较短的导管构成。腺泡无腺腔,外层为扁平或立方形细胞,周围有基底膜带和结缔组织包裹,腺体细胞破裂后,细胞内成分(包括脂滴)释出并经导管排出。导管由复层鳞状上皮构成,开口于毛囊上部,位于立毛肌和毛囊的夹角之间,立毛肌收缩可促进皮脂排泄。皮脂腺广泛分布于除掌跖和指(趾)屈侧以外的全身皮肤。头面部和胸背上部等处因皮脂腺较多,称为皮脂溢出部位。在颊黏膜、唇、妇女乳晕、大小阴唇、眼

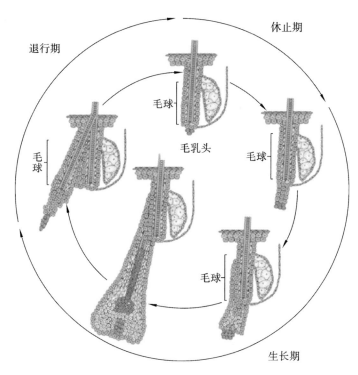

图 1-7 毛发生长周期示意图

Figure 1-7   Illustration showing the hair growth cycle

睑、包皮内侧等无毛皮肤区域,腺导管直接开口于皮肤表面。皮脂腺也有生长周期,但与毛囊的生长周期无关,主要由雄激素水平控制。

（三）汗腺

根据结构和功能不同,人体汗腺可分为小汗腺和顶泌汗腺。

小汗腺也称为外泌汗腺,为单曲管状腺,由分泌部和导管构成。分泌部位于真皮深部和皮下组织,由单层细胞构成,呈管状排列并盘绕呈球状;导管部由两层小立方形细胞组成,管径较小,穿过真皮,直接开口于汗孔。除唇、鼓膜、甲床、乳头、包皮内侧、龟头、小阴唇及阴蒂外,小汗腺遍布全身,以掌跖、腋窝、额部较多,背部较少。小汗腺主要调节体温,手掌、足底部位的小汗腺还有提高触觉敏感度以及增强黏附性的作用。小汗腺受交感神经系统支配,神经递质是乙酰胆碱。

顶泌汗腺也称为大汗腺,属于大管状腺体,由分泌部和导管构成,主要分布在腋窝、乳晕、脐周、会阴部,偶见于面部、头皮和躯干。此外,外耳道耵聍腺、眼睑的睫腺也属于顶泌汗腺。其分泌部位于皮下脂肪层,腺体为一层扁平、立方形或柱状分泌细胞,其外有肌上皮细胞和基底膜带。导管的结构与小汗腺相似,但其直径约为小汗腺导管的 10 倍;开口于毛囊上部皮脂腺开口的上方,偶尔直接开口于皮肤表面。顶泌汗腺的分泌主要受性激素影响,青春期分泌旺盛。顶泌汗腺也受交感神经系统支配,神经递质为去甲肾上腺素。

（四）甲

甲是人体最大的皮肤附属器,覆盖于指（趾）末端伸面,由多层紧密排列的角质形成细胞构成。甲的主要功能包括保护指（趾）尖、提高感觉辨别能力、辅助手指完成精细动作、搔抓及美学功能。甲的外露部分称为甲板,呈外凸的长方形,甲近端的新月状淡色区称为甲半月;甲板周围的皮肤称为甲廓,深入近端皮肤中的甲板部分称为甲根;甲板下方的皮肤称为甲床,其中位于甲根下方者称为甲母质,是甲板的生发结构。甲下真皮富含血管。指甲生长速度约为每3个月1 cm,趾甲生长速度约为每9个月1 cm。甲的性状和生长速度受到疾病、营养状况、环境和生活习惯等因素的影响。

五、皮肤的神经、脉管及肌肉

(一) 神经

皮肤中有丰富的神经纤维,可分为感觉神经和运动神经。通过与中枢神经系统联系感受各种刺激,支配靶器官活动,完成各类神经反射。皮肤的神经支配具有节段性,但相邻的节段间有部分重叠。神经纤维多分布在真皮和皮下组织中。

1. 感觉神经

皮肤的感觉神经极其复杂,丰富的感觉神经末梢主要分布在表皮下及毛囊周围。感觉神经可分为神经小体和游离神经末梢。游离神经末梢呈细小树枝状分布。神经小体分为囊状小体和非囊状小体(如梅克尔细胞-轴突复合体),囊状小体由有结缔组织包裹的神经末梢构成,包括以下部分。

(1)触觉感受器:又名 Meissner 小体,呈椭圆形。分布于真皮乳头层内,小儿指尖皮肤内最多见。

(2)痛觉感受器:结构简单,位于表皮内。其有髓神经纤维进入表皮后即失去神经膜,并分支成网状或小球状,散布于表皮细胞的间隙中。

(3)温度觉感受器:呈圆形、卵圆形或梭形,外围有一薄层结缔组织包膜。感觉神经末梢进入包膜后,分成很多小支盘绕成球状。接受冷觉者为球状小体,又名 Krause 球,位于真皮浅层;接受热觉者为梭形小体,又名 Ruffini 球,位于真皮深部。

(4)压觉感受器:又称 Pacini 小体,呈同心圆形,其切面可呈环层结构,甚似洋葱,故又名环层小体。其直径为 0.5 mm 或以上,位于真皮较深部和皮下组织内。

感觉神经可单独或与囊状小体一起作为受体,感受触、痛、痒、温度和机械等刺激。

2. 运动神经

皮肤中运动神经末梢呈细小树枝状分布,来源于交感神经节后纤维。肾上腺素能神经纤维支配立毛肌、血管、血管球、顶泌汗腺、小汗腺及皮脂腺基底膜的肌上皮细胞,发挥血管收缩、顶泌汗腺分泌、竖毛肌收缩或肌上皮收缩等功能。胆碱能神经纤维主要支配小汗腺分泌细胞。面部横纹肌由面神经支配。

(二) 血管

皮下组织的小动脉和真皮深部较大的微动脉具有 3 层结构:内膜、中膜和外膜。真皮中有微动脉和微静脉构成的乳头下血管丛以及真皮下部血管丛;这些血管丛大致呈层状分布,与皮肤表面平行;浅丛和深丛之间由垂直走向的血管相连,形成丰富的吻合支。皮肤的毛细血管大多由连续的内皮细胞构成管壁,相邻的内皮细胞间有细胞连接。皮肤中静脉系统总体上与对应的动脉系统相平行。真皮血管系统在附属器部位尤其丰富。皮肤血管的上述结构特点有助于其发挥营养代谢和调节体温等作用。

（三）淋巴管

皮肤中的淋巴管较少，在正常皮肤组织内一般不易辨认。皮肤的淋巴管网与几个主要的血管丛平行，皮肤毛细淋巴管盲端起始于真皮乳头层，逐渐汇合为管壁较厚的具有瓣膜的淋巴管，形成乳头下浅淋巴管网和真皮淋巴网；再连通到皮肤深层和皮下组织的更大淋巴管，然后进入全身的大循环。淋巴管的构造与静脉相同，也可分为三层。与静脉不同的是，淋巴管管壁更薄，腔内无红细胞，中膜内平滑肌纤维的排列不规则，外膜较厚。毛细淋巴管与毛细血管的结构也相同，其不同点为毛细淋巴管管腔不规则，呈窦状，周围没有外周细胞（即 Rouget 细胞）。

（四）肌肉

皮肤内最常见的肌肉是竖毛肌，由纤细的平滑肌纤维束构成。其一端起自真皮的乳头层，而另一端插入毛囊中部的纤维鞘内。此外，阴囊肌膜和乳晕等处具有平滑肌，其在血管壁上也可见到。汗腺周围的肌上皮细胞也有平滑肌的功能。面部皮肤内尚可见横纹肌，即表情肌。

第二节　皮肤的功能

皮肤被覆于人体表面，直接与外界环境接触，能够维持体内环境稳定，具有屏障、吸收、感觉、分泌和排泄、体温调节、物质代谢及免疫等多种功能。

一、皮肤的屏障功能

皮肤可以保护体内各种器官和组织免受外界有害因素（如物理、化学和微生物因素）的损伤，也能防止体内水、电解质和营养物质的流失，维持内环境的稳定。角质形成细胞、桥粒、角质形成细胞间脂质、角质层内水分和适宜的 pH 以及角质形成细胞脱落相关的酶对维持皮肤的屏障功能至关重要。

1. 对物理性损伤的防护

皮肤对外界的各种机械性损伤（如摩擦、冲击、挤压和牵拉等）具有一定的防护能力。角质层致密而柔韧，是主要的防护结构。表皮在受到损伤后具有自身修复能力。真皮内含有胶原纤维、弹性纤维和网状纤维，使皮肤具有弹性和伸展力。皮下脂肪层对机械外力具有缓冲作用。皮肤对电的屏障作用主要位于角质层，且与角质层的含水量有关。皮肤通过对光线的吸收，促进黑素的产生，起到光防护作用。

2. 对化学性损伤的防护

角质层是皮肤防护化学性损伤的主要结构，正常皮肤具有缓冲酸、碱的能力。

3. 对微生物侵入的防护

完整而排列致密的角质层细胞可机械性防御微生物的侵入。皮肤角质层含水量较少，且表面 pH 在弱酸性范围，不利于某些微生物的生长、繁殖。通过角质层生理性脱落可清除一些寄生于体表的微生物。此外，角质形成细胞产生的抗菌肽具有广谱抗菌作用（见扩展阅读 3）。

4. 防止水、电解质及营养成分流失

正常皮肤角质层具半透膜性质，可防止体内营养物质、电解质和水的丢失。

二、皮肤的吸收功能

皮肤具有吸收功能,是皮肤科外用药物治疗的基础。经角质层吸收是经皮吸收的主要途径,其次为经毛囊、皮脂腺和汗腺吸收途径。皮肤的吸收功能主要受到以下因素的影响。

1. 全身及皮肤的状况

(1)年龄、性别:有人认为婴儿和老年人的皮肤相对于其他年龄组更易吸收。但大多数研究显示,新生儿和婴儿的皮肤吸收能力降低或正常。性别之间无差异。

(2)部位和结构:皮肤的吸收能力与角质层的厚薄、完整性和通透性有关,吸收能力随角质层增厚而递减。其吸收能力为阴囊>前额>大腿屈侧>上臂屈侧>前臂>掌跖。

(3)时期:角质层在生长、脱落的不同周期内功能上的差异可导致其吸收能力的变化,其次,温度和湿度的改变也可影响其吸收。如温度从 26 ℃升至 35 ℃时,表皮的水扩散能力可增加 1 倍。

(4)皮肤的水合程度:角质层的水合程度越高,皮肤的吸收能力越强。若角质层的水分含量低于 10%,角质层即变脆易裂,吸收能力降低。

2. 被吸收物质的理化性质

(1)分子量及分子结构:分子量小的氨气极易透入皮肤,分子量大的物质,如汞软膏、葡聚糖分子也可透入皮肤。这种情况可能与分子结构、形状、溶解度有关。

(2)浓度:一般认为透入物质的浓度越高,皮肤吸收越多。但也有少数物质在高浓度时对角蛋白产生凝固作用反而影响了皮肤通透性,导致吸收不良,如苯酚。

(3)解离度:一般能解离的物质比不能解离的物质易透入皮肤,如水杨酸钠相比水杨酸更易被皮肤吸收。

3. 外界因素

(1)环境温度升高可使皮肤血管扩张、血流速度变快,加快已透入组织内的物质弥散,从而使皮肤的吸收能力提高。

(2)当环境湿度增加时,角质层水合程度增加,皮肤的吸收能力也会增强。

(3)外用药剂型:剂型对物质的吸收有明显的影响。同一种药物,由于剂型不同,皮肤吸收的情况不同。粉剂、水溶液等很难被皮肤吸收。霜剂中的药物可被少量吸收。软膏剂及硬膏剂可促进药物的吸收。有机溶媒(如二甲基亚砜、月桂氮䓬酮)可增加脂溶性及水溶性物质的吸收。

4. 病理情况

皮肤充血时,血流速度变快,物质也易于透入;理化损伤后的皮肤通透性增加,物质易于透入;影响角质层的皮肤疾病可影响其屏障作用,影响皮肤吸收能力。角化不全的疾病如银屑病和湿疹会使皮肤屏障功能减弱、吸收能力增强。

三、皮肤的感觉功能

皮肤内感觉、运动神经末梢和特殊感受器广泛分布于表皮、真皮和皮下组织,可感知体内外的各种刺激,产生各种感觉,引起相应的神经反射。皮肤的感觉可分为单一感觉和复合感觉两大类。由神经末梢或特殊的囊状感受器接受体内外单一性刺激,转换为一定的动作电位;沿相应的神经纤维传入中枢,产生触觉、压觉、冷觉、热觉、痛觉和痒觉等感觉,称为单一感觉;由皮肤中不同类型的感觉神经末梢或感受器共同感受的刺激传入中枢,由大脑皮质进行综合分析,产生如潮湿、干燥、平滑、粗糙、坚硬及柔软等感觉,称为复合感觉。此外,皮肤还有形体觉、两点辨别觉和定位觉等。

四、皮肤的分泌和排泄功能

人体皮肤主要通过富含的汗腺和皮脂腺分泌、排泄汗液和皮脂,完成皮肤的分泌和排泄功能。

(1)小汗腺:小汗腺的分泌和排泄功能主要受体内外温度、精神因素和饮食的影响。正常情况下小汗腺分泌的汗液无色透明、呈酸性,大量出汗时汗液碱性增强。汗液中水分占99%,其他成分仅占1%,后者包括无机离子、乳酸和尿素等。小汗腺的分泌功能对维持体内电解质平衡非常重要。

(2)顶泌汗腺:青春期顶泌汗腺分泌旺盛,情绪激动和环境温度升高时,其分泌也增加。顶泌汗腺新分泌的汗液是一种无味液体,经细菌酵解后可发出臭味。有些人的顶泌汗腺可分泌一些有色物质,使局部皮肤或衣服变色,称为色汗症。

(3)皮脂腺:皮脂是多种脂类的混合物,皮脂腺的分泌功能主要受各种激素(如雄激素、孕激素、雌激素、糖皮质激素、垂体激素等)的影响,其中雄激素可加快皮脂腺细胞的分裂,使其体积增大、皮脂合成增加;雌激素可抑制内源性雄激素的产生或直接作用于皮脂腺,减少皮脂分泌。

五、皮肤的体温调节功能

一方面,皮肤通过遍布全身的外周温度感受器来感受外界环境温度变化,并向下丘脑发送信息;另一方面,皮肤作为体温调节的效应器可接受中枢信息,通过血管舒缩、寒战或出汗等反应调节体温。皮肤覆盖全身,且动静脉吻合丰富。冷应激时交感神经兴奋,血管收缩,动静脉吻合关闭,皮肤血流量减少,皮肤散热减少;热应激时动静脉吻合开启,皮肤血流量增加,皮肤散热增加。体表散热主要通过辐射、对流、传导和汗液蒸发实现。环境温度过高时主要通过汗液蒸发散热。

六、皮肤的物质代谢功能

与其他组织器官相比,皮肤的代谢功能具有其特殊性,主要包括以下代谢。

(1)糖代谢:皮肤中的糖主要为糖原、葡萄糖和黏多糖等。真皮中黏多糖含量丰富,主要包括透明质酸、硫酸软骨素等。黏多糖的合成及降解主要通过酶促反应完成,但某些非酶类物质也可降解透明质酸。此外,内分泌因素也可影响黏多糖的代谢。

(2)蛋白质代谢:皮肤蛋白质包括纤维性蛋白质和非纤维性蛋白质,前者包括角蛋白、胶原蛋白和弹性蛋白等,后者包括细胞内的核蛋白以及调节细胞代谢的各种酶类。皮肤中蛋白质的降解是在蛋白水解酶作用下,通过催化多肽链的水解完成的。蛋白水解酶分为肽链内切酶和肽链外切酶两类;酶作用缺乏严格的底物特异性。皮肤中的蛋白水解酶除在正常情况下参与细胞外的结构物质代谢外,也参与皮肤的炎症过程和细胞功能的调节。

(3)脂类代谢:皮肤中的脂类包括脂肪和类脂质。表皮细胞在分化的各个阶段,其类脂质的组成有显著差异,由基底层到角质层,胆固醇、脂肪酸、神经酰胺含量逐渐增多,而磷脂则逐渐减少。表皮中较丰富的必需脂肪酸为亚油酸和花生四烯酸,后者在日光作用下可合成维生素 D。

(4) 水、电解质代谢:皮肤中的水分主要分布于真皮内。当机体脱水时,皮肤可提供其水分的 5%~7%,以维持循环血容量的稳定。皮肤中含有的各种电解质主要储存于皮下组织,它们对维持细胞间的晶体渗透压和细胞内外的酸碱平衡具有重要作用。

七、皮肤的免疫功能

皮肤是人体最大的组织器官,构成机体和外界环境间的免疫屏障,同时也是重要的免疫器官。皮肤免疫系统的功能如下:①参与固有免疫应答,如角质形成细胞间紧密连接构成细胞屏障,巨噬细胞等吞噬、溶解和杀灭病原微生物以及补体溶细胞作用等;②参与适应性免疫应答,如角质形成细胞、朗格汉斯细胞和真皮树突状细胞等的抗原呈递作用、T 细胞及其亚群的效应以及免疫分子(如细胞因子和抗体等)的效应等。研究表明,真皮中的血管内皮细胞、成纤维细胞也能参与皮肤免疫应答。皮肤能有效地启动免疫应答并及时恢复和维持免疫稳态以避免免疫病理损伤,皮肤免疫功能紊乱会导致疾病状态。皮肤通过多种免疫细胞成分及大量的免疫分子来完成免疫功能。

(一) 皮肤免疫系统的细胞

皮肤免疫系统的细胞根据功能可分为专职免疫细胞和非专职免疫细胞。专职免疫细胞包括朗格汉斯细胞、树突状细胞、淋巴细胞、巨噬细胞和肥大细胞;非专职免疫细胞包括角质形成细胞、成纤维细胞和内皮细胞等(表 1-1)。

表 1-1 皮肤中主要免疫细胞的分布和功能

细 胞 种 类	分 布 部 位	主 要 功 能
专职免疫细胞		
朗格汉斯细胞	表皮	抗原呈递,合成、分泌细胞因子,免疫监视等
树突状细胞	真皮	抗原呈递,合成、分泌细胞因子,免疫监视等
淋巴细胞	真皮	介导免疫应答、抗皮肤肿瘤、参与炎症反应、创伤修复、维持皮肤自身稳定等
巨噬细胞	真皮浅层	创伤修复、防止微生物入侵
肥大细胞	真皮乳头层血管周围	Ⅰ型超敏反应
非专职免疫细胞		
成纤维细胞	真皮	参与维持皮肤免疫系统的自稳
角质形成细胞	表皮	合成、分泌细胞因子,参与抗原呈递
内皮细胞	真皮血管	分泌细胞因子、参与炎症反应、组织修复等

角质形成细胞是表皮屏障的第一道防线,可通过识别病毒核酸、脂多糖、鞭毛蛋白和酵母聚糖等在早期监视病原体中发挥重要作用。同时,角质形成细胞和朗格汉斯细胞一样,能摄取、加工和向 T 细胞呈递抗原,还能释放多种细胞因子和趋化因子,调节免疫应答和参与炎症反应。角质形成细胞表达多种膜分子。①黏附分子:包括细胞间黏附分子-1(ICAM-1)、淋巴细胞功能相关抗原-3(LFA-3)、整合素 $\alpha_2\beta_1/\alpha_6\beta_4$ 及钙黏附素(E-cadherin、P-cadherin)等。整合素 $\alpha_5\beta_1$ 与受体结合可介导内吞及杀灭病原体;ICAM-1 与 LFA-1 结合可诱导免疫细胞向表皮迁移,同时提供共刺激信号,调节细胞间相互作用。②MHC 分子:稳态时角质形成细胞主要表达 MHC I 类分子,炎症条件下(如盘状红斑狼疮、银屑病和湿疹等),MHC I 类和 II 类分子表达上调,参与适应性免疫应答。③表面受体:包括多种细胞因子受体和模式识别受体,可监测外界环境的变化,并在病原体入侵时向免疫细胞提供促炎和趋化信号。此外,角质形成细胞能分泌多种免疫效应分子如细胞因子(IL-1、IL-6、IL-7、IL-17、IL-23、TNF-α 和 TGF-β 等)、趋化因子(CXCL8、CCL17 和 CCL20 等)和多种抗微生物物质参与炎症反应,调节免疫应答。

朗格汉斯细胞是来源于骨髓的树突状非色素性细胞,占表皮细胞总数的 3%~5%。朗格汉斯细胞膜分子包括 CD1a、MHC I 类和 II 类分子、CD45 及 CD45RO、整合素 β_1 和 β_2、Langerin(即 CD207,为朗格汉斯细胞标志物,可诱导朗格汉斯细胞内伯贝克颗粒的形成)、趋化因子受体(如 CCR6 等)。CD1a 在未成熟朗格汉斯细胞中高表达,而在成熟和培养的朗格汉斯细胞中表达明显降低。朗格汉斯细胞可分泌多种细胞因子(IL-1、IL-4、IL-6、IL-10、IL-15 和 TNF-α 等)和趋化因子,如巨噬细胞衍生的趋化因子、巨噬细胞炎性蛋白-α 和单核细胞趋化蛋白-1 等,介导朗格汉斯细胞从外周血向皮肤归巢以及摄取抗原后从表皮迁移至真皮淋巴结。朗格汉斯细胞还可调控 T 细胞的增殖和迁移,并参与免疫调节、免疫监视、免疫耐受、皮肤移植物排斥反应和接触性超敏反应等(见扩展阅读 4)。

皮肤树突状细胞包括以下几种:①表皮树突状细胞,即朗格汉斯细胞(如前所述);②真皮定居的树突状细胞,是常驻真皮的树突状细胞,具有摄取和呈递抗原能力,表面标志为 CD1c;③"炎症性"真皮树突状细胞,来源于血液循环 DC 前体细胞,在炎症和趋化因子信号刺激下迁移至皮肤,表面标志为 CD11c⁺ CD1c⁻,可激活 Th17 细胞;④浆细胞样树突状细胞,一类特殊的常驻(皮肤)树突状细胞,表面标志为 BDCA-2,病毒感染时可产生高水平 1 型 IFN。皮肤树突状细胞的功能如下:①借助表面 Toll 样受体(Toll-like receptor,TLR)识别病原相关分子模式(pathogen-associated molecular pattern,PAMP)而被激活,分泌 TNF-α 等,促进与病原体接触的角质形成细胞产生 TNF-α 和 IL-1;②激活的树突状细胞迁移至皮肤引流淋巴结,启动适应性免疫应答。

巨噬细胞包括组织定居的巨噬细胞和由循环中单核细胞渗出血管进入皮肤分化发育而来的巨噬细胞,可杀灭病原体、吞噬异物及衰老变性的组织细胞和杀伤肿瘤细胞,并能作为抗原呈递细胞参与适应性免疫应答。

皮肤肥大细胞主要分布于真皮血管、毛囊、神经和皮脂腺周围。肥大细胞不仅参与 IgE 介导的 I 型超敏反应,而且在抗感染固有免疫和适应性免疫应答中发挥重要作用,也参与炎症性自身免疫性疾病的发生。

皮肤中的淋巴细胞主要为 T 细胞,表皮中 T 细胞约占淋巴细胞总数的 2%,多为表达 TCRαβ 的 CD4⁺ 或 CD8⁺ T 细胞。绝大多数(90% 以上)T 细胞位于真皮,多为 CD4⁺ CD45RO⁺ 记忆性 T 细胞,其余为 CD8⁺ T 细胞。参与 T 细胞归巢的黏附分子主要为皮肤淋巴细胞相关抗原(CLA)和 E-选择素,以及 VLA-4、LFA-1 与 ICAM-1/2 等(见扩展阅读5)。

(二) 皮肤免疫系统的体液成分

皮肤免疫系统的体液成分包括细胞因子、免疫球蛋白、补体、抗微生物多肽和神经多肽等。

细胞因子是一类小分子可溶性多肽介质,表皮内多种细胞可合成和分泌细胞因子。细胞因子分为六大类:白细胞介素、干扰素、造血克隆刺激因子、肿瘤坏死因子、生长因子与转化因子以及趋化因子。细胞因子既可在局部发挥作用,也可通过激素样方式作用于全身。

正常皮肤中通常无补体存在,皮肤发生炎症时,补体系统被激活。补体可通过溶解细胞、免疫吸附、杀菌和过敏毒素及促进介质释放等方式,参与固有免疫应答和适应性免疫应答。补体缺陷与某些皮肤疾病相关,例如:C1r、C1s、C2 和 C4 缺陷与系统性红斑狼疮(SLE)、红斑狼疮样综合征及皮肌炎相关;C1 抑制剂缺陷与遗传性血管性水肿、系统性红斑狼疮和盘状红斑狼疮(DLE)相关;C4 缺陷能增加患白癜风的风险。

免疫球蛋白是指具有抗体活性或化学结构上与抗体相似的球蛋白,在适应性免疫应答中起作用。正常皮肤中免疫球蛋白含量很低,某些自身免疫性皮肤疾病(如红斑狼疮、硬皮病、天疱疮、类天疱疮及疱疹性皮炎)患者体内自身抗体水平明显升高,后者与相应自身抗原形成免疫复合物,沉积于皮肤及其他组织器官中,导致疾病发生。

抗微生物多肽有 20 余种,包括抗菌肽、β-防御素、P 物质和趋化因子等。抗菌肽是一类能直接杀灭多种病原体的小分子多肽,在正常皮肤固有免疫中起重要作用,同时对中性粒细胞、巨噬细胞和 T 细胞具有趋化作用。此外,皮肤神经末梢受外界刺激后可释放感觉神经肽如降钙素基因相关肽、P 物质、神经激酶 A 等,对中性粒细胞、巨噬细胞等产生趋化作用,导致局部产生炎症反应。

第三节　挑战与展望

皮肤具有独特的解剖结构和层次,是人体的第一道防线。根据皮肤独特的解剖结构与层次可设计出高效的高分子透皮药物以提高传统药物的透皮效率,进而提高疗效。同时,高分子材料还有望应用于皮肤疾病的无创性检测和诊断,例如自身免疫性疾病常伴有真表皮交界处免疫复合物沉积,若能根据皮肤的结构特点设计相应的高分子材料,则可替代皮肤活组织病理检查,大大减轻临床工作的负担。此外,皮肤免疫系统在多种皮肤疾病的发生和发展中发挥重要作用。通过对各种免疫细胞在不同皮肤疾病中功能的深入研究,可设计特异性靶向特定免疫细胞亚群的高分子载药材料以实现皮肤疾病的精准治疗。组织工程皮肤近年来取得了里程碑式的进展,能显著改善皮肤创面修复的质量,对皮肤组织结构的深入研究和认识将有助于选择和设计更为合适的天然高分子材料,用于组织工程皮肤的研发。综上所述,皮肤的解剖结构和功能是皮肤病学的基石,通过对皮肤解剖结构和功能的深入认识,将高分子材料与皮肤的结构和功能紧密结合,将会开创皮肤疾病诊断与治疗的新纪元。

思　考　题

1. 根据表皮的结构特点如何设计更为高效的高分子透皮药物?

2. 请概括参与表皮和真皮免疫应答的主要免疫细胞的特点,并思考如何设计可特异性靶向特定免疫细胞亚群的高分子载药材料。

3. 根据真表皮交界处的结构特点能否设计相应的高分子材料替代皮肤活组织病理检查，用于以真表皮交界处免疫复合物沉积为特点的自身免疫性疾病的无创性检测和诊断？

4. 结合皮肤的结构与功能，能用于组织工程皮肤的天然高分子材料有哪些？

5. 如何设计一种能在促进皮肤屏障修复的同时兼具抗菌效能的高分子材料，以用于皮肤创面的修复？

扩 展 阅 读

[1] Kaplan D H. Ontogeny and function of murine epidermal Langerhans cells[J]. Nat Immunol,2017,18(10):1068-1075.

[2] Egami S,Yamagami J,Amagai M. Autoimmune bullous skin diseases,pemphigus and pemphigoid[J]. J Allergy Clin Immunol,2020,145(4):1031-1047.

[3] Grice E A,Segre J A. The skin microbiome[J]. Nat Rev Microbiol,2011,9(4):244-253.

[4] Nestle F O,Di Meglio P,Qin J Z,et al. Skin immune sentinels in health and disease[J]. Nat Rev Immunol,2009,9(6):679-691.

[5] Kabashima K,Honda T,Ginhoux F,et al. The immunological anatomy of the skin[J]. Nat Rev Immunol,2019,19(1):19-30.

参 考 文 献

[1] 张学军,郑捷. 皮肤性病学[M]. 9 版. 北京:人民卫生出版社,2018.

[2] 赵辨. 中国临床皮肤病学[M]. 南京:江苏科学技术出版社,2010.

[3] 张建中,高兴华. 皮肤性病学[M]. 北京:人民卫生出版社,2015.

[4] 龚非力. 医学免疫学[M]. 4 版. 北京:科学出版社,2014.

[5] 朱学骏,王宝玺,孙建方,等. 皮肤病学[M]. 2 版. 北京:北京大学医学出版社,2015.

[6] Someya T,Amagai M. Toward a new generation of smart skins[J]. Nat Biotechnol,2019,37(4):382-388.

[7] Prausnitz M R,Langer R. Transdermal drug delivery[J]. Nat Biotechnol,2008,26(11):1261-1268.

[8] Quevedo W C,Fleischmann R D. Developmental biology of mammalian melanocytes[J]. J Invest Dermatol,1980,75(1):116-120.

[9] Lin J Y,Fisher D E. Melanocyte biology and skin pigmentation[J]. Nature,2007,445(7130):843-850.

[10] Breathnach S M. The Langerhans cell[J]. Br J Dermatol,1988,119(4):463-469.

[11] Atmatzidis D H,Lambert W C,Lambert M W. Langerhans cell:exciting developments in health and disease[J]. J Eur Acad Dermatol Venereol,2017,31(11):1817-1824.

[12] Blanpain C,Fuchs E. Epidermal homeostasis:a balancing act of stem cells in the skin[J]. Nat Rev Mol Cell Biol,2009,10(3):207-217.

[13] Zimmerman A,Bai L,Ginty D D. The gentle touch receptors of mammalian skin[J]. Science,2014,346(6212):950-954.

[14] Asgari M M, Sokil M M, Warton E M, et al. Effect of host, tumor, diagnostic, and treatment variables on outcomes in a large cohort with Merkel cell carcinoma[J]. JAMA Dermatol, 2014, 150(7):716-723.

[15] Delevoye C. Melanin transfer: the keratinocytes are more than gluttons[J]. J Invest Dermatol, 2014, 134(4):877-879.

[16] van Smeden J, Janssens M, Boiten W A, et al. Intercellular skin barrier lipid composition and organization in Netherton syndrome patients[J]. J Invest Dermatol, 2014, 134(5):1238-1245.

[17] Bruckner-Tuderman L, Has C. Disorders of the cutaneous basement membrane zone—the paradigm of epidermolysis bullosa[J]. Matrix Biol, 2014, 33:29-34.

[18] Deckers J, Hammad H, Hoste E. Langerhans cells: sensing the environment in health and disease[J]. Front Immunol, 2018, 9:93.

[19] Egawa G, Kabashima K. Role of lymphoid structure in skin immunity[J]. Curr Top Microbiol Immunol, 2020, 426:65-82.

[20] Kobayashi T, Naik S, Nagao K. Choreographing immunity in the skin epithelial barrier [J]. Immunity, 2019, 50(3):552-565.

[21] Skabytska Y, Kaesler S, Volz T, et al. How the innate immune system trains immunity: lessons from studying atopic dermatitis and cutaneous bacteria[J]. J Dtsch Dermatol Ges, 2016, 14(2):153-156.

[22] Nakamizo S, Egawa G, Honda T, et al. Commensal bacteria and cutaneous immunity [J]. Semin Immunopathol, 2015, 37(1):73-80.

[23] Nowarski R, Jackson R, Flavell R A. The stromal intervention: regulation of immunity and inflammation at the epithelial-mesenchymal barrier[J]. Cell, 2017, 168(3):362-375.

[24] Stenn K S, Paus R. Controls of hair follicle cycling[J]. Physiol Rev, 2001, 81(1):449-494.

[25] Panteleyev A A. Functional anatomy of the hair follicle: the secondary hair germ[J]. Exp Dermatol, 2018, 27(7):701-720.

[26] Lane M E. Skin penetration enhancers[J]. Int J Pharm, 2013, 447(1-2):12-21.

[27] Bhattacharya N, Sato W J, Kelly A, et al. Epidermal lipids: key mediators of atopic dermatitis pathogenesis[J]. Trends Mol Med, 2019, 25(6):551-562.

[28] Gonzales K A U, Fuchs E. Skin and its regenerative powers: an alliance between stem cells and their niche[J]. Dev Cell, 2017, 43(4):387-401.

[29] Takeo M, Lee W, Ito M. Wound healing and skin regeneration[J]. Cold Spring Harb Perspect Med, 2015, 5(1):a023267.

[30] Fuchs E. Scratching the surface of skin development[J]. Nature, 2007, 445(7130):834-842.

[31] Kanitakis J. Anatomy, histology and immunohistochemistry of normal human skin[J]. Eur J Dermatol, 2002, 12(4):390-399.

[32] Arda O, Göksügür N, Tüzün Y. Basic histological structure and functions of facial skin

［J］. Clin Dermatol,2014,32(1):3-13.

［33］ Schneider M R,Schmidt-Ullrich R,Paus R. The hair follicle as a dynamic miniorgan ［J］. Curr Biol,2008,19(3):R132-R142.

［34］ Honda T,Egawa G,Kabashima K. Antigen presentation and adaptive immune responses in skin［J］. Int Immunol,2019,31(7):423-429.

［35］ Lappin M B,Kimber I,Norval M. The role of dendritic cells in cutaneous immunity ［J］. Arch Dermatol Res,1996,288(3):109-121.

［36］ Delamarre L,Mellman I. Harnessing dendritic cells for immunotherapy［J］. Semin Immunol, 2011,23(1):2-11.

［37］ Girardi M. Cutaneous perspectives on adaptive immunity［J］. Clin Rev Allergy Immunol, 2007,33(1-2):4-14.

［38］ Igyártó B Z,Kaplan D H. Antigen presentation by Langerhans cells［J］. Curr Opin Immunol,2013,25(1):115-119.

［39］ Mildner A,Jung S. Development and function of dendritic cell subsets［J］. Immunity, 2014,40(5):642-656.

［40］ du Pré M F,Samsom J N. Adaptive T-cell responses regulating oral tolerance to protein antigen［J］. Allergy,2011,66(4):478-490.

［41］ Vukmanovic-Stejic M,Rustin M H,Nikolich-Zugich J,et al. Immune responses in the skin in old age［J］. Curr Opin Immunol,2011,23(4):525-531.

［42］ Belkaid Y,Segre J A. Dialogue between skin microbiota and immunity［J］. Science, 2014,346(6212):954-959.

［43］ Pasparakis M,Haase I,Nestle F O. Mechanisms regulating skin immunity and inflammation［J］. Nat Rev Immunol,2014,14(5):289-301.

［44］ Eyerich S,Eyerich K,Traidl-Hoffmann C,et al. Cutaneous barriers and skin immunity:differentiating a connected network［J］. Trends Immunol,2018,39(4): 315-327.

［45］ Belkaid Y,Tamoutounour S. The influence of skin microorganisms on cutaneous immunity［J］. Nat Rev Immunol,2016,16(6):353-366.

［46］ Kupper T S,Fuhlbrigge R C. Immune surveillance in the skin:mechanisms and clinical consequences［J］. Nat Rev Immunol,2004,4(3):211-222.

［47］ Lee D H,Oh J H,Chung J H. Glycosaminoglycan and proteoglycan in skin aging［J］. J Dermatol Sci,2016,83(3):174-181.

（李军　陶娟）

Chapter 1
Structure and Function of the Skin

1.1 Structure of the Skin

Skin covers the body surface and directly contacts the external environment. It is the first line of defense of the human body and has very important functions. The skin structure is usually divided into three parts: epidermis, dermis, and subcutaneous tissue. The epidermis and dermis are connected by a basement membrane zone. In addition to various skin appendages (e. g. , hair, sebaceous glands, sweat glands, and nails), skin also contains abundant blood vessels, lymphatic vessels, nerves, and muscles. Skin is the largest organ of the human body, and its total weight accounts for about 16% of an individual's body weight. The total area of an adult skin is about 1.5 m², and that of newborns is about 0.21 m². The thickness of the skin varies with the individual, age, and location, and is usually 0.5-4.0 mm. The skin on the eyelids, vulva, and breast is thin, with a thickness of 0.8-1.4 mm, while the palm and the plantar area is thick, with a thickness of 3-4 mm. Skin color varies with the race, age, gender, nutritional status, and location.

1.1.1 Epidermis

The epidermis belongs to the stratified squamous epithelium, mainly composed of keratinocytes, melanocytes, Langerhans cells, and Merkel cells.

1.1.1.1 Keratinocytes

Keratinocytes originated from the ectoderm, are the main cells of the epidermis, and they can produce keratin which is one of the main structural proteins of keratinocytes. It serves as a cytoskeleton to maintain cell structure and participate in physiological and pathological processes such as epidermal differentiation and keratinization. According to the differentiation stage and characteristics of keratinocytes, the epidermis can be divided into 5 parts from deep to shallow, i. e. , stratum basale, stratum spinosum, stratum granulosum, stratum lucidum, and stratum corneum, respectively (Figure 1-1).

(1) Stratum basale: It is located at the bottom of the epidermis. Stratum basale consists of a layer of cylindrical basal cells, usually arranged neatly, like a fence. Its long axis is perpendicular to the boundary line between the epidermis and the dermis. The cytoplasm is deeply basophilic, the nucleus is oval, the nucleolus is obvious, and the mitosis is common. The melanin granules can be seen on the top of the nucleus to gather or arrange in a cap. The basal cells and the spinous cells above it are connected by intercellular bridges. The bottom of the basal cells are attached to the basement membrane zone under the epidermis by hemidesmosomes. This zone is not easy to be identified during HE staining and can only be revealed by special staining, e. g. , periodic acid schiff (PAS) staining. Basal cells express keratin K5/K14.

It is a precisely regulated process for the basal cells to divide, differentiate, mature into stratum corneum, and finally fall off from the skin surface. Under normal circumstances, about 30% of the basal cells are in the mitotic phase. The new keratinocytes move up in an orderly manner. It takes about 14 days to migrate from the basal layer to the granular layer, and another 14 days to migrate to the surface of the stratum corneum and fall off. The whole 28 days are termed as the cuticle transit time or replacement time.

(2) Stratum spinosum: It is located above the basal layer. Stratum spinosum is usually composed of 4-8 layers of polygonal cells. The closer to the surface, the flatter the cells shape. Each cell has many cytoplasmic processes, called spinous processes, so this layer of cells is also called spinous cells. The spinous processes of normal skin are not clearly visible under high magnification but are visible when there is intercellular edema. Under the electron microscope, it can be seen that there are many tension filaments in the cytoplasm gathered in bundles and attached to the desmosomes. In the cytoplasm of the upper spinous layer, there are scattered coated particles with a diameter of 100-300 nm, called keratinocytes or Odland bodies. Spinous cells express keratin K1/K10.

(3) Stratum granulosum: It is located above the spinous layer. Stratum granulosum is usually composed of 1-3 layers of flat or diamond-shaped cells, with the long axis paralleling to the skin surface. The cytoplasm is filled with large, deeply basophilic transparent keratinous granules. The thickness of the stratum granulosum of normal skin is directly proportional to the thickness of the stratum corneum. Where the stratum corneum is thin, there are only 1-3 layers of stratum granulosum. While where the stratum corneum is thick (e. g. , palm and plantar), the stratum granulosum can be up to 10 layers. The nucleus and organelles are dissolved, and a large number of transparent keratinous particles with irregular shapes can be seen in the cytoplasm deposited between the tension filaments.

(4) Stratum lucidum: It is located between the granular layer and the stratum corneum. Stratum lucidum is only seen in areas with thicker epidermis (e. g. , palm and plantar), especially in the skin tissue sections of the heel area, where this layer is the most obvious. This layer is composed of 2-3 layers of relative flat cells. The cell boundaries are unclear and

easily stained by eosin. The cytoplasm is homogeneous and highly refractive under light microscope.

(5) Stratum corneum: It is located at the uppermost layer of the epidermis. Stratum corneum is composed of 5-20 layers of dead flat cells (40-50 layers at the palm and plantar area). In the stratum corneum, the normal structure of the cell disappears, the staining is eosinophilic, and the cytoplasm is full of keratin formed by the combination of tension filaments and homogeneous substances. The desmosomes between cells in the upper stratum corneum disappear or form residues, thus they are easy to fall off. Since the outer layer of the stratum corneum is constantly falling off, it is difficult to determine its thickness. In formalin-fixed specimens, the stratum corneum has large intracellular and extracellular spaces, so it is often reticulated.

1.1.1.2　Melanocytes

Melanocytes originate from the neural crest of the ectoderm and are located in the stratum basale and hair follicle of the epidermis, accounting for about 10% of the cells in stratum basale. The number of melanocytes varies with different parts of the body and age, and it can increase after repeated exposure to ultraviolet light. There is no significant difference in the number and distribution of melanocytes among different ethnic groups. Therefore, the difference of their skin color is mainly ascribed to the difference in the amount and distribution of melanin produced by melanocytes. In HE stained sections, melanocytes have a small and densely stained nucleus and transparent cytoplasm, so they are also called clear cells. However, not all clear cells seen in conventional slices are melanocytes, because basal cells can occasionally shrink artificially, which make it difficult to distinguish from melanocytes. Melanocytes have the function of forming melanin, thus the dopa response is positive; moreover, they contain melanin, thus the silver staining is positive. Melanin is transported into basal cells through dendritic processes of melanocytes. Under the electron microscope, characteristic melanosomes can be seen in the cytoplasm of melanocytes. Melanosomes are organelles containing tyrosinase and are the place where melanin is synthesized. One melanocyte can provide melanin to the surrounding 10-36 keratinocytes through its dendritic processes, called epidermal melanin unit. Melanin can block and reflect ultraviolet rays, thereby protecting the dermis and deep tissues (Figure 1-2).

1.1.1.3　Langerhans cells

Langerhans cells are immunocompetent cells that originated from bone marrow mononuclear-macrophages and are distributed in the epidermis and hair follicle epithelium above the stratum basale, accounting for 3%-5% of the total number of epidermal cells. The density of Langerhans cells varies with the location. Generally, there are comparatively more Langerhans cells in the skin of the face and neck, while less in the palm and plantar regions. When impregnated with gold chloride, the Langerhans cells may appear as the shape of dendritic cells; however, the dopa response is negative and ATPase response is positive. Under the optical microscopy investigation, Langerhans cells are polygonal in shape, with clear cytoplasm, smaller nuclei and lobulated, abundant mitochondria, golgi bodies and endoplasmic reticulum, and lysosomes. Electron microscopy investigation demonstrates that the cytoplasm of the cells contains unique Birbeck granules, which are used to distinguish from melanocytes (Figure 1-3). At present, it is believed that Birbeck granules are formed by the invagination of the envelope during the phagocytosis of foreign antigens by Langerhans cells, which is a phagocytic or antigen storage form for the digestion of extracellular substances. Langerhans cells can recognize, ingest, process, and present antigens to T cells. Langerhans cells also play an important role in tumor immunity. Langerhans cells have a variety of surface markers, including FcR of IgG and IgE, C3b receptors, MHC class Ⅱ antigens (HLA-DR, DP, DQ) and CD4, CD45, S-100, etc. The specific surface markers of Langerhans cells are CD1a and Langerin (CD207) (see extended reading 1).

1.1.1.4　Merkel cells

Merkel cells are tactile sensory cells located at the stratum basale of the epidermis. They are mostly found in the palms, plantar, oral cavity and genital mucosa, nail bed, and hair follicle funnel. Merkel cells have short finger-like protrusions and are connected to the surrounding keratinocytes by desmosomes. They are often fixed to the basement membrane and do not migrate upward with keratinocytes. Merkel cells cannot be identified under the optical microscope. In mammalian hairy skin, Merkel cells uniquely clusters into a discoid-shape, named as hairy disc or Merkel disc. In the silver-stained section, there is a meniscus-like nerve ending close to the base of each Merkel cell, called the Merkel disc, and a sensory nerve fiber terminates at the disc. Merkel cells are denser in sensitive areas (e. g. , finger tips and nose tips) where nerve fibers near the epidermis lose myelin sheaths and their flat disc-shaped axon ends combine with the base surface of Michael cells to form a Merkel cell-neurite complex, which may have a non-neural terminal-mediated sensory effect.

1.1.1.5　The connection between keratinocytes and the dermis

(1) Desmosomes: The epidermal keratinocytes are mainly connected by desmosomes. Other connection methods include adhesion connections, gap connections, and tight connections. Desmosomes are the main structure of the connection between keratinocytes, formed by the dense and thickened local cell membranes of adjacent cells. Under the electron microscope, the desmosomes are disc-shaped and have a paired button-like structure with a diameter of 0. 2-0. 5 μm and a thickness of 30-60 nm. There is a 20-30 nm wide electronic transparent gap in the center, containing low-density tension filaments. The dense layer with higher electron density in the center of the gap is called the central layer; a deeper dyed interline can be seen in the middle of the central layer, which is a highly osmiophilic layer. There is a thickened disc-shaped attachment plate on the inner side of adjacent cell membranes constituting desmosomes, with a length of 0. 2-0. 3 μm and a thickness of about 30 nm. Many tension filaments with a diameter of about 10 nm are attached to the attachment plate in loops and then folded back into the cytoplasm. In addition, there are

thinner filaments (transmembrane filaments) that emerge from the inside of the attachment plate, extend into the intercellular space, and are interlaced with the filaments in the central layer (Figure 1-4). The main proteins that make up desmosomes include: ①transmembrane proteins, mainly composed of desmoglein and desmocolin, which form the electronically transparent intercellular space and intercellular contact layer of desmosomes; ②desmoplakin in the cytoplasm is a component of the disc-shaped attachment plate, mainly composed of desmoplakin and desmosomal porphyrin. Desmosomes themselves have a strong resistance to tension, and the continuous network of tension filaments between adjacent cells strengthens the connection between cells. The destruction of desmosome structure can cause keratinocytes to separate from each other, forming dermal blisters or bullous skin diseases, such as pemphigus.

(2) Hemidesmosome: It is the main connection structure between the basal cells and the underlying basement membrane zone. It is formed by the irregular protrusions of the basal keratinocytes and the basement membrane zone interlocking with each other to form a similar structure of a half desmosomes, but its constituent proteins are very different from desmosomes. Under the electron microscope, the inner part of the hemidesmosome is a high-density adhesion spot, and the keratin tension filaments of the basal cells are attached to it; the outer part of the cell membrane is a subbasal dense spot. The dense spots on both sides and the central cell membrane form a sandwich-like structure. The dense spots contain bullous pemphigoid antigen 1/2 (BPAG1/BPAG2), integrin, and other proteins (Figure 1-5).

(3) Basement membrane zone: Basement membrane zone is located between the dermis and the epidermis. Under the optical microscope, Basement membrane zone is dyed by PAS as a 0.5-1.0 μm purple-red homogeneous band, and the silver dip dyeing method can dye it to black. There are also basement membrane bands between the skin appendages and the dermis and around the blood vessels. The basement membrane zone under the electron microscope is composed of 4 layers: cell membrane layer, transparent layer, dense layer, and dense lower layer.

① Cell membrane layer: It is mainly composed of the cytoplasmic membrane on the dermis side of the basal keratinocytes, with a thickness of about 8 nm. The hemidesmosomes span between them. The hemidesmosomes are connected with the tension filaments in the cytoplasm through attachment spots. The other side adhere to the transparent layer with the help of a variety of transmembrane proteins (e. g. , BPAG2, integrin $\alpha_6\beta_4$), to form a rivet-like connection in the basement membrane band.

② Transparent layer: Transparent layer is located under the cell membrane at the bottom of hemidesmosomes and basal cells, with the thickness of 35-40 nm. It appears transparent due to low electron density. The main components are the extracellular matrix composed of laminin and its isomers and anchor filaments. The anchor filaments can pass through the transparent layer to a dense layer, which has a connection and fixation effect.

③ Dense layer: It is a ribbon-like structure with a thickness of 35-45 nm. The main component is type Ⅳ collagen and a small amount of laminin. Type Ⅳ collagen molecules are cross-linked to form a highly stable continuous three-dimensional grid, which is an important supporting structure of the basement membrane zone.

④ Dense lower layer: Dense lower layer, called mesh plate as well, can migrate with the dermis without obvious boundaries; the main component is type Ⅶ collagen. Anchor fibrils traverse in the dense lower layer, combine with anchor spots, connect the dense layer and the underlying dermis, and maintain the connection between the epidermis and the underlying connective tissue.

The four-layer structure of the basement membrane zone is organically combined through various mechanisms. In addition to tightly connecting the dermis and the epidermis, it also has the functions of penetration and barrier. There is no blood vessel distribution in the epidermis. Nutrients in the blood can enter the epidermis through the basement membrane zone, and the epidermal metabolites can enter the dermis through the basement membrane zone. Under normal circumstances, the basement membrane zone restricts the passage of macromolecules with a molecular weight greater than 40000. But when it is damaged, inflammatory cells, tumor cells, and other macromolecular substances can also enter the epidermis through the basement membrane zone. The abnormal structure of the basement membrane zone can cause the dermis to separate from the epidermis, forming sub-epidermal blisters or bullae. The representative disease is pemphigoid (see extended reading 2).

1.1.2　Dermis

The dermis develops from the mesoderm, which is mainly composed of connective tissue, containing nerves, blood vessels, lymphatic vessels, muscles, and skin appendages. The dermis can be divided into the papillary layer and the reticular layer from shallow to deep, but there is no clear boundary between the two layers. The papillary layer is a papillary bulge that protrudes toward the bottom of the epidermis and is connected to the epidermal process in a crisscross shape. The reticular layer is thicker, is located below the papillary layer, and has larger blood vessels, lymphatic vessels, and nerves.

The dermis connective tissue is composed of collagen fibers, elastic fibers, matrix, and many cells. Collagen fibers and elastic fibers are interwoven with each other and buried in the matrix. The cells in the normal dermis include fibroblasts, tissue cells, and mast cells, etc. Collagen fibers, elastic fibers, and matrix are all produced by fibroblasts.

1.1.2.1　Collagen fibers

Among dermal connective tissues, collagen fiber is the most abundant. HE staining of the collagen fiber shows a light red color, with a diameter between 2 and 15 μm. The collagen fibers in the dermal papilla layer, epidermal appendages, and the vicinity of blood vessels are fine and do not go in a certain direction, while collagen fibers in other parts are combined into bundles. In the collagen bundles, there are a few fibroblasts scattered, the nucleus of which is stained darkly and the longitudinal section of which is diamond-shaped. The collagen bundles in the dermis gradually thicken from top to bottom, and the directions of the lower and middle collagen bundles are almost parallel to the leather surface and interweave with each other, extending in all directions on a horizontal surface. The collagen bundles in the lower dermis are the thickest one. Collagen fibers are formed by polymerization of collagen fibrils with a diameter of 70-140 nm. The main component is type I collagen, and a few are type III collagen. Collagen fibers are poorly stretchable, but are tough and resistant to parallel tension.

1.1.2.2 Reticular fibers

Reticular fibers (diameter: 0.2-1.0 μm) are not independent fiber components, but immature and slender immature collagen fibers. HE staining is difficult to show reticular fibers. However, due to the silver-philic nature, they can be blacked with silver nitrate solution, which are therefore called silver-philic fibers as well. In the embryonic period, reticular fibers appear the earliest. Reticular fibers are mainly distributed in the nipple layer and skin appendages, and surrounding of blood vessels. In wound healing, fibroblast hyperplasia or new collagen formation lesions, reticular fibers tend to massive hyperplasia.

1.1.2.3 Elastic fibers

HE staining is not easy to recognize elastic fibers, and aldehyde magenta dyeing of elastic fibers is purple. After staining, it can be seen that the elastic fibers are entangled between the collagen bundles, which are wavy and interwoven into a net, with the diameter being 1-3 μm. The elastic fibers are the thickest under the dermis, and they are arranged in the same direction as the collagen bundle, parallel to the epidermis. The number of elastic fibers in the normal dermis is small, accounting for 2%-4%. Elastic fibers have strong elasticity.

1.1.2.4 Matrix

The matrix is an amorphous substance. The main components are proteoglycans, glycoproteins, and glycosaminoglycans. They exist in the spaces between fibers and fiber bundles and between cells, and are rarely found in normal skin. Proteoglycan and glycosaminoglycan complexes have strong water absorption and play an important role in regulating bound water and dermal plasticity. The matrix is involved in the connection of cell components and fiber components, affecting cell proliferation and differentiation, tissue repair, and structural reconstruction.

1.1.2.5 Cells

The resident cells in the dermis mainly include fibroblasts, macrophages, and mast cells. They are mainly distributed in the papillary layer of the dermis, around the blood vessels under the papillary layer, and between the collagen fiber bundles. The dermis also contains a small amount of dermal dendritic cells and lymphocytes. Fibroblasts are derived from the mesoderm and can synthesize and degrade fiber and matrix components. They play an important role in dermal network construction and epidermal connection. Macrophages are derived from bone marrow hematopoietic stem cells and differentiate into circulating monocytes and migrate to the dermis to differentiate into macrophages, which have the effects of phagocytosis, antigen presentation, killing pathogenic microorganisms and tumor cells. Mast cells can synthesize and release inflammatory mediators, such as histamine, heparin, trypsin, and participate in type I hypersensitivity. Dermal dendritic cells are specialized antigen-presenting cells in the dermis. They can efficiently recognize and present antigens, synthesize and secrete cytokines, and migrate to local draining lymph nodes to activate T cells to induce immune responses.

1.1.3　Subcutaneous tissue

Subcutaneous tissue, also known as the subcutaneous fat layer, is located below the dermis. It is connected to the muscle membrane and other tissues underneath. It consists of loose connective tissue and fat leaflets. The connective tissue wraps the fat leaflets to form the leaflet interval. The subcutaneous tissue contains blood vessels, lymphatic vessels, nerves, small glands, and apocrine sweat glands. Its thickness varies with location, gender, and nutritional status. It is thicker at the hip and abdomen, while thinner at the nose and sternum. The subcutaneous tissue has the functions of providing skin elasticity, participating in fat metabolism and sugar metabolism, storing energy, and endocrine.

1.1.4　Cutaneous appendages

Skin appendages include hair, hair follicles, sebaceous glands, sweat glands, nails, etc. All of them are differentiated from ectoderm.

1.1.4.1　Hair and hair follicles

The hair is made up of keratinocytes arranged concentrically and keratinized. Palms, soles, flexion of fingers (or toes) and their nodal extensions, lips, nipples, glans, medial foreskin, labia minora, medial labia majora, clitoris are hairless, called hairless skin; other parts with hairs of different lengths, diameters and colors are called hairy skin. Generally, hair can be divided into two types: bristles and vellus hair. The bristles are hard, medulla, and dark in color. There are two types of bristles:① long hair, such as hair, beard, armpit hair, and pubic hair; ② short hair, such as eyebrows, eyelashes, nose hair and ear hair, is usually shorter compared with long hair. The vellus hair is soft, without medulla, and lighter in color, mainly seen on the face, limbs, and trunk. The part of the hair that is visible on the body surface is the hair shaft, and the part that is located inside the skin is the hair root. The ends of the hair roots swell in the shape of onions and are called hair bulbs. From the longitudinal section, the hair shaft can be divided into medulla, cortex, and hair scalp from inside to outside. The medulla is the central part of the hair, which is composed of 2-3 layers of cubic cells, and the cytoplasm is lightly stained. At the end of the hair, there is usually no medulla; the cortex is the main part of the hair, which is composed of several layers of fusiform epithelial cells; the hair coat is a thin and transparent layer of keratinocytes, overlapping each other like a roof tile (Figure 1-6).

Hair follicles are located in the dermis and subcutaneous tissues. They are necessary structures for hair growth and are composed of epithelial cells and connective tissue. The sebaceous gland ducts usually open up into the upper part of a hair follicle, called the infundibulum. The part below the opening of the sebaceous gland ducts to the place where the hairy muscles attach is called the hair follicle isthmus; the end of the hair follicle is mostly spherical, called the hair bulb. The hair follicles are composed of inner and outer hair root sheaths and connective tissue sheaths. The cells of the first two layers of hair root sheaths all originate from the epidermis, while the connective tissue sheaths originate from the dermis.

The hair growth cycle can be divided into anagen, catagen, and telogen, corresponding to about 3 years, 3 weeks, and 3 months, respectively(Figure 1-7). Hair in all parts does not grow and fall at the same time. About 80% of all hairs are in the anagen. Normal people can lose 70-100 hairs per day, and there is also an equal amount of hair regeneration. Hair traits are related to a variety of factors including genetics, health, hormone levels (e. g., sex hormones, thyroid hormones, glucocorticoids), drugs, and climate.

1.1.4.2　Sebaceous glands

The sebaceous glands produce sebum and belong to the alveolar glands, which are composed of acinus and shorter ducts. The acinus has no glandular cavity, and the outer layer is flat or cuboid cells, surrounded by a basement membrane band and connective tissue. After rupture of the glandular cells, intracellular components including lipid droplets are released and discharged through the catheter. The catheter is composed of a stratified squamous epithelium, which is opened in the upper part of the hair follicle and is located in the angle between the hairy muscle and the hair follicle. The sebaceous glands are widely distributed on the whole body skin except the palms, soles and flexor side of the digit. There are many sebaceous glands in the head and face and the upper part of the chest and back, which is called the sebum overflow site. In areas of hairless skin such as buccal mucosa, lips, women's areola, labia majora, eyelids, and inner foreskin, the glandular duct directly opens to the skin surface. The sebaceous glands also have a growth cycle, but it has nothing to do with the hair follicle growth cycle, which is mainly controlled by androgen levels.

1.1.4.3　Sweat glands

According to different structures and functions, human sweat glands are usually divided into small glands and apocrine sweat glands.

Small glands, also known as eccrine sweat glands, are single-curved tubular glands composed of secretory parts and ducts. The secretory part is located in the deep part of the dermis and the subcutaneous tissue. It is composed of a single layer of cells, arranged in a tube and coiled into a spherical shape. The ducts are composed of two layers of small cubic cells with relatively smaller diameter, pass through the dermis, and directly opens to the sweat pores. Except for lips, eardrum, nail bed, nipple, medial foreskin, glans, labia minora, and clitoris, the small glands are all over the body, with relatively more in the palms, soles, armpits and forehead, and fewer in the back. The main function of the small glands is to regulate body temperature. The small glands in the palms and soles of the feet also have the effect of improving tactile sensitivity and increasing adhesion. The small glands are dominated by the sympathetic nervous system, and the neurotransmitter is acetylcholine.

The apocrine sweat glands, also known as the large glands, are large tubular glands composed of a secretory part and a duct. They are mainly distributed in the armpits, areola, periumbilical, and perineum, occasionally found in the face, scalp, and trunk. In addition, ceruminous glands of the external auditory canal and eyelid ciliary glands are also apocrine sweat glands. The secretory part is located in the subcutaneous fat layer. The gland is a layer of flat, cubic, or columnar secretory cells with myoepithelial cells and basement membrane zone. The structure of the duct is similar to that of the small glands, but its diameter is about 10 times that of the small glands. It opens above the opening of the sebaceous glands in the upper part of the hair follicles and occasionally directly on the skin surface. The secretion of apocrine sweat glands is mainly affected by sex hormones, so the secretion is strong in adolescence. The apocrine sweat glands are also dominated by the sympathetic nervous system, and the neurotransmitter is norepinephrine.

1.1.4.4　Nail

The nail is the largest skin appendage of the human body, covering the extended side of the end of the fingers (or toes), consisting of multiple layers of tight keratinocytes. The main functions of the nail include protecting the tip of the finger, improving the sense of discrimination, assisting the finger to complete fine movements, scratching, and aesthetic functions. The exposed part of the nail is called nail plate, shaped like a convex rectangle. The crescent-shaped light-colored area at the proximal end of the nail is called nail lunula. The skin around the nail plate is called nail wall, and the portion of the nail plate deep into the proximal skin is called nail root. The skin beneath the nail plate is called nail bed, and those below the nail root are called nail matrix, which is the germinal structure of the nail. The subdermal dermis is rich in blood vessels. The fingernail growth rate is about 1 cm every 3 months, and the toenail growth rate is about 1 cm every 9 months. The trait and growth rate are affected by factors such as disease, nutritional status, environment, and lifestyle.

1.1.5　The nerves, vessels, and muscles of the skin

1.1.5.1　Nerves

There are abundant nerve fibers in the skin, which can be divided into sensory nerves and motor nerves. By contacting with the central nervous system, various stimuli can be felt, which can control the activities of target organs and complete various types of nerve reflexes. The innervation of the skin is segmental, but there is a partial overlap between adjacent segments. Nerve fibers are mostly distributed in the dermis and subcutaneous tissues.

1. Sensory nerves

The sensory nerves of the skin are extremely complex, and the rich sensory nerve endings are mainly distributed under the epidermis and around the hair follicles. Sensory nerves can be divided into nerve bodies and free nerve endings. The free nerve endings are distributed in small branches. Nerve bodies are divided into cystic bodies and non-cystic bodies (e. g. , Merkel cell-axon complex). The cystic bodies are composed of nerve endings wrapped with connective tissue, including:

①Tactile receptors, also known as Meissner bodies, are oval. They are distributed in the dermal papillary layer, most commonly seen in the skin of the fingertips of children.

②Pain receptors is located in the epidermis with simple structure. The myelinated nerve fiber loses the nerve membrane after entering the epidermis, and branches into a mesh or small spherical shape, scattered in the gaps of epidermal cells.

③Temperature sensors are round, oval, or fusiform, with a thin layer of connective tissue envelope. After the sensory nerve endings enter the envelope, it develops into many small branches and coils into a spherical shape. Those which receive cold sensations are spherical bodies, also known as Krause balls, located in the superficial dermis; those which receive heat sensations are fusiform bodies, also known as Ruffini balls, located in the deep dermis.

④Pressure receptors, also known as Pacini bodies, are in concentric circles, and their cut surfaces can have a ring-layer structure, much like an onion, so they are also called ring-layer corpuscles. Their diameters are 0. 5 mm or more. They are located in the deeper part of the dermis and subcutaneous tissue.

Sensory nerves act as receptors alone or with cystic bodies to feel touch, pain, itching, temperature, and mechanical stimulation.

2. Motor nerves

The motor nerves in the skin are distributed in small branches, derived from the fibers of the sympathetic ganglia. Adrenergic nerve fibers innervate the myoepithelial cells of the erectile muscles, blood vessels, glomus, apocrine sweat glands, small glands, and sebaceous glands basement membranes, and play roles of vasoconstriction, apocrine sweat gland secretion, erector muscle contraction or myoepithelial contraction. Cholinergic nerve fibers innervate small gland secretory cells. The facial striated muscle is innervated by the facial nerve.

1. 1. 5. 2　Blood vessels

The small arteries of the subcutaneous tissue and the large arteries deep in the dermis have three layers: intima, media, and adventitia. There are subpapillary vascular plexus and subdermal vascular plexus composed of arterioles and venules in the dermis. These vascular plexuses are roughly layered and parallel to the skin surface. There is a vertical blood vessel connection between the shallow plexus and the deep plexus, forming a rich anastomosis. The capillaries of the skin are mostly continuous, with continuous endothelium forming the wall of the vessels, and there are cell connections between adjacent endothelial cells. The venous system in the skin is generally parallel to the corresponding arterial system. The dermal vascular system is particularly abundant in the appendages. The above-mentioned structural characteristics of skin blood vessels contribute to nutrient metabolism and body temperature regulation.

1.1.5.3   Lymphatic vessels

There are relatively fewer lymphatic vessels in the skin which are generally difficult to identify in normal skin tissues. The lymphatic network of the skin is parallel to several major vascular plexuses. The blind end of the skin capillary lymphatic vessels starts in the dermal papilla layer and gradually merges into a thicker wall with valve-like lymphatic vessels, forming a shallow lymphatic network under the papillary layer and the lymphatic network of the dermis. Then, they join and connect to the larger lymphatic vessel in deep skin and subcutaneous tissues, and subsequently enter the systematic circulation of the whole body. The structure of lymphatic vessels is the same as that of veins, and can also be divided into three layers. Different from the veins, the tube walls of lymphatic vessels are thinner, there are no red blood cells in the cavity, the smooth muscle fibers in the media are arranged irregularly, and the adventitia is thicker. The structures of lymphatic capillaries and capillaries are also the same. The difference is that the lumens of lymphatic vessels are irregular and sinus-shaped, and there are no surrounding cells(namely Rouget cells).

1.1.5.4   Muscles

The most common one in the skin is the arrector pili muscle, composed of slender smooth muscle fiber bundles, one end of which reaches the papillary layer of the dermis and the other end is inserted into the fiber sheath in the middle of the hair follicle. In addition, there are smooth muscles of the scrotum's sarcolemma and areola, as well as smooth muscles on the blood vessel wall. The muscle epithelial cells around sweat glands also function as smooth muscle. There are striated muscles in the facial skin, that is, mimetic muscle.

1.2   Function of the Skin

The skin covers the surface of the human body and directly contacts the external environment, which can maintain the stability of the internal environment of the body, and has various functions such as barrier, absorption, sensation, secretion and excretion, body temperature regulation, metabolism, and immunity.

1.2.1   Barrier function

The skin can protect various organs and tissues in the body from damages of external harmful factors (e. g. , physical factors, chemical factors, and microbial factors), and can also prevent the loss of water, electrolytes, and nutrients in the body and maintain the stability of the internal environment. Keratinocytes, keratin desmosomes, keratinocyte lipids, water in the stratum corneum and maintaining an appropriate pH, and enzymes related to keratinocytes shedding are essential for maintaining skin barrier function.

1. Protection against physical damage

The skin has a certain degree of protection against external mechanical damage (e. g. , friction, impact, squeezing, and pulling). The stratum corneum is dense and flexible, and is the main protective structure. The epidermis can repair itself after being damaged. The dermis contains collagen fibers, elastic fibers, and mesh fibers, which make the skin elastic and stretchable. The subcutaneous tissue has a buffering effect on mechanical external forces. The skin's barrier to electricity is mainly in the stratum corneum and is related to the water content of the stratum corneum. The skin absorbs light and promotes the production of melanin to play a role in light protection.

2. Protection against chemical damage

The stratum corneum is the main structure for protecting the skin from chemical stimuli. In addition, the hydrogen ion concentration on the surface of normal skin can buffer acids and bases.

3. Protection against microbial invasion

The stratum corneum cells are densely arranged, and the intact skin can mechanically defend against the invasion of microorganisms. The stratum corneum has less water and the surface pH is weakly acidic, which is not conducive to the growth and reproduction of certain microorganisms. The stratum corneum is physiologically shed so as to clear some microorganisms parasitic on the body surface; the antibacterial peptides produced by keratinocytes have a broad-spectrum antibacterial effect (see extended reading 3).

4. Prevention of the loss of water, electrolytes and nutrients

The stratum corneum of normal skin is a semi-permeable membrane, which can prevent the loss of nutrients, electrolytes, and water in the body.

1.2.2 Absorption function

The skin has an absorption function which is the basis of external dermatological medicine treatment. The stratum corneum is the main route of transdermal absorption, followed by hair follicles, sebaceous glands, and sweat glands. The absorption function of the skin is mainly affected by the following factors.

1. The condition of the whole body and skin

(1) Age and gender: Some people think that the skin of babies and the elderly is easier to absorb than other age groups. However, most studies have shown that the skin of newborns and infants has reduced or normal transdermal absorption capacity. There is no difference between genders.

(2) Part and structure: The absorption capacity of the skin is related to the thickness, integrity and permeability of the stratum corneum. The absorption capacity decreases along with the thickness of the stratum corneum: scrotum>forehead>flexed thigh>flexed upper arm>forearm>palmoplantar area.

(3) Period: Primarily, the difference in the function of the stratum corneum in different periods of growth and shedding can lead to the changes in its absorption capacity. Secondarily, changes in temperature and humidity can also affect its absorption capacity. If the temperature rises from 26 ℃ to 35 ℃, the water dispersion of the epidermis can double.

(4) The degree of hydration of the skin: The higher the degree of hydration of the stratum corneum, the stronger the absorption capacity of the skin. If the moisture content of the stratum corneum is less than 10%, the stratum corneum becomes brittle and easily cracked, and the absorption capacity is reduced.

2. Physical and chemical properties of the absorbed substance

(1) Molecular weight and molecular structure: Ammonia with a small molecular weight can easily penetrate into the skin, and substances with a large molecular weight such as mercury ointment and dextran molecules can also penetrate into the skin. This situation may be related to the structures, shapes and solubilities of the molecules.

(2) Concentration: It is generally believed that the higher the concentration of the penetrating substance, the more the skin absorbs. However, there are also a few substances with high concentration have a coagulation effect on keratin, which affects the permeability of the skin and causes malabsorption, such as carbolic acid.

(3) Electrolysis: Generally, substances that can be dissociated are easier to penetrate into the skin than those cannot. For example, the skin absorbs sodium salicylate better than salicylic acid.

3. External factors

(1) The increase in ambient temperature can cause skin blood vessels to dilate, increase blood flow speed, and accelerate the diffusion of substances that have penetrated into the tissues, thereby improving skin absorption capacity.

(2) When the environmental humidity increases, the stratum corneum hydrates, and the skin absorption capacity increases.

(3) External dosage form: The dosage form has an obvious influence on the absorption of the substance. The same drug has different skin absorption conditions due to different dosage forms. Powders, aqueous solutions, etc., are difficult to be absorbed. The medicine in the cream can be absorbed in small amounts. Ointment and plaster can promote the absorption of drugs. Organic solvents (e. g., dimethyl sulfoxide, azone) can increase the absorption of fat-soluble and water-soluble substances.

4. Pathological conditions

It is easy to penetrate for substances when skin is congested with faster blood flow or is physically or chemically damaged with increased skin permeability. Skin diseases that affect the stratum corneum can affect its barrier function and affect skin absorption capacity. Diseases of hypokeratosis such as psoriasis and eczema will weaken the barrier function and increase the absorption capacity.

1. 2. 3　Sensory function

Sensory nerves endings, motor nerves endings and special receptors are widely distributed in the epidermis, dermis, and subcutaneous tissues. They can sense various stimuli inside and outside the body, produce various sensations, and cause corresponding nerve reflexes. The sensation of the skin can be divided into two categories: single sensation and compound sensation. The nerve endings or special cystic receptors receive a single stimulus in and out of the body, convert into a certain action potential, pass into the center along with the corresponding nerve fiber, and finally produce sensations of tactile, pressure, cold, thalposis, pain, or itching, called single sensations; the stimuli co-sensed by different types of sensory nerve endings or receptors in the skin are introduced into the center and are comprehensively analyzed by the cerebral cortex. The sensations (e. g. , moisture, dryness, smoothness, roughness, hardness, and softness) are called compound sensations. In addition, the skin also has body sense, two-point discrimination, and localization sense.

1. 2. 4　Secretory and excretory functions

Human skin mainly secretes and excretes sweat and sebum through rich sweat glands and sebum to complete skin secretion and excretion functions.

(1) Small glands: The secretion and excretion functions of the small glands are mainly affected by internal and external temperature, mental factors, and diet. In normal settings, the sweat secreted by the small sweat glands is colorless, transparent, and acidic, and the sweat becomes more alkaline when sweating a lot. The moisture in sweat accounts for 99%, and other components only account for 1%. The latter includes inorganic ions, lactic acid, and urea. The secretion of small sweat glands is very important to maintain electrolyte balance in the body.

(2) Apocrine sweat glands: The secretion of apocrine sweat glands during adolescence is strong, and when the emotion is agitated and the ambient temperature increases, its secretion also increases. The newly secreted sweat from the apocrine sweat glands is an odorless liquid, which can emit a foul smell after bacterial fermentation. Some people's apocrine sweat glands can secrete some colored substances, causing local skin or clothing to change color, which is called chromidrosis.

(3) Sebaceous glands: Sebum is a mixture of various lipids. Sebaceous gland secretion is mainly affected by various hormones (e. g., androgens, progesterone, estrogen, glucocorticoids, pituitary hormones), among which androgens can accelerate the division of sebaceous gland cells, making their volume increase and cortical synthesis increase. Estrogen can inhibit endogenous androgen production or directly induce sebaceous glands to reduce

sebum secretion.

1. 2. 5　Temperature regulation function

On the one hand, the skin senses changes of the external environment temperature through the peripheral temperature sensors throughout the body, and sends information to the hypothalamus; on the other hand, the skin acts as a body temperature regulating effector to regulate body temperature via vasomotion, chills, or sweating after receiving central information.

The skin covers the whole body, and arteriovenous anastomosis is abundant. During cold stress, sympathetic nerves are excited, blood vessels contract, arteriovenous anastomosis are closed, skin blood flow and skin heat dissipation are reduced. When arteriovenous anastomosis are gently opened during heat stress, skin blood flow and skin heat dissipation are increased. Body surface heat dissipation is mainly achieved through radiation, convection, conduction, and sweat evaporation. When the ambient temperature is too high, the main method of heat dissipation is the evaporation of sweat.

1. 2. 6　Metabolic function

Compared with other tissues and organs, the metabolic function of skin has its particularity and mainly encompasses the following metabolism.

(1) Glycometabolism: The sugars in the skin are mainly glycogen, glucose, and mucopolysaccharides. The dermis is rich in mucopolysaccharides, mainly including hyaluronic acid and chondroitin sulfate. The synthesis and degradation of mucopolysaccharides are mainly accomplished through enzymatic reactions, but certain non-enzymatic substances can also degrade hyaluronic acid. In addition, endocrine factors can also affect the metabolism of mucopolysaccharides.

(2) Protein metabolism: Skin proteins include fibrous proteins and non-fibrous proteins. The former includes keratin, collagen, and elastin, and the latter includes nuclear proteins in cells and various enzymes that regulate cell metabolism. The degradation of proteins in the skin is accomplished by catalyzing the hydrolysis of polypeptide chains under the action of proteolytic enzymes. Proteolytic enzymes are divided into two types: endopeptidase and exonuclease. The enzyme action lacks strict substrate specificity. The proteolytic enzymes in the skin not only participate in the metabolism of extracellular structural substances under normal circumstances, but also participate in the inflammatory process of the skin and the regulation of cell functions.

(3) Lipid metabolism: Lipids in the skin include fats and lipoids. Epidermal cells differ significantly in their lipid composition at various stages of differentiation. From the basal layer to the stratum corneum, the contents of cholesterol, fatty acids, and ceramide gradually increase, while the content of phospholipids gradually decreases. The abundant essential fatty acids in the epidermis are linoleic acid and arachidonic acid, the latter can

synthesize vitamin D under the influence of sunlight.

(4) Water and electrolyte metabolism: The water in the skin is mainly distributed in the dermis. When the body is dehydrated, the skin can provide 5%-7% of water content to maintain the stability of the circulating blood volume. The skin contains various electrolytes, mainly stored in the subcutaneous tissue. They play important roles in maintaining the crystal osmotic pressure between cells and the acid-base balance inside and outside the cells.

1.2.7 Immune function

The skin is the largest tissue organ of the human body, constituting the immune barrier between the body and the external environment, and is also an important immune organ. The functions of the skin immune system include: ①innate immune function, such as tight junctions between keratinocytes to form a cell barrier; phagocytosis, dissolution and killing of pathogenic microorganisms of macrophages; cytolysis of complement; ②adaptive immune function, refers to the antigen presentation effect of keratinocytes, Langerhans cells, and dermal dendritic cells; the effect of T cells and their subgroups; and the effect of immune molecules (e.g., cytokines and antibodies). It has been discovered that vascular endothelial cells and fibroblasts in the dermis can also participate in the skin immune response. The skin can effectively initiate an immune response and restore and maintain immune homeostasis in time to avoid immune pathological damage, and skin immune function disorders can lead to disease states. The skin completes its immune function with a variety of immune cell components and a large number of immune molecules.

1.2.7.1 Cells of the skin's immune system

The cells of the skin's immune system can be divided into professional immune cells and non-professional immune cells according to their functions. Professional immune cells include Langerhans cells, dendritic cells, lymphocytes, macrophages, and mast cells; non-professional cells include keratinocytes, fibroblasts, and endothelial cells (Table 1-1).

Table 1-1 Distributions and functions of major immune cells in the skin

Cell type	Distributions	Functions
Professional immune cells		
Langerhans cells	Epidermis	Antigen presentation, synthesis and secretion of cytokines, immune monitoring, etc.
Dendritic cells	Dermis	Antigen presentation, synthesis and secretion of cytokines, immune monitoring, etc.
Lymphocytes	Dermis	Mediation of immune response, anti-skin tumors, participation in inflammatory response, wound repair, maintain skin's own stability, etc.

Continued

Cell type	Distributions	Functions
Macrophages	Upper dermis	Wound repair, prevent microbial invasion
Mast cells	Around the dermal papilla blood vessels	Type I hypersensitivity

Non-professional immune cells

Fibroblasts	Dermis	Maintain immune homeostasis
Keratinocytes	Epidermis	Synthesis and secretion of cytokines, involved in antigen presentation
Endothelial cells	Dermal blood vessels	Secretion of cytokines, participation in inflammation, tissue repair, etc.

Keratinocytes are the first line of defense in the epidermal barrier. They play important roles in the early surveillance of pathogens by identifying viral nucleic acids, lipopolysaccharides, flagellin, and zymosan. At the same time, keratinocytes, like Langerhans cells, can ingest, process and present antigens to T cells, and can also release a variety of cytokines and chemokines, regulate immune responses and participate in inflammatory responses. Keratinocytes express a variety of membrane molecules: ① Adhesion molecules, including intercellular adhesion molecule -1 (ICAM-1), lymphocyte function-associated antigen-3 (LFA-3), integrin $\alpha_2\beta_1/\alpha_6\beta_4$ and cadherin (E-cadherin, P-cadherin), etc. The binding of integrin $\alpha_5\beta_1$ to the receptor can mediate endocytosis and kill pathogens; the combination of ICAM-1 and LFA-1 can induce immune cells to migrate to the epidermis, provide costimulatory signals, and regulate cell-cell interactions. ② MHC molecules. In normal circumstances, keratinocytes mainly express MHC class I molecules. In inflammatory conditions (e. g. , discoid lupus erythematosus, psoriasis, and eczema), the expression of MHC class I and class II molecules can be up-regulated and participate in adaptive immune responses. ③ Surface receptors, including a variety of cytokine receptors and pattern recognition receptors, which can monitor changes in the external environment and provide pro-inflammatory and chemotactic signals to immune cells when pathogens invade. In addition, keratinocytes can secrete a variety of immune effector molecules such as cytokines (IL-1, IL-6, IL-7, IL-17, IL-23, TNF-α, and TGF-β, etc.), chemokines (CXCL8, CCL17, and CCL20, etc.), and a variety of antimicrobial substances to participate in the inflammatory response and regulate the immune response.

Langerhans cells are dendritic non-pigmented cells derived from bone marrow, accounting for 3%-5% of epidermal cells. Langerhans cell membrane molecules include CD1a, MHC class I and class II molecules, CD45 and CD45RO, integrins β_1 and β_2, Langerin (i. e. , CD207, which is a marker of Langerhans cells that can induce the formation of Birbeck particles in Langerhans cells), chemokines body (e. g. , CCR6). CD1a is highly expressed in immature Langerhans cells, while its expression in the mature and cultured Langerhans cells is significantly reduced. Langerhans cells can secrete a variety of cytokines (IL-1, IL-4, IL-6, IL-10, IL-15, and TNF-α, etc.) and chemokines, such as macrophage-derived chemokines, macrophage inflammatory protein-α, and monocyte chemoattractant protein-1, to mediate the homing of Langerhans cells from the peripheral blood to the skin and the migration from the epidermis to the dermal lymph nodes after ingesting antigens. Langerhans cells can regulate the proliferation and migration of T cells, and participate in immune regulation, immune surveillance, immune tolerance, skin graft rejection and contact hypersensitivity (see extended reading 4).

Skin dendritic cells include: ①epidermal dendritic cells, that is, Langerhans cells (as described above); ②dermal-resident dendritic cells, which are dendritic cells that reside in the dermis, have the capacity of antigen-uptaking and presenting, the surface marker of which is CD1c; ③"inflammatory" dermal dendritic cells, derived from circulating DC precursor cells, migrate to the skin under the stimulation of inflammation and chemokine signals, and the surface marker is $CD11c^+CD1c^-$, which can activate Th17 cells; ④plasmacytoid dendritic cells (pDC), which are a special type of resident (skin) dendritic cells with a surface marker of BDCA-2, which can produce high levels of type 1 IFN during virus infection. The functions of skin DC include: ①recognize PAMP (pathogen-associated molecular patterns) with the help of surface TLR (Toll-like receptor) and get activated, secreting TNF-α, etc., to promote keratinocytes in contact with pathogens to produce TNF-α and IL-1; ②activated dendritic cells migrate to the skin to drain lymph nodes initiating the adaptive immune response.

Macrophages include tissue colonized macrophages and macrophages derived from circulating monocytes infiltrating blood vessels into the skin to differentiate and develop. They can kill pathogens, phagocytosis of foreign bodies, senescent and degenerated tissue cells, and kill tumor cells, and it can be used as an antigen-presenting cell to participate in adaptive immune response.

Skin mast cells are mainly distributed around dermal blood vessels, hair follicles, nerves, and sebaceous glands. Mast cells not only participate in IgE-mediated type Ⅰ hypersensitivity, but also play an important role in the anti-infective innate immunity and adaptive immune response, and participate in the occurrence of inflammatory autoimmune diseases.

The lymphocytes in the skin are mainly T cells, and the T cells in the epidermis account for about 2% of the total number of lymphocytes. Most of them are $CD4^+$ or $CD8^+$ T cells that express TCRαβ. The vast majority (over 90%) of T cells are located in the dermis, most of which are $CD4^+CD45RO^+$ memory T cells, and the rest are $CD8^+$ T cells. The adhesion molecules involved in T cells homing are mainly skin lymphocyte-associated antigen (CLA) and E-selectin, as well as VLA-4, LFA-1 and ICAM-1/2 (see extended reading 5).

1.2.7.2　The humoral components of the skin's immune system

The humoral components of the skin's immune system include cytokines, immunoglobulins, complement, antimicrobial peptides, neuropeptides, etc.

Cytokines are a class of small-molecule soluble peptide mediators. A variety of cells in the epidermis can synthesize and secrete cytokines. Cytokines are divided into six categories: interleukin, interferon, hematopoietic clone stimulating factor, tumor necrosis factor, growth factor and transforming factor, and chemokine. Cytokines can act locally, or act systematically in a hormone-like manner.

Normal skin usually has no complement. The complement system is activated when the skin is inflamed. Complement can participate in natural immunity and acquired immunity by dissolving cells, immunoadsorption, sterilization, and allergic toxins and promoting the release of mediators. Complement deficiency is associated with certain skin diseases. For example, C1r, C1s, C2, and C4 deficiency are associated with systemic lupus erythematosus, lupus-like syndrome, and dermatomyositis; C1 inhibitor deficiency is associated with hereditary angioedema, SLE, and discoid to lupus erythematosus; C4 deficiency can increase the risk of vitiligo.

Immunoglobulin refers to a globulin with antibody activity or chemical structure similar to that of an antibody and plays the role in acquired immunity. The content of immunoglobulin in normal skin is very low. Patients with certain autoimmune skin diseases (e. g., lupus erythematosus, scleroderma, pemphigus, pemphigoid, and herpetic dermatitis) have significantly higher levels of autoantibodies. The latter forms immune complexes with corresponding autoantigens and deposits in the skin and other tissues and organs, leading to diseases.

There are more than 20 kinds of antimicrobial peptides, including antibacterial peptides, β-defensins, substance P, and chemokines. Antibacterial peptides are a kind of small molecule peptides that can directly kill a variety of pathogens and play an important role in normal skin innate immunity. Moreover, antibacterial peptides have chemotactic effects on neutrophils, macrophages, and T cells. In addition, skin nerve endings can release sensory neuropeptides such as calcitonin gene-related peptides, substance P, and neurokinase A after being stimulated by the external environment, causing chemotaxis to neutrophils and macrophages and resulting in local inflammation.

1.3　Challenges and Perspectives

Skin covers the body surface with unique anatomical structures, and is the first line of defense of the human body. In the future, according to the unique structure of the skin, high-efficiency polymer transdermal drugs can be designed to make up for the shortcomings of traditional treatments and improve curative effects. At the same time, polymer materials are also expected to be used in non-invasive detection and diagnosis of skin diseases. For example, autoimmune diseases are often accompanied by the deposition of immune complexes at the dermal-epidermal junction. If the corresponding polymer materials can be designed according to the structural characteristics of the skin, and then it can replace the skin biopsy, greatly reducing the burden of clinical work. Furthermore, skin immune system plays an important role in the pathogenesis of many skin diseases. In the future, through in-depth research on the functions of various immune cells in different skin diseases, drug-encapsulated polymers that specifically target specific subgroups of immune cells can be designed to help precise treatment of skin diseases. Finally, tissue engineered skin has made milestone progress in recent years, which can significantly improve the quality of skin wound repair. In the future, detailed and in-depth research on skin tissue structure can further help us find and design more suitable natural polymer materials for the research and development of tissue engineered skin. In summary, the anatomical structure and function of the skin are the cornerstones of dermatology. Through in-depth exploration of the anatomical structure and function of the skin, the combination of polymer technology and the structure and function of the skin will create the new era of diagnosis and treatment of skin diseases.

Questions

1. How to design more efficient polymer transdermal drugs based on the structural characteristics of the epidermis?

2. Please summarize the characteristics of the main immune cells involved in the epidermal and dermal immune responses, and think about how to design polymer drug-carrying materials that can specifically target specific immune cell subgroups.

3. According to the structural characteristics of the dermal-epidermal junction, can the corresponding polymer materials be designed to replace the skin biopsy and be used for the non-invasive detection and diagnosis of autoimmune diseases characterized by the deposition of immune complexes at the dermal-epidermal junction?

4. Considering the structure and function of the skin, which natural polymer materials can be used for tissue engineered skin?

5. How to design a polymer material with skin barrier function restoration and antibacterial properties to promote its application in skin wound repair?

Extended Reading

[1] Kaplan D H. Ontogeny and function of murine epidermal Langerhans cells[J]. Nat Immunol,2017,18(10):1068-1075.

[2] Egami S, Yamagami J, Amagai M. Autoimmune bullous skin diseases, pemphigus and pemphigoid[J]. J Allergy Clin Immunol,2020,145(4):1031-1047.

[3] Grice E A, Segre J A. The skin microbiome[J]. Nat Rev Microbiol,2011,9(4):244-253.

［4］ Nestle F O，Di Meglio P，Qin J Z，et al. Skin immune sentinels in health and disease
［J］. Nat Rev Immunol，2009，9(6):679-691.

［5］ Kabashima K，Honda T，Ginhoux F，et al. The immunological anatomy of the skin
［J］. Nat Rev Immunol，2019，19(1):19-30.

(Li Jun   Tao Juan)

第二章
皮肤健康与
代表性皮肤疾病

健康、完整的皮肤作为第一道屏障,能保护机体以抵御外部各种物理性、化学性损伤以及微生物的入侵。如果皮肤受到破坏,屏障功能受损,会导致皮肤炎症、过敏等相应的皮肤疾病。本章将对皮肤屏障的组成、功能、稳态调节进行介绍,并讲述皮肤屏障损伤与几种常见的皮肤疾病之间的联系。

第一节　皮肤健康

一、皮肤屏障

皮肤直接与外界环境接触,在内环境与外界环境之间形成保护性屏障,以抵御有害物质(如极端温度、紫外线、过敏原、毒素和微生物)的侵袭。皮肤屏障的损伤会导致皮肤干燥、瘙痒、脱皮和渗液等,也与多种皮肤疾病的发生密切相关。

（一）皮肤屏障的组成

皮肤屏障通常指表皮,尤其是角质层的物理或机械屏障结构(图 2-1)。从生化组成和功能作用方面来看,表皮的物理屏障结构与表皮的脂质、各种蛋白质、水、无机盐以及其他代谢产物密切相关。

1. 角质层

角质层主要由角质形成细胞和脂质构成。细胞外脂质可作为渗透、抗氧化和抗菌屏障,角质形成细胞可作为抗紫外线和机械屏障。角质层由角质形成细胞的分化和不断更新形成。角质化的过程中,角质形成细胞经历了不同的发育阶段,从基底层的循环角质形成细胞,到棘层和颗粒层的早期到晚期分化细胞,再到角质层中死亡的角质形成细胞。细胞角蛋白和角蛋白中间丝相关蛋白参与了角质化过程。

角质形成细胞会形成富含蛋白质和脂质的外围包膜,即角质化的细胞套膜。在角质化细胞套膜的最外层,神经酰胺和其他脂质共价结合形成脂质包膜。脂质包膜的主要功能是防止经皮水分散失(TEWL),以及 Na^+、K^+、Ca^{2+} 等溶质的流失。

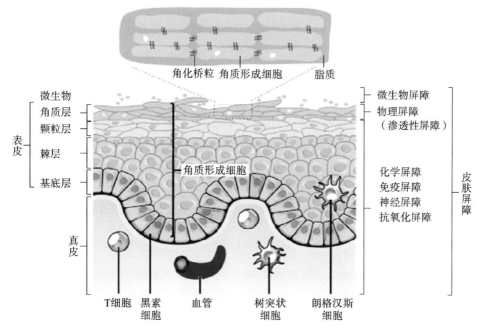

图 2-1　皮肤屏障示意图

Figure 2-1　Illustration showing the skin barrier

2. 桥粒和紧密连接

桥粒是角质形成细胞间连接的主要结构,由附着板和一些重要的桥粒蛋白构成。桥粒将外侧细胞膜的顶端封闭,因此细胞外液被分成两个部分,维持不同的离子强度和溶质浓度。

除了桥粒之外,紧密连接也参与了皮肤屏障的构成。紧密连接包括多种跨膜蛋白和胞内蛋白,主要有 Claudin 家族、Occludin 家族、ZO 家族、黏附分子家族等。这些蛋白质在细胞产生极性及分化的过程中相互交联,最终形成致密网状结构,封锁细胞间隙。它不仅是物理屏障,还具有离子选择性和粒子大小选择性。根据不同的细胞类型和生理需求,屏障功能的紧密程度也不同,从而能够动态调节物质运输。

3. 朗格汉斯细胞

朗格汉斯细胞作为免疫屏障发挥重要功能。朗格汉斯细胞是皮肤的抗原呈递细胞,能识别、结合和处理侵入皮肤的抗原,并把抗原呈递给 T 细胞,在人体的防御系统中起着极为重要的作用。在机体处于稳态时,朗格汉斯细胞的树突朝向外侧,位于紧密连接的内侧。被激活时,朗格汉斯细胞的树突穿过紧密连接的屏障,从外侧环境中摄取抗原。

4. 其他

角质形成细胞合成并分泌多种抗菌肽(AMPs),具有抗菌特性。AMPs 可以与脂质包膜相互作用并结合在一起,当微生物与表皮接触时,共同提供杀死或灭活微生物的功能。表皮有一个钙离子浓度梯度,在基部和增殖层中钙离子浓度较低,而在外层分化层中钙离子浓度逐渐升高。这种表皮的钙离子浓度梯度在皮肤屏障功能中起着非常重要的作用。表皮钙离子浓度梯度调节表皮分化过程和表皮通透性屏障的稳态。

人的皮肤表面 pH 为 4.5~5.5,与正常生理 pH 相比略呈酸性。角质层的酸度对建立表皮通透性屏障、产生表皮抗菌屏障和控制角质层的完整性和凝聚力至关重要。角质层中存在大量的蛋白质降解酶和蛋白酶,每种蛋白酶都有其最适 pH。

蛋白酶也参与表皮的屏障功能。持续的更新过程是由表皮表面的"老"角质形成细胞脱落来平衡的,这被称为脱屑。

(二) 皮肤屏障的保护功能

1. 抗物理性损伤

表皮具有一定的机械强度,对各种机械力如摩擦、挤压等有防护作用,并在受到损伤后具有一定的修复能力。表皮中的黑素屏障和角质层的蛋白质屏障可以通过吸收紫外线辐射发挥屏障作用。

2. 防化学性损伤

正常皮肤对各种化学物质具有一定的屏障作用。皮肤表面的弱酸性环境具有缓冲酸、碱的能力。

3. 防生物性入侵

完整的皮肤屏障能够机械性地防御微生物入侵。一方面,皮肤产生的抗微生物多肽可以杀伤细菌、病毒、真菌等微生物;另一方面,皮肤的弱酸性环境和角质层的生理性脱落也不利于微生物的生长繁殖。

4. 防止水、电解质及营养物质的流失

角质层的半透膜性可以防止体内水、电解质和营养物质的流失。皮肤表面的皮脂膜也可大大减少水分丢失。正常情况下,成人每天经皮肤丢失的水分为 $240\sim480$ mL(不显性出汗);但如果角质层完全丧失,每天通过皮肤丢失的水分将增加 10 倍以上。

(三) 皮肤屏障稳态的调节

皮肤屏障稳态的维持涉及以下几种机制:皮肤表面 pH、角质层的水合作用、表皮中的钙离子浓度梯度及核激素受体等。

1. 皮肤表面 pH

正常皮肤表面 pH 为 $4.5\sim5.5$。皮肤表面微生物代谢产物、来源于毛囊皮脂腺的游离脂肪酸、乳酸、表皮丝聚蛋白的降解产物(吡咯烷酮羧酸和尿酸)等参与皮肤表面酸性环境的形成。酸性皮肤表面环境在预防感染、表皮屏障的损伤修复以及角质形成细胞脱落中都发挥着重要作用。皮肤表面 pH 的变化与一些皮肤疾病的发病密切相关,如刺激性接触性皮炎、特应性皮炎、鱼鳞病、寻常痤疮和白色念珠菌感染等。

2. 角质层的水合作用

角质层的含水量与皮肤弹性、角质形成细胞的脱落和皮肤屏障的损伤修复有关。角质层含水量较少的皮肤弹性差。调节角质形成细胞脱落的酶,如丝氨酸蛋白酶和糖苷酶,其功能的正常发挥需要角质层中的水。角质层的水合作用对皮肤屏障的修复也很重要。在高湿度条件下,屏障破坏后脂质的生物合成作用降低,皮肤屏障损伤修复得更慢。

3. 钙离子浓度梯度

在表皮中存在钙离子浓度梯度,基底层、棘层和角质层的钙离子浓度较低,颗粒层的钙离子浓度最高。钙离子浓度梯度在皮肤屏障破坏后的修复过程中非常重要,细胞连接形成的过程也需要钙离子的参与。表皮钙离子浓度梯度异常具有临床意义。在 X 连锁鱼鳞病和银屑病等皮肤屏障异常的疾病中存在表皮钙离子浓度梯度异常。

4. 核激素受体

核激素受体的功能与转录过程密切相关,在调节表皮发育和皮肤屏障稳态时发挥重要作用。脂质及其代谢产物结合并激活核激素受体,调节板层小体分泌脂质并进行脂质的进一步加工,从而形成砖墙结构。因此,核激素受体在表皮屏障的形成和损伤修复过程中的作用不容忽视。

(四) 屏障损伤相关疾病

皮肤屏障稳态的维持需要上述多种机制共同发挥作用,其中任何一种机制异常都会造成皮肤屏障损伤,从而导致皮肤疾病的发生。此外,遗传因素、年龄、不恰当地使用去污剂和化妆品等也会损伤皮肤屏障。皮肤屏障在多种皮肤疾病中都会遭到破坏,如特应性皮炎、刺激性皮炎、银屑病和葡萄球菌性烫伤样皮肤综合征等。下面以特应性皮炎和接触性皮炎为例进行介绍。

1. 特应性皮炎(AD)

丝聚蛋白(FLG)参与上皮屏障的形成,编码丝聚蛋白的 FLG 基因突变是 AD 的重要危险因素。FLG 基因突变后丝聚蛋白合成减少,上皮屏障形成障碍;过敏原、刺激物和微生物能透过该屏障进入皮肤环境中,导致上皮细胞因子(如胸腺基质淋巴细胞生成素(TSLP)、IL-4、IL-13 和 IL-33)的释放,它们在 2 型免疫反应和炎症反应的发生中起着关键作用。IL-4 和 IL-13 可以抑制表皮功能,加之丝聚蛋白和丝聚蛋白降解产物的减少,共同促进了金黄色葡萄球菌的侵袭和定植。在 AD 患者中,皮肤屏障和皮肤免疫之间存在恶性循环,所以皮肤屏障的恢复对治疗 AD 以及阻止其发展都很重要。

研究表明,使用润肤剂改善皮肤屏障可以预防 AD 的发生。研究结果表明,润肤剂的使用使 AD 的发生率降低了 50%,但并非所有的润肤剂使用后都能预防 AD 的发生,其原因仍需要进一步研究。

2. 接触性皮炎

接触性皮炎通常是由接触具有刺激性或毒性的物质引起,这些物质破坏皮肤屏障,造成皮肤黏膜组织损伤。产生刺激的主要病理机制包括皮肤屏障破坏、细胞因子级联反应和氧化应激网络的参与。表皮屏障的完整性在人类皮肤对刺激的响应中起关键作用,不同刺激引起皮肤屏障障碍的机制不同,但无论何种刺激,都会打破皮肤屏障的稳态。受损的角质层释放更多的水从而使颗粒层中钙离子浓度降低,诱导板层小体分泌脂质,引起皮肤修复反应的发生。

对某些职业来说,长期接触溶剂、水和清洁剂是不可避免的,这可能会破坏皮肤屏障,使有害物质进入皮肤,从而导致接触性皮炎的发生。润肤剂的使用可以有效地预防接触性皮炎。

二、光老化

皮肤老化是皮肤科的常见病,与遗传、环境等因素相关。皮肤内在老化是由基因决定的,皮肤内在老化相关的临床特征包括皮肤萎缩、弹性丧失、细纹、干燥以及血管突出等。外在老化与环境因素(如紫外线辐射、吸烟、污染、营养和生活方式因素)相关。与环境因素相关的临床特征包括深度皱纹、粗糙纹理、毛细血管扩张、皮疹和不规则的色素沉着等。紫外线引起的皮肤老化称为光老化,紫外线是最常见的环境因素。由于人们对皮肤年轻化的追求,光老化逐渐成为人们关注的焦点。本节将从光老化的发病机制、临床表现、组织学特征和防治等方面来对光老化进行阐述。

（一）发病机制

1. 紫外线诱导皮肤胶原蛋白降解

（1）活性氧（ROS）：紫外线可增加 ROS 的产生。过量的 ROS 会对细胞造成氧化损伤，从而导致胶原蛋白降解。

（2）促分裂原活化蛋白激酶（MAPK）：MAPK 在细胞生长和前胶原Ⅰ形成的调控中发挥着关键作用。紫外线上调 MAPK 信号转导通路，引起下游信号转导和激活蛋白 1（AP-1）的形成。AP-1 能抑制胶原蛋白合成并促进胶原蛋白分解。

（3）基质金属蛋白酶（MMPs）：基质金属蛋白酶的表达升高，促使真皮细胞外基质降解（尤其是前胶原Ⅰ和Ⅲ），胶原蛋白合成也减少。

2. 紫外线导致皮肤细胞的基因和分子改变

紫外线可通过直接和间接（激活 ROS）的方式损伤脱氧核糖核酸（DNA）和线粒体 DNA（mtDNA），从而引起 DNA 的端粒缩短，以及 mtDNA 的 ATP 生成减少，从而加速皮肤老化。

3. 紫外线对血管产生双重作用

紫外线可以诱导皮肤新生血管的形成。然而，这些新生血管渗透性较高，可产生炎症因子渗出到细胞间质引发皮肤炎症，导致细胞外基质降解，真皮血管减少，从而加速光老化。

（二）临床表现和组织学特征

1. 临床表现

光老化在临床分型上可以分为两大类：萎缩性光老化和肥厚性光老化。前者表现为皱纹减少和增生异常的癌前病变，如光线性角化病。后者表现为较深的皱纹、皮肤粗糙、雀斑和古铜色外观，也可表现出黄色鹅卵石样外观。

2. 组织学特征

光老化的组织学特征包括真表皮交界处的弹性组织变性和胶原断裂，表皮厚度和表皮细胞的形态均不规则。随着增生性成纤维细胞数量的增加，糖胺聚糖和蛋白多糖的生成也增加，包括肥大细胞、嗜酸性粒细胞和单核细胞在内的炎症细胞增多。紫外线损伤还会导致黑素生成的上调。

（三）防治

光老化有两种防治措施，包括光防护和药物治疗。

1. 光防护

光防护是一项主要的预防策略，包括穿防晒服、适当涂抹防晒霜、在紫外线最强的时候避免晒太阳等。

2. 药物治疗

（1）外用维 A 酸：维 A 酸和他扎罗汀是目前美国 FDA 批准用于治疗光老化的两种外用维生素 A 衍生物。它们能促进胶原纤维的生成，改善临床症状。

（2）5-氟尿嘧啶乳膏：尽管没有被美国 FDA 批准，但外用 5-氟尿嘧啶乳膏对光老化治疗是有益的。研究表明，5-氟尿嘧啶可以促进伤口愈合和皮肤重塑。

（3）药妆：药妆对光老化有一定的疗效，包括抗氧化剂、大豆、茶、银杏、人参等。其中抗氧化剂可以清除自由基，从而保护细胞免受损害，比如辅酶 Q、硫辛酸、维生素 C 和维生素 E。

三、色素和皮肤颜色

皮肤作为机体的保护性屏障,可以使机体免受外界环境刺激如紫外线、毒素、病原微生物等的侵袭。其中,皮肤色素在抵御紫外线的过程中发挥着重要的作用。皮肤色素的生成是一个受严格调控的复杂过程,多种内源性和外源性因素参与黑素生成的调节;许多生理和外部事件都可以改变皮肤色素沉着过程,导致色素沉着过多或不足,从而引起皮肤疾病。

(一)皮肤颜色

正常的皮肤颜色主要由两个因素决定:一是皮肤内色素的含量,包括黑素、胡萝卜素等;二是皮肤的解剖学差异,主要是皮肤的厚薄,尤其是角质层和颗粒层的厚薄。黑素是决定皮肤颜色的主要色素。

(二)皮肤色素的生成过程及调节

皮肤色素沉着主要是由于角质形成细胞中黑素颗粒的积聚。黑素细胞分泌的黑素进入黑素小体中,然后黑素小体转移到角质形成细胞内,并在核上区域运输和重组、形成黑素帽,从而保护角质形成细胞核免受紫外线损伤。

皮肤色素沉着调节过程精细而复杂,多种途径(包括细胞内信号通路、非编码 RNA (miRNAs 和 lncRNAs)和循环外泌体等)共同作用,并通过表皮的黑素细胞和角质形成细胞以及真皮的成纤维细胞相互作用,分泌细胞因子(如 α-MSH、SCF、KGF、bFGF)来调节皮肤色素沉着。

(三)色素沉着相关疾病

皮肤色素沉着易受许多生理和外界条件的影响。遗传因素、长期暴露于紫外线、雌激素水平升高是引起黄褐斑的常见原因。近年来,人们也发现皮肤常驻细胞、肥大细胞、成纤维细胞、真皮血管数量增加与黄褐斑色素沉着有关。miRNA 在黄褐斑黑素生成和黑素小体转移过程中具有潜在作用。随着年龄的增长,局部皮肤色素沉着可出现老年斑。一些皮肤疾病可引起局部炎症后色素沉着,如痤疮、特应性皮炎、扁平苔藓等。内分泌疾病(如原发性肾上腺功能不全)也可引起皮肤色素沉着。皮肤色素生成障碍或不足也会导致疾病,如后天性色素脱失性皮肤黏膜疾病——白癜风和先天性色素生成障碍性疾病——白化病。

四、皮肤的无创检测

皮肤疾病的诊断常常依赖于医生的肉眼观察和临床经验,因此视觉判断对疾病的诊断有着重要意义。皮肤组织病理学、免疫组织化学、电镜等技术的发展提高了皮肤疾病诊断的准确度,并且提高了对疾病发病机制的认识。对大多数皮肤疾病来说,皮肤组织病理仍为疾病诊断的金标准。然而,皮肤活检为有创的侵入性检查,常伴随疼痛,存在感染及瘢痕的风险。

近年来,皮肤无创成像技术飞速发展,包括皮肤镜(dermoscopy)、反射式共聚焦显微镜(reflectance confocal microscope,RCM)、高频超声(high-frequency ultrasound,HFUS)和光学相干断层扫描(optical coherence tomography,OCT)等各种技术。皮肤无创成像技术可应用于皮肤肿瘤、炎症性皮肤疾病、感染性皮肤疾病、毛发和甲病等的诊断和监测。它们具有无创、可重复性、实时监测皮损变化等优点,能够减少不必要的活检,受到广大患者及临床医生的青睐。

(一) 皮肤镜

皮肤镜是一种非侵入性的诊断工具,可以放大皮肤病变,观察肉眼不可见的微结构。有手持式皮肤镜,能够提供 20 倍的放大率;也有连接电子系统的皮肤镜工作站,包含摄像头、光纤及镜头,能够放大至 200 倍。皮肤镜能够通过"透明"介质或(和)偏振光源,消除皮肤表面的反射、折射、衍射光,从而使皮损结构更为明显。

皮肤镜分为非接触式(图 2-2(a))与接触式(图 2-2(b))两种。接触式皮肤镜使用玻璃镜片直接接触皮肤,并使用酒精或成像凝胶等介质来降低皮肤和皮肤镜镜头之间的折射率。而在非接触式皮肤镜中,镜片不会与皮肤接触,使用的是偏振光源,交叉偏振透镜吸收所有散射光,只允许单一平面的光通过(图 2-3)。皮肤镜可用于诊断皮肤肿瘤、色素性皮肤疾病、炎症性皮肤疾病、感染性皮肤疾病、自身免疫性皮肤疾病,以及观察毛发和指(趾)甲等。

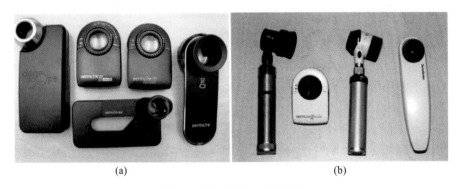

(a)   (b)

图 2-2　常见手持式皮肤镜

(a)常见非接触式偏振光皮肤镜;(b)常见接触式非偏振光皮肤镜

Figure 2-2　Common handheld dermoscopes

(a)Common non-contact polarized dermoscopes;(b)Common contact non-polarized dermoscopes

(二) 共聚焦显微镜

20 世纪 50 年代,激光扫描共聚焦显微镜成像原理被提出。第一台商用的激光扫描共聚焦显微镜仪器由 Rajadhyaksha 等人在哈佛医学院搭建,它基于 830 nm 激光发射器进行水平扫描,形成多层面的平扫图像。组织的可视化是基于不同组织发光团(特别是黑素、胶原蛋白和角蛋白之间)的折射指数的内在差异来创建图像的。黑素的折射率最强为 1.7,角蛋白的折射率为 1.5,胶原蛋白和炎症细胞也是高度折射的结构。当反射光到达探测器时,这些结构出现明亮的白色,而非反射结构出现黑暗。高度、中度和非反射结构之间的相互作用产生了一个在细胞水平上代表该区域的黑白图像。不同于在组织病理学上垂直于皮肤表面的图像,反射式共聚焦显微镜(RCM)生成的图像是水平和平行于皮肤表面的。它的横向分辨率为 $1\ \mu m$,放大率相当于 30 倍的显微镜物镜。这项技术的局限性在于它的穿透深度仅有 $200\ \mu m$。它可以探测真表皮交界处和真皮浅层,但不能探测更深的层次,并且需要经过大量训练才能获取和分析图像。皮肤共聚焦显微镜检查主要的适应证包括浅部真菌病、色素增加及减退性疾病、皮肤肿瘤、炎症或病毒性疾病等。

(三) 高频超声

高频超声使用超声波从具有不同声阻抗的界面的反射波生成图像。探头放在皮肤上,反射的声波由计算机分析并生成图像。图像亮度取决于到达换能器的回波幅度。高强度回声

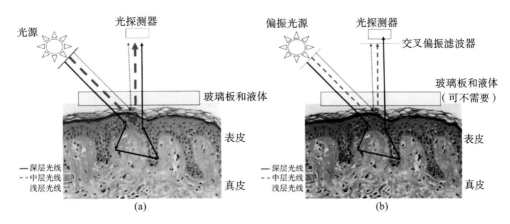

图 2-3 皮肤镜原理

（a）接触式皮肤镜使用时的光学特性示意图。大部分光在表皮浅层被角质层反射,从而使观察者看不到皮肤深层反射的光。使用玻璃板和液体后,少量光线被反射离开角质层（蓝线）,极少量光线散射（粗红线）。一些入射光可以穿透得更深,经过多次散射后被吸收及反射回来（黑线）。（b）偏振光皮肤镜使用时的光学特性示意图。皮肤镜光源发出的光通过交叉偏振滤波器。从角质层反射的光线（蓝线）和表皮浅层吸收的光线（红线）都减少了,从而使观察者能够看到皮肤镜下的结构。偏振光皮肤镜一般不需要与皮肤接触及液体界面,但部分设备可以在接触式与非接触式中进行切换

Figure 2-3　Principles of dermoscopy

（a）The schematic representation of optical properties of light during the use of contact dermoscopy. Most of the light is reflected off the stratum corneum, and thereby precluding the observer from visualizing the light reflected from the deeper layer of the skin. With the use of a glass plate or liquid interface, less light is reflected off the stratum corneum (blue line), minimal light scattered (thick red line). Some of the light penetrates more deeply and is absorbed and reflected back after multiple scattering events (black line). (b) The schematic representation of optical properties of light during the use of polarized dermoscopy. Light emitted from the dermoscopy source passes through a cross-polarized filter. Both the light reflected from the stratum corneum (blue line) and the light absorbed at the superficial layers of the epidermis (red line) reduced, thus allowing the observer to visualize dermoscopic structures (black line). While polarized dermoscopy does not require direct contact and a liquid interface, some of the devices have the option for contact and non-contact types

（或大振幅）产生高回声图像（白色）,而低强度回声（或小振幅）产生低回声图像（灰色）,消声图像是黑色图像。在超声检查中,声波的频率与穿透深度成反比,与图像分辨率成正比。因此,HFUS 的波长越短,分辨率越高,但穿透力越小。在皮肤病学中,常用的频率是 20～25 MHz,但也可以高达 100 MHz。在约 20 MHz 的频率下,分辨率达到 50～200 μm,穿透深度为6～7 mm。如果频率增加到 50 MHz,则分辨率增加到 39～120 μm,但穿透深度仅为 4 mm。目前,高频超声主要用于识别皮肤肿瘤的类型和程度。手术前,它可以提供有关肿瘤类型和大小的信息,确定周围血管的位置,确定切口的最佳位置,并在与患者实时查看超声屏幕时设置范围。它还可以帮助临床医生评估手术后肿瘤是否被完全切除。但使用高频超声区分各种低回声组织（即肿瘤、脂肪和炎症浸润）仍是一个挑战。

五、皮肤毛发

毛发是皮肤附属器,由露出皮面的毛干和深入皮肤的毛根组成。除了提供保护作用,毛发还具有传递社会心理信号和性别信号的功能。尽管毛发疾病一般不会危及生命,但随着人们对生活品质和美的追求日益提高,人们也越来越重视毛发健康问题。常见的毛发疾病有毛囊

炎、雄激素性脱发、斑秃等。

毛发的生长呈周期性,一般分为生长期、退行期和休止期(图 2-4)。相邻毛囊呈非同步生长,处于不同的生长周期。身体各部分毛发生长周期是有差异的,头发的生长周期最长,生长期可长达 5 年,退行期约 2 周,休止期约 3 个月。正常人平均有 100000 根头发,85%～90%的头发处于生长期,小于 1%的头发处于退行期,10%～15%处于休止期。每日脱落 100 根以内的头发是正常的。病理性脱发是指头发异常或过度脱落,其原因很多,包括遗传因素、激素水平、精神压力、药物因素等。其中最常见的类型是雄激素性脱发,表现为毛发密度进行性降低,困扰着近 80%的男性和 42%的女性,其发病机制尚未完全阐明。遗传倾向(例如基因位点的单核苷酸多态性和体内激素水平)导致患者局部头皮毛囊对雄激素敏感性增加,终末期毛囊转变为毳毛毛囊,毛囊逐渐微小化、萎缩。尽管雄激素性脱发的治疗手段有很多,包括口服、外用药物,光疗、手术植发、富含血小板的自体血浆局部注射疗法(PRP)等,但都不能达到完全治愈的效果。目前非那雄胺(选择性Ⅱ型 5α-还原酶抑制剂)和米诺地尔治疗男性雄激素性脱发,米诺地尔治疗女性雄激素性脱发仍然是具有最高证据水平的选择,但药物治疗往往需要较长的维持时间。如何选择性降低毛囊对雄激素的敏感性,逆转毛发微囊化,是目前治疗的难点。

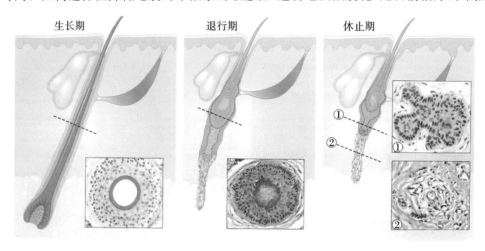

图 2-4　毛发的生长周期(生长期、退行期和休止期)示意图

Figure 2-4　Illustration showing hair growth cycle (growth period, regression period, and resting period)

除了毛发疾病的治疗外,毛发健康管理还包括毛发的日常护理。人们对毛发的护理需求不亚于面部皮肤。各种洗发、护发、生发产品层出不穷,毛发的日常护理具有非常广阔的发展前景。

第二节　皮　肤　伤　口

一、皮肤伤口概述

皮肤伤口是指外力或其他因素导致皮肤组织出现离断或缺损,造成皮肤组织的外观形态、结构功能等的改变。

（一）皮肤伤口愈合机制

皮肤受到损伤（物理、化学、光热等）后立即开始精细、复杂、连续的愈合进程以恢复皮肤完整结构与功能。皮肤伤口愈合包括四个阶段：止血期、炎症期、增殖期、组织重塑期（图 2-5）。此过程涉及多种细胞因子、信号通路和生长因子，它们协同促进皮肤伤口愈合。

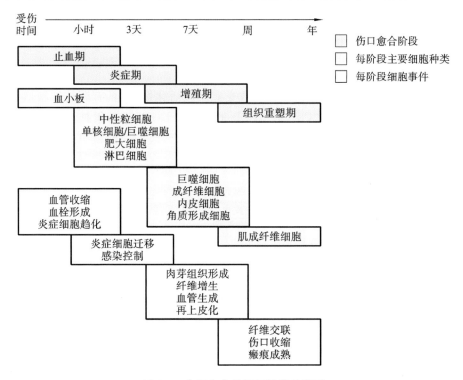

图 2-5 伤口愈合的不同阶段示意图

Figure 2-5 Illustration showing the different stages of wound healing

1. 止血期

皮肤屏障破坏后，血管迅速收缩，外源凝血系统被激活，产生凝血酶，促进纤维蛋白原转化为纤维蛋白。红细胞、血小板与交联排列的胶原纤维聚集在伤口局部形成血凝块封闭受损血管。聚合的血小板活化，诱导糖蛋白及多种生长因子释放。糖蛋白可使更多血小板黏附，形成血栓，产生止血作用。表皮生长因子（EGF）、转化生长因子-β（TGF-β）、成纤维细胞生长因子（FGF）和血小板源性生长因子（PDGF）等通过刺激成纤维细胞产生胶原蛋白和弹性蛋白。

2. 炎症期

随着血管舒张和血管通透性增加，大量白细胞和巨噬细胞浸润到伤口局部清除坏死组织，预防伤口感染。首先，中性粒细胞迁移到伤口局部，通过吞噬作用清除伤口内细菌等病原微生物，分泌蛋白酶降解坏死组织。随后，巨噬细胞浸润伤口，清除细菌和污染物。大量的生长因子、白细胞介素（IL）和肿瘤坏死因子（TNF）等也参与伤口愈合炎症期环节。

3. 增殖期

肉芽组织由增生的成纤维细胞及新生薄壁的毛细血管组成，伴有炎症细胞浸润。巨噬细胞分泌 TGF-β 和 PDGF 诱导成纤维细胞增殖，并产生大量Ⅲ型胶原蛋白，内皮细胞在沉积的胶原蛋白上增殖并促进微血管形成。成纤维细胞合成、分泌Ⅰ型和Ⅲ型胶原蛋白，其中Ⅲ型胶原蛋白比较重要。基质金属蛋白酶(MMPs)、生长因子和白细胞介素具有调节成纤维细胞迁移的功能。研究表明脂肪细胞可迁移至伤口周围,促进表皮细胞覆盖伤口,促进伤口愈合。

4. 组织重塑期

角质形成细胞、成纤维细胞和巨噬细胞等分泌多种基质降解酶,分解多余细胞外基质,组织强度更高的Ⅰ型胶原逐渐代替Ⅲ型胶原,平行排列的Ⅰ型胶原蛋白束能增强组织强度。在组织重塑期,皮肤组织变厚、变坚韧,恢复正常的皮肤屏障功能,整个过程可长达2年。

（二）影响伤口愈合的因素

1. 生长因子对伤口愈合的影响

生长因子是来源于造血系统、免疫系统或炎症反应活化细胞,具有调控细胞增殖分化、促进生长代谢的生物活性多肽,包括 EGF、TGF-β、FGF、PDGF、胰岛素样生长因子(IGF)等。TGF-β 可促进胶原纤维的合成与沉积,具有加速伤口愈合、改变局部组织张力,进而影响瘢痕形成等功能(图 2-6)。

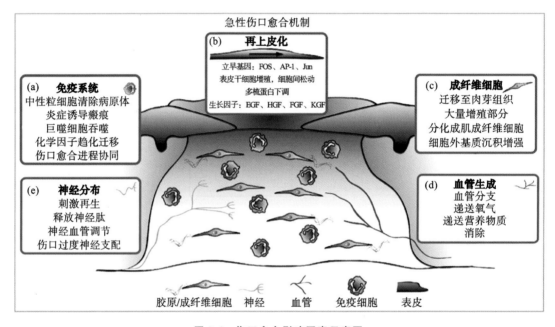

图 2-6　伤口愈合影响因素示意图
(a)免疫系统;(b)再上皮化;(c)成纤维细胞;(d)血管生成;(e)神经分布
Figure 2-6　Illustration showing the factors affecting wound healing
(a)Immune system;(b)Re-epithelization;(c)Fibroblasts;(d)Angiogenesis;(e)Innervation

FGF 可诱导毛细血管的新生,加速上皮和肉芽组织生长。PDGF 是血小板 α 颗粒分泌的多肽,具有刺激处于细胞分裂间期的细胞进入分裂期、促进组织细胞增殖分化等功能。当组织受到损伤时,内皮细胞、平滑肌细胞、成纤维细胞和巨噬细胞合成并分泌 PDGF,趋化炎症细胞浸润伤口、促进肉芽组织形成。目前,国内批准用于创面治疗的生长因子制剂有重组牛碱性成纤维细胞生长因子外用凝胶、重组人碱性成纤维细胞生长因子、重组人表皮生长因子外用溶液等。

2. 基质金属蛋白酶对伤口愈合的影响

基质金属蛋白酶(MMPs)是以 Ca^{2+}、Zn^{2+} 为辅助的肽键内切酶,其活性受金属蛋白酶组织抑制因子(TIMPs)的抑制,参与胶原蛋白等细胞外基质的降解。研究表明,完整皮肤中 MMPs 的表达很低,皮肤损伤后其表达上调;此外,TIMPs 可使伤口愈合延迟,这表明 MMPs 是促进伤口愈合的关键分子。成纤维细胞分泌 MMPs 促进细胞迁移、降解不稳定的细胞外基质。此外,MMPs 可促进巨噬细胞浸润伤口,清除坏死组织,促进血管内皮快速建立伤口区微循环,加速肉芽组织形成。

3. 炎症相关微小 RNA 对伤口愈合的影响

伤口区炎症应答对伤口愈合有关键作用,炎症应答失调会延缓伤口愈合,引起感染,产生增生性瘢痕和瘢痕疙瘩。微小 RNA(miRNA)是来源于真核生物,长度为 21~23 个核苷酸的非编码单链 RNA。miRNA 与转录后的 mRNA 结合,抑制转录后水平基因表达。炎症相关 miRNA 是炎症应答与组织修复的关键调节因子。多种伤口愈合相关 miRNA 已被识别出来,其调节功能失常导致病理性伤口愈合,即愈合缓慢和产生瘢痕等。

4. 氧分子对伤口愈合的影响

临床观察发现,出血较多的伤口大部分愈合良好,而出血较少的伤口愈合较差或不愈合,任何类型的伤口愈合都需要充足的血流灌注和氧气供应。一项临床研究证明,对结直肠切除的患者术前采用氧疗法可使术后伤口感染的发生率降低一半,对慢性延迟愈合的伤口采用高压氧疗法也取得了较好的效果。因此,氧疗法对伤口愈合和预防感染起到了非常重要的作用。

5. 伤口湿性环境对伤口愈合的影响

White 等在猪模型上研究发现,伤口在潮湿环境下比在干燥状态下愈合得快,进而提出了伤口湿性愈合理论。其后多项研究证实了伤口湿性愈合理论,伤口湿性环境可使伤口基底潮湿,刺激血管新生、肉芽组织形成,缩短愈合时间并降低瘢痕形成的可能。

伤口湿性愈合理论指出,采用保湿敷料给伤口保湿可加速伤口愈合。这类保湿敷料使伤口局部形成湿润环境,促进成纤维细胞增殖、毛细血管形成及内源性胶原酶释放和激活,特别是溶解坏死组织的蛋白酶和尿激酶。伤口微环境的改善可吸引大量炎症细胞,分泌多种生长因子,促进伤口愈合。此外,保湿敷料能减少敷料与创面的粘连,减轻换药时的疼痛与二次损伤。目前,伤口湿性愈合理论在我国临床应用中尚存在争议,部分学者认为封闭潮湿环境会造成伤口区病原微生物繁殖,使伤口感染。

二、皮肤伤口修复的并发症及治疗

(一)伤口感染

皮肤作为身体最外层屏障易受到病原微生物侵袭。此外,皮肤表面存在大量常驻菌群,皮肤损伤时易发生感染。感染造成过度持续炎症是伤口难愈合的主要原因之一。据统计,超过 2% 的美国人患有难愈合伤口,每年约花费 200 亿美元用于治疗伤口相关感染。

临床传统治疗皮肤伤口的方法包括外用抗生素软膏、生长因子制剂、纱布等伤口敷料。然而,该方法常伴有抗生素耐药、更换敷料时强烈疼痛及需要专业医护人员换药等问题。随着伤口湿性愈合理论的提出及新材料的合成,水凝胶因含有大量水分可保持伤口湿润、吸收组织渗液及良好的生物安全性,在医学领域发展迅速。目前,越来越多的研究聚焦在载抗菌药物的水凝胶上。

(二)慢性难愈合伤口

皮肤慢性难愈合伤口(溃疡)包括创伤性溃疡、下肢静脉性溃疡、压迫性溃疡以及糖尿病性溃疡等。其具有病程长、影响美观及存在多种严重并发症等特点,对患者的生活质量造成极大的影响。发达国家与发展中国家在皮肤慢性难愈合伤口的发病率、发生部位、年龄以及易患人群方面存在不同。在中国,由创伤所致的皮肤慢性难愈合伤口常见于青少年和青壮年,糖尿病性、压迫性和静脉性溃疡常见于60岁以上的老年人。

皮肤慢性难愈合伤口的病因、发病机制尚未完全阐明。不同皮肤慢性难愈合伤口的发病机制有所差异(图2-7)。研究表明,创伤性溃疡细胞外纤维连接蛋白的基因表达下调,导致组织修复细胞支架破坏,延缓伤口愈合。成纤维细胞的过度凋亡减少真皮胶原纤维的产生,延缓创面修复。伤口内生长因子浓度改变及愈合调控网络发生障碍延缓伤口愈合。相关研究表明,Ca^{2+}信号通路、丝裂原激活的蛋白激酶(MAPKs)、Jaks-STATs、蛋白激酶C(PKC)在慢性难愈合伤口的治疗过程中起介导作用。相关研究有待进一步验证。

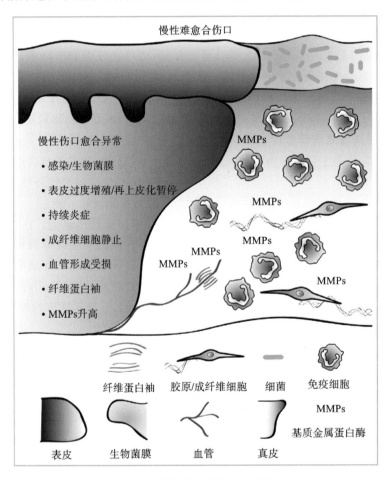

图 2-7　慢性难愈合伤口示意图

Figure 2-7　Illustration showing chronic refractory wound healing

由于病因和发病机制不完全相同,慢性难愈合伤口的治疗方式存在较大差异。创伤性溃疡需首先进行创面的外科处理(清创),其次,采用某些措施和方法来促进创伤性溃疡愈合。糖尿病性溃疡治疗首先必须控制血糖和治疗糖尿病;下肢静脉曲张性溃疡首先必须处理静脉曲张问题等。

近年来,治疗皮肤慢性难愈合伤口的方法包括新型敷料类、生长因子制剂及干细胞与组织工程产品等。水凝胶是亲水性三维网络高分子聚合物,可以吸收大量的水分或液体,具有良好的弹性、溶胀性、表面特性、机械特性和生物安全性,是组织工程、伤口敷料的优良材料。生长因子参与了伤口愈合每一个阶段的调控过程,外源性补充生长因子可调控细胞增殖、分化以及创面愈合的信号转导。美国食品药品监督管理局(FDA)批准上市应用于临床的生长因子制剂包括重组人血小板源性生长因子、重组人和重组牛成纤维细胞生长因子以及重组人表皮生长因子等。伤口愈合的转基因方法将生长因子的基因以裸露的 DNA 形式,通过注射或基因枪等方法转移到伤口局部,促进细胞增殖或血管新生,达到促进伤口愈合的目的。

(三)病理性皮肤瘢痕

皮肤瘢痕是创伤所引起的正常皮肤组织的外观形态和组织病理学改变的统称。据统计,发达国家每年新发一亿以上的瘢痕患者。瘢痕引起机体外观和功能的改变,会影响患者的身心健康,降低患者的生活质量。病理性皮肤瘢痕包括增生性瘢痕、瘢痕疙瘩、萎缩性瘢痕和瘢痕癌等。

瘢痕发病机制还未被阐明,不同类型瘢痕的发生和发展机制也有不同(图 2-8)。公认的观点是成纤维细胞的异常增殖分化与细胞外基质的异常沉积是疾病的中心环节,参与其过程的主要分子有 TGF-β、炎症相关细胞因子、金属基质蛋白酶家族等。此外,机械力相关信号通路也被认为在调控瘢痕形成的过程中发挥重要效应。

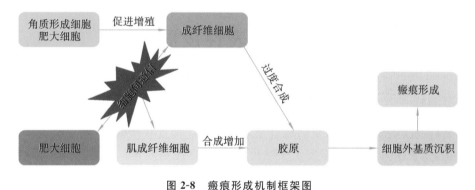

图 2-8 瘢痕形成机制框架图

Figure 2-8 The pathogenic mechanism of scar formation

瘢痕现有的治疗方式繁多,主要可以分为五大类:①手术切除;②瘢痕内药物注射,包括肉毒素 A、博来霉素、糖皮质激素和 5-氟尿嘧啶(5-FU)等;③光电技术治疗,包括点阵激光、脉冲染料激光、射频消融和强脉冲光等;④外用药物,包括洋葱提取物、丝裂霉素 C 和咪喹莫特等;⑤物理治疗,包括硅酮凝胶、压力服、冷冻治疗、放射治疗及微针治疗等。治疗方式的选择与瘢痕的类型、患者既往治疗史以及患者依从性密切相关。

手术切除可单独用于治疗瘢痕疙瘩,鉴于单纯手术切除瘢痕疙瘩的复发率高达 40%~100%,现通常与瘢痕内药物注射、放射治疗、光电技术治疗、物理治疗、外用药物等治疗方式联合进行。

瘢痕内药物注射也是目前的主流治疗方式之一,可注射的药物种类繁多,如糖皮质激素、博来霉素、5-氟尿嘧啶、雷帕霉素、维拉帕米、多柔比星、肉毒素 A 和维 A 酸等,其中有一定临床证据的药物是 5-氟尿嘧啶、糖皮质激素和博来霉素。

由于具有致癌的可能性,放射治疗通常不作为一线治疗措施,而是用于其余方法均无效的难治性瘢痕疙瘩和增生性瘢痕的治疗。放射治疗皮肤瘢痕的潜在机制:诱导成纤维细胞凋亡,诱导基因突变和结缔组织干细胞的损伤。不同类型的激光治疗皮肤瘢痕在临床实践中多有尝试,如剥脱性激光(Er:YAG 点阵激光、CO_2 点阵激光)、强脉冲光和脉冲染料激光(585 nm、595 nm)等。

冷冻治疗皮肤瘢痕的原理是通过制冷剂(通常是液氮)迅速降温导致细胞被冷冻破坏,及解冻后血液淤滞,诱导瘢痕组织的破坏。此外,冷冻使患者局部感觉麻木,能减轻患者的疼痛感,增加患者接受治疗的依从性。

常用的外用药物包括洋葱提取物、丝裂霉素 C 和咪喹莫特等。洋葱提取物在临床上多用于瘢痕的预防或者辅助治疗。洋葱提取物能抑制成纤维细胞和肥大细胞增殖,并且减轻炎症反应,进而减少瘢痕形成。丝裂霉素 C 治疗增生性瘢痕的临床试验较少,证据不足。咪喹莫特多用于耳郭瘢痕疙瘩的切除后复发。

微针治疗瘢痕的机制尚不明确,有研究者认为微针治疗瘢痕后,产生轻微的炎症反应,导致瘢痕组织内基质金属蛋白酶(MMPs)被激活,诱导异常排列的胶原蛋白降解,以达到瘢痕组织重塑的目的。此外,微针被认为是通过影响间隙连接蛋白,改变成纤维细胞感受的机械力,从而改变成纤维细胞中胶原蛋白生成和相关细胞因子分泌的过程。微针接触细胞引起细胞膜电位变化导致细胞活性显著升高,引起蛋白质、钾和生长因子的释放增加,从而刺激成纤维细胞向受伤区域的迁移,并促进胶原蛋白、弹性蛋白和蛋白多糖的产生。

第三节　代表性皮肤疾病

一、银屑病

银屑病(psoriasis)是一种常见的易复发的慢性炎症性皮肤疾病,典型皮损为鳞屑性斑块和丘疹,可发生于任何年龄,但多发生于青壮年,无明显性别差异。自然人群发病率为 0.1%～3%,我国发病率为 0.123%。春冬季节易复发或加重,而夏秋季节多缓解。

（一）病因

银屑病的确切病因尚不清楚。目前认为,银屑病是遗传因素与环境因素等多种因素相互作用的多基因遗传病。

1. 遗传因素

人口调查、家系、遗传学(如双胞胎研究)及 HLA 研究均支持银屑病的遗传倾向。20% 左右的银屑病患者有家族史,且有家族史者发病早于无家族史者。父母一方患有银屑病,其子女银屑病的发病率在 16% 左右;而父母同患银屑病时,其子女银屑病的发病率为 50%。HLA 系统中 Ⅰ 类抗原 A1、A13、A28、B13、B17、B37 及 Cw6 和 Ⅱ 类抗原 DR7 在银屑病患者中表达的频率高于正常人,其中 Cw6 位点与银屑病的相关性最显著。

2. 环境因素

流行病学研究显示,双生子中同卵双生子共患银屑病的概率为 70%,异卵双生子共患银屑病的概率仅为 20%,表明仅有遗传因素不足以引起发病,环境因素在诱发银屑病中起重要作用。易促发或加重银屑病的因素有感染、精神紧张、外伤、手术、妊娠、吸烟和某些药物作用等。

3. 免疫因素

寻常型银屑病皮损处淋巴细胞和单核细胞浸润明显,尤其 T 细胞真皮浸润是银屑病的重要病理特征,说明 T 细胞参与该病的发生与发展过程,虽然其在银屑病病理过程中的确切作用还不清楚。

（二）发病机制

免疫系统参与银屑病的发病。对银屑病相关基因的全基因组扫描已经确定了主要的免疫相关基因,这为遗传学与免疫之间的联系提供了证据。银屑病皮损源于免疫系统(固有免疫和适应性免疫)与皮肤常驻细胞相互作用失调。关于银屑病免疫发病机制的研究有多种理论,包括固有免疫和适应性免疫之间的相互作用以及 TNF-α 的中心作用;白细胞介素-23(IL-23)/辅助性 T 细胞 17(Th17)轴等（图 2-9）。

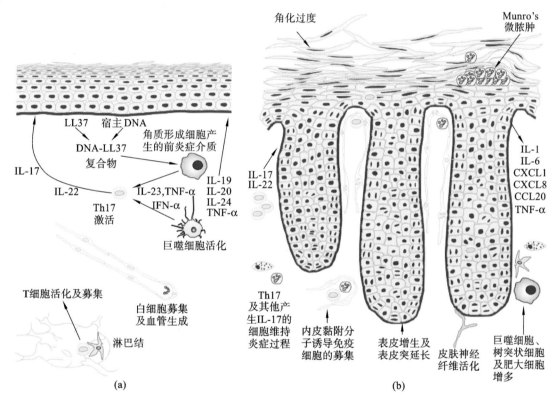

图 2-9　树突状细胞通过 IL-23 刺激 Th1 与 Th17 的分化;适应性免疫与固有免疫系统产生多种炎症介质,在表皮及真皮中诱导和维持银屑病的病理学特征

（a）银屑病前皮肤;（b）银屑病皮损

Figure 2-9　Illustration showing the differentiation of Th1 and Th17 is stimulated by dendritic cells through IL-23;pathogenic cells of the adaptive and the innate immune systems produce several mediators that induce and maintain psoriatic hallmark features in both dermis and epidermis

（a）Pre-psoriatic skin;（b）Psoriatic skin

1. 固有免疫与适应性免疫之间的相互作用

银屑病主要是一种树突状细胞和 T 细胞介导的疾病,具有从抗原呈递细胞、中性粒细胞、角质形成细胞、血管内皮细胞到皮肤神经系统的复杂反馈回路。TNF-α、INF-γ 和 IL-1 等细

胞因子介导的固有免疫系统和适应性免疫系统之间的相互作用是一个重要的研究热点。宿主DNA与表皮产生的抗菌肽 LL-37 复合物被认为可以刺激皮肤浆细胞样树突状细胞产生INF-α。银屑病发病时,激活的树突状细胞产生 TNF-α 和 IL-23。TNF-α 是一种促进炎症的细胞因子,它通过几种不同的途径来放大炎症反应。TNF-α 由多种类型的细胞产生,包括巨噬细胞、淋巴细胞、角质形成细胞和内皮细胞,并对几种不同类型的细胞发挥作用。TNF-α 诱导继发性介质和黏附分子,这些都与银屑病有关。因此,TNF 阻断剂在治疗银屑病中能获得成功。

2. IL-23/Th17 轴

Th17 是表达 IL-17 的 T 细胞亚群,它们的扩增和存活依赖于髓系细胞产生的 IL-23,IL-23驱动 Th17 的分化。IL-23 主要作用于记忆性 T 细胞,因为原始 T 细胞不表达 IL-23 受体。一旦激活,Th17 会产生多种介质,如 IL-17A、IL-17F 和 IL-22,这些介质可诱导角质形成细胞增殖。在银屑病皮损中,IL-17 是由 $CD4^+$ T 细胞、表皮 $CD8^+$ T 细胞、中性粒细胞、肥大细胞和巨噬细胞产生的,这解释了为什么特异性靶向抑制 IL-17 可迅速产生广泛的临床疗效。

(三) 临床表现

根据银屑病的临床特征,银屑病可分为寻常型、关节病型(银屑病关节炎)、红皮病型及脓疱型,其中寻常型占 90% 以上。

1. 寻常型银屑病(psoriasis vulgaris)

初期皮损为红色丘疹或斑丘疹,逐渐扩展成为边界清楚的红色斑块,有多种形态(如点滴状、钱币状、地图状、蛎壳状等),上覆厚层银白色鳞屑,刮除成层鳞屑,犹如轻刮蜡滴(蜡滴现象),刮去银白色鳞屑可见淡红色发光半透明薄膜(薄膜现象),剥去薄膜可见点状出血(Auspitz 征)。蜡滴现象、薄膜现象和点状出血对银屑病有诊断价值。瘙痒程度因人而异。

2. 关节病型银屑病(psoriasis arthropathica)

关节病型银屑病又称为银屑病关节炎,有 5%~8% 的银屑病患者可出现关节炎症状。关节病型银屑病病程为慢性,关节病变常在皮损后出现。任何关节均可受累,尤其是下肢的大关节和指(趾)远端关节,甚至脊椎和骶髂关节。伴有明显甲损害者更易出现指(趾)关节炎;大关节可出现关节畸形,类似类风湿关节炎,但与后者不同的是,银屑病关节炎的类风湿因子常为阴性。脊椎及骶髂关节受累患者常与 HLA-B27 存在密切关联。

3. 红皮病型银屑病(erythrodermic psoriasis)

红皮病型银屑病表现为全身大部分皮肤广泛的炎症和脱屑,皮肤呈弥漫性潮红、浸润肿胀并伴有大量糠状鳞屑,其间可有正常皮肤(皮岛),可伴有发热、全身淋巴结肿大等全身症状。病程较长,易复发。

4. 脓疱型银屑病(pustular psoriasis)

脓疱型银屑病分为泛发性和局限性两型。①泛发性脓疱型银屑病:常急性发病,皮损可迅速发展至全身,在寻常型银屑病皮损或正常皮肤上迅速出现黄色或黄白色的针尖至粟粒大小浅表性无菌性小脓疱,常密集分布融合成"脓湖",有疼痛感,常伴有寒战、高热等全身症状。经过 1~2 周,脓疱可干燥结痂,病情缓解,但可反复发作。患者可因继发感染、全身衰竭而死亡。②局限性脓疱型银屑病:皮损局限于手掌及足跖,对称分布,皮损为成批发生在红斑基础上的无菌性小脓疱。经 1~2 周,脓疱破裂、结痂、脱屑,新脓疱又可在鳞屑下出现,病程较长,经久不愈,仅少数显著消退。甲常受累,可出现点状凹陷、横沟、纵嵴、甲剥离及甲下积脓等。

（四）治疗

小面积的轻度银屑病常采用局部治疗,中度或重度银屑病常需要光疗联合系统治疗。局部疗法通常适用于局限性的斑块。对于广泛的银屑病,光疗的效价比高。传统的免疫抑制剂中,环孢素起效快,但一般不适用于持续治疗。甲氨蝶呤依然是最有效的系统性治疗药物。生物制剂疗效好,但费用昂贵。具有不同毒性的药物联合治疗,常可降低系统总的毒性,并可降低英夫利昔单抗(infliximab)等药物产生中和抗体的发生率。

1. 局部治疗

（1）糖皮质激素:外用糖皮质激素的霜剂、软膏、洗剂、泡沫以及喷剂是治疗银屑病常用的药物。低中效的霜剂适用于间擦部位及面部。对于较厚的角化性鳞屑,为了增强局部糖皮质激素的疗效,在用药之前应将局部浸湿,用药后用聚乙烯薄膜(商品名 Saran Wrap)或桑拿服封包。遗憾的是,当停用激素后皮损会很快复发,且长期使用激素软膏会产生多种不良反应,包括表皮萎缩、类固醇痤疮、栗丘疹和脓皮病。

（2）他扎罗汀(tazarotene):他扎罗汀是维 A 酸的非同分异构体,是一种受体特异性维 A酸。它通过调节角质形成细胞的分化和过度增殖,同时抑制炎症反应来治疗银屑病。

（3）钙泊三醇(calcipotriene):维生素 D_3 通过调节表皮细胞对钙的反应而在一定程度上影响角质形成细胞的分化。使用维生素 D_3 的类似物钙泊三醇软膏、霜剂或溶液治疗斑块型和头皮银屑病非常有效。钙泊三醇和高效能激素制剂的联合应用可达到更好的效果,不良反应更少,激素用量减少。

（4）大环内酰胺类(钙调神经磷酸酶抑制剂)(macrolactams, calcineurin inhibitors):对于容易发生萎缩或类固醇痤疮的部位,或皮肤较薄的部位,局部应用大环内酰胺类如他克莫司或吡美莫司特别有效。初始使用时的烧灼感是这类药物最常见的不良反应,在使用前先应用糖皮质激素软膏,且用于干燥而非沐浴后的皮肤,常可缓解这种烧灼感。

（5）水杨酸:水杨酸的香波、霜剂和凝胶可用作角质溶解剂,能促进其他局部药物的吸收。大面积外用可能导致水杨酸中毒,表现为耳鸣、急性精神紊乱和顽固性低血糖,特别是对糖尿病和肾功能损害的患者。

（6）紫外线疗法:在大多数情况下,日光可改善银屑病病情。但是,严重的皮肤晒伤可能引起同形反应和病情加重。荧光灯泡可产生宽谱或窄谱的人工紫外线(UVB)。通常在最小红斑量(MED)时获得最大效应。在皮损消退后继续维持 UVB 治疗有助于延长病情缓解的时间,这在许多患者身上得到了证实。

（7）PUVA 疗法:患者服用 8-甲氧补骨脂素(商品名 Oxsoralen Ultra),2 h 后给予高强度的长波紫外线照射,每周 2 次,即使对于严重的银屑病患者也非常有效。大多数患者经过 20～25 次治疗后皮损被清除,但仍需维持治疗。尽管 PUVA 疗法非常有效,但是对皮损面积不超过全身 50% 的患者来说,UVB 疗法与 PUVA 一样好。PUVA 疗法是皮肤恶性肿瘤(如鳞癌和黑素瘤)的危险因素。未采取生殖器保护而进行 PUVA 治疗的男性发生阴茎和阴囊鳞状细胞癌的危险性增加。尽管发生癌症的风险与剂量相关,但是累积的 PUVA 照射量超过多少即可预测致癌还没有一个确切的阈剂量。

2. 系统治疗

（1）维 A 酸类药物:维 A 酸类药物适用于各型银屑病,如阿维 A 酯 0.75～1.0 mg/（kg·d）口服。但其"致畸"的副作用以及会导致甘油三酯、总胆固醇和肝酶水平的增高,严重限制了其在育龄期女性、老年人及儿童中的应用。维 A 酸类药物在孕妇中禁用。

(2) 免疫抑制剂:免疫抑制剂主要用于红皮病型、脓疱型、关节病型银屑病,常用药物为甲氨蝶呤,成人剂量为每周 10～25 mg,口服,每周剂量不超过 50 mg,也可用环孢素、他克莫司等;甲氨蝶呤起效慢,疗效常在 12 周或 16 周明显,用药期间须定期检测血常规、肝肾功能。若连续累积剂量大于 1500 mg,须预防及监测肝纤维化。环孢素常用推荐剂量为 3～5 mg/(kg·d),其起效快,症状控制后逐渐减量。长期使用时须监测肾功能及血压。

(3) 生物制剂:生物制剂对银屑病患者能产生很满意的疗效,但价格昂贵。主要有三类生物制剂,包括 TNF-α 抑制剂、IL-12/23 抑制剂及 IL-17 抑制剂。英夫利昔单抗(infliximab)是一种针对 TNF-α 的嵌合单克隆抗体,需静脉输注。依那西普(etanercept)是人 TNF-α Ⅱ 型受体及 IgG1 Fc 区的融合蛋白。阿达木单抗(adalimumab)是一种针对 TNF-α 的重组全人源 IgG1 单克隆抗体。阿法西普(alefacept)是 LFA-3 的胞外区和 IgG1 Fc 区的融合蛋白,可阻断 T 细胞活化并引发致病性 T 细胞的凋亡。依那西普提供了良好的安全性和有效性的平衡。除英夫利昔单抗外,所有用于治疗银屑病的生物制剂均采用皮下注射。总的来说,在使用生物制剂治疗的银屑病患者中,严重感染或内部恶性肿瘤的发生率没有增高,不良反应发生率略高于安慰剂组,且在所有生物制剂中都很常见,包括注射部位反应、鼻咽炎和上呼吸道感染。

(五)治疗难点

前述多种外用药、光化学疗法及传统免疫抑制剂能减轻皮损,缓解症状;系统性使用 IL-23 单克隆抗体、IL-17A 单克隆抗体等多种生物制剂直接阻断 IL-23/Th17 细胞途径均能快速清除银屑病皮损。尽管如此,停止治疗后皮损常复发,这是现阶段银屑病治疗的难点。

银屑病作为一种炎症性疾病,常与多种疾病共同存在,影响患者的生活质量。关节损害是银屑病最常见的并发症。大约有 1/3 的银屑病患者最终发展成关节病型银屑病。严重的银屑病及早年发病的银屑病患者患心血管等代谢性疾病的风险增加,例如糖尿病、高脂血症、肥胖、动脉粥样硬化斑块等。此外,银屑病患者患神经精神疾病的风险更高,例如抑郁、焦虑等。银屑病患者患炎症性肠病的风险也是普通人群的 4 倍。这些共患病与银屑病的确切关系及共患病的治疗也是目前银屑病治疗的难点。

二、黑素瘤

(一)概述

1. 病因及发病机制

(1) 危险因素:紫外线照射是主要的环境危险因素。宿主方面的危险因素包括黑素细胞痣或发育不良性痣、黑素瘤病史、黑素瘤家族史,以及表型特征,如浅色的头发、眼睛、肤色和雀斑。小部分黑素瘤病例由基因突变导致。

(2) 黑素瘤的发生:紫外线(UVA)通过两种不同的机制诱导黑素细胞的恶性转化。原癌基因和抑癌基因(TP53、NF1、PTEN 等)的突变可使正常黑素细胞直接转化为肿瘤细胞。BRAF 基因突变是良性痣形成的典型特征,BRAF 基因在 80% 的良性痣患者中发生了突变。免疫监视作用可使良性痣长期处于惰性,进一步发展为中间病变、原位癌、浸润癌和肿瘤转移需要更多突变。最常见的体细胞突变涉及调控细胞基本生命活动的基因,如增殖(BRAF、NRAS 和 NF1)、生长和代谢(PTEN 和 KIT)、抗凋亡(TP53)、细胞周期调控(CDKN2A)和复制周期(TERT)。这些基因突变导致黑素瘤中细胞信号通路的异常激活,以 MAPK 通路和

PI3K-AKT 通路为主。

（3）肿瘤微环境改变：黑素瘤的扩散是基因突变和肿瘤微环境改变共同导致的结果。肿瘤微环境中，基质金属蛋白酶（MMPs）的过度表达发挥了关键作用，MMPs 可诱导细胞外基质降解，有利于肿瘤细胞的浸润和血流扩散。

（4）黑素瘤细胞的免疫逃逸：黑素瘤细胞还可以逃避机体免疫系统的监控。当 T 细胞识别肿瘤抗原时，释放的干扰素可触发 JAK-STAT 通路介导的 PD-1 配体（PD-L1 和 PD-L2）在黑素瘤细胞表面的表达。PD-1 与 PD-L1 和 PD-L2 的结合，抑制了 T 细胞活性和抗肿瘤免疫反应。其他免疫抑制机制还包括肿瘤相关抗原和 I 类主要组织相容性复合物表达的下调，以及 TGF-β 等抑制因子的表达。

2. 临床表现、分型与分期

（1）临床表现、分型：典型的特征是病灶不对称、边缘不规则、颜色不均匀、直径在 5 mm 以上等。

①浅表扩散型黑素瘤（57.4%）：好发于男性背部和女性腿部。起初为局限于表皮的斑块，呈放射状，生长缓慢，后发展为丘疹或结节，垂直生长迅速。皮肤镜下可见增粗的网状结构，多发的棕色小点，色调多变不一，可出现色素脱失。组织学上以异型黑素细胞在表皮内 Paget 样播散为特点（图 2-10）。

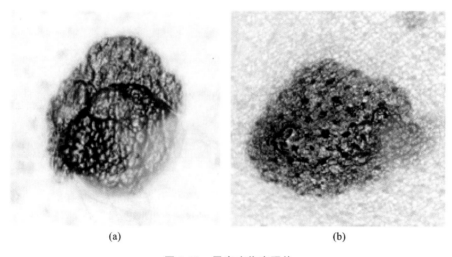

(a) (b)

图 2-10 黑素瘤临床照片
(a)浅表扩散型黑素瘤：发生于发育不良痣；(b)原位黑素瘤
Figure 2-10 Clinical images of melanoma
(a) Superficial spreading melanoma：arising within a dysplastic nevus；(b) Melanoma *in situ*

②结节性黑素瘤（21.4%）：常见于躯干、头颈，男性多于女性。起初为蓝黑色或粉红色结节，可有溃疡或出血，缺乏放射性水平生长而一直处于快速的侵袭性垂直生长状态。皮肤镜下可见不同颜色小球状结构、白色条纹、不规则血管。组织学特征是巢状异型黑素细胞增生。

③恶性雀斑样黑素瘤（8.8%）：好发于鼻、脸颊或任何晒伤的皮肤。表现为颜色不均匀棕黑色斑点，边界不规则。皮肤镜下可见毛囊开口处色素沉着。组织学特征是真表皮交界处非典型性黑素细胞雀斑样增生和日光性弹性组织变性。

④肢端雀斑样黑素瘤（4%）：好发于足底和手掌。早期表现为不规则、边界不清的斑块损

害,后侵袭性生长为结节。皮肤镜下可见不规则、灰褐色多边形及多个色素减退区。甲下黑素瘤可表现为甲床出现纵行色素带或黑色条纹以及 Hutchinson 现象,即甲皱襞和周围皮肤色素沉着。组织学上以基底层异型性黑素细胞雀斑样或团巢状增生为特点。

(2) TNM 分期:2017 年 AJCC 第 8 版黑素瘤分期见表 2-1。

表 2-1　黑素瘤 TNM 分期

分　期		表　现
Tx		原发肿瘤无法评估
T0		无原发肿瘤证据
Tis		原位癌
T1		厚度≤1.0 mm
T2		厚度 1.1~2.0 mm
	T2a	不伴溃疡
	T2b	伴溃疡
T3		厚度 2.1~4.0 mm
	T3a	不伴溃疡
	T3b	伴溃疡
T4		厚度>4.0 mm
	T4a	不伴溃疡
	T4b	伴溃疡
Nx		区域淋巴结无法评估
N0		无淋巴结转移
N1		1 个淋巴结转移
	N1a	1 个淋巴结临床隐匿转移(无区域淋巴结转移的临床或影像学证据,但淋巴结活检发现肿瘤累及的区域发生淋巴结转移),不伴卫星灶、局部复发或移行转移
	N1b	1 个淋巴结临床显性转移(临床或影像学检查发现肿瘤累及的区域发生淋巴结转移),不伴卫星灶、局部复发或移行转移
	N1c	无淋巴结转移,伴卫星灶、局部复发或移行转移
N2		2~3 个淋巴结转移
	N2a	2~3 个淋巴结临床隐匿转移,不伴卫星灶、局部复发或移行转移
	N2b	2~3 个淋巴结转移,其中至少 1 个淋巴结临床显性转移,不伴卫星灶、局部复发或移行转移
	N2c	1 个淋巴结临床隐匿转移或临床显性转移,伴卫星灶、局部复发或移行转移

分　期		表　现
N3	≥4 个淋巴结转移	
	N3a	≥4 个淋巴结临床隐匿转移,不伴卫星灶、局部复发或移行转移
	N3b	≥4 个淋巴结转移,其中至少 1 个淋巴结临床显性转移,不伴卫星灶、局部复发或移行转移
	N3c	≥2 个淋巴结临床隐匿转移或临床显性转移,伴卫星灶、局部复发或移行转移
M0	无远处转移	
M1a	皮肤、皮下组织,或远处淋巴结转移	
	M1a(0)	LDH 正常
	M1a(1)	LDH 升高
M1b	肺转移	
	M1b(0)	LDH 正常
	M1b(1)	LDH 升高
M1c	其他内脏转移	
	M1c(0)	LDH 正常
	M1c(1)	LDH 升高
M1d	脑转移	
	M1d(0)	LDH 正常
	M1d(1)	LDH 升高

（3）临床分期和病理分期:见表 2-2。

表 2-2　黑素瘤临床分期和病理分期

分　期	T	N	M
临床分期			
0 期	Tis	N0	M0
ⅠA 期	T1a	N0	M0
ⅠB 期	T1b	N0	M0
	T2a	N0	M0
ⅡA 期	T2b	N0	M0
	T3a	N0	M0
ⅡB 期	T3b	N0	M0
	T4a	N0	M0

续表

分　　　期	T	N	M
ⅡC 期	T4b	N0	M0
Ⅲ 期	任何 T	≥N1	M0
Ⅳ 期	任何 T	任何 N	M1

病理分期

分期	T	N	M
0 期	Tis	N0	M0
Ⅰ A 期	T1a	N0	M0
Ⅰ A 期	T1b	N0	M0
Ⅰ B 期	T2a	N0	M0
Ⅱ A 期	T2b	N0	M0
Ⅱ A 期	T3a	N0	M0
Ⅱ B 期	T3b	N0	M0
Ⅱ B 期	T4a	N0	M0
Ⅱ C 期	T4b	N0	M0
Ⅲ A 期	T1a/b～T2a	N1a 或 N2a	M0
Ⅲ B 期	T0	N1b,N1c	M0
Ⅲ B 期	T1a/b～T2a	N1b/c 或 N2b	M0
Ⅲ B 期	T2b/T3a	N1a～N2b	M0
Ⅲ C 期	T0	N2b,N2c,N3b/c	M0
Ⅲ C 期	T1a～T3a	N2c 或 N3a/b/c	M0
Ⅲ C 期	T3b/T4a	≥N1	M0
Ⅲ C 期	T4b	N1a～N2c	M0
Ⅲ D 期	T4b	N3a/b/c	M0
Ⅳ 期	任何 T	任何 N	M1

3. 诊断及鉴别

（1）临床和皮肤镜诊断：大多数黑素瘤根据其显著的色素沉着和形态学特征,有经验的医生视诊即可发现和诊断。黑素瘤高风险人群应定期进行筛查。需要筛查或监测的高危因素包括黑素细胞痣、发育不良性痣以及黑素瘤的病史和家族史。黑素瘤的筛查包括借助皮肤镜或其他成像技术进行全身皮肤检查。

根据 ABCD 法则视诊：A 病灶不对称(asymmetry),B 边缘不规则(irregular borders),C 颜色不均匀(inhomogeneous colour),D 直径≥5 mm,可早期诊断可疑黑素瘤。

皮肤镜是诊断色素瘤及非色素瘤,以及发现黑素瘤的重要工具。黑素瘤的特异性诊断标准包括不典型色素网、不规则的点/球、不规则的条纹、蓝白结构、退行性改变、不规则血管、斑点、白色条纹、菱形结构等。

黑素瘤的鉴别诊断包括其他黑素细胞色素性皮损(先天性、非典型、常见的黑素细胞痣和日光性雀斑样痣)、非黑素细胞色素性皮损(脂溢性角化病、血管瘤、皮肤纤维瘤和色素性基底细胞癌)和其他非色素性肿瘤(血管瘤、基底细胞癌、鳞状细胞癌)。

（2）组织病理学诊断：可获得临床和病理分期、肿瘤厚度、有无溃疡、分裂活性、卫星灶、切缘情况、有无血管或神经累及等。

（3）免疫组化检测：常用的黑素细胞特征性标志物包括 S100、SOX10、MART1/Melan-A、HMB45、酪氨酸酶、MITF 和 Ki67 等。同时选用其中 2 个或多个标志物用于免疫组化可提高检测黑素细胞的灵敏度。黑素细胞分化程度的指标包括 S100、MART1/Melan-A、HMB45、酪氨酸酶、MITF 和 SOX10。S100 蛋白灵敏度很高，是黑素瘤的过筛指标，但其特异性较差。MART1/Melan-A、HMB45 和酪氨酸酶的特异性较高。MITF 和 SOX10 可用于鉴别日光性角化病和原位黑素瘤。黑素瘤的预后指标包括 Ki67 和磷酸化组蛋白 H3。在黑素瘤中，Ki67 增殖指数为 5%～50%，病灶中可见有丝分裂象大量分布。

（4）分子诊断：分子诊断的靶点主要是 BRAF V600 突变，来指导 BARF 抑制剂和 MEK 抑制剂的临床治疗。在部分病例中，分子诊断的靶点还有 NRAS 突变、NF1 突变和 CKIT 突变。用于黑素瘤诊断的细胞学和分子方法包括比较基因组杂交(CGH)、荧光原位杂交(FISH)、质谱成像(IMS)、qRT-PCR、多重连接探针扩增(MLPA)。

（5）影像学诊断：区域淋巴结超声和 CT、MRI 可用于判断是否有肿瘤转移。

（6）其他成像技术：其他成像技术可用于帮助医生鉴别黑素瘤及其前体与良性病变，包括体内反射式共聚焦显微镜、计算机辅助多光谱数字分析、电阻抗图谱(EIS)、光声成像(PAI)、光学相干断层扫描等。

（二）治疗现状

黑素瘤是来源于黑素细胞的高度恶性肿瘤，其特征是高度侵袭性、早期易转移，并且对常规放疗、化疗和免疫治疗等抵抗能力强。现就黑素瘤的治疗现状及展望进行概述。

1. 传统治疗手段

（1）手术治疗：黑素瘤确诊后，应尽早经手术完整切除原发灶。手术切除的范围原则上根据肿瘤的 Breslow 厚度决定，且应包括皮下组织，并深达筋膜。且对于黑素瘤患者，建议进行预防性淋巴结清扫和前哨淋巴结活检。然而，手术治疗只能对部分早期黑素瘤患者有效，仍有约 60% 的黑素瘤患者死于黑素瘤的复发和转移。因此对于无转移但复发风险高的黑素瘤患者，手术切除后，应给予系统的免疫治疗，这能有效抑制临床无法检测的微小病灶和转移的形成。

（2）化疗和放疗：化疗是针对转移性黑素瘤的首选方案。2011 年，美国 FDA 批准达卡巴嗪作为治疗转移性黑素瘤的化疗药物，目前，其仍是最有效的药物，但是其治疗有效率仅为 20%。放疗虽然能缓解黑素瘤患者的梗阻症状以及抑制远处的转移灶，但是不能延长患者的生存期。而且黑素瘤细胞存在放疗抵抗性，可能是由于黑素瘤细胞因反复受到 DNA 损伤而具备有效的 DNA 修复能力。

（3）细胞因子：①干扰素：大量临床研究证明，早期黑素瘤患者术后联合大剂量干扰素治疗，可有效降低复发率，延长生存期。但是该疗法有较强的副作用，而且价格昂贵。②重组白细胞介素-2(IL-2)：IL-2 是一种炎症细胞因子，是美国 FDA 批准的用于治疗转移性黑素瘤的第一种免疫治疗剂。在 8 项 Ⅱ 期临床试验，共 270 例患者中，大剂量 IL-2 给药后，约有 15% 的患者发生了总体缓解，而这些患者中有 4%～6% 的患者出现长期完全缓解。但是，大剂量

IL-2治疗可导致如血流动力学休克和呼吸功能不全等严重的不良反应。

(4)肿瘤疫苗：大多数用于肿瘤疫苗研究的肿瘤相关抗原可以分成以下两类。①自身抗原，在肿瘤组织中分布并且肿瘤抗原过度表达的分子；②癌睾抗原，在睾丸和胎盘中表达受限的肿瘤相关抗原。接种疫苗可以诱导免疫系统排斥肿瘤，但是黑素瘤的总体反应率较低，为4%~5%。

2. 系统免疫疗法

(1)细胞过继治疗：即肿瘤浸润淋巴细胞的回输治疗，通常是分离黑素瘤患者的肿瘤浸润淋巴细胞，在体外进行处理(如加入抗原和细胞因子刺激)，并筛选和扩增具有肿瘤杀伤活性的免疫效应细胞，然后回输到患者体内。该方法对一些晚期黑素瘤患者有效，而且完全反应者很少复发，甚至可达到完全临床缓解。但是，经过手术切除的黑素瘤患者中只有40%~50%的患者可获得肿瘤浸润淋巴细胞。此外，该方法存在很强的个性化且准备周期较长，临床应用仍然是一个挑战。另一种方法是使用具有嵌合抗原受体(CARs)的工程化外周血淋巴细胞。CARs是T细胞受体(TCR)和共刺激分子或者具有TCR高亲和力的肿瘤相关抗原结合的单联抗体。CARs识别肿瘤相关抗原不受HLA限制，在造血系统恶性肿瘤以及实体肿瘤中，临床反应率很高。但是，由于存在交叉反应，该治疗方法容易在重要的正常组织中出现严重的毒性反应。

(2)分子靶向治疗：近年来，通过对黑素瘤发病机制的研究，人们认识到黑素瘤的形成与一些信号通路的异常激活相关。例如，有40%~60%的黑素瘤发生了BRAF基因突变，从而导致丝裂原激活的蛋白激酶(MAPK)途径对下游信号进行组成性激活。因此，一系列针对信号通路的新型药物的出现为黑素瘤靶向治疗开辟了新局面，如威罗非尼和达拉非尼等先后获得美国FDA批准。BRAF和MEK抑制剂进入2019版美国NCCN黑素瘤诊治指南，中国黑素瘤BRAF、NRAS基因突变率低，主要基因谱待研究。对于转移性黑素瘤，不能耐受免疫治疗者，首选BRAF/MEK靶向治疗；该方法初始应答率高，患者生存期可得到延长，局限性是应答期平均时长短、复发率高。

(3)免疫检查点抑制剂：免疫检查点是指参与维持免疫稳态的分子，有助于维持外周对自身分子的耐受性，并可抑制或增强免疫反应。其中，广为人知的抑制性免疫检查点是CTLA-4和PD-1，它们已在临床取得重要突破。美国FDA近年来批准用于黑素瘤免疫治疗的药物包括2011年批准的伊匹单抗(抗CTLA-4)、2014年批准的帕博利珠单抗(抗PD-1)、2016年批准的纳武单抗(抗PD-1)。免疫治疗的出现大幅提高了黑素瘤患者的生存率，为黑素瘤的临床治疗带来了希望。帕博利珠单抗成为晚期黑素瘤一线治疗标准方案，能够长期阻断疾病进展、提高总生存率，85%的患者在停药后2年仍无进展。免疫治疗从根本上改变了黑素瘤过去的窘境，使患者看到了"治愈"的希望。欧美黑素瘤患者以皮肤型为主，我国黑素瘤患者中肢端、黏膜型比例超过50%。帕博利珠单抗被证明对肢端、黏膜黑素瘤同样有效。对于转移性黑素瘤，抗PD-1$^{+/-}$CTLA-4治疗改善了总生存率、反应率和反应持久性，是首选的一线治疗方案。免疫检查点阻断(ICB)治疗的优势包括总生存期明显延长，应答持久。其局限性是只有部分患者对ICB治疗应答，免疫相关副作用不可忽视。

(4)免疫治疗新策略(纳米、微针等)：常规疗法(如达卡巴嗪、干扰素和白细胞介素-2)受限于低应答率，并且不会提高总生存率。新型靶向疗法(如威罗非尼、达拉非尼和曲美替尼)具有较高的初始应答率，对总体生存率有明显改善，但通常在6~9个月发生复发。虽然免疫疗法(如伊匹单抗、帕博利珠单抗和纳武单抗)可以获得长期和持久的反应,但仅对部分患者有效,且不良事件发生率非常高。因此,虽然在过去 10 年里,随着分子靶向治疗和免疫治疗的出现,黑素瘤治疗领域出现了前所未有的临床进展,但是,黑素瘤的临床治疗仍然面临着巨大的挑战。随着纳米技术用于癌症治疗的迅速发展,纳米疗法为克服这些缺点带来了希望,纳米药物的抗肿瘤应用是多种多样的,包括纳米药物直接杀伤肿瘤细胞,或者作为化学疗法和基因疗法的载体起作用,还有基于纳米材料的光热疗法(PTT)和光动力疗法(PDT)的应用。此外,纳米药物可通过被动或主动靶向将效应结构递送到肿瘤部位,从而增加治疗特异性和减少副作用。几种纳米药物已获得美国 FDA 的批准用于临床治疗,以及目前正在进行临床前或临床试验的其他纳米药物已显示出可用于肿瘤治疗的潜力。我们预期纳米药物载体的应用将在可预见的未来改变黑素瘤治疗的格局(见扩展阅读 1)。

(5)联合治疗:与单独使用任何一种疗法相比,将抗 CTLA-4 单抗和抗 PD-1 单抗联合用于抗肿瘤效果更好。联合治疗与无进展生存期(PFS)及总体生存期相关。此外,晚期黑素瘤是少数常转移到大脑的癌症之一,联合免疫疗法可减少黑素瘤脑转移。目前已有几个新型的免疫检查点抑制剂处于临床前和临床研究阶段,包括针对 LAG-3、TIM3、IDO、FOXP3、CSF1R 的抑制剂。它们可用于 PD-L1 水平发生变化、对 ICB 单一用药反应不佳的黑素瘤患者,还可与不同检查点抑制剂联合应用。溶瘤病毒联合 ICB 能促进肿瘤内 T 细胞浸润,提高免疫治疗应答率。抗 PD-(L)1 联合 BRAF/MEK 靶向治疗在早期临床试验中已显示反应率改善,但不良反应发生率增高。PD-1 或 BRAFi/MEKi 是当前黑素瘤切除后辅助治疗的一线选择,抗 CTLA-4 单抗和抗 PD-1 单抗被批准用于辅助治疗Ⅲ期和低转移的Ⅳ期可切除黑素瘤。BRAFi/MEKi(达拉非尼/曲美替尼)被批准用于Ⅲ期黑素瘤的辅助治疗。

三、非黑素瘤性皮肤癌

（一）概述

1. 基底细胞癌(basal cell carcinoma, BCC)

基底细胞癌是常见的皮肤癌之一,多见于中年以上的浅肤色人群,恶性度较低,极少发生转移。

(1)病因与发病机制:基底细胞癌的发病率随着日光照射量和年龄的增加而增高;此外,基底细胞癌的发生与肤色和遗传等因素有关,慢性砷中毒、电离辐射以及免疫抑制也能促进基底细胞癌的发生。

(2)临床表现与分型。

① 结节型:基底细胞癌最常见的亚型,也称经典型基底细胞癌,占 50%～80%,病变常见于头颈部,表现为结节,随病灶的增大,肿瘤可破溃出血。

② 浅表型:基底细胞癌第二常见的亚型,占 10%～30%。平均发病年龄相对年轻。病变常见于躯干和四肢,头颈部少见,表现为单个或数个浅表性红斑,边缘隆起,表面具有鳞屑。

③ 色素型:除具有结节型基底细胞癌的所有特征外,有色素沉着于病变部位。

④ 纤维上皮瘤型:本型较少见,常发生于躯干,表现为皮色或红色的高于皮肤的无蒂斑块。

⑤ 漏斗状囊型:多发生于老年人头颈部,表现为界限分明的珍珠样丘疹。

⑥ 硬斑病样型:表现为白色、质硬斑块,伴有明显的毛细血管。

(3)诊断与鉴别诊断:依据临床表现与组织学特征,基底细胞癌较易诊断,但要注意与鳞状细胞癌、日光性角化病、角化棘皮瘤、Bowen病、Paget病、脂溢性角化病等鉴别。

2. 鳞状细胞癌(squamous cell carcinoma, SCC)

鳞状细胞癌是仅次于基底细胞癌的常见皮肤癌,是来源于表皮及其附属器角质形成细胞的恶性肿瘤,通常发生在日光照射部位,以头颈部为主,多见于60岁及以上人群。

(1)病因与发病机制:鳞状细胞癌的发生主要与长期日光照射有关,紫外线引起DNA损伤,导致角质形成细胞发生基因突变和恶变。辐射、化学致癌因素、长期HPV感染、长期不愈合的慢性溃疡、盘状红斑狼疮等也与鳞状细胞癌有关。此外,鳞状细胞癌的发生还与机体的免疫状态有关,免疫抑制患者(如器官移植患者)的鳞状细胞癌发病率较一般人群增高。

(2)临床表现:鳞状细胞癌常见于头颈部等日光照射部位,非日光照射部位也可发生,60岁以上人群多见。典型的鳞状细胞癌表现为不愈合、生长迅速的皮肤颜色的结节,基底坚硬,表面可伴有鳞屑或硬痂,中央可破溃形成溃疡。病变部位疼痛,触之易出血。

(3)诊断及鉴别诊断:当头颈部等好发部位出现生长迅速、基底坚硬的结节,触之易出血,易形成溃疡时应尽早行病理组织活检,皮肤病理组织学检查是确诊鳞状细胞癌的主要依据。病变早期,鳞状细胞癌与日光性角化病难以区分。此外,鳞状细胞癌还应与基底细胞癌、角化棘皮瘤以及孢子丝菌病等鉴别。

(二)治疗现状

非黑素瘤性皮肤癌的治疗方式应综合考虑患者年龄、肿瘤的分期和部位、复发的风险、患者的期望以及潜在的副作用等因素进行选择。非黑素瘤性皮肤癌的治疗方式可分为外科手术治疗和非手术治疗,外科手术治疗包括标准切除术、Mohs显微手术、电烧灼法和刮除术。非手术治疗包括放疗、冷冻治疗、局部外用药物治疗、系统药物治疗和光动力治疗等。其中,外科手术治疗是非黑素瘤性皮肤癌的基石疗法。肿瘤的风险评估指南见表2-3。

表 2-3 美国国家综合癌症网络(NCCN*)肿瘤风险评估指南

指 标	低 风 险	高 风 险
部位		
躯干和四肢	任何<20 mm 的皮损	任何≥20 mm 的皮损
头皮,前额,脸颊,颈部,胫前	任何<10 mm 的皮损	任何≥10 mm 的皮损
面部"面具区"+,生殖器,手,足	N/A	任何大小的皮损
边界	边界清晰	边界模糊
原发或复发	原发	复发
是否出现免疫抑制	否	是
是否为接受过放疗的区域	否	是
周围神经侵袭/神经症状	否	是
侵袭性组织分型‡	否	是
鳞状细胞癌特有的特点	否	是
是否有慢性炎症	否	是

续表

指　标	低　风　险	高　风　险
肿瘤是否迅速发展	否	是
是否是低分化肿瘤	否	是
深度≥2 mm	否	是
Clark 分级 Ⅳ/Ⅴ	否	是
淋巴管血管侵袭	否	是

* National Comprehensive Cancer Network. National clinical practice guidelines in oncology：squamous cell skin cancer (version Ⅰ.2017).

†面部"面具区"是指面部中央、眼睑、眉毛、眼眶周围、鼻、嘴唇、下巴、下颌骨、耳朵、耳前/耳后和太阳穴。

‡基底细胞癌的侵袭性组织学亚型包括硬斑状、基底鳞状、硬化、混合浸润和微结节；鳞状细胞癌的侵袭性组织学亚型包括腺样（棘膜溶解）、腺鳞状、间质增生（黏蛋白产生）和化生（癌肉瘤）。

1. 低风险肿瘤

（1）手术治疗：低风险肿瘤首选标准切除术，并在术后进行切缘活检（基底细胞癌建议对切缘 4 mm 处进行活检，鳞状细胞癌建议对切缘 4～6 mm 处进行活检）。若出现切缘阳性则需根据情况扩大切除范围并辅以放疗。

电烧灼法和刮除术也可用于治疗低风险肿瘤，利用手术刀或电凝刀彻底瓦解并清除肉眼可见的肿瘤，优势在于手术过程快且成本低。但是电烧灼法和刮除术的效果与手术者的技术熟练程度和肿瘤的部位高度相关。此外，电烧灼法和刮除术对皮肤的创伤大，会遗留明显的瘢痕。因此，位于影响美观部位的肿瘤不适宜使用电烧灼法和刮除术。

（2）非手术治疗：若患者由于自身情况无法进行手术治疗，可选择非手术治疗，包括放疗、局部外用药物治疗、光动力治疗、冷冻治疗等。

放疗是普遍使用的非手术疗法，可用于治疗无法进行手术的高/低风险患者，并可用作手术治疗的辅助治疗。但由于放疗的远期慢性毒副作用，一般只推荐老年患者（＞60 岁）使用。

局部外用药物治疗是目前最常用的非手术疗法，在肿瘤皮损局部外用 5-氟尿嘧啶和咪喹莫特，这两种药物可以通过抑制 DNA 合成并激活细胞免疫进而促进肿瘤细胞的凋亡。局部外用药物治疗对原位浅表性低风险肿瘤的效果显著，且特别适用于全身多发皮损的患者，相较手术治疗，其对皮肤损伤小。局部外用药物治疗的缺点在于需要长时间多疗程治疗，因此对患者的依从性要求非常高。

光动力治疗也是目前常用的非手术治疗方法之一，对于原位浅表性低风险的肿瘤效果显著。光动力治疗由于疼痛、慢性伤口和色素沉着等反应常造成患者无法耐受。

冷冻治疗是指在－50 ℃的液氮条件下，使用重复的冻融循环来局部破坏肿瘤细胞，同样可以有效治疗原位浅表性低风险肿瘤。冷冻治疗过程快、成本低且不需要局部麻醉。然而，冷冻治疗可造成局部持续性水肿、神经痛并遗留瘢痕和色素沉着，因此其使用范围没有上述两种方法广泛。

2. 高风险肿瘤

对于高风险非黑素瘤性皮肤癌，治疗的金标准是 Mohs 显微手术。研究证明 Mohs 显微手术具有极高的治愈率、低死亡率，并能最大限度地保留组织的完整性。若 Mohs 显微手术无法实施，也可考虑使用标准切除术，但要将切缘活检扩大至 10 mm 处。对于无法实行手术的患者,可考虑前述的非手术治疗方案,但需接受效果不佳和肿瘤复发的风险。

3. 复发、转移性和晚期肿瘤

对于局部复发而无远处转移证据的肿瘤,应按照高风险肿瘤处理。对于局部复发和远处转移的肿瘤,应通过多学科协作共同制订治疗方案,在尽可能手术治疗的基础上,进行多种辅助治疗,辅助治疗选择包括放疗、化疗和 Hedgehog 通路抑制剂等。对于无法进行手术的晚期肿瘤患者,应充分考虑患者自身情况,以最大限度地缓解症状、保证生存质量为目的,为患者选择合适的系统治疗方案,如放化疗、Hedgehog 通路抑制剂等。

第四节　挑战与展望

皮肤伤口发病率高,治疗方法的不当及治疗延迟易造成伤口出血、感染,形成难愈合伤口及病理性瘢痕,影响患者的生活质量。目前,皮肤伤口及并发症的发病机制尚未完全阐明,还需进一步研究。随着高分子材料的发展,智能响应型水凝胶、抗菌水凝胶及微针等已在皮肤伤口的动物模型上取得良好的治疗效果。

高分子材料可单独使用,或与传统治疗方式等联用来治疗皮肤伤口。抗菌水凝胶作为一种新型皮肤伤口敷料,具有抗菌和伤口保湿双重特性,可缩短伤口愈合炎症期,促进伤口愈合。随着对抗菌材料的进一步研究,抗菌水凝胶的种类将进一步丰富。未来关于抗菌水凝胶促进皮肤伤口愈合的作用机制及针对皮肤伤口愈合不同阶段抗菌水凝胶的选择等基础研究会进一步完善。目前临床应用的微针技术有滚轮微针和射频微针,微针技术可单独使用,也可与放疗、激光和外用药物联合使用。微针应用于皮肤瘢痕的优势在于微痛、方便、安全和高效,但关于微针作用于皮肤瘢痕的机制研究亟待加强。

严重类型的银屑病常需要联合治疗。例如,应用甲氨蝶呤(MTX)治疗的同时外用药物以减少其剂量。甲氨蝶呤可与英夫利昔单抗联合应用以降低中和抗体的发生率;对于严重的泛发性脓疱型银屑病患者也可与阿维 A 联合使用。每种药物的毒性不同,系统的联合治疗常可降低总的毒性。然而,由于存在潜在的蓄积毒性或者药物之间的相互作用,新的治疗策略应谨慎使用。随着研究的深入,经皮药物递送技术日趋完善,使用微针贴片无痛地穿透表皮,并形成皮肤微通道,将甲氨蝶呤、阿维 A 或生物制剂等药物,透过角质层成功地递送到皮损病变部位,再通过不同的刺激响应功能,按需按时给药,既减轻了传统给药引起的胃肠道不适(如恶心、呕吐、腹泻、腹痛等)、口腔炎、骨髓抑制、肝肾毒性等不良反应,还减少了注射可能带来的疼痛和出血等副作用。因此,改变传统药物递送途径,在未来会为患者提供更安全、更简便的治疗体验。

尽管在过去的 10 年中,由于免疫治疗和靶向治疗的发展,黑素瘤的临床疗效有了显著改善,但并非所有患者都能从现有的治疗方法中获益,而进一步的优化则需要对肿瘤免疫生物学机制进行深入的了解。因此,需要进行广泛的临床前、转化和临床研究,以更好地了解对黑素瘤当前疗法的反应和耐药机制,开发合理的下一代疗法和组合疗法,并建立更复杂有效的黑素瘤模型,以支持进一步的临床前和临床转化研究。目前,非黑素瘤性皮肤癌以手术治疗为金标准;但手术治疗存在很大的局限性,并不是所有的患者都能进行手术治疗,且手术治疗存在创伤大、影响组织功能和美观性等问题。常用的非手术治疗方法如局部外用药物、光动力治疗等,虽然创伤小,但存在药物渗透能力差、治疗范围窄的问题,只能有效治疗原位、浅表性的肿瘤。生物化学技术与传统治疗的结合有望为皮肤肿瘤的治疗指出新的方向,如:利用微针、经皮给药技术促进局部药物和光敏剂的渗透,提高局部外用药物治疗和光动力治疗的疗效;设计纳米靶向药物精准靶向癌组织来减少系统治疗的副作用等。

思 考 题

1. 目前雄激素性脱发首选的治疗手段有哪些?

2. 银屑病的传统系统治疗有哪些不足?

3. 目前生物制剂包括哪些类型? 作用的靶点是什么?

4. 目前银屑病治疗的难点是什么?

5. 黑素瘤等皮肤肿瘤的传统治疗存在哪些问题? 高分子材料对于解决这些问题将发挥怎样的作用?

扩 展 阅 读

[1] Griffiths C, Barker J, Bleiker T, et al. Rook's textbook of dermatology[M]. 9th ed. New Jersey: Wiley-Blackwell, 2016.

[2] Wolff K, Johnson R A. Fitzpatrick's color atlas and synopsis of clinical dermatology [M]. 6th ed. New York: McGraw-Hill, 2009.

[3] Yamada M, Prow T W. Physical drug delivery enhancement for aged skin, UV damaged skin and skin cancer: translation and commercialization[J]. Adv Drug Deliv Rev, 2020, 153: 2-17.

[4] William J, Dirk E, James T, et al. Andrews' diseases of the skin[M]. 13th ed. Amsterdam: Elsevier, 2019.

[5] Baltzis D, Eleftheriadou I, Veves A. Pathogenesis and treatment of impaired wound healing in diabetes mellitus: new insights[J]. Adv Ther, 2014, 31(8): 817-836.

参 考 文 献

[1] Donald Y M L, Evgeny B, Elena G. Cutaneous barrier dysfunction in allergic diseases [J]. J Allergy Clin Immun, 2020, 145(6): 1485-1497.

[2] Kabashima K, Izuhara K. Barrier dysfunction in the skin allergy[J]. Allergol Int, 2018, 67(1): 3-11.

[3] Baroni A, Buommino E, Gregorio V D, et al. Structure and function of the epidermis related to barrier properties[J]. Clin Dermatol, 2012, 30(3): 257-262.

[4] Han H W, Roan F, Ziegler S F. The atopic march: current insights into skin barrier dysfunction and epithelial cell-derived cytokines[J]. Immunol Rev, 2017, 278(1): 116-130.

[5] Kobayashi T, Naik S, Nagao K. Choreographing immunity in the skin epithelial barrier [J]. Immunity, 2019, 50(3): 552-565.

[6] Zhu T H, Zhu T R, Tran K A, et al. Epithelial barrier dysfunctions in atopic dermatitis:

a skin-gut-lung model linking microbiome alteration and immune dysregulation[J]. Brit J Dermatol,2018,179(3):570-581.

[7] Yosipovitch G,Misery L,Proksch E,et al. Skin barrier damage and itch:review of mechanisms,topical management and future directions[J]. Acta Derm-Venereol,2019, 99(13):1201-1209.

[8] Naidoo K,Hanna R ,Birch-Machin M A. What is the role of mitochondrial dysfunction in skin photoaging? [J]. Exp Dermatol,2018,27(2):124-128.

[9] Thornton M J. Shedding more light on photoageing[J]. Brit J Dermatol,2020,182(5): 1086-1087.

[10] Sachs D L,Varani J,Chubb H,et al. Atrophic and hypertrophic photoaging:clinical, histologic,and molecular features of 2 distinct phenotypes of photoaged skin[J]. J Am Acad Dermatol,2019,81(2):480-488.

[11] Schneider S L,Kohli I,Hamzavi I H,et al. Emerging imaging technologies in dermatology: part Ⅰ:basic principles[J]. J Am Acad Dermatol,2019,80(4):1114-1120.

[12] Nischal K C,Khopkar U. Dermoscope[J]. Indian J Dermatol Venereol Leprol,2005,71 (4):300-303.

[13] Koehler M J,Lange-Asschenfeldt S,Kaatz M. Non-invasive imaging techniques in the diagnosis of skin diseases[J]. Expert Opin Med Diagn,2011,5(5):425-440.

[14] Marghoob N G,Liopyris K,Jaimes N. Dermoscopy:a review of the structures that facilitate melanoma detection[J]. J Am Osteopath Assoc,2019,119(6):380-390.

[15] Oh B H,Kim K H,Chung K Y. Skin imaging using ultrasound imaging, optical coherence tomography,confocal microscopy,and two-photon microscopy in cutaneous oncology[J]. Front Med (Lausanne),2019,6:274.

[16] Kanti V,Messenger A,Dobos G,et al. Evidence-based (S3) guideline for the treatment of androgenetic alopecia in women and in men-short version[J]. J Eur Acad Dermatol Venereol,2018,32(1):11-22.

[17] Profyris C,Tziotzios C,Vale I D. Cutaneous scarring:pathophysiology, molecular mechanisms,and scar reduction therapeutics:part Ⅰ. The molecular basis of scar formation[J]. J Am Acad Dermatol,2012,66(1):13-24.

[18] Adam J,Singer R,Clerk A F. Cutaneous wound healing[J]. New Engl J Med,1999,1 (1):738-746.

[19] Gill S E,Parks W C. Metalloproteinases and their inhibitors:regulators of wound healing[J]. Int J Biochem Cell Biol,2008,40(6-7):1334-1347.

[20] Gottrup F. Oxygen in wound healing and infection[J]. Wound J Surg,2004,28(3), 312-315.

[21] Junker J P E,Caterson E J,Eriksson E. The microenvironment of wound healing[J]. J Craniofac Surg,2013,24(1):12-16.

[22] Metcalf D G,Bowler P G. Biofilm delays wound healing:a review of the evidence[J]. Burn Trauma,2013,1(1):5-12.

[23] Drury J L, Mooney D J. Hydrogels for tissue engineering: scaffold design variables and applications[J]. Biomaterials, 2003, 24(24): 4337-4351.

[24] Fu X, Sheng Z, Guo Z, et al. Healing of chronic cutaneous wounds by topical treatment with basic fibroblast growth factor[J]. Chin Med J (Engl), 2002, 115: 331-335.

[25] Berman B, Maderal A, Raphael B. Keloids and hypertrophic scars: pathophysiology, classification, and treatment[J]. Dermatol Surg, 2016, 43(1): S3-S18.

[26] Davis M, McEvoy M T, Camilleri M, et al. Goeckerman treatment: neglected in the consensus approach for critically challenging case scenarios in moderate to severe psoriasis[J]. J Am Acad Dermatol, 2010, 62(3): 508.

[27] Doherty S D, Voorhees A V, Lebwohl M G, et al. National psoriasis foundation consensus statement on screening for latent tuberculosis infection in patients with psoriasis treated with systemic and biologic agents[J]. J Am Acad Dermatol, 2008, 59(2): 209-217.

[28] Duffin K C, Chandran V, Gladman D D, et al. Genetics of psoriasis and psoriatic arthritis: update and future direction[J]. J Rheumatol, 2008, 35(7): 1449-1453.

[29] Weiss S C, Rehmus W, Kimball A B. An assessment of the cost-utility of therapy for psoriasis[J]. Ther Clin Risk Manag, 2006, 2(3): 325-328.

[30] Wozel G. Psoriasis treatment in difficult locations: scalp, nails, and intertriginous areas[J]. Cin Dermatol, 2008, 26(5): 448-459.

[31] Zell D, Hu S, Kirsner R. Genetic alterations in psoriasis[J]. J Invest Dermatol, 2008, 128(7): 1614.

[32] Wang C, Ye Y, Hochu G, et al. Enhanced cancer immunotherapy by microneedle patch-assisted delivery of anti-PD1 antibody[J]. Nano Lett, 2016, 16(4): 2334-2340.

[33] Zhu Z, Luo H, Lu W, et al. Rapidly dissolvable microneedle patches for transdermal delivery of exenatide[J]. Pharm Res, 2014, 31(12): 3348-3360.

[34] Nolan B V, Yentzer B A, Fe Ldman S R. A review of home phototherapy for psoriasis[J]. Dermatol Online, 2010, 16(2): 1.

[35] Papp K A. Monitoring biologics for the treatment of psoriasis[J]. Clin Dermatol, 2008, 26(5): 515-521.

[36] Boehncke W H, Schön M P. Psoriasis[J]. Lancet, 2015, 386(9997): 983-994.

[37] Armstrong A W, Read C. Pathophysiology, clinical presentation, and treatment of psoriasis: a review[J]. JAMA, 2020, 323(19): 1945-1960.

[38] Schadendorf D, van Akkooi A C J, Berking C, et al. Melanoma[J]. Lancet, 2018, 392(10151): 971-984.

[39] Robert C, Ribas A, Schachter J, et al. Pembrolizumab versus ipilimumab in advanced melanoma (KEYNOTE-006): post-hoc 5-year results from an open-label, multicentre, randomised, controlled, phase 3 study[J]. Lancet Oncol, 2019, 20(9): 1239-1251.

[40] Jenkins R W, Fisher D E. Treatment of advanced melanoma in 2020 and beyond[J]. J Invest Dermatol, 2021, 141(1): 23-31.

［41］ Amaria R N，Reddy S M，Tawbi H A，et al. Neoadjuvant immune checkpoint blockade in high-risk resectable melanoma［J］. Nature Med，2018，24(11)：1649-1654.

［42］ Tawbi H A，Forsyth P A，Algazi A，et al. Combined nivolumab and ipilimumab in melanoma metastatic to the brain［J］. New Engl J Med，2018，379(8)：722-730.

［43］ Ribas A，Dummer R，Puzanov I，et al. Oncolytic virotherapy promotes intratumoral T cell infiltration and improves anti-PD-1 immunotherapy［J］. Cell，2017，174（4）：1031-1032.

［44］ Smith H，Wernham A，Patel A. When to suspect a non-melanoma skin cancer［J］. Brit Med J，2020，368：m692.

［45］ Keyal U，Bhatta A K，Zhang G，et al. Present and future perspectives of photodynamic therapy for cutaneous squamous cell carcinoma［J］. J Am Acad Dermatol，2019，80(3)：765-773.

［46］ 《中国黑色素瘤规范化病理诊断专家共识(2017 年版)》编写组. 中国黑色素瘤规范化病理诊断专家共识(2017 年版)［J］. 中华病理学杂志，2018，47(1)：7-13.

［47］ 张建中，高兴华. 皮肤性病学［M］. 北京：人民卫生出版社，2015.

（杨柳　安湘杰　索慧男　杨井　董励耘）

Chapter 2
Skin Health and
Representative Skin Diseases

Healthy and intact skin acts as the first barrier, protecting the body against a variety of external physical and chemical damages, and microbial invasion. If the skin is damaged, the barrier function is impaired, which will lead to skin inflammation, allergy and other corresponding skin diseases. This chapter will introduce the composition, function and homeostasis regulation of the skin barrier, and explain the relationship between skin barrier damage and several common skin diseases.

2.1 Skin Health

2.1.1 Skin barrier

The skin directly interfaces with the external environment, the most important function of which is to provide a protective barrier against the outside world, protecting organisms from environmental dangers such as extreme temperatures, ultraviolet, allergens, toxins, and microbes. Impaired barrier function has been linked to dry skin, itching, peeling, and exudation, and is closely related to the occurrence of skin disease.

2.1.1.1 Composition of skin barrier

Skin barrier usually refers to the physical or mechanical barrier structure of epidermis, especially stratum corneum (Figure 2-1). In terms of biochemical composition and function, the physical barrier structure of epidermis is related to the lipid of epidermis, and also to various proteins, water, inorganic salts and other metabolites.

1. Stratum corneum

Stratum corneum is mainly composed of keratinocytes and lipids. The extracellular lipids act as permeability, antioxidant, and antimicrobial barriers, and the keratinocytes act as ultraviolet and mechanical barriers. The stratum corneum is formed by differentiation and renewal of keratinocytes. During the cornification, keratinocytes undergo different developmental stages from cycling keratinocytes in the stratum basale, through early to late differentiating cells in the stratum spinosum and the stratum granulosum to dead keratinocytes in the stratum corneum. Keratin and keratin intermediate filaments-associated protein are involved in the process of cornification.

The keratinocytes develop a protein- and lipid-rich peripheral envelope, called the cornified envelope. In the outermost layer of the cornified envelope, ceramides and other lipids are covalently bound and form the so-called lipid envelope. The main function of the lipid envelope is to prevent trans-epidermal water loss (TEWL) and the loss of solutes, such as Na^+、K^+ and Ca^{2+}.

2. Desmosomes and tight junctions

Desmosomes seal the apical end of the lateral cell membrane and the extracellular fluid is compartmentalized into two parts by desmosomes maintaining different ionic strengths and solute concentrations.

In addition to desmosomes, tight junctions also contribute to the formation of the skin barrier. Tight junctions include a variety of transmembrane and intracellular proteins, mainly including Claudin family, Occludin family, ZO family, adhesion molecule family and so on. These proteins cross-link each other in the process of cell polarity and differentiation, and eventually form a dense network structure, blocking the intercellular space. Tight junctions are not just physical barriers; they exhibit ion and size selectivity and their barrier function varies significantly in tightness, depending on cell type and physiological requirements, enabling dynamic regulation of substances that traffic between compartments.

3. Langerhans cells

Langerhans cells (LCs) play an important role as an immune barrier. They are antigen-presenting cells of the skin, which can recognize, bind and process antigens invading the skin and deliver them to T cells. When the body is in homeostasis, the dendrites of Langerhans cells are outwards, on the medial side of the tight junctions. When activated, dendrites of Langerhans cells cross the tight junction barrier and take up antigens from the outer environment.

4. Others

Keratinocytes synthesize and secrete diverse antimicrobial peptides (AMPs), which have antimicrobial properties. AMPs can interact with and bind to the lipid envelope and together provide the functions to kill or inactivate microorganisms when the microorganisms come into contact with the epidermis. There is an epidermal calcium ion gradient with low calcium ion concentrations in the basal, proliferating layers, and a progressively higher concentration as one proceeds to the outer differentiated layers. This epidermal calcium ion gradient plays a crucial role in skin barrier function. The epidermal calcium ion gradient regulates the epidermal differentiation process and the homeostasis of the epidermal permeability barrier.

Skin surface pH ranges from 4.5 to 5.5 in humans, which is slightly acidic compared to the normal physiologic pH. The acidity of stratum corneum is crucial for establishing the epidermal permeability barrier, as well as producing the epidermal antimicrobial barrier and controlling the integrity and cohesion of stratum corneum. Moreover, a lot of protein degrading enzymes and proteases exist in the stratum corneum and each protease has its optimal pH.

Protease also participates in the barrier function of epidermis. The continuous renewing process is balanced by shedding of the "old" keratinocytes from the surface of the epidermis, which is referred to desquamation.

2.1.1.2 Function of skin barrier

1. Defense physical damages

The skin has a certain mechanical strength, which can protect various mechanical forces such as friction and extrusion. The skin also has the ability to repair after being damaged. The melanin barrier in epidermis and protein barrier in stratum corneum can play a role of barrier by absorbing ultraviolet radiation.

2. Defense chemical damages

The skin has a certain barrier to various chemicals. The weak acidic environment on the surface of skin has the ability of buffering acids and bases.

3. Defense biological damages

A complete skin barrier can be mechanically resistant to microorganisms. Antimicrobial peptides produced by the skin can kill bacteria, viruses, fungi and other microorganisms. In addition, the weak acidity of the skin and physiological desquamation of stratum corneum are not conducive to the growth and reproduction of microorganisms.

4. Prevent the loss of water, electrolyte and nutrients

The semi-permeable nature of the stratum corneum can prevent the loss of water, electrolyte and nutrients in the body. The sebaceous membrane on the skin's surface can also greatly reduce water loss. Under normal conditions, adults lose 240-480 mL of water through their skin every day (non-overt sweating). However, if the stratum corneum is completely lost, the amount of water lost through the skin increases by more than 10 times each day.

2.1.1.3 Regulation of skin barrier homeostasis

Several mechanisms are involved in the regulation of skin barrier homeostasis, including skin surface pH, hydration of the stratum corneum, calcium ion gradient in the epidermis, nuclear hormone receptors and so on.

1. Skin surface pH

The normal skin surface pH is 4.5-5.5. Microbial metabolites, free fatty acid of pilosebaceous origin, lactic acid, breakdown products of epidermal filaggrin (pyrrolidone carboxylic acid and urocanic acid) contribute to the formation of acidic environment on the surface of the skin. The acidity of the skin surface is essential in preventing infection, epidermal barrier recovery and regulation of the exfoliation of keratinocytes. Changes in the pH may play a role in the pathogenesis of some skin diseases, such as irritant contact dermatitis, atopic dermatitis, ichthyosis, acne vulgaris, and *Candida albicans* infection.

2. Hydration of the stratum corneum

Water content of the stratum corneum is related to skin elasticity, the process of keratinocytes desquamation on the skin surface and the repair of disrupted barrier. The skin with low stratum corneum hydration shows reduced elasticity. Several enzymes that regulate keratinocytes desquamination such as serine proteases and glycosidases, need the water in the stratum corneum to perform their normal function. Hydration of the stratum corneum is also important for skin barrier recovery. Under high humidity conditions, lipid biosynthesis decreases after barrier disruption, and the barrier recovery is slower.

3. Calcium ion gradient

There exists calcium ion gradient in the epidermis. In basal layer, spinous layer and stratum corneum, the calcium ion concentrations are very low, whereas the calcium ion concentration in the granular layer is the highest. Calcium ion gradient is important in the repair process after the destruction of the skin barrier, and the participation of calcium ions is also required in the formation of cell-to-cell junctions. Epidermal calcium ion gradient abnormality has clinical significance. X-linked ichthyosis and psoriasis demonstrate dysfunctions in the epidermal calcium ion gradient.

4. Nuclear hormone receptors

The function of nuclear hormone receptors is closely related to the transcription process and plays an important role in regulating epidermal development and skin homeostasis. Lipids and their metabolites bind and activate nuclear hormone receptors, and then regulate the lipids secretions and further processing of lamellar bodies. Thus, the role of nuclear hormone receptors that regulate the formation of bricks-and-mortar during epidermal development and recovery of the impaired skin barrier should not be ignored.

2.1.1.4 Skin barrier disturbance related dermatoses

Above-mentioned mechanisms need to work together to maintain the homeostasis of skin barrier, any dysfunction of which can cause barrier damage, finally leading to the occurrence of skin diseases. In addition, genetic factors, age, inappropriate use of detergents and cosmetic products can also induce the skin barrier disturbance. The skin barriers are damaged in a variety of skin diseases, such as atopic dermatitis, irritant dermatitis, psoriasis, and staphylococcus scaled skin syndrome. The followings introduce atopic dermatitis and contact dermatitis as examples.

1. Atopic dermatitis (AD)

Epidermal barrier disturbance is closely related to the occurrence and development of AD. Filaggrin (FLG) is important in the formation of skin barriers, and the mutation of the FLG gene that encodes filaggrin is the most famous risk factor for atopic dermatitis. FLG gene mutation leads to the reduction of FLG expression, thus damages the information of skin barrier, which allows the tissue penetration of allergens, irritants and microbes. These then lead to the release of epithelial cytokines such as thymic stromal lymphopoietin (TSLP) 、IL-4、IL-13 and IL-33, which play important roles in inducing type 2 immune and inflammatory. It has been proved that IL-3 and IL-4 can inhibit the epidermal barrier function, accompanied by the reduced levels of filaggrin and filaggrin degradation products, creating a permissive environment for *S. aureus* growth and attachment to AD skin. In AD patients, there is an exacerbation loop between the epidermal barrier and epidermal immunity, which suggests that the repair of skin barrier function is important for treating AD and preventing its development.

Studies have shown that improving the skin barrier with emollients can prevent the occurrence of AD, and in some successful studies, the uses of emollients have reduced the incidence of AD by approximately 50%. However, not all emollients application has the same effect, and the reason for which still requires further studies.

2. Contact dermatitis

Contact dermatitis is usually caused by exposure to irritating or toxic substances, which disturb the skin barrier and thus cause damage to the skin's mucous membrane tissue. The main pathological mechanisms of irritancy include skin barrier damage, cytokine cascade reactions, and oxidative stress networks. The integrity of the epidermal barrier plays a key role in the human skin's response to stimuli. Different mechanisms of skin barrier impairment responses to various stimuli, but no matter what kind of stimulation, the skin barrier homeostasis will be broken. Damaged stratum corneum release more water and consequently the concentration of calcium ions in the stratum granulosum decreased, which induces lamellar body to secrete lipids, and finally lead to the occurrence of skin repair process.

In many occupation, long-term exposure to solvents, water and detergents is inevitable, which can damage the skin barrier and allow hazardous substances to enter the skin, leading to the occurrence of contact dermatitis. The use of emollients can effectively prevent contact dermatitis.

2.1.2　Photoaging

Skin aging is a common dermatological disease related to heredity and environment. The intrinsic aging of the skin is determined by gene. Age-related clinical features include skin atrophy, loss of elasticity, fine wrinkles, dryness and prominence of vasculature. External aging is related to the environment (e. g. , solar radiation, smoking, pollution, nutrition and lifestyle factors). Extrinsically aged skin clinical features include deep wrinkles, rough textures, telangiectasia, rashes, and irregular pigmentation. Skin aging caused by ultraviolet is called photoaging, and ultraviolet is the most common environmental factor. Because of people's pursuit of skin rejuvenation, photoaging has become more and more concerned. In this part, we will discuss the pathogenesis, clinical manifestations, histological features, and management of photoaging.

2.1.2.1　Pathogenesis

1. Ultraviolet can induce degration of skin collagen

（1）Reactive oxygen species（ROS）：Ultraviolet can cause an increase of ROS. Excessive ROS can cause oxidative damage to cells, which resultantly contributes to collagen breakdown.

（2）Mitogen-activated protein kinase（MAPK）：MAPK holds a key role in the regulation of cell growth and procollagen Ⅰ formation. Ultraviolet radiation upregulates the MAPK signal transduction pathway, which causes downstream signal transduction and the formation of activator protein 1（AP-1）. AP-1 can inhibit the synthesis of collagen and promotes its breakdown.

（3）Matrix metalloproteinases（MMPs）：The expression of metalloproteinases is increased, instigating the degradation of the dermal extracellular matrix, especially procollagens Ⅰ and Ⅲ. Collagen synthesis is also reduced.

2. Ultraviolet can lead to genetic and molecular changes of the cells in the skin

Ultraviolet can damage deoxyribonucleic acid（DNA）and mitochondrial DNA（mtDNA）in direct and indirect ways. This causes telomere shortening in DNA and ATP generation reduction in mtDNA, which induce acceleration of skin aging.

3. Ultraviolet has paradoxical effects on blood vessels

Ultraviolet can induce the skin neovascularization. However, these new blood vessels are hyperpermeable, producing inflammatory factors that leak into the intercellular stroma and trigger cutaneous inflammation. This leads to extracellular matrix degradation and reduces dermal vasculature, accelerating photoaging.

2.1.2.2　Clinical manifestations and histological features

1. Clinical manifestations

Clinical classification of photoaging can be divided into two categories: atrophic photoaging and hypertrophic photoaging. The former shows signs with fewer wrinkles and dysplastic premalignant changes such as actinic keratosis. The latter displays features with thick wrinkles, leathery skin, lentigines, and bronzed appearance; a yellow cobblestone appearance of the skin may also be present.

2. Histological features

The histological features of photoaging include elevated elastosis and collagen fragmentation beneath the dermal-epidermal junction. The epidermal thickness and the morphology of epidermal cells can be irregular. There is an increase in the amount of glycosaminoglycans and proteoglycans with increased numbers of hyperplastic fibroblasts. The number of inflammatory cells also increases, such as mast cells, eosinophils, and mononuclear cells. Melanogenesis is upregulated following ultraviolet insult.

2.1.2.3　Management

There are two kinds of photoaging prevention measures, i. e. , photoprotection and medications that reverses skin damage.

1. Photoprotection

Photoprotection is a key primary preventative strategy, including wearing sun protective clothing, appropriate sunscreen application, and sun avoidance during peak ultraviolet times.

2. Medications

(1)Topical retinoids: Tretinoin and tazarotene are the two topical vitamin A derivatives that are currently approved by the US FDA for the treatment of photoaging. They can promote collagen fiber production and improve clinical symptoms.

(2) 5-fluorouracil cream: Topical 5-fluorouracil cream can be beneficial although it is not approved by the US FDA for photoaging management. It was reported that 5-fluorouracil could stimulate wound healing and subsequent dermal remodeling.

(3) Cosmeceuticals: Cosmeceuticals include antioxidants, soy, tea, ginkgo biloba, and ginseng. Antioxidants can scavenge free radicals and thus protect cells from damage, which include coenzyme Q, lipoic acid, and vitamins C and E.

2.1.3　Pigment and skin color

As the protective barrier of our body, the skin protects organisms from environmental stimuli, such as ultraviolet, toxins, and microbes. Skin pigmentation plays an important role in the defense against ultraviolet. In human skin, melanogenesis is a tightly regulated process. Many internal and external factors are involved in the melanogenesis process, and many physiological and external events can modify skin melanogenesis, leading to hyperpigmentation or hypopigmentation, and finally resulting in dermatosis.

2.1.3.1　Skin color

Normal skin color is mainly determined by two factors. One is the pigment content in the skin, including melanin, carotene, etc. , and the other is the anatomical difference of the skin, mainly including the thickness of the skin, especially the thickness of the stratum corneum and stratum granulosum. Melanin is the main pigment that determines the color of the skin.

2.1.3.2　Generation and regulation of pigment

Skin pigmentation is mainly due to the accumulation of melanin granules in keratinocytes. Melanocytes secrete melanin into the melanosome, which then moves into the keratinocyte and reassembles in the supranuclear area to form a melanin cap, protecting the keratinocyte nucleus from ultraviolet damage.

Skin pigmentation is a delicate and complex process, which includes many regulatory mechanisms in intracellular signalling pathways, non-coding RNAs (miRNAs and lncRNAs) and circulating exosomes. Skin pigmentation is regulated by the secretion of cytokines (such as α-MSH, SCF, KGF and bFGF) through the interaction of melanocytes and keratinocytes in the epidermis and fibroblasts in the dermis.

2.1.3.3 Pigmentation related diseases

Skin pigmentation is subject to many physiological and external conditions. Genetic factors, long-term exposure to ultraviolet, and elevated estrogen levels are common causes of chloasma. In addition, it has also been found that the increase in the number of dermal resident cells, mast cells, fibroblasts and dermal blood vessels is related to chloasma pigmentation. miRNAs has a potential role in the generation of melanin in chloasma and the transfer of melanosome. With age, local skin pigmentation may appear age spots. Some skin diseases can cause located post-inflammatory pigmentation, such as acne, atopic dermatitis and lichen planus. Endocrine diseases such as primary adrenal insufficiency can also cause skin pigmentation. Skin melanin production disorder or deficiency can also lead to diseases, such as acquired depigmentation skin and mucous membrane disease, vitiligo and congenital pigmentation disorder, albinism.

2.1.4 Non-invasive techniques in skin imaging

Dermatological diagnosis has often strongly relied on the observation of naked eyes and clinical experience, therefore the visual perception is of outstanding significance. The development of histological inspection of tissue, immunohistochemistry or electron microscopy have further increased the diagnostic validity thereby gaining new insights into potential pathological mechanisms. The routine histology remains the gold standard for the majority of skin diseases, but the excision biopsy of tissue for evaluation is inherently invasive and procedures are associated with pain, the risk of skin infection and scar formation.

With the fast development of dermoscope, reflectance confocal microscope (RCM), high-frequency ultrasound (HFUS) and optical coherence tomography (OCT), non-invasive skin imaging techniques are now widely applied for the diagnosis and monitoring of skin diseases, such as skin tumors, inflammatory dermatosis, infectious dermatosis, diseases of hair and nails. The non-invasive skin imaging techniques are popular among dermatologists and patients, because they are non-invasive, repeatability and real-time, to avoid unnecessary biopsies.

2.1.4.1 Dermoscopy

Dermoscopy is a non-invasive technique that allows microscopic visualization of subsurface skin structures not visible to the naked eye. It may be performed with manual devices and allow magnifications up to ×20, or with digital systems requiring a video camera equipped with optic fibers and lenses that ensure magnifications of up to ×200. Dermoscopy can eliminate the reflection, refraction, diffraction of light by adding a "clearing" medium or/and a polarized light, so as to visualize the structures of cutaneous lesions.

Dermoscope has two types: non-contact type (Figure 2-2(a)) and contact type (Figure

2-2(b)). Contact dermoscopy uses a glass window with alcohol or imaging gel in contact with the skin to reduce the refractive index between the skin and dermoscope lens. In the non-contact dermoscopy, there is no contact of the lens with the skin. The cross-polarized lens absorbs all the scattered light and hence allows only light in a single plane to pass through it (Figure 2-3). Dermoscopy can be applied to diagnose skin tumor, pigmented skin disease, inflammatory dermatosis, infectious dermatosis and autoimmune dermatosis, as well as to observe hair and nails.

2.1.4.2　Confocal microscope

The principle of confocal laser scanning microscope was first described in the 1950s. The first commercially available system was realized by Rajadhyaksha et al. at the Harvard Medical School in 1995 based on an 830 nm diode laser that is used as a point light source in a scanning mode providing horizontal tomographic images. The visualization of tissues is based on the different refraction indices of the distinct tissue chromophores and cell structures, especially melanin, collagen, and keratin. Melanin has the strongest refractive index of 1.7, and keratin's refractive index is 1.5. Collagen and inflammatory cells are other highly refractive structures. These structures appear bright white when reflected light reaches the detector whereas non-reflective structures appear dark. The interplay between highly, moderately, and non-reflective structures generates a black and white image representing the area at the cellular level. Generated images by reflectance confocal microscope (RCM) are horizontal and parallel to the skin surface, which contrasts with the perpendicular images viewed on histopathology. It has a lateral resolution of 1 μm and magnification equivalent to a $\times$30 microscope objective. The limit of this technique is that its penetration depth is about 200 μm. It allows the visualization of the dermal-epidermal junction and the superficial dermis, but not the deeper layers. Moreover, it requires extensive training to operate the device and analyze images. The main indications for RCM include superficial fungal infections, hyperpigmentation and hypopigmentation, skin tumors, inflammation and viral diseases of the skin.

2.1.4.3　High-frequency ultrasound(HFUS)

HFUS involves the creation of images using the reflection of ultrasound waves off interfaces with different acoustic impedances. The probe is placed on the skin, and reflected sound waves are interpreted by a computer and generate images. Image brightness is determined by the amplitude of the echo reaching the transducer. High-intensity echoes (or large amplitudes) create hyperechoic images (white), whereas low-intensity echoes (or small amplitudes) produce hypoechoic images (gray). Anechoic images are black images. In ultrasonography, the frequency is inversely proportional to the depth of penetration and directly proportional to image resolution. Thus, HFUS has a shorter wavelength, providing a better resolution but less penetration. In dermatology, the commonly used frequencies are 20-25 MHz, but can be as high as 100 MHz. With frequency is about 20 MHz, resolution reaches 50-200 μm with a depth of penetration of 6-7 mm. If frequency increases to 50 MHz, resolution reaches 39-120 μm, but the depth of penetration is only 4 mm. It is mainly used to differentiate benign and malignant tumors. Before surgery, it can provide information about tumor type and size and surrounding vessels, helping identify the best area for incision. Doctors can discuss with the patients in front of the ultrasound screen about the range of skin lesion in real time. It can also help the clinician evaluate whether the tumor was completely removed or not. However, it is still a challenge to differentiate various tissues (e. g., tumor, fat, and inflammatory infiltrates) under HFUS.

2.1.5　Hair

Hair is skin appendage, consisting of the hair shaft outside the skin and the hair root that penetrates into the skin. In addition to providing protection, hair also transmits psychosocial and gender signals. Though hair diseases scarcely endanger a life, people attach more and more great attention to hair health. Common hair diseases include folliculitis, androgenetic alopecia (AGA), alopecia areata (AA), etc.

Hair grows periodically. There are three phases of hair cycle: growth stage (anagen), regression stage (catagen) and resting stage (telogen) (Figure 2-4). Each hair follicle is growing independent of its neighbors. The duration of each stage varies from regions. The hair cycle of scalp is the longest, with the anagen lasting for up to 5 years, catagen for about 2 weeks and telogen for about 3 months. The scalp contains an average of 100000 hairs averagely, in which about 85% are normally in the anagen, 10%~15% in the telogen, and less than 1% in the catagen. Shedding less than 100 hairs a day is considered normal. Excessive hair loss or abnormal hair loss are considered as pathologic alopecia, which may be due to various factors, including genetic factors, hormone levels, mental stress, medication, and so on. The most common type of alopecia is androgenetic alopecia, affecting at least 80% of men and at least 42% of women, and its pathogenesis remains obscure. Genetic factors (single nucleotide polymorphisms of gene loci and hormone levels) could lead to increase of sensitivity to androgen of scalp hair follicles, and the terminal hair follicles turn into vellus hair, with hair follicles gradually miniaturize and atrophy. There are many treatments for androgenetic alopecia, such as oral medication, topical medication, phototherapy, hair transplantation and platelet rich autologous plasma injection therapy (PRP); however, none of them achieves a complete cure. Finasteride (selective type Ⅱ 5α-reductase inhibitors) and minoxidil are still the best choice in the treatment of AGA for male, and minoxidil is the best choice in the treatment of AGA for female, with high level of evidence. However, the drug treatment often needs a long course of treatment. How to reduce the sensitivity to androgen of hair follicles and reverse the miniaturization of hair follicles remain challenges currently.

Except for the treatment of hair diseases, hair health management include daily care of hair. Hair care is as much in demand as skin care. A variety of shampoo, conditioner and germinal products emerge in endlessly, hair daily care has a very broad market prospect.

2.2   Skin Wound

2.2.1   Overview of skin wound

Skin wound is the skin rupture or defect caused by external force or other factors, resulting in the damage of the skin structure and function.

2.2.1.1   The mechanism of skin wound healing

Sophisticated and consecutive wound healing process starts immediately after the skin is damaged (physical, chemical and photo-thermal damage). This process includes four stages: hemostatic phase, inflammation phase, proliferation phase and maturation/reconstruction phase(Figure 2-5). It involves a variety of cytokines, signal pathways and growth factors, which promote the skin wound healing collaboratively.

1. Hemostatic phase

Blood vessels contracted and exogenous coagulation system are activated promptly after the skin is damaged. The secreted thrombin promote fibrinogen transforming into fibrin. Red blood cells, platelets and crosslinking collagen fibers aggregate in the local wound site and block the impaired vessel via the formation of blood clots. Then the aggregated platelets are activated and induced the production of glycoproteins and various growth factors. Glycoproteins can promote the formation of thrombus, exerting hemostatic effect. Epidermal growth factor (EGF), transforming growth factor-β (TGF-β), fibroblast growth factor (FGF) and platelet derived growth factor (PDGF) stimulate fibroblasts to produce more collagen and elastin.

2. Inflammation phase

As the vasodilation of blood vessels and increased vascular permeability, a large number of white blood cells and macrophages infiltrate into the wound site and remove necrotic tissue, preventing wound infection. At first, neutrophils migrate into the wound site, remove microorganisms by phagocytosis and degrade necrotic tissue by protease. Subsequently, macrophage infiltrates into the wound site and remove the bacteria and contaminants. A large variety of interleukins (ILs), growth factors and tumor necrosis factor (TNF) participate in the inflammation phase of skin wound healing process.

3. Proliferation phase

Granulation tissue consists of fibroblasts, newborn thin-walled capillary and inflammatory cells. Macrophages secrete TGF-β and PDGF to induce the proliferation of fibroblasts and the production of type Ⅲ collagen. Endothelial cells proliferate on the collagen and promote the formation of microvessels. Fibroblasts synthesize and secrete the type Ⅰ and type Ⅲ collagen, of which type Ⅲ collagen is prominent. The migration of fibroblasts is mediated by matrix metalloproteinases (MMPs), growth factors and interleukins. Studies have shown that fat cells can migrate into the surrounding wound sites, induce epidermal cells covering wounds, and promote wound healing.

4. Maturation/reconstruction phase

Keratinocytes, fibroblasts and macrophages secrete various kinds of matrix degrading enzymes to degrade the excessive extracellular matrix. Type Ⅲ collagen is replaced by the more intensive type Ⅰ collagen. During the maturation/reconstruction phase, the skin tissue thickened and the skin barrier function is recovered. This stage could last for 2 years or more.

2.2.1.2 The factors affecting skin wound healing

1. Growth factors affecting wound healing process

Growth factors are the bioactive peptides derived from the hematopoietic system, immune system and activated inflammatory cells, which could regulate the proliferation and differentiation of cells and promote metabolism. Growth factors include EGF, TGF-β, FGF, PDGF, and insulin-like growth factor (IGF). TGF-β could promote the synthesis and deposition of collagen fibers, accelerate wound healing, change the tension of local tissue and affect the formation of scarring(Figure 2-6).

FGF could induce the production of capillaries and accelerate the growth of epithelium and granulation tissue. PDGF is the peptide secreted by platelet α particle, which could promote the cells from interphase into mitotic phrase, and promote cell proliferation and differentiation. PDGF is synthesized and secreted by endothelial cells, smooth muscle cells, fibroblast cells and macrophages, which enables inflammatory cells infiltrating into the wound site and promotes the formation of granulation tissue when skin tissue is damaged. Currently, the growth factor agents approved by China Food and Drug Administration include recombinant bovine basic fibroblast growth factor for external use gel, recombinant human basic fibroblast growth factor and recombinant human epidermal growth factor external solution.

2. Matrix metalloproteinases affecting wound healing process

Matrix metalloproteinases (MMPs) are intrapeptidase assisted by Ca^{2+} and Zn^{2+}, whose activity is inhibited by tissue inhibitor of metalloproteinases (TIMPs). MMPs are involved in the degradation of extracellular matrix such as collagen. Studies have shown that the expression of MMPs is very low in intact skin tissue and is up-regulated after skin injury. In addition, TIMPs can delay wound healing, suggesting that MMPs are key molecules in wound healing. Fibroblasts secrete MMPs to promote cell migration and degrade unstable extracellular matrix. Moreover, MMPs can promote macrophages infiltration in the wound to remove necrotic tissue, promote establishing microcirculation in the wound area, and accelerate granulation tissue formation.

3. Inflammation-related mircoRNA affecting wound healing process

Inflammation response in wound area plays a key role in wound healing. The disruption of inflammation response can delay wound healing, lead infection, and generate hyperplastic scar and keloid. MircoRNA (miRNA), 21-23 nucleotide noncoding single-stranded RNA, is derived from eukaryotes. miRNA is bond with mRNA and inhibit the gene expression of transcription level. Inflammation-related miRNA is the key regulator of the inflammatory response and tissue repair. Multiple kinds of miRNA related to wound healing have been identified, and the dysfunction of miRNA could lead pathological wound healing, such as slow healing process and scarring.

4. Oxygen affecting wound healing process

Clinical studies found that more bleeding wounds heal well while less bleeding wounds suffer poor healing. Any kind of wound healing requires sufficient blood perfusion and oxygen supply. A clinical study have demonstrated that oxygen therapy prior to surgery could reduce 50% of postoperative wound infections in patients with colorectal resection. Hyperbaric oxygen therapy also achieves satisfactory results in chronic delayed healing wound. Thus, oxygen therapy plays very important roles in wound healing and preventing infection.

5. Wet wound environment affecting wound healing process

White et al. observed that wound healed faster in humid environment than in dry conditions through the pig experimental models, and proposed the theory of wet wound healing. Subsequently, a number of studies have confirmed this theory. The wet environment of the wound can make the wound base moist, stimulate the formation of vessels and granulation tissue, shorten the healing period and reduce the possibility of scar formation.

The theory of wet wound healing suggests that wet dressings could keep wound moist and accelerate wound healing. The wet dressings could keep wound moist, promote fibroblasts proliferation and capillary formation, and release and activate the collagen enzyme, especially protease and urokinase dissolving necrotic tissue. The improvement of wound microenvironment can attract a large number of inflammatory cells to secrete a variety of growth factors, promoting wound healing. In addition, wet dressings could reduce the adhesion between dressings and wound, and reduce patients' pain during dressings change and secondary injury. At present, the theory of wet wound healing is still controversial in China. Some scholars believed that the closed moist environment would cause the proliferation of pathogenic bacteria in the wound area and lead wound infection.

2.2.2 Complications and treatment of skin wound repair

2.2.2.1 Skin wound infection

Skin acts as the external barrier of body, which is susceptible to the insult of pathogenic microorganisms. In addition, there are a lot of resident flora on the skin surface. Skin wounds are likely to be infected when the integrity of skin is destroyed. Excessive sustained inflammation process caused by infection is one of the main factors in non-healing wounds. It is estimated that more than 2% of the American population suffer non-healing wounds and more than \$20 billion annually poured into treating wound related infections.

Conventional therapies of skin wounds include topical antibiotic ointments, growth factor agents and wound dressings. However, this method is often accompanied by antibiotic-resistance, intensive pain during dressing change, and professional operations. As the proposal of the theory of wet wound healing and the synthesis of new materials, hydrogel which contain many water is developing rapidly in the medical field. Hydrogel could keep the wound moist, absorb exudate of tissue and possess well biological safety. Currently, more studies focus on hydrogel with antibacterial drugs, combined the antibacterial properties and the advantages of promoting wound healing.

2.2.2.2　Chronic refractory wound

Chronic refractory wound (ulcer) includes traumatic ulcer, variceal ulcer of lower extremities, pressure ulcer and diabetic ulcer. It has long duration period, affects esthetics, and is accompanied with serious complications, which affect the patients' quality of life significantly. The incidence, lesion location, age and susceptible population of chronic refractory skin is different between developed and developing countries. In China, chronic refractory wound caused by trauma is given priority to adolescents and young adults, and diabetic, oppressive, venous ulcers are prominent in the elderly over the age of 60.

The etiology and pathogenesis of chronic refractory wound has not yet been fully elucidated. The pathogenesis differs among different kinds of chronic refractory wounds (Figure 2-7). Studies have shown that the down expression of extracellular protein fiber connection gene lead to the damage of tissue repair cell scaffold and delay wound healing. The excessive apoptosis of the fibroblast reduce the generation of dermal collagen fibers and delay wound healing. The concentration change of growth factors in wound site and dysfunction of regulation network delay wound healing. Ca^{2+} signaling pathways, mitogen-activated protein kinases (MAPKs), Jaks-STATs, and protein kinase C (PKC) are shown to mediate the healing process of chronic refractory wound. The relevant studies need to be further verified.

Due to the differences in etiology and pathogenesis, the therapies are differed among different kinds of chronic refractory wounds. At first, performing surgical treatment (debridement) for skin ulcers; second, adopting some measures to promote traumatic ulcer healing. Blood sugar and varicose problems need to be first treated in the treatment for diabetic ulcer and variceal ulcer of lower extremities, respectively.

Recently, treatment for chronic refractory wound include new types of dressing materials, growth factor agent as well as stem cells and tissue engineering. Hydrogel, hydrophilic three-dimensional network, can absorb a large amount of water or liquid, and has good elasticity, swelling and surface properties, and biological safety, which is a good material for wound dressings and tissue engineering. Growth factors are involved in the whole stages of wound healing. Adding exogenous growth factors could promote proliferation and differentiation of cells and regulate signal transduction. Commercially growth factor agents approved by Food and Drug Administration (FDA) of the United States include human recombinant platelet derived growth factor (PDGF), recombinant human/bovine fibroblast growth factor and epidermal growth factor (EGF), etc. Transgenic method of wound healing transfers the naked DNA of growth factors gene into local wound sites through injection and gene gun, promoting cell proliferation, angiogenesis and wound healing.

2.2.2.3 Pathologic skin scars

Skin scar is the change of skin tissue morphology and histopathological features caused by trauma. According to the statistics, it is estimated that there are more than one hundred million new cases of scar patients annually in developed countries. Skin scar causes the changes of appearance and function, affects the mental health of patients and reduces the quality of life of patients. Pathologic skin scars includes hyperplastic scar, keloid, atrophic scar, and the scar cancer, etc.

The pathogenesis of skin scar has not been fully elucidated, and the pathogenesis differs among different kinds of skin scars (Figure 2-8). It has been widely accepted that abnormal proliferation and differentiation of fibroblasts and deposition of extracellular matrix are the central parts of the disease. These processes mainly involve TGF-β, inflammatory cytokines and MMP family, etc. In addition, mechanical force related signaling pathway is also thought to play an important role in regulating the formation of skin scar.

There are various therapies for treating scars, which can be divided into five categories: ① surgical resection; ② intrascar injection, including botulinum toxin A, bleomycin, glucocorticoid and 5-fluorouracil (5-FU); ③ electro-optical technology treatment, including dot matrix laser, pulsed dye laser, radiofrequency ablation and intense pulsed light; ④ topical drugs, including onion extract, mitomycin C and imiquimod; ⑤ physical therapy, including silicone gel pressure therapy, cryotherapy, radiation therapy and microneedle therapy. The choice of therapies is closely related to the type of scar, the patient's previous treatment history and the patient's compliance.

Surgical resection can treat keloid alone. However, due to the recurrence rate of keloid is as high as 40%-100%, surgical resection is usually combined with radiotherapy, frozen therapy, silicone gel and intrascar injection. There are several types of injection drugs, such as glucocorticoid, bleomycin, 5-fluorouracil, rapamycin, verapamil, doxorubicin, botulinum toxin A and tretinoin. Among them, 5-fluorouracil, bleomycin and glucocorticoid have been supported by clinical studies.

Due to the possibility of oncogenicity, radiation therapy is usually not recommended as the first-line treatment, but for the refractory keloid and hyperplastic scar. Radiation therapy could induce fibroblast apoptosis and gene mutation, and damage the stem cell of connective tissue. Striping laser (Er: YAG laser, CO_2 laser), intense laser and pulsed dye laser (585 nm and 595 nm), etc., has been studied in clinical trials.

The mechanism of cryotherapy for skin scar is that low temperature cause the damage of cells through the rapidly cooling of refrigerant (usually liquid nitrogen) and blood stasis after thawing damage the scar tissue. In addition, frozen can make patients numb, reduce the pain and increase the compliance of treatment.

Commonly used topical drugs include onion extract, mitomycin C and imiquimod. Onion extraction is commonly used in preventing scar formation or as the adjunct therapy. Onion extraction can inhibit the proliferation of fibroblasts and mast cells, reduce inflammation, and prevent scar formation. Clinical trials of mitomycin C in treating hyperplastic scar are insufficient and lack of evidence. Imiquimod is used for the recurrence of auricular keloid.

The mechanism of microneedle in treating skin scar is unclear. Some scholars believe that the moderate inflammatory response after microneedle therapy can activate MMPs, degrade the collagen fibers with abnormal arrangement and remodel the skin tissues. Besides, it is considered that microneedle can affect the gap-junction protein, change the mechanical force of fibroblasts, so as to intervene the production of collagen and secretion of cytokines. The change of membrane potential after exposure to microneedle improves the viability of cells, promotes the production of protein, potassium and growth factors, stimulates the migration of fibroblasts to the injured area, and increases the production of collagen, elastin and proteoglycan.

2.3 Representative Skin Diseases

2.3.1 Psoriasis

Psoriasis is a common, chronic and recurring inflammatory skin disease. The typical lesions are scaly plaques and papules. The disorder may occur at any age without gender predominance, but it is more common in young adults. The prevalence of natural population varies between 0.1% and 3.0%, and the incidence of psoriasis in China is 0.123%. Psoriasis is prone to relapse or aggravate in spring and winter, and tend to relieve in summer and autumn.

2.3.1.1 Etiology

The etiology of psoriasis is not yet fully elucidated. Currently, psoriasis is recognized as polygenic disease mediated by genetic and environmental factors.

1. Genetic factors

All studies on demographic survey, pedigree, genetics (e. g. , twin studies), and HLA strongly suggest a genetic predisposition to psoriasis. About 20% of psoriatic patients report a positive family history, of whom psoriasis occurs at an earlier age than those without family history. The chance for an offspring to develop psoriasis is about 16% if one parent is affected by the disease and the likelihood goes up to 50% when both parents are affected. Histocompatibility antigen studies have shown that the class I antigens A1, A13, A28,

B13, B17, B37, and Cw6 (in which Cw6 shows the strongest association with this disease), and the class Ⅱ antigen DR7 are more likely to be expressed in psoriatic patients compared to normal individuals.

2. Environmental factors

Epidemiological studies for the prevalence of psoriasis in monozygotic twins suggest a 70% chance of one twin developing psoriasis if the other has developed the condition, but only a 20% chance for dizygotic twins. These findings indicate that the hereditary factors are insufficient to trigger psoriasis independently, while the environmental factors play an important role in its occurrence. The common environmental factors triggering or aggravating psoriasis include infection, emotional stress, trauma, surgical incision, pregnancy, cigarette smoking, and certain kinds of drugs.

3. Immune factors

Abundant lymphocytes and monocytes infiltrate lesions of psoriasis vulgaris, especially T cells. It is an important pathological feature of psoriasis, indicating T cells involved in the occurrence and development of the disease. However, the role of T cells in the pathogenesis remains unclear.

2.3.1.2　Pathogenesis

Involvement of the immune system in psoriasis is now widely accepted. Genome-wide scans for psoriasis associated genes have identified predominantly immunerelated genes providing a mechanistic link between genetics and immunity. Psoriatic skin lesions originate as a result of dysregulated interactions of innate and adaptive components of the immune system with resident cutaneous cell types. Research about the immunopathogenesis of psoriasis has resulted in several highly specific therapies that target components of the immune system. Now there are several mechanisms of the disease: cross-talk between innate and adaptive immunities and the central role of TNF-α; the interleukin-23(IL-23)/T helper cell 17 (Th17) axis (Figure 2-9).

1. Cross-talk between innate and adaptive immunities

Psoriasis is mainly a dendritic cell- and T cell-mediated disease with complex feedback loops from antigen-presenting cells, neutrophilic granulocytes, keratinocytes, vascular endothelial cells, to the cutaneous nervous system. Cross-talk between the innate and the adaptive immune systems mediated by cytokines including TNF-α, interferon-γ, and interleukin-1 is a major research focus. Complexes of host DNA and the epidermis-produced antimicrobial peptide LL-37 (cathelicidin) are thought to stimulate dermal plasmacytoid dendritic cells to produce interferon-α. On exacerbation or onset of psoriasis, activated dendritic cells produce, among other mediators, TNF-α and interleukin-23. TNF-α is a pro-inflammatory cytokine that amplifies inflammation through several distinct pathways. TNF-α is produced by a broad range of cell types including macrophages, lymphocytes, keratinocytes, and endothelial cells, and exerts its activities on several different cell types. TNF-α induces secondary mediators and adhesion molecules, all of which have been implicated in psoriatic disease. The clinical success of TNF-blocking agents is therefore not surprising.

2. IL-23/Th17 axis

Interest is rising in the IL-23/Th17 axis in psoriasis, which has resulted in several novel targeted therapies. Th17 are a subset of T cells expressing IL-17, distinct from the classical Th17 that play a predominant role in the pathogenesis of psoriasis and other inflammatory disorders. Expansion and survival of these T cells depends on myeloid cell-produced IL-23, which drives the differentiation of Th17. IL-23 acts mainly on memory T cells, because naive T cells do not express the IL-23 receptor. Once activated, Th17 produce several mediators such as IL-17A, IL-17F, and IL-22, which induce keratinocytes proliferation and other hallmark features of psoriasis. In psoriatic skin, IL-17 is produced by $CD4^+$ T cells, epidermal $CD8^+$ T cells, neutrophils, mast cells, and macrophages, which might explain the broad and rapid clinical efficacy of specifically targeting IL-17.

2.3.1.3 Clinical manifestations

Psoriasis could be categorized into psoriasis vulgaris, psoriasis arthropathica (psoriatic arthritis), erythrodermic psoriasis, and pustular psoriasis according to their respective clinical patterns. Psoriasis vulgaris accounts for more than 90% of cases, and the other two types listed above (except psoriatic arthritis) are frequently the exacerbation of psoriasis vulgaris caused by triggers such as strongly irritating topical treatments, the sudden withdrawal of systemic glucocorticoids or immunosuppressants, infection, or even mental stress.

1. Psoriasis vulgaris

This type of psoriasis begins with red papules or maculopapules that gradually becomes well-demarcated red plaques in a variety of morphologic patterns (e. g. , guttate, nummular, geographic, ostraceous), covered with thick silvery scales. Scraping off these lamellar scales is similar to scraping off wax drippings (candle wax phenomenon), which then exposes a shiny reddish translucent film on the surface of the lesion (film phenomenon). When the film is removed completely, punctuate spots of bleeding appear within a few seconds(Auspitz's sign). The candle wax phenomenon, the film phenomenon, and the punctate bleeding are all important diagnostic clues for psoriasis. The degree of pruritus vary from patients to patients.

2. Psoriasis arthropathica

It is also known as psoriatic arthritis. 5%-8% of psoriatic patients eventually develop psoriatic arthritis. Psoriatic arthritis typically has a chronic course. Psoriasis lesions usually precede the onset of joint symptoms. Psoriatic arthritis can affect any particular joint, but is more common affecting large joints of the lower extremities, the distal joints of the fingers and toes, and even the back and sacroiliac joints. Marked nail damage often accompanies digital joint arthritis. The involved large joints may resemble rheumatoid arthritis with joint malformation. However, unlike rheumatoid arthritis, the rheumatoid factor in psoriatic arthritis is usually negative. Patients with spine and sacroiliac joint involvement show a strong correlation with HLA-B27 antigen.

3. Erythrodermic psoriasis

This type of psoriasis appears as inflammation and exfoliation of the skin over most of the body surface, in which the small normal-appearing areas look like islands. There is generalized redness and swelling of the skin covered with bran-like scales which may be accompanied with fever and lymphadenopathy. The course of this condition is more persistent and also is more likely to recur.

4. Pustular psoriasis

There are two forms of pustular psoriasis, i. e., generalized pustular psoriasis and localized pustular psoriasis. ① Generalized pustular psoriasis: Here the pustules have a sudden onset and can spread quickly over the entire body. The yellow or yellow-white, pinhead to milium-sized, superficial, sterile, and small pustules occur in groups around old lesions of psoriasis vulgaris or in normal skin, and may coalesce, thereby forming "large lakes" of pus. The skin around the pustules is often red, inflamed and can be painful. Attacks are often preceded by chills, high fever, and other constitutional signs. The patients may present fissured tongue, and thickened and turbid fingernails or toenails when the tongue and nails are involved. Usually the pustules dry up to form crusts within 1-2 weeks, but recurrent attacks can take place. The conditions can be progressive in some patients, presenting with severe symptoms and death from secondary infection and multiple organ failure. ②Localized pustular psoriasis: The sterile pustules are distributed symmetrically at the palms and soles only, especially in the thenar or hypothenar eminences or in the central portion of the palms and soles. For each episode, crops of small pustules develop on the erythematous areas and may rupture and crust or desquamate within 1-2 weeks, but new pustules will keep appearing under the scales. The process runs a chronic course with only a slight chance of significant remission. Nails are often involved in these patients, with punctate depressions, transverse grooves, longitudinal ridges, onycholysis, and subungual pus.

2.3.1.4　Treatment

Topical therapy is generally recommended for small area of plaques, and moderate or severe psoriasis often requires phototherapy combined with systemic treatment. Phototherapy remains highly cost-effective for widespread psoriasis. Cyclosporin has a rapid onset of action, but is generally not suitable for continuous therapy. Methotrexate remains the most effective systemic agent. Biological agents can produce dramatic responses at the high cost. Rotating therapeutic agents with varying toxicities have conceptual appeal, and combination therapy may reduce toxicity and reduce the incidence of neutralizing antibodies to agents such as infliximab.

1. Topical treatment

（1）Corticosteroids: Topical application of corticosteroids in creams, ointments, lotions, foams, and sprays is the most frequent prescribed therapy for psoriasis. Low-to-mid strength creams are preferred in the intertriginous areas and on the face. To augment effectiveness of topical corticosteroids in areas with thick keratotic scale, the area should be hydrated by soaking prior to application, and covered with an occlusive dressing of a polyethylene film (Saran Wrap) or a sauna suit. Unfortunately, there is typically rapid recurrence of disease when corticosteroid therapy is discontinued. Side effects include epidermal atrophy, steroid acne, miliaria, and pyoderma.

(2) Tazaroten: Tazarotene is a nonisomerizable retinoic acid receptor specific retinoid. It appears to treat psoriasis by modulating keratinocytes differentiation and hyperproliferation, as well as by suppressing inflammation.

(3) Calcipotriene: Vitamin D_3 affects keratinocytes differentiation partly through its regulation of epidermal responsiveness to calcium. Treatment with the vitamin D_3 analog calcipotriene (Dovonex) in ointment, cream, or solution form has been shown to be very effective in the treatment of plaque-type and scalp psoriasis. Combination therapy with calcipotriene and high-potency steroids may provide greater response rates, fewer side effects, and steroid sparing.

(4) Macrolactams(calcineurin inhibitors): Topical macrolactams such as tacrolimus and pimecrolimus are especially helpful for thin lesions in areas prone to atrophy or steroid acne. The burning commonly associated with these agents can be problematic, but may be avoided by prior treatment with a corticosteroid, and by application to dry skin, rather than after bathing.

(5) Salicyclic acid: Salicylic acid is used as a keratolytic agent in shampoos, creams and gels. It can promote the absorption of other topical agents. Widespread application of salicyclic acid may lead to salicylate toxicity manifesting with tinnitus, acute confusion, and refractory hypoglycemia, especially in patients with diabetes and those with compromised renal function.

(6) Ultraviolet therapy: In most instances, sunlight can improve psoriasis. However, burning of the skin may cause Koebner's phenomenon and an aggravation. Artificial UVB is produced by fluorescent bulbs in broad- or narrow-band spectrums. Maximal effect is usually achieved at minimal erythemogenic doses (MED). Maintenance UVB therapy after clearing contributes to the duration of remission and is justified for many patients.

(7) PUVA therapy: High-intensity longwave UV radiation (UVA) given 2 h after ingestion of 8-methoxypsoralen (Oxsoralen Ultra), twice a week, is highly effective, even in severe psoriasis. Most patients clear within 20-25 treatments, but maintenance treatment is needed. Although PUVA therapy is highly effective, in patients with less than 50% of the skin surface affected, UVB may be as good. PUVA therapy is a risk factor for skin cancer, including squamous cell carcinoma and melanoma. Men treated without genital protection are at an increased risk of developing squamous cell carcinomas of the penis and scrotum. Although the risk of cancer is dose related, there is no definitive threshold dose of cumulative PUVA exposure above which carcinogenicity can be predicted.

2. Systemic treatment

(1) Retinoids: Retinoids are suitable for the treatment of all types of psoriasis, such as etretinate administered orally in dosages of 0.75-1.0 mg/(kg • d). However, retinoids have severe teratogenic effects, cause an increase in the levels of triglycerides, total cholesterolcan and liver enzymes. These side effects limit the application of retinoids in women of childbearing age, the elderly and children. Retinoids are contraindicated in pregnant patients.

(2) Immunosuppressants: Immunosuppressants are prescribed mostly for erythrodermic psoriasis, pustular psoriasis, and psoriasis arthropathica. The medication frequently used in this group is methotrexate given orally in a dosage of 10-25 mg/week for an adult patient, but the weekly dosage may not exceed 50 mg. Other choices include cyclosporine and tacrolimus. Methotrexate takes effect slowly, and the effect is usually obvious after 12 or 16 weeks treatment. Blood test, liver and kidney function should be tested regularly during the treatment. If the cumulative dose is more than 1500 mg, it is necessary to monitor liver fibrosis. Commonly recommended dose of cyclosporine is 3-5 mg/(kg • d), and should gradually reduce the dose after symptom control. Nephrotoxicity and hypertension should be monitored during long-term use.

(3) Biological agents: Several biological agents are available that can produce dramatic responses in some patients with psoriasis; while all are expensive. There are 3 classes of biological agents used to treat psoriasis: TNF inhibitors, IL-12/23 inhibitors, IL-17 inhibitors. Infliximab is a chimeric monoclonal antibody to TNF-α and requires intravenous infusion; etanercept is a fusion protein of human TNF-α Ⅱ receptor and the Fc region of IgG1; adalimumab is a recombinant fully human IgG1 monoclonal antibody to TNF-α. Alefacept is a fusion protein of the external domain of LFA-3 and the Fc region of IgG1, and blocks T-cell activation and triggers apoptosis of pathogenic T-cells. Etanercept provides a good balance of safety and efficacy. All biological agents used to treat psoriasis are administered subcutaneously except infliximab. Overall, there are no increased rates of serious infections or internal malignancies in patients with psoriasis who are treated using biological agents. Adverse effects that occur at slightly higher rates than placebo and are common to all biological agents include injection site reaction, nasopharyngitis, and upper respiratory tract infections.

2.3.1.5　Treatment difficulties

A variety of topical therapies, photochemical therapy and traditional immunosuppressants can reduce skin lesions and relieve symptoms; systemic using of IL-23 monoclonal antibody, IL-17A monoclonal antibody and other biological agents that directly block the IL-23/Th17 cell pathway can quickly remove psoriasis lesions. However, skin lesions of psoriasis often recur after stopping treatment, which is the difficulty of psoriasis treatment.

Psoriasis is an inflammatory skin disease that is associated with multiple comorbidities and substantially diminishes patients' quality of life. Joint damage is the most common complication of psoriasis. About 1/3 of psoriasis patients eventually develop into psoriatic arthritis. Patients with severe psoriasis and early onset psoriasis have an increased risk of cardiovascular and other metabolic diseases, such as diabetes, hyperlipidemia, obesity and atherosclerotic plaque. In addition, patients with psoriasis have a higher risk of mental diseases, such as depression, anxiety and suicidality. The risk of inflammatory bowel disease in patients with psoriasis is four times that of the general population. The exact relationships between these comorbidities and psoriasis and the treatments of comorbidities are also the difficulties in the treatment of psoriasis.

2.3.2 Melanoma

2.3.2.1 Introduction

1. Etiology and pathogenesis

(1) Risk factors: Ultraviolet (UV) radiation is the main environmental risk factor. Host risk factors for melanoma include the presence of melanocytic or dysplastic naevi, a personal history of melanoma, a family history of melanoma, and phenotypic characteristics including fair hair, eye and skin colors, and the tendency to freckle. Gene mutations account for only a small proportion of melanoma cases.

(2) The genesis of melanoma: UVA radiation induces melanocytes malignant transformation through two different mechanisms. The direct transformation of normal melanocytes in neoplastic cells through the occurrence of several mutations affecting both proto-oncogene and tumor suppressor genes (TP53, NF1, PTEN, etc.). The activating BRAF mutation is a typical feature of benign nevi formation and BRAF is mutated in up to 80% of benign nevi. These nevi remain indolent for decades due to immune surveillance. Further progression into intermediate lesions, melanomas *in situ*, invasive potential and metastasis requires additional mutations. The most frequent somatic mutations affect genes that control central cellular process, such as proliferation (BRAF, NRAS and NF1), growth and metabolism (PTEN and KIT), resistance to apoptosis (TP53), cell cycle control (CDKN2A) and replicative lifespan (TERT). These genetic alterations yield a reciprocal overstimulation of the affected cellular pathways in melanoma, mainly the MAPK pathway and the PI3K/AKT pathway.

(3) Tumor microenvironmental alterations: Melanoma spreading is the result of genetic mutations and tumor microenvironmental alterations. A key role is played by the overexpression of matrix metalloproteinases (MMPs) that induces the degradation of the components of the extracellular matrix to favor tumor cell infiltration and spreading through the bloodstream.

(4) Immune escape of melanoma cells: Melanoma cells also evade the immune system. Upon tumor antigen recognition by T cells, released interferons trigger JAK-STAT-mediated expression of PD-1 ligands PD-L1 and PD-L2 on the surface of melanoma cells. Binding of PD-L1 and PD-L2 to PD-1 leads to the suppression of T cell activity and inhibits the

antitumor immune response. Further immunosuppressive mechanisms include the down regulation of tumor-associated antigens and class Ⅰ major histocompatibility complex, and the secretion of inhibitory factors like tumor growth factor-β.

2. Clinical presentations, subtypes and staging

(1) Clinical presentations and subtypes: Typical features are asymmetry of the lesion, irregular borders, inhomogeneous color, diameter of 5 mm and more.

①Superficial spreading melanoma(57.4%): Common in trunk in men and lower legs in women. It begins as macule with slow radial growth phase limited to epidermis or focally in papillary dermis and then develops into papule or nodule with a rapid vertical growth phase. On dermoscopy, it exhibits broad network of multiple brown dots, color variation and possible depigmentation. Histologically, the feature is pagetoid spread of malignant melanocytes throughout the epidermis (Figure 2-10).

②Nodular melanoma(21.4%): Typically arises on trunk, head and neck in men more than women. It begins as a blue black, or pink nodule which may ulcerate or bleed with an aggressive vertical phase and a short or absent horizontal growth phase. On dermoscopy, it exhibits individual globules with color variation, white streaks and irregular vessels. Microscopically, there are irregular nests of melanocytes.

③Lentigo maligna melanoma (8.8%): Common in nose, cheek, or any sun-damaged skin. It begins as a brownish black macule with variegated color and irregular indented border. On dermoscopy, it exhibits hyperpigmented follicular openings slowly overgrown by irregular pigmented dots. It is characterized histologically by a lentiginous proliferation of atypical melanocytes at the dermal-epidermal junction and histological features of solar elastosis.

④Acral lentiginous melanoma (4%): Commonly arises on soles and palms. In its initial intraepidermal phase, there is irregular and poorly circumscribed macule; therewith a nodular region reflects the invasive growth pattern. On dermoscopy, it exhibits irregular, gray-brown polygons and multiple hypopigmented areas. When involving the nail bed, it can present with longitudinal melanonychia extending onto the hyponychium or beyond the lateral or proximal nail fold, the latter referred to as Hutchinson's sign. Histologically, there are proliferating and atypical melanocytes within basal layer of hyperplastic dermis either arranged solitary or in irregular nests.

(2) TNM classification: AJCC 8th edition TNM staging categories for melanoma, see Table 2-1.

Table 2-1　TNM staging for melanoma

Stages	Manifestations
Tx	Primary tumor cannot be assessed
T0	No evidence of primary tumor
Tis	Melanoma *in situ*

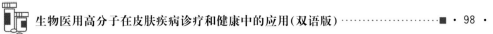

Continued

Stages	Manifestations	
T1	Thickness≤1.0 mm	
T2	Thickness 1.1-2.0 mm	
	T2a	Without ulceration
	T2b	With ulceration
T3	Thickness 2.1-4.0 mm	
	T3a	Without ulceration
	T3b	With ulceration
T4	Thickness >4.0 mm	
	T4a	Without ulceration
	T4b	With ulceration
Nx	Regional nodes cannot be assessed	
N0	No regional metastases detected	
N1	1 node	
	N1a	1 node, clinically occult without satellites, local recurrence, or in-transit metastasis. ("Clinically occult" nodal metastasis: patients without clinical or radiographic evidence of regional lymph node metastasis but who have tumor-involved regional nodal metastasis found at SLN biopsy.)
	N1b	1 node, clinically detected without satellites, local recurrence, or in-transit metastasis. ("Clinically detected" nodal metastasis: patients with tumor-involved regional lymph nodes detected by clinical or radiographic examination.)
	N1c	No nodes with satellites, local recurrence, or in-transit metastasis
N2	2-3 nodes	
	N2a	2-3 nodes, clinically occult without satellites, local recurrence, or in-transit metastasis
	N2b	2-3 nodes, at least one node clinically detected without satellites, local recurrence, or in-transit metastasis
	N2c	1 node, clinically occult or detected with satellites, local recurrence, or in-transit metastasis
N3	≥4 nodes	
	N3a	4 or more nodes, all clinically occult without satellites, local recurrence, or in-transit metastasis present
	N3b	4 or more nodes, at least one node clinically detected or matted without satellites, local recurrence, or in-transit metastasis present
	N3c	2 or more nodes, clinically occult or detected with satellites, local recurrence, or in-transit metastasis present

Continued

Stages	Manifestations	
M0	No detectable evidence of distant metastasis	
M1a	Metastases to skin, subcutaneous, or distant lymph	
	M1a(0)	Normal LDH
	M1a(1)	Elevated LDH
M1b	Lung metastasis	
	M1b(0)	Normal LDH
	M1b(1)	Elevated LDH
M1c	Other visceral metastasis	
	M1c(0)	Normal LDH
	M1c(1)	Elevated LDH
M1d	Brain metastasis	
	M1d(0)	Normal LDH
	M1d(1)	Elevated LDH

（3）Clinical staging and pathologic staging of melanoma see Table 2-2.

Table 2-2　Clinical staging and pathologic staging of melanoma

Stage	T	N	M
Clinical stage			
0	Tis	N0	M0
I A	T1a	N0	M0
I B	T1b	N0	M0
	T2a	N0	M0
II A	T2b	N0	M0
	T3a	N0	M0
II B	T3b	N0	M0
	T4a	N0	M0
II C	T4b	N0	M0
III	Any T	≥N1	M0
IV	Any T	Any N	M1
Pathologic stage			
0	Tis	N0	M0
I A	T1a	N0	M0
	T1b	N0	M0

Continued

Stage	T	N	M
ⅠB	T2a	N0	M0
ⅡA	T2b	N0	M0
	T3a	N0	M0
ⅡB	T3b	N0	M0
	T4a	N0	M0
ⅡC	T4b	N0	M0
ⅢA	T1a/b-T2a	N1a or N2a	M0
ⅢB	T0	N1b,N1c	M0
	T1a/b-T2a	N1b/c or N2b	M0
	T2b/T3a	N1a-N2b	M0
ⅢC	T0	N2b,N2c,N3b/c	M0
	T1a-T3a	N2c or N3a/b/c	M0
	T3b/T4a	≥N1	M0
	T4b	N1a-N2c	M0
ⅢD	T4b	N3a/b/c	M0
Ⅳ	Any T	Any N	M1

3. Diagnosis and differential diagnosis

(1) Clinical and dermoscopic diagnosis: Most melanomas are readily detected and diagnosed by visual inspection by an experienced physician because of their prominent pigmentation and morphological pattern. People at an increased risk for melanoma should be screened at regular intervals. High-risk characteristics that prompt screening or surveillance include melanocytic naevi, dysplastic naevi, and personal and family histories of melanoma. Screening for melanoma includes a total body skin examination supported by dermoscopy or other imaging techniques.

Examination with the naked eye assesses the so-called A (asymmetry), B (irregular borders), C (inhomogeneous color) and D (diameter ≥ 5 mm) criteria, which point to suspicious melanocytic lesions (ABCD rule).

Dermoscopy is an essential tool for the examination of pigmented and non-pigmented skin tumors to detect melanoma. Melanoma-specific criteria includes atypical pigment network, irregular dots/globules, irregular streaks, blue-whitish veil, regression structures, irregular vascular structures, blotches, shiny white streaks and rosettes.

The differential diagnosis of melanoma involves other melanocytic pigmented lesions (congenital, atypical, common melanocytic naevi and actinic lentigo), non-melanocytic pigmented lesions (seborrheic keratosis, hemangioma, dermatofibroma, and pigmented basal cell carcinoma), and other non-pigmented tumors (hemangioma, basal cell carcinoma, squamous cell carcinoma).

（2）Histopathologic diagnosis: Histological examination can provide information about clinic-pathologic type, tumor thickness, presence or absence of ulceration, mitotic activity, microsatellites, lateral and deep excision margins, vascular or perineural involvement.

（3）Immunohistochemical stains: Characteristic markers commonly used for melanocytes include S100, SOX10, MART1/Melan-A, HMB45, tyrosinase, MITF and Ki67. A mixture of two or more markers can be used in immunohistochemistry to increase the sensitivity for the detection of melanocytes. The markers of melanocytic differentiation include S100, MART1/Melan-A, HMB45, tyrosinase, MITF and SOX10. The sensitivity of S100 in melanomas is very high, which makes it a screening index, but the specificity of S100 is not high. MART1/Melan-A, HMB45 and tyrosinase have high specificity. MITF and SOX10 are useful markers for the distinction of pigmented actinic keratosis from melanoma *in situ*. Prognostic markers of melanoma include Ki67 and phosphohistone H3 (PHH3). In melanomas, the Ki67 proliferation index ranges from 5%-50%, with mitotic figures distributed throughout the lesion.

（4）Molecular diagnosis: The main molecular diagnosis test performed involves the BRAF V600 mutational status, to identify patients eligible for treatment with BRAF inhibitors and MEK inhibitors. NRAS mutations, NF1 mutations and CKIT mutations have also been identified in a proportion of cases. Cellular and molecular methods that have been applied to the diagnosis of melanoma include comparative genomic hybridization (CGH), fluorescence *in situ* hybridization (FISH), imaging mass spectrometry (IMS), quantitative real-time polymerase chain reaction (qRT-PCR), multiplex ligation-dependent probe amplification (MLPA).

（5）Imaging diagnosis: Ultrasonography of the regional lymph-node and radiographic imaging using CT or MRI should be done to exclude metastatic spread.

（6）Other imaging techniques: Other imaging techniques are available to assist the physicians in the differentiation of melanoma and its precursors from benign lesions, which include *in vivo* reflectance confocal microscopy, computer-aided multispectral digital analysis, electrical impedance spectroscopy (EIS), photoacoustic imaging (PAI), and optical coherence tomography.

2.3.2.2 Current treatment

Melanoma is a highly malignant tumor derived from melanocytes, which characterized by high invasiveness, early metastasis, and strong resistance to conventional radiotherapy, chemotherapy and immunotherapy. Now the current status and prospects of melanoma treatment are summarized.

1. Traditional treatment

（1）Surgical treatment: After the diagnosis of melanoma, the primary lesion should be completely removed by surgery as soon as possible. The scope of surgical resection is determined in principle according to the Breslow thickness of the tumor, and should include subcutaneous tissue and reach the fascia. And for patients with melanoma, it is recommended to perform preventive lymph node dissection and sentinel lymph node biopsy. However, surgical treatment can only be effective for some early melanoma patients. Nearly 60% of melanoma patients still die of recurrence and metastasis. Therefore, for melanoma patients without metastasis but with a high risk of recurrence, systemic immunotherapy is needed after surgical resection, which can effectively suppress the formation of clinically undetectable microscopic lesions and metastases.

(2) Chemotherapy and radiotherapy: Chemotherapy is the first choice for metastatic melanoma. In 2011, the US FDA approved dacarbazine, which is still the most effective drug, as the chemotherapy drug for metastatic melanoma. However, the efficiency of dacarbazine is only 20%. Although radiotherapy can relieve the obstruction symptoms and inhibit distant metastases of melanoma, it cannot prolong the survival time of patients. Moreover, melanoma cells are resistant to radiotherapy, which may be due to DNA damage have been repeatedly happened to melanoma cells, and therefore have effective DNA repair capabilities.

(3) Cytokines: ① Interferon: Many clinical trials have proved that the melanoma patients combined with high-dose interferon after early excision can effectively reduce the recurrence rate and prolong the survival period. However, this therapy is expensive and has serious side effects. ②Recombinant interleukin-2 (IL-2): IL-2 is an inflammatory cytokine and is the first immunotherapeutic agent approved by the US FDA for the treatment of metastatic melanoma. In eight phase Ⅱ clinical trials, a total of 270 patients, approximately 15% of the patients experienced overall remission after high-dose IL-2 administration, and approximately 4%-6% of the patients experienced long-term complete remission. However, high-dose IL-2 treatment can cause serious adverse effects such as hemodynamic shock and respiratory failure.

(4) Tumor vaccines: Most tumor-associated antigens used in tumor vaccine research can be classified as follows: ① autoantigens, molecules distributed in tumor tissues and overexpressed tumor antigens; ② cancer testis antigens, tumor-associated antigens with restricted expression in the testis and placenta. Vaccination can induce the immune system to reject tumors, but the overall response rate is 4%-5% for melanoma.

2. Systemic immunotherapy

(1) Adoptive cell therapy: The reinfusion therapy of tumor-infiltrating lymphocytes. Tumor-infiltrating lymphocytes of melanoma patients are isolated and modified *in vitro* (such as adding some antigen and cytokines to stimulate), thereafter screening and expanding the active immune effector cells that can kill cancer cells, and then reinfuse them back to the patients. This method is effective for some patients with advanced melanoma, and complete responders rarely relapse, even complete clinical remission can be reached. However, only 40%-50% of the patients with surgery can obtain tumor-infiltrating lymphocytes. Moreover, the method has strong personalization and a long preparation period, thus clinical application

is still a challenge. Another method is to use engineered peripheral blood lymphocytes with chimeric antigen receptors (CARs). CARs are T cell receptors, costimulatory molecules or single-chain antibodies that bind to tumor-associated antigens with high TCR affinity. CARs' recognition of tumor-associated antigens is not restricted by HLA, and the clinical response rate is high in hematopoietic malignant tumors and solid tumors. However, due to the presence of cross-reactions, this treatment method has serious toxic effects in important normal tissues.

(2) Molecular targeted therapy: In recent years, with the improvement insight on the pathogenesis of melanoma, it has been found that the formation of melanoma is related to the abnormal activation of some signaling pathways. For example, 40%-60% of melanomas have BRAF gene mutation, which subsequently causes the mitogen-activated protein kinase (MAPK) pathway to constitutively activate the downstream signals. Therefore, the emergence of a series of new drugs targeting signaling pathways, such as vemurafenib and dabrafenib, has opened new insights for targeted therapy of melanoma. BRAF and MEK inhibitors entered the 2019 edition of the US NCCN guidelines for the diagnosis and treatment of melanoma. The BRAF and NRAS genes mutation rates among Chinese melanoma patients are low, and the main gene profiles are to be studied. For patients with metastatic melanoma who cannot tolerate immunotherapy, targeted therapy with BRAF/MEK is preferred. This method has a high initial response rate and improved survival. The limitations are the short average length of the response period and the high recurrence rate.

(3) Immune checkpoint inhibitors: Immune checkpoints are the molecules involved in maintaining immune homeostasis, which help maintain the tolerance of the periphery to own molecules, and can suppress or enhance immune responses. The well-known inhibitory immune checkpoints are CTLA-4 and PD-1, which have made important breakthroughs in clinical practice. The US FDA has approved melanoma immunotherapy drugs in recent years including ipilimumab (anti-CTLA-4) in 2011, pembrolizumab (anti-PD-1) in 2014, and nivolumab (anti-PD-1) in 2016. Immunotherapy has greatly improved that raised the survival rate of melanoma patients and brought hope to the clinical treatment of melanoma. Pembrolizumab has become the standard first-line treatment for advanced melanoma, as it can block disease progression for a long time and improve overall survival, and 85% of the patients still do not progress 2 years after drug withdrawal. Immunotherapy has fundamentally changed the past dilemma of melanoma, making patients see the hope of "healing". In Europe and the United States, skin melanoma is more likely to be found, whereas the proportion of extremity and mucosal melanoma in China exceeds 50%. It has been proved that pembrolizumab has equal effect for extremities and mucosal melanoma. For current metastatic melanoma, anti-PD-1$^{+/-}$ CTLA-4 treatment improves overall survival, response rate, and durability of response and is the first-line treatment. The advantages of immune checkpoint blockade (ICB) treatment include significant improvement in overall survival and long-lasting response. The limitation is that only some patients respond to ICB

and immune-related side effects cannot be ignored.

(4) New immunotherapy strategies (nano, microneedles, etc.): Conventional therapies (e. g. , dacarbazine, interferon, and interleukin-2) are limited by low response rates and will not improve overall survival. New targeted therapies (e. g. , vemurafenib, dabrafenib, and trametinib) have a high initial response rate and significantly improve overall survival, but usually relapse within 6-9 months. Although immunotherapy (e. g. , ipilimumab, pembrolizumab, and nivolumab) can obtain long-term and long-lasting responses, it is only effective for some patients, and the incidence of adverse events is very high. For all this, in the past decade, with the advent of molecular targeted therapy and immunotherapy, there has been unprecedented clinical progress in the field of melanoma therapy. However, the clinical treatment of melanoma still faces huge challenges. With the rapid development of nanotechnology for cancer treatment, nanotherapy provides important prospects for overcoming these shortcomings. The antitumor applications of nanomedicine are diverse, including nanomedicine directly killing tumor cells, or as a carrier of chemotherapy and gene therapy. There are also applications of photothermal therapy (PTT) and photodynamic therapy (PDT) based on nanomaterials. In addition, nanomedicines can passively or actively deliver effect structures to tumor sites, thereby increasing treatment specificity and reducing side effects. Several nanomedicines have been approved by the US FDA for clinical treatment, and other nanomedicines currently in preclinical or clinical trials have shown potential for tumor therapy. We expect that the application of nanocarriers will change the landscape of melanoma treatment in the future (see extended reading 1).

(5) Combination therapy: Compared with the use of any one therapy alone, the combination of anti-CTLA-4 and anti-PD1 antibodies has a better antitumor response. Combination therapy is associated with progression-free survival (PFS) and overall survival. In addition, advanced melanoma is one of the few cancers that often metastasize to the brain, and combined immunotherapy can reduce melanoma brain metastases. There are several new immune checkpoint inhibitors are currently undergoing preclinical and clinical stages, including LAG-3, TIM3, IDO, FOXP3, CSF1R inhibitors, etc. They can be used for melanoma patients who associated with changes in PD-L1 levels and show poor response to ICB single medication. They can also be used in combination with different checkpoint inhibitors. Oncolytic virus combined with ICB can promote T cell infiltration in the tumor and improve the response rate of immunotherapy. Anti-PD-(L)1 combined with BRAF/MEK targeted therapy has shown improved response rates in early clinical trials, but the incidence of adverse effects has increased. PD-1 or BRAFi/MEKi is the current first-line option for adjuvant therapy after melanoma resection. Anti-CTLA-4 monoclonal antibody and anti-PD-1 monoclonal antibody are approved for adjuvant treatment of stage Ⅲ and low metastatic stage Ⅳ resectable melanoma. BRAFi/MEKi (dabrafenib and trametinib) is approved for the adjuvant therapy of stage Ⅲ melanoma.

2.3.3 Non-melanoma skin cancers

2.3.3.1 Introduction

1. Basal cell carcinoma

Basal cell carcinoma (BCC) is one of the common skin cancers, with low malignancy, and its metastasis is extremely rare. It occurs more commonly in the people above middle age with fair skin.

(1) Etiology and pathogenesis: The incidence of BCC increases with increasing sun exposure and age. In addition, a fair complexion, a positive family history of BCC, chronic arseniasis, radiation and immunosuppression are risk factors of BCC.

(2) Clinical features and classfication.

①Nodular BCC: As the most common subtype, nodular BCC also known as classic BCC, accounts for 50%-80% of all BCCs. It favors the head and neck. The lesion typically presents as nodule. As the lesion becomes larger, ulcer and bleeding can occur on the tumor.

②Superficial BCC: Superficial BCC is the second most common subtype of BCC, accounting for approximately 10%-30% of tumors. The average age of onset is younger than other subtypes. Superficial BCC always presents as single or multiple erythematous plaque with superficial flat growth, which have clear thin rolled borders and scale on it. This type of BCC is most commonly found on the trunk and distal extremities, whereas head and neck are less common to be found.

③Pigmented BCC: This subtype is similar to nodular BCC, but in addition, the lesion contains melanin.

④Fibroepithelial BCC: It is also known as fibroepitheliomas of Pinkus. This uncommon subtype has a predilection for the trunk, which presents as an elevated, skin-colored or erythematous sessile plaque.

⑤Infundibulocystic BCC: This subtype of BCC presents as well-circumscribed pearly papules, which is commonly found on the head and neck of the elderly.

⑥Morpheaform BCC: It clinically presents as white sclerotic plaque with smooth surface and poorly defined borders. It resembles the plaque of morphea, and telangiectasia is present.

(3) Diagnosis and differential diagnosis: According to the clinical presentation and histopathological features, BCC is easy to be diagnosed. It is frequently mistaken for BCC in squamous cell carcinoma, hypertrophic actin keratosis, keratoacanthoma, Bowen's disease, Paget's disease, and seborrheic keratosis.

2. Squamous cell carcinoma

Squamous cell carcinoma (SCC) is the second most common form of skin cancer after basal cell carcinoma. It is a malignant tumor of keratinocytes originating within the epidermis or its appendages, which commonly occurs on the areas that have had sun exposure, especially the head and neck. SCC favors the people aged 60 years or over.

（1）Etiology and pathogenesis：Long-term sun exposure is the major risk factor of SCC，UV damages DNA，which induces gene mutations in keratinocytes and subsequently malignant change happens. Radiation and chemical carcinogens such as 3,4-benzpyrene and arsenic can promote the development of SCC. Long-term HPV infection，primarily HPV 16，18，31，and 35，play a role in SCC that develops on genitalia. Chronic non-healing ulcers，lesions of discoid LE can develop into SCC. In addition，immunosuppression (e. g. ，organ transplantation) enhances the risk of SCC.

（2）Clinical features：SCC commonly occurs on sun exposed sites，mostly the head and neck，and non-sun-exposed areas are less favored. It is more likely to be found in people over 60 years. The typical appearances present as a non-healing，usually rapidly growing，and skin colored nodule with indurated base and sometimes with adherent surface，crust or central ulceration. Lesions are painful and bleed on contact.

（3）Diagnosis and differential diagnosis：Diagnosis biopsy should be performed when lesions with indurated base and central ulceration that grow rapidly and bleed on contact occur on the head and neck. Skin biopsy is the main evidence to diagnose SCC. In the early stages，it is difficult to distinguish SCC from hypertrophic actin keratosis. In addition，SCC also may be confused with basal cell carcinoma，keratoacanthoma，and sporotrichosis.

2.3.3.2 Treatment

The treatment plan of non-melanoma skin cancer should be selected based on factors such as age，tumor stage and location，risk of recurrence，patient expectations，and potential adverse effects. The treatment of non-melanoma skin cancer can be divided into surgical treatment and non-surgical treatment. Surgical treatment includes standard excision，Mohs micrographic surgery，electrodesiccation and curettage. Non-surgical treatments include radiotherapy，cryotherapy，topical therapy，systemic therapy，and photodynamic therapy. Among them，surgery is cornerstone of non-melanoma skin cancer treatment. Table 2-3 shows the cancer risk assessment.

Table 2-3　Differentiating low-risk and high-risk basal and squamous cell
carcinomas based on guidelines from the NCCN*

Characteristics	Low-risk	High-risk
Location		
Trunk and extremities	Any lesion<20 mm	Any lesion≥20 mm
Scalp, forehead, cheeks, neck, pretibias	Any lesion<10 mm	Any lesion≥10 mm
Mask area† of face, genitalia, hands, feet	N/A	Any sized lesion
Borders	Well-defined	Poorly defined
Primary vs. recurrent	Primary	Recurrent
Immunosuppression	No	Yes

Continued

Characteristics	Low-risk	High-risk
Site of prior radiation therapy	No	Yes
Perineural involvement/neurologic symptoms	No	Yes
Aggressive histologic subtypes‡	No	Yes
Unique to squamous cell carcinoma	No	Yes
Chronic inflammatory process	No	Yes
Rapidly growing tumors	No	Yes
Poorly differentiated	No	Yes
Depth≥2 mm	No	Yes
Clark level Ⅳ or Ⅴ	No	Yes
Lymphovascular invasion	No	Yes

* National Comprehensive Cancer Network. National clinical practice guidelines in oncology: squamous cell skin cancer (version Ⅰ. 2017).

†Mask area of face refers to central face, eyelids, eyebrows, periorbital, nose, lips, chin, mandible, ears, preauricular/postauricular, and temple.

‡Aggressive histologic subtypes for basal cell carcinoma include morpheaform, basosquamous, sclerosing, mixed infiltrative, and micronodular. Aggressive histologic subtypes for squamous cell carcinoma include adenoid (acantholytic), adenosquamous, desmoplastic (showing mucin production), and metaplastic (carcinosarcomatous).

1. Low-risk tumors

(1) Surgical treatment: Standard excision is preferred for low-risk tumors, with postoperative margin assessment (4 mm for basal cell carcinomas and 4-6 mm for squamous cell carcinomas). If there is a positive margin, the resection should be expanded according to the situation and supplemented with radiotherapy.

Electrodesiccation and curettage can also be used to treat low-risk tumors. Using mechanical debridement and electrocoagulation to completely disintegrate and remove visible tumors, the advantage is that the surgical procedure is fast and costeffective. However, the effects of electrodesiccation and curettage highly depend on operator and location. For example, tumors in the hair-bearing area (scalp, pubic, axilla, and beard area) may invade the hair follicle. The electrodesiccation may result in incomplete removal of the tumor and cause tumor recurrence. In addition, electrodesiccation and curettage have great trauma to the skin, leaving obvious scars. Therefore, tumors located in cosmetically sensitive areas are not suitable for electrodesiccation and curettage.

(2) Non-surgical treatment: If surgical treatment cannot be performed according to the patients' condition, non-surgical treatment can be selected, including radiotherapy, topical therapy, photodynamic therapy, cryotherapy, etc.

Radiotherapy is a commonly used non-surgical therapy, which can be used to treat high-

and low-risk tumors when surgery can't be performed, and can be used as adjuvant therapy to surgical treatment. However, due to the long-term chronic toxic side effects of radiotherapy, radiotherapy is generally recommended for elderly patients ($>$60 years old).

Topical therapy is currently the most commonly used non-surgical therapy. 5-fluorouracil and imiquimod are used topically in tumor lesions. These two drugs can promote the apoptosis of tumor cells by inhibiting DNA synthesis and activating cell-mediated immune response. Topical therapy has significant effect on superficial low-risk primary tumors, and is particularly suitable for patients with multiple skin lesions throughout the body. In addition, topical therapy has less damage to the skin than surgical treatment, and retains the aesthetic function of the skin to the greatest extent. However, the drawbacks to topical therapy are that they require long and multiple treatments, so the compliance requirements of patients are very high.

Photodynamic therapy is also one of the commonly used non-surgical therapies, and it has a significant effect on superficial low-risk primary tumors. Photodynamic therapy often causes patient intolerance due to pain, chronic open wounds, and pigmentation.

Cryotherapy refers to the use of repetitive freeze-thaw cycles to locally destroy malignant skin cells under liquid nitrogen at -50 ℃. It can also effectively treat superficial low-risk primary tumors. The cryotherapy process is fast, costeffective and does not require local anesthesia. However, cryotherapy can cause localized persistent edema, neuralgia, scarring and pigmentation, so the use of cryotherapy is not as extensive as the above two therapies.

2. High-risk tumors

For high-risk non-melanoma skin cancers, the gold standard of treatment is Mohs micrographic surgery. Studies have shown that Mohs micrographic surgery has a very high cure rate and low mortality, and can preserve the integrity of the tissue to the greatest extent. If Mohs micrographic surgery cannot be performed, standard excision can also be considered, but the margin assessment should be expanded to 10 mm. For patients who cannot perform surgery, the aforementioned non-surgical treatment options can be considered, but the risk of poor efficacy and tumor recurrence needs to be accepted.

3. Recurrence, metastatic and advanced tumors

Tumors with local recurrence without evidence of distant metastasis should be treated as high-risk tumors. For locally and distantly metastasized tumors, treatment plans should be jointly developed through multidisciplinary collaboration. On the basis of surgical treatment as much as possible, a variety of adjuvant therapy are carried out. Adjuvant therapy options include radiotherapy, chemotherapy and Hedgehog pathway inhibitors. For patients with advanced tumors that cannot be operated, full consideration should be given to the patient's own situation, with the purpose of maximizing symptom relief and ensuring quality of life, and selecting appropriate systemic treatment options for patients, such as radiotherapy, chemotherapy, and Hedgehog pathway inhibitors.

2. 4　Challenges and Perspectives

The incidence of skin wound is high. Improper and delay treatment could cause the wound bleeding, infection, refractory healing and pathological scar formation, affecting the patients' quality of life. At present, the pathogeneses of skin wound and its complications have not been fully elucidated, and need to be further explored. With the development of polymer materials, intelligent-response hydrogel, antibacterial hydrogel and microneedles have achieved satisfactory therapeutic effects in the experimental animal model of skin wound.

Polymer materials can be used alone, or be combined with conventional therapy in treating skin wound. Antimicrobial hydrogel, a new type of skin wound dressings, has antibacterial property and can keep wound moisture, which could shorten inflammation phase of wound healing process. With the further research of antibacterial materials, the kinds of antibacterial hydrogel will enlarge. Moreover, the molecular mechanism of antibacterial hydrogel in promoting skin wound healing and the selection of antibacterial hydrogel in different stages of skin wound healing need to be further improved in the future. Available microneedle technology in clinical practice include roller microneedle and radio-frequency microneedle, which can be used alone or in combination with radiotherapy, laser and external drugs. The advantages of microneedle in treating skin scar are hypodynia, convenient, safe and efficient. Studies on the mechanism of microneedles in treating skin scars need to be strengthened.

In more severe forms of psoriasis, a combination of treatment modalities may be employed. In treating patients with methotrexate (MTX), for example, concomitant topical agents may be used to minimize the dose. Methotrexate has been combined with infliximab to reduce the incidence of neutralizing antibodies, and has been used with acitretin in managing patients with severe and generalized pustular psoriasis. Combination systemic therapy has the potential to reduce overall toxicity if the toxicities of each agent are different. However, new regimens should be used with caution because the potential for cumulative toxicity or drug interaction exists. With the development of scientific progress, the transdermal drug delivery technology is becoming more and more perfect, using a micrometer-sized needle-like structure to penetrate the epidermis painlessly, and form a reversible skin microchannel to convert methotrexate. Drugs such as MTX, acitretin, or biological agents are successfully delivered to the lesions through the stratum corneum, and then delivered on time according to different stimulus response functions, which reduces the gastrointestinal discomfort (nausea, vomiting, diarrhea, abdominal pain, etc.), stomatitis, bone marrow suppression, liver and kidney toxicity and other adverse reactions caused by traditional administration, but also reduces the pain and bleeding caused by the syringe. Therefore, changing the traditional drug delivery route will provide patients with a safer and easier treatment experience in the future.

In the past decade, due to the development of immunotherapy and targeted therapy, the clinical efficacy of melanoma has been improved significantly, but not all patients can benefit from the existing treatment methods, and further optimization requires an in-depth understanding of tumor immunobiology mechanisms. Therefore, extensive pre-clinical, translational, and clinical studies are needed to better understand the response to current therapies and drug resistance mechanisms, develop rational next-generation therapies and combination therapies, and establish more complex and effective melanoma models to support further pre-clinical and clinical translation studies. Currently, surgical treatment is the gold standard for non-melanoma skin cancers. However, surgical treatment has great limitations, not all patients can undergo surgery, and surgical treatment has problems such as great trauma, affecting tissue function and aesthetics. The commonly used non-surgical treatment such as topical therapy and photodynamic therapy, although the trauma is small, but there are problems of poor drug penetration and narrow treatment range, which can only effectively treat primary and superficial tumors. The combination of biochemical technology and traditional treatment may bring new directions for the treatment of skin tumors, such as the use of microneedle and transdermal drug delivery technology to promote the penetration of local drugs and photosensitizers and improve the efficacy of topical therapy and photodynamic therapy; design nano-targeted drugs to precisely target cancer tissues, so as to reduce the side effects of systemic treatment.

Questions

1. What are the preferred treatment methods for androgen alopecia currently?

2. What are the shortcomings of traditional systematic treatment for psoriasis?

3. What types of biological agents are recommended at present? What is the target of action?

4. What are the difficulties in the treatment for psoriasis?

5. What are the limitations in traditional treatment for skin tumors such as melanoma? How to fix them by application of polymer materials?

Extended Reading

[1] Griffiths C,Barker J,Bleiker T,et al. Rook's textbook of dermatology[M]. 9th ed. New Jersey:Wiley-Blackwell,2016.

[2] Wolff K,Johnson R A. Fitzpatrick's color atlas and synopsis of clinical dermatology [M]. 6th ed. New York: McGraw-Hill,2009.

[3] Yamada M,Prow T W. Physical drug delivery enhancement for aged skin,UV damaged skin and skin cancer:translation and commercialization[J]. Adv Drug Deliv Rev,2020, 153:2-17.

［4］ William J, Dirk E, James T, et al. Andrews' diseases of the skin［M］. 13th ed. Amsterdam：Elsevier,2019.

［5］ Baltzis D, Eleftheriadou I, Veves A. Pathogenesis and treatment of impaired wound healing in diabetes mellitus：new insights ［J］. Adv Ther,2014,31(8):817-836.

（Yang Liu　An Xiangjie　Suo Huinan　Yang Jing　Dong Liyun）

第三章
生物医用高分子简介

第一节　生物医用高分子简史

　　生物医用高分子是指基于高分子化合物在临床医学、医疗等领域的实际应用需求,有针对性地设计开发的,在生物及医学等领域使用的高分子功能材料及其制品,是生命科学、材料科学、医学与高分子化学等多学科交叉的研究领域(见扩展阅读1和2)。生物医用高分子材料泛指应用于诊断、治疗和器官修复与再生等生物医学领域的高分子材料,致力于满足生物医用领域的产业需求,服务于人们对健康美好生活的更高追求。生物医用高分子材料在生物材料中占有不可替代的重要地位,其应用有助于改善人体健康、延长患者生存期、提高人类生活品质。

一、生物医用高分子的发展历程

　　经过约一个世纪的发展,生物医用高分子材料及其相关器件已成为现代医学多种诊疗技术领域的重要辅助工具和功能材料,在现代医学中占有不可替代的重要地位,并不断推动各种诊疗技术的推陈出新和持续发展。生物医用高分子材料的组成基础是高分子化合物。因此,为了阐述生物医用高分子的发展历程,下面首先对高分子科学的相关基础知识进行简单介绍。

　　高分子科学及人工合成高分子技术是20世纪20—30年代开始萌芽的。发展至今,高分子材料已成为人类日常生活和工业生产必不可少的一部分,高分子材料与金属材料、陶瓷材料并称为现代社会的三大材料。高分子化合物简称为高分子、大分子、聚合物或高聚物,是由许多相同的结构单元,通过共价键重复键合链接而成,分子量达几千甚至几百万,并具有一定力学性能的大分子化合物。组成高分子化合物的每一个重复结构单元称为该高分子化合物的单体,即合成高分子化合物的原料,单体能够通过聚合反应形成一定分子量的化合物。与小分子化合物相比,高分子化合物具有以下显著特点:①分子量大,分子似"长链";②具有一定的长径比;③若分子链上有分支,则可形成星形、超支化、网状等拓扑结构;④分子量具有不均一性,即多分散性;⑤分子间作用力大,所以只有液态和固态,不能汽化;⑥固体高分子化合物具有一定的机械强度,可用作承力材料,能成块、能抽丝、能制膜。其中,应用于人工器官、组织工程、再生医学、理疗康复、体内外诊断、药物缓控释、血液制剂和医疗器械等领域的高分子材料,称为生物医用高分子材料。

早在"高分子科学"概念、"人工合成高分子"技术出现之前,一些天然高分子制品,如棉花纤维、马鬃等已被古代人类应用于伤口缝合;竹片、木板等用于骨折固定。这些天然的高分子制品被公认为最早的生物医用高分子材料。此外,组成动植物体的关键物质,如蛋白质、肌肉、纤维素、淀粉、生物酶和果胶等都是高分子化合物。因此可以说,天然高分子是生命体的基础,生物界是天然高分子的巨大产地。高分子化合物在生物界的普遍存在,决定了它们在医学领域中的特殊地位。在各种材料中,人工合成的高分子材料的分子结构、化学组成及理化性质与生物体组织有重要的相似之处,因此可广泛用作生物医用材料。

现代意义上的生物医用高分子材料是伴随着"高分子科学"概念、"人工合成高分子"技术的提出而诞生的。之后高分子领域发生了多次巨大变革,高分子科学与技术得到迅速发展,新的高分子合成材料不断涌现,为医学领域提供了更多的选择,也使得临床应用的生物医用高分子材料不断推陈出新,见表 3-1。

表 3-1　生物医用高分子的发展与进步

年　代	高分子领域的发明	临床应用
20 世纪 30 年代	聚甲基丙烯酸甲酯(有机玻璃,PMMA)	假牙和补牙
20 世纪 40 年代	赛璐珞(Celluloid)薄膜	血液透析
20 世纪 50 年代	有机硅橡胶(organosilicon rubber)	人工肾脏
20 世纪 50 年代	聚氨酯(polyurethane,PU)	人工心脏
20 世纪 50 年代	膨体聚四氟乙烯(铁氟龙/特氟隆/特氟龙/特富隆/泰氟龙)	人工血管
20 世纪 60 年代	聚甲基丙烯酸羟乙酯(PHEMA)交联水凝胶(水溶胀的柔软透明弹性胶体)	软角膜接触镜、动脉血管、手术修补材料
20 世纪 60 年代	聚羟基乙酸(poly(glycolic acid),PGA,Dexron®)、聚乳酸(poly(lactic acid),PLA)	可吸收缝合线
20 世纪 70 年代	聚乳酸-羟基乙酸(poly(lactic-co-glycolic acid),PLGA)	可吸收缝合线
20 世纪 80 年代	海藻酸钠/钙离子交联水凝胶包埋胰岛素	人工胰腺
20 世纪 80 年代	胶原-糖胺聚糖交联水凝胶用作仿细胞外基质	皮肤再生和修复
20 世纪 90 年代	功能化、智能响应性生物医用高分子	人工透镜、创伤敷料、组织工程、再生医学、药物控释
21 世纪	个性化、精准化、仿生智能化、功能集成化	动态结构可调高分子支架、组织工程和可植入器械/器官、响应性高分子纳米药物精准诊疗体系

二、生物医用高分子的进步与皮肤美容、皮肤疾病的诊疗

生物医用高分子材料发展至今,已成为现代医学领域必不可少的材料,特别是在过去的30 年时间里,其在全球范围内经历了一个高速发展的阶段。生物医用高分子作为学科交叉的

结晶与典范,融合了高分子化学与物理、生物化学、合成材料工艺学、病理学、药理学、解剖学和临床医学等多领域知识,还涉及诸多工程学问题,如各种医疗器械的设计、制造等。上述学科的相互交叉、渗透,促使生物医用高分子材料的品种越来越丰富,性能越来越完善,功能越来越齐全,因此,越来越多的生物医用高分子材料被研究开发并应用于临床医疗和日常防护。生物医用高分子材料是与在什么场合使用及如何使用相关联的,同时不同的应用领域,材料需要有特定的功能。在皮肤美容、皮肤健康、皮肤疾病诊疗及日常防护等领域,生物医用高分子材料已得到广泛应用。

皮肤包在身体表面,是人体最大的器官。成年人皮肤总面积为 $1.5 \sim 2 \ m^2$,占总体重的 $5\% \sim 15\%$。皮肤直接与外界环境接触,本教材第一章"皮肤结构与功能"中已阐述了皮肤在保护人体免受各种理化刺激和病原体的侵害、保护人体深层组织和器官、排泄、调节体温和感受外界刺激等方面的重要作用。而伴随着年龄的增长,人们的皮肤会逐渐松弛、下垂、弹性降低,并出现皱纹。此时,将高分子支撑材料/填充剂注射到真皮层或皮下组织以填充、增加组织容积,有助于在临床上矫正或增加软组织的功能,达到皮肤美容的功效。

理想的面部填充剂需要具有良好的生物相容性、安全性及优异的美容效果。面部填充剂可分为不可吸收和可吸收填充剂两类。不可吸收填充剂是由不可降解高分子材料制备得来,包括聚甲基丙烯酸甲酯(poly(methyl methacrylate),PMMA)、聚丙烯酰胺(polyacrylamide,PAM)、膨体聚四氟乙烯(polytetrafluoroethylene,PTFE)和硅胶(silica gel)等。可吸收填充剂由可降解的生物医用高分子材料制备得到,包括胶原蛋白(collagen)、透明质酸(hyaluronic acid,HA)和左旋聚乳酸(poly(L-lactic acid),PLLA)等。其中膨体聚四氟乙烯是聚四氟乙烯经双向拉伸工艺,形成的"纤维结节",呈多孔状,空隙一般小于 $1 \ \mu m$,细胞易于长入,生物相容性好,是优良的面部填充材料。其用于整形材料时具有自然逼真、安全永久、可塑性强等优点,通常用于隆鼻、软组织修补、面部填充、下颌假体、鼻唇沟填充等。此外,可吸收注射填充剂则是新一代的医用植入物的发展方向,注入体内一定时间后可以自发降解,且降解产物具有良好的生物相容性,可被人体经代谢排出体外。目前除用于皮肤除皱外,可吸收整形用植入物还广泛用于凹陷填充、瘢痕修复、面部塑性等,其主要使用的高分子材料有透明质酸钠凝胶、胶原蛋白植入剂、肉毒素及3D聚乳酸微球材料等。

此外,皮肤还是人体的第一道生理防线,同时还参与机体的各项功能活动,因此机体的异常情况甚至病变也可以通过皮肤反映出来。若皮肤的生理功能受到影响、引起损害,就会引起皮肤疾病。皮肤疾病中常见的致病因素是感染与过敏等,随着年龄增长引起退行性变化,老年性皮肤疾病、皮肤癌等也作为重要的皮肤疾病出现。另外,皮肤完整性的损伤或丧失都可能影响皮肤的功能,进而导致严重的残疾甚至死亡。因此伤口的愈合对人体而言至关重要,是科研及临床医学共同面临的一大挑战。关于皮肤疾病的详细介绍,请参见第二章"皮肤健康与代表性皮肤疾病"。生物医用高分子在皮肤疾病的诊疗中发挥着巨大作用且已获得广泛应用,包括皮肤创伤敷料、药用辅料、复合材料人工皮肤等。

皮肤伤口的修复是整个人类及医学界所共同面临的重要基本问题之一。伤口修复过程复杂,良好的敷料可起到保护伤口、防止感染、促进愈合的作用,近年来皮肤伤口的治疗方法和产品种类日益增多(见扩展阅读3)。传统敷料(如棉纱布等)仅具有简单保护、减少感染的功能,起到覆盖伤口和吸收渗液等有限的保护作用;由生物医用高分子化合物构建的新型合成敷料(如水凝胶、海藻酸盐敷料、泡沫敷料等),对皮肤创面的护理更加有效,能与伤口相互作用。除具有吸收渗液的作用外,还具有允许气体交换、防止外环境微生物侵入、预防伤口感染的功效。敷料不仅创造了一个有助于伤口愈合的环境,还可减轻患者痛苦、减少瘢痕与收缩,同时敷料自身能够加速伤口愈合。随着表皮细胞培养方法的建立与完善,在生物材料与合成材料研究的基础上,活性人工皮肤即组织工程皮肤也逐渐诞生。生物医用高分子敷料及组织工程皮肤凭借着为创面所提供的"湿"性环境、良好的促进愈合功能等显著优点而在临床的应用日益广泛。

天然生物医用高分子材料(如藻酸盐、壳聚糖敷料等)已广泛用于皮肤伤口的修复。从天然海藻中提取的敷料含有藻酸钙成分,敷料中的钙离子与血液中和伤口分泌的钠离子发生离子交换,形成凝胶起到凝血止血、稳定生物膜的功效,保护创面,促进肉芽组织生长。市售的藻酸盐敷料产品有 AlgiSite、Sorbsan 及 Kaltostat 等,适用于中到大量渗液的伤口、轻度出血伤口以及黄色腐肉、坏死组织伤口,但不能用于干的、有焦痂的伤口,且大多数产品不具有自黏性,需要二级辅助敷料加以固定,成本相对较高。许多合成生物医用高分子材料,如维纶、丙纶、聚酰胺(尼龙)、聚氨酯、聚乙烯醇、聚丙烯腈、聚己内酯、聚乳酸、聚氨基酸、聚四氟乙烯、聚硅氧烷弹性体等均可作为敷料使用,其中较重要的有聚氨酯、有机硅等。

聚氨酯制成的膜状敷料如 OpSite 及 Tegaderm 等,有一定的弹性,体现出较好的黏附性能,水蒸气能顺利通透,但水和细菌却不能通透。同时,该类敷料不会干扰创面正常愈合过程,制成的膜透明度高,便于观察;并且具有良好的生物相容性,不会引起免疫反应,可留在创面直至伤口愈合。其缺点是水蒸气通透率虽比正常皮肤高,但低于创面的液体渗出率,易产生膜下积液,诱发感染,因此薄膜型敷料适用于浅表溃疡或擦伤。有时,该类敷料需与其他材料结合使用,如有报道黑素细胞移植治疗白癜风时,在将细胞移植到去表皮的病灶磨削面之后,随即贴附一层硅胶及浸过 F12 培养基(Ham's F12 nutrient medium)的敷料,外面采用 Tegaderm 覆盖。英国 S&N 公司生产的 FlexiGrid 单方向透气膜,其主要成分是聚氨酯和聚丙烯酸,优点是具有"分子阀门"功效,创面中坏死组织分解的腐臭气体等能够顺利渗透到膜外,而膜外的细菌、空气等无法透过该薄膜侵入皮肤创面,使得创面具有良好的通透性。此外,聚醚型聚氨酯由于其膜透水性强,创面渗出液的水分能透过析出,蛋白质等成分在敷料下转变成凝胶,可缓解疼痛。

根据不同状态可将高分子合成敷料分为薄膜型、泡沫型、水凝胶、水胶体及复合型。商品化的多为复合型产品。常见敷料的优缺点以及适用范围如表 3-2 所示。

表 3-2 常见敷料的优缺点以及适用范围

敷料类型	优 点	缺 点	适 用 范 围
透明膜敷料	1. 可渗透气体和水蒸气,细菌和液体不能通过; 2. 提供湿性愈合环境,促进自溶清创; 3. 透明,容易观察伤口; 4. 可作为内敷料或外敷料使用; 5. 有弹性、顺应性好	1. 吸收渗液能力差,可能浸渍周围皮肤; 2. 不能用于感染伤口; 3. 移除时可能撕伤周围脆弱皮肤	1. 伤口免受外来污染; 2. 伤口渗液少或无时; 3. 也常用作二级敷料,如与水凝胶结合用于黑色坏死或黄色腐肉伤口

续表

敷料类型	优 点	缺 点	适用范围
水胶体敷料（主要成分为羧甲基纤维素钠）	1. 提供湿性愈合环境,促进自溶清创; 2. 吸收少量渗液; 3. 防水防菌保湿、促进上皮细胞爬行; 4. 移除时不易损伤肉芽组织; 5. 片状敷料具有自黏性、无须外固定	1. 不能用于感染伤口和骨头、筋腱暴露的伤口; 2. 不能用于深部潜行和渗液过多的伤口; 3. 容易撕伤伤口周围脆弱的皮肤,容易卷边	1. 部分皮层损伤的伤口; 2. 少量渗液的伤口; 3. 黄色腐肉和黑色坏死伤口; 4. 可作为外用敷料使用
水凝胶敷料	1. 保持伤口湿润,提供湿性愈合环境,促进自溶清创; 2. 无黏性、容易清除; 3. 可填充窦道及腔隙,保护外露骨膜、肌腱等; 4. 具有柔和性,可减轻疼痛	1. 容易造成伤口浸渍; 2. 不能涂抹在正常皮肤上; 3. 需要二级敷料固定; 4. 不主张用于渗液多的伤口和感染伤口	1. 真皮层和全皮层损伤伤口; 2. 黄色腐肉或黑色坏死伤口; 3. 烧伤和电疗的伤口
藻酸盐敷料	1. 提供湿性愈合环境,促进自溶清创; 2. 钙钠离子交换,可止血; 3. 形成凝胶,保护创面; 4. 促进肉芽组织生长,可无创性去除; 5. 吸收渗液量是自身重量的17～20倍	1. 不能用于干的、有焦痂的伤口; 2. 需要二级敷料固定	1. 中到大量渗液的伤口; 2. 轻度出血伤口; 3. 黄色腐肉、坏死组织伤口
泡沫敷料	1. 气体和水蒸气可自由通过; 2. 提供湿性愈合环境; 3. 保护创面,减轻疼痛; 4. 促进肉芽组织生长; 5. 溶解坏死组织; 6. 吸收大量渗液,防止肉芽组织水肿,不浸渍周围皮肤; 7. 使过长的肉芽变平; 8. 柔软,可在压力下使用	1. 不能用于干的、有焦痂的伤口; 2. 是无黏胶的敷料,需二级敷料固定; 3. 不透明,不方便观察伤口; 4. 顺应性相对较差	1. 用于腔洞伤口时可配合使用清创胶、藻酸盐敷料; 2. 用于静脉溃疡的伤口时,最好外加弹力绷带

续表

敷料类型	优　点	缺　点	适用范围
硅酮敷料	1. 更换时无创,保护伤口及周围的皮肤; 2. 专利技术实现垂直吸收,有效避免浸渍; 3. 提供更适宜的湿性愈合环境; 4. 快速上皮化; 5. 贴敷柔顺,能很好地贴合皮肤; 6. 有自黏性,可以随意裁剪; 7. 可反复粘贴	1. 不能用于感染伤口; 2. 不适用干的、有焦痂的伤口; 3. 如果无渗出液将导致干燥	1. 撕脱伤口; 2. 周围皮肤易损的伤口; 3. 压疮的预防
硅胶泡沫	1. 3D 树枝状发泡结构,超级吸水; 2. 柔软纤薄,顺应性好,自粘自固,可反复粘贴	1. 皮肤破损处,开放性伤口禁用; 2. 外壳未拆线伤口禁用; 3. 有皮炎、湿疹时停用,或症状缓解后再用	1. 多种渗出性伤口; 2. 周围皮肤脆弱的伤口及老年人和儿童的伤口; 3. 薄型可应用于需要更多活动的患者和关节部位的伤口
高渗盐敷料(美盐,组成成分为聚酯纤维和28%的NaCl)	1. 吸收大量渗液和坏死组织,具有清创作用; 2. 减轻水肿,促进伤口愈合; 3. 操作方便,无异物残留; 4. 可任意裁剪,美盐填充条可填充腔隙; 5. 可提供高渗环境,抑制细菌生长	1. 不能用于干燥伤口; 2. 不能与正常组织接触,不能用在干的、有焦痂的伤口和健康肉芽上; 3. 需要外层敷料	1. 渗液很多的伤口; 2. 水肿的肉芽; 3. 黄色腐肉的清创; 4. 已化脓或有恶臭的感染伤口
亲水性纤维素敷料(主要成分为羧甲基纤维素钠)	1. 具有强效渗液管理能力,强吸收、强锁定、防浸渍; 2. 独特的柔软性和顺应性; 3. 不粘连创面、无痛	1. 不能用于干的伤口; 2. 需要外固定敷料	多种渗出性伤口

瘢痕(scar)是各种创伤(包括皮肤的切割伤、烧伤,皮肤感染,外科手术等)所引起的正常皮肤组织的外观形态和组织病理学改变的统称。瘢痕是人体创伤修复过程中必然的产物。瘢痕生长超过一定的限度就会引发各种并发症,诸如外形的破坏及功能活动障碍等,给患者带来巨大的生理和心理痛苦,尤其是烧伤、烫伤等严重外伤后遗留的瘢痕。常用的治疗瘢痕的高分子材料有交联的多聚二甲基硅氧烷(俗称硅酮),它可以形成具有与人体皮肤一样的柔软性和伸展性的覆盖层。用于瘢痕治疗的硅酮通常有油膏、贴膜及凝胶三种形态,能预防新瘢痕形

成,对已有的肥厚性瘢痕减轻其症状体征,如红斑、硬化、增大、瘙痒等。单独使用聚氨酯贴膜或结合加压疗法也可减轻瘢痕的颜色、硬度、厚度等,使用方法与硅酮制品类似,每天贴附 12~24 h,连续 2~4 个月,其优点在于透明的外观,适用于头面部及手等暴露部位,且不易发生浸渍。

交联的多聚二甲基硅氧烷薄膜还能很好地帮助皮肤保湿,可用于护肤品或化妆品,也可应用于医用皮肤。美国麻省理工学院 Robert Langer 联合麻省总医院、Living Proof 和 Olivo Laboratories 两家公司共同研发出名为"第二层皮肤"的弹性薄膜材料,该材料是一种以多聚二甲基硅氧烷作为基底的交联聚合物,构建的薄膜具有良好的透气性,贴在皮肤上"没有感觉",且目前尚未发现对人体的副作用。最重要的是,该薄膜能有效地恢复皮肤原有的力学性能,能有效地消除使用者面部的眼袋,同时具有一定的补水性。若该类产品成功上市,未来有望直接用于医治患者的皮肤(如治疗湿疹等皮肤疾病)或添加防晒成分后,长期防止紫外线照射带来的皮肤伤害等方面。

皮肤封包疗法是指采用无渗透作用的薄膜(如保鲜膜、塑料袋、绷带、手套、医用敷料等)对涂敷药物的患处表面进行封闭式包裹,从而达到治疗目的的一种疗法。局部外用糖皮质激素封包是治疗慢性炎症性皮肤疾病,如慢性肥厚性皮炎、角化增生性皮肤疾病、疣状增生性皮肤疾病等的传统方法。封包材料从最初的聚乙烯塑料发展到现在的水胶体贴膜,糖皮质激素可与封包材料一起制成复合制剂,也可以分开先后使用。局部外用糖皮质激素加水胶体贴膜 DuoDerm 进行封包治疗对银屑病有很好的治疗效果,该方法也用于特应性皮炎的难治性皮损及其他一些慢性炎症性皮肤疾病的治疗。此外,水胶体贴膜 Actiderm 加中效激素外用治疗掌跖脓疱病,效果远优于单纯用强效激素;水胶体贴膜 3M AcneDressing 可以通过减少手接触及紫外线照射明显改善痤疮患者的病情。这些方法都利用了水胶体外用材料的强黏附性及封闭性,既能促进药物吸收,又能减少患者搔抓。搔抓会促进局部皮肤炎症慢性化,故减少搔抓具有治疗作用。

三、生物医用高分子在皮肤美容、皮肤疾病诊疗中的应用

高分子材料是现代社会的三大材料之一,是人类生产和生活必不可少的物质基础。伴随着高分子科学与技术的诞生,几乎同时发展的生物医用高分子及其制品,已经获得广泛的临床应用,医疗工作中的每个环节都可见高分子材料及其制品的身影。近年来,高分子材料在皮肤领域的应用,主要包括皮肤疾病的诊疗、皮肤美容、可穿戴皮肤器件与电子皮肤,及皮肤修复与再生等,通过科研攻关和临床实践,已取得显著成效和较完整的认知。

皮肤疾病是发生在皮肤以及皮肤附属器的多种疾病的总称。皮肤疾病种类繁多,目前可以命名的具有不同临床特点的皮肤疾病达 2000 余种。个体从出生至死亡的各个年龄段皆可患皮肤疾病,全身任何部位均可累及。从医学角度讲,人的一生几乎没有不被皮肤疾病困扰的个体,因此皮肤疾病属于最常见、最多发的疾病。同时,内脏发生的病变在皮肤上也经常有所表现,此外由感染因素引起的皮肤疾病(如麻风,疥疮,皮肤细菌、真菌病等)通常具有传染性,不仅影响身体健康,还会导致社会歧视和心理问题等。皮肤疾病中较常见的是感染性疾病与过敏性皮炎,随着年龄增长引起的退行性变化,老年性皮肤疾病、皮肤癌也成为重要的皮肤疾病。随着人们对健康美好生活的追求,皮肤疾病的诊疗越来越受到人们的重视。皮肤疾病的确诊与鉴别诊断包括体格检查、实验室检查等。同时,为明确生物体组织结构,阐明生物体各

种生理功能,生物成像技术在皮肤疾病的研究及临床诊断中已获得广泛应用,详细内容请参见第五章"皮肤影像学诊断技术"。

皮肤疾病的传统治疗大多使用外用药,存在皮肤吸收率低、多耐药性等不足。近年来的研究表明,使用高分子纳米粒子作为药物载体可实现靶向递送、缓控释给药的目的,并逐渐发展为皮肤疾病治疗的有效途径,详细内容请参见第六章"高分子纳米药物载体及其在皮肤疾病治疗中的应用"。黑素瘤是由皮肤及其他器官黑素细胞产生的肿瘤,其转移发生早、恶性度高、死亡率高,是皮肤疾病治疗中非常重要的内容,详细介绍请参见第七章"生物医用高分子在黑素瘤免疫治疗中的应用"。与传统给药方式相比,新型给药技术如透皮给药是指在皮肤表面给药,使药物以可控速率或程序,穿过皮肤进入体内循环,实现局部或全身治疗的崭新技术。透皮给药技术在皮肤疾病的治疗中具有显著优势:不受消化道内强酸性、饮食、转运时间等因素干扰;可避免肝脏首过效应;避免因药物吸收过快而产生血药浓度过高引起的不良反应;可持续控制给药速度,个性化灵活给药。透皮给药的最新研究进展与临床应用,请参见第八章"透皮给药技术"。

皮肤美容中的生物医用高分子按照填充材料的持续时间分类,有短效性(6～12个月)、半永久性(18～30个月)和永久性(5年以上)3类。重要的皮肤填充基础材料有胶原蛋白、聚乳酸和透明质酸等,如表3-3所示。关于皮肤美容中的生物医用高分子材料,详细内容参见第九章"生物医用高分子在皮肤美容中的应用"。

表 3-3 皮肤美容中的生物医用高分子简介

生物医用高分子	美国 FDA 批准时间	持续时间	代表性产品	优 点	缺 点
胶原蛋白	1981 年	短效性	双美Ⅰ号	生物安全性	有效期短
透明质酸	2003 年	短效性、半永久性	瑞蓝、乔雅登、伊婉、爱芙莱、艾莉薇、海薇	广泛存在于生物体内,是组成细胞外基质的主要成分,安全可靠	注射后皱纹加深、交联剂存在残留
聚乳酸	2009 年	半永久性	Sculptra、AestheFill、Derma Veil	生物安全性高,作用时间长、温和、自然	注射后易形成结节

此外,可穿戴电子皮肤是一种可测量人体健康生理指标,如心率、脉搏、血压、体温、肌肉群振动等的检测技术,其优势在于可对人体健康数据变化做出及时感应和反馈甚至实现疾病的前期预防和诊断,此部分内容请参见第十章"可穿戴电子皮肤器件"。生物体对组织损伤和缺损具有巨大的修补及恢复能力,既包括皮肤组织结构不同程度的修复,也体现为组织机体功能的重建。对皮肤损伤而言,表皮损伤通常可以再生,损伤一旦到达真皮及皮下组织,通常很难完全修复。皮肤修复及再生用的生物医用高分子材料包括传统的创伤敷料及近期发展的人工皮肤。创伤敷料的特点是追求伤口的快速良好修复,而人工皮肤主要致力于皮肤的结构和功能的彻底恢复,即皮肤再生。天然皮肤的结构和功能是很复杂的,因此在皮肤结构和功能的知识基础上,研究并透彻地理解皮肤创伤修复及愈合的机制,对设计构建新型面部填充剂、创伤

敷料和人工皮肤有重要的意义。有关皮肤伤口愈合的生理过程、皮肤伤口修复的并发症及治疗,以及皮肤修复和再生用的生物医用高分子材料,请参见第十一章"生物医用高分子在皮肤伤口修复中的应用"。

第二节 皮肤美容、皮肤疾病诊疗中的生物医用高分子基础知识

一、生物医用高分子的必备条件和特殊性能要求

生物医用高分子用于皮肤美容和皮肤疾病的诊疗时,材料作用于人体内或皮肤表面,必然与人体组织、血液及体液接触;由于人体的自然保护性反应,将产生排斥反应,往往产生极严重的后果,甚至危及患者生命。因此,与通用高分子材料相比,生物医用高分子材料的要求非常严格,同时对其性能有具体的特殊要求。医用高分子材料进入临床使用之前,都必须对材料本身的物理化学性能、机械性能、材料与生物体及人体的相互适应性进行翔实和全面的评价,然后经国家管理部门批准才能进入临床应用。通常,生物医用高分子材料必须具备如下性能。

1. 生物安全性

材料必须无毒或毒副作用极小。生物医用高分子材料与人体组织接触后,会产生一系列复杂的生物、物理及化学反应,并由此产生多种暂时或深远的影响。因此,一方面要求高分子化合物纯度高,生产加工环节环境清洁,各种杂质残留少,确保无病、无菌、无毒传播。另一方面要求高分子材料与体液接触后,无致敏性、无刺激性、无遗传毒性、无三致(致癌、致畸和致突变),体现生物惰性;在体内不发生任何结构和组成的变化、不可降解,或在体内可降解,但不发生不良反应,不产生对人体有害的副产物。可降解生物医用高分子材料最初的应用就是可吸收缝合线,如表 3-1 所述,其中具代表性的有聚羟基乙酸(PGA)、聚乳酸(PLA)和聚乳酸-羟基乙酸(PLGA)。

人体环境对高分子材料主要有以下常见影响:体液可引起高分子的降解、交联和相变化;体内的自由基可引起材料的氧化降解反应;生物酶可引起聚合物的分解反应。此外,在体液作用下,高分子材料中的添加剂可能会溶出,同时血液、体液中的类脂质、类固醇及脂肪等物质渗入高分子材料,使其增塑,导致力学强度下降。但对生物医用高分子材料来说,在某些情况下,人体环境对高分子材料的老化、分解、降解等反应,并不一定都是负面的,有时甚至具有积极的意义。如作为医用手术缝合线时,在发挥了相应的效用后,反倒不希望手术缝合线有太好的化学稳定性和生物惰性,使它们长期停留在体内,而是希望它们尽快地被组织所分解、吸收或迅速排出体外,无须通过二次手术取出。在这种情况下,对生物医用高分子材料的附加要求是在分解过程中,不应产生对人体有害的副产物。

2. 物理、化学和力学性能

材料应满足皮肤美容、皮肤疾病诊疗所需设计和功能的要求。不同于较高强度的牙科、骨科用高分子材料,皮肤美容、伤口修复中使用的高分子材料强度要求不高,但必须具有一定的柔软性,特别是皮肤填充剂,应体现与正常皮肤相似甚至一致的伸缩性和弹性等力学性能,并

且应与皮肤具有一定的粘接性和适应性，才能与皮肤相配合，融为一体。皮肤损伤部位的修复材料是与人体皮肤组织进行物理结合。该类软组织修复材料应具有一定的活性，能促进损伤部位的修复，并在伤口修复后发生降解反应，最终被人体吸收和代谢。

3. 较低的临床应用成本

材料不能过分昂贵，应适用于平民消费，且容易获取及制备，最终实现生物医用高分子材料的广泛应用。

二、生物医用高分子的组成和分类

根据来源不同，生物医用高分子材料可分为天然和人工合成生物医用高分子材料两大类。这两类材料各有优缺点，通常天然高分子的生物相容性好，而合成高分子的机械力学性能好。其中，天然生物医用高分子材料通常是从生物体内提取或自然环境中直接得到的一类大分子材料，主要包括天然多糖类和天然蛋白质类材料，还包括动物或人体自身的脱细胞基质材料，以及来源于微生物发酵的天然高分子材料；合成生物医用高分子材料还可细分为不可降解和可降解生物医用高分子材料。

一些常见天然生物医用高分子的化学结构如图 3-1 所示。天然多糖类材料主要包括淀粉/纤维素/壳聚糖及它们的衍生物、海藻酸盐、透明质酸、肝素和硫酸软骨素等；天然蛋白质类材料主要包括胶原、明胶、丝素蛋白、白蛋白及大豆蛋白等；动物或人体自身的脱细胞基质材料则可来源于小肠、膀胱、皮肤、骨骼、心脏、心脏瓣膜等；来源于微生物发酵的天然高分子材料有聚(3-羟基丁酸酯)、聚(γ-谷氨酸)、聚(ε-赖氨酸)等。天然的生物医用高分子材料来源广泛、容易获取，而且一般都具有良好的生物相容性和生物可降解性，已被广泛应用于药用辅料、可吸收缝合线、医用隔离膜、创伤修复膜、创伤敷料、医用黏合剂、人工皮肤、可降解组织工程支架以及纳米药物载体等。然而，天然生物医用高分子材料也存在一定的缺陷，如蛋白质类和脱细胞基质材料存在潜在的免疫原性、结构复杂、不易化学修饰以及机械性能不佳等缺陷。

人工合成的高分子材料中，不可降解材料是最早应用于生物医学领域的高分子材料。它们的特点是在机体生理环境中能长期稳定存在，不易发生降解、交联反应或物理磨损，并具有优良的机械力学性能；普遍具有与细胞、组织黏附性差，力学性能与周围组织匹配性、适应性差等显著缺点。它们主要应用于各类医疗器械和耗材中，常见的有医疗产品包装材料、体外诊断设备、一次性医疗产品、医用防护用品、介入栓塞材料、血液袋、眼科透镜、人工组织、人工器官等。一些常见的人工合成的不可降解生物医用高分子的化学结构如图 3-2 所示。

相对于不可降解高分子材料，人工合成的可降解高分子材料是新一代医用材料，也是当今科研领域的热点，近年来已被广泛应用于医学领域中，并在临床上取得了成功，是未来发展的重要方向。可降解生物医用高分子材料是指在生理环境中经水解、酶解等反应过程，逐渐降解成低分子量化合物或单体，降解产物能被排出体外或能参加体内正常新陈代谢而消失的一类高分子材料，常见的包括聚乳酸(PLA)、聚羟基乙酸(PGA)、聚乳酸-羟基乙酸(PLGA)、聚碳酸酯(polycarbonate，PC)、聚对二氧环己酮(poly(p-dioxanone)，PPDO)，聚(ε-己内酯)(poly(ε-carprolactone)，PCL)、聚氨基酸(poly(amino acid)，PA)、聚磷酸酯(polyphosphoester，PPE)、聚原酸酯(poly(ortho ester)，POE)、聚酸酐(polyanhydride)、聚磷腈(polyphophazene)等。这些高分子相应的化学结构如图 3-3 所示。

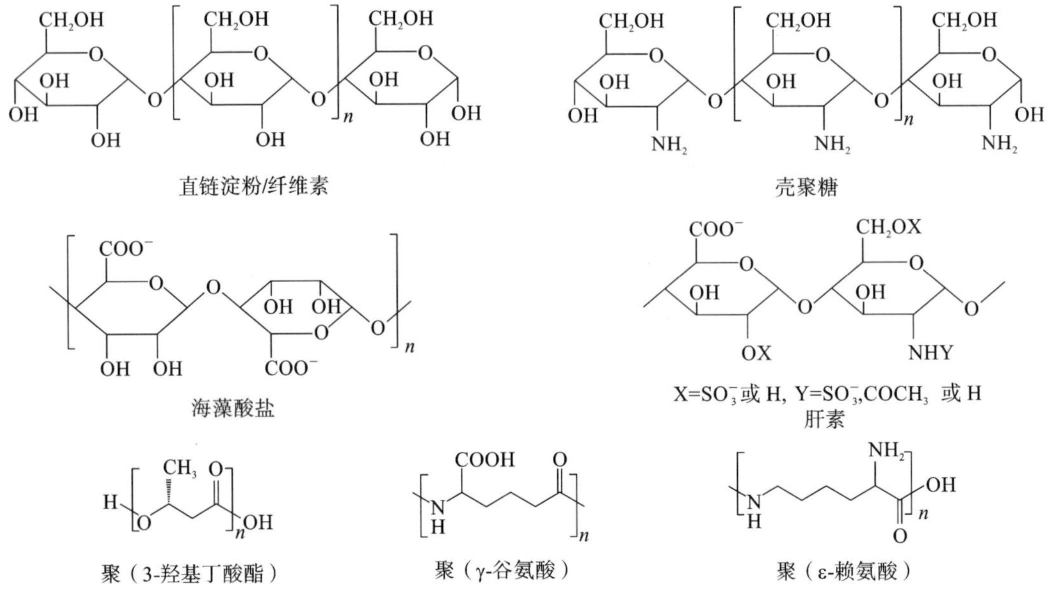

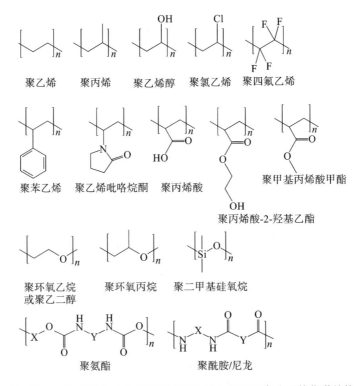

直链淀粉/纤维素

壳聚糖

海藻酸盐

X=SO₃⁻或 H, Y=SO₃⁻,COCH₃ 或 H
肝素

聚（3-羟基丁酸酯）

聚（γ-谷氨酸）

聚（ε-赖氨酸）

图 3-1　一些常见天然生物医用高分子的化学结构

Figure 3-1　Chemical structures of some common natural biomedical polymers

聚乙烯　　聚丙烯　　聚乙烯醇　　聚氯乙烯　　聚四氟乙烯

聚苯乙烯　　聚乙烯吡咯烷酮　　聚丙烯酸

聚甲基丙烯酸甲酯

聚丙烯酸-2-羟基乙酯

聚环氧乙烷
或聚乙二醇　　　聚环氧丙烷　　聚二甲基硅氧烷

聚氨酯　　　聚酰胺/尼龙

图 3-2　一些常见的人工合成的不可降解生物医用高分子的化学结构

Figure 3-2　Chemical structures of some common synthetic non-degradable biomedical polymers

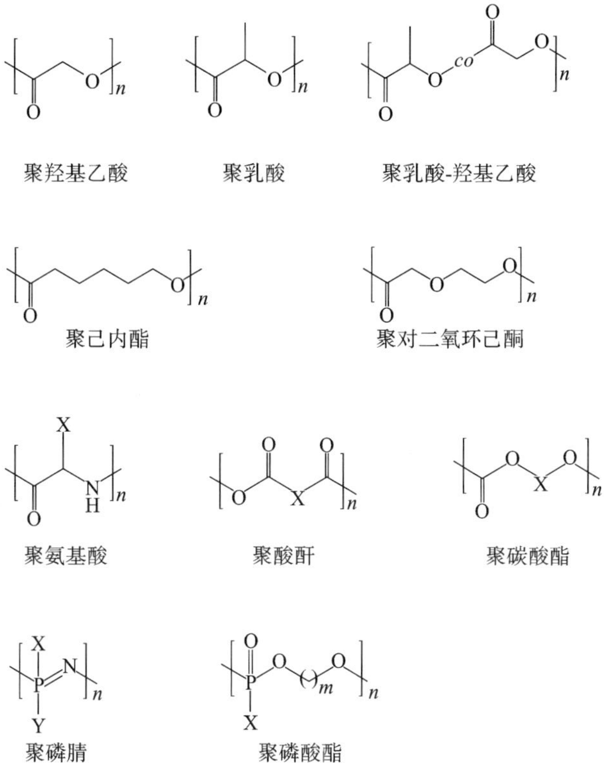

图 3-3 常见人工合成可降解生物医用高分子的化学结构

Figure 3-3 Chemical structures of common synthetic degradable biomedical polymers

此外,生物医用高分子根据结构特征,也可分为软性即橡胶状、半结晶和其他有关生物医用高分子,如表 3-4 所示。

表 3-4 软性、半结晶和其他有关生物医用高分子

高分子分类	聚合物名称	主 要 用 途
软性生物医用高分子	硅橡胶	组织代用品、药物释放器件、黏合剂、管形材料、接触镜等
	聚醚氨酯	血液泵、储血袋、人工心脏、管形材料
	聚氯乙烯	管形材料、储血袋
	橡胶	管形材料
半结晶生物医用高分子	聚酯	脉管接枝物、缝合线、心脏瓣膜缝合环
	聚四氟乙烯	脉管接枝物、血液和氧合器膜
	尼龙 66	缝合线、敷料
	聚乙烯	人工关节、宫内节育器、药物释放器件
	纤维素	血液透析膜、药物释放器件、接触镜

续表

高分子分类	聚合物名称	主 要 用 途
其他相关生物医用高分子	聚甲基丙烯酸烷基酯	硬和软接触镜、牙科填料、骨粘固粉、眼内镜
	聚甲基丙烯酸 β-羟乙酯	软接触镜、烧伤敷料、涂抹类药物的释放基质
	聚甲基丙烯酸	软接触镜、生物功能细珠
	聚丙烯酰胺	软接触镜、生物功能细珠
	聚 N-乙烯基吡咯烷酮	软接触镜、前期代血浆扩张剂
	聚氰基丙烯酸酯	组织黏合剂、血管闭合剂
	聚丙烯酸锌盐	牙科粘固粉

第三节 生物医用高分子的制备与修饰

一、生物医用高分子的制备与修饰的目的和意义

在生物实验研究和长期的临床实践中,人们逐渐意识到,直接使用单一的高分子材料往往很难达到预期的使用效果。例如,高分子材料的力学强度与人体组织的力学强度不一致或不匹配,高分子材料与组织界面间的黏附力微弱,降解过程中材料力学性能损耗过快,降解时间与体内服役工作时间差距较大,非特异性吸附组织或血液成分进而引发局部炎症反应等棘手问题。此外,考虑到纳米药物需要克服体内多重生理壁垒才能最终实现体内药物的成功递送,这就要求制备的高分子药物载体能体现多种功能性,具备多重响应性。而制备这些功能性或响应性高分子,需要设计新的合成思路、探索新的合成方法,或对传统高分子材料进行修饰与改进。因此,通过分子设计的途径,合成出具有生物医用功能的理想高分子材料的前景是十分广阔的,最终制备出性能优良的生物医用高分子材料是未来发展的重要方向之一。

二、生物医用高分子的设计思路

与通用高分子材料不同,生物医用高分子材料由于直接与生物体相互接触、相互作用,除需具备如前所述的一般高分子材料的物理化学性能外,还要满足生物医学领域的特殊性能需求。因此,生物医用高分子材料的设计方案需从原料选择、合成策略、材料构造与物理形态等多方面综合考虑。同时,生物医用高分子的合成目标是带来全新的功能如智能型、靶向性、响应性、可视化等;优化材料性能,如生物相容性、亲疏水性、机械力学性能等。目前,生物医用高分子的设计思路主要包括新型生物医用高分子的合成及对传统高分子的修饰与改性。无论是针对新型生物医用高分子的设计与合成,还是针对现有高分子的修饰及改进,都可以丰富现有

材料的结构与组成,填补现有材料的空缺,获得具有崭新性能和体现特殊功能的生物医用高分子材料。

为了制备生物医用高分子,常见的合成方法主要有聚合反应、有机合成及物理共混等。近年来,得益于"活性"可控聚合技术的高速发展,由功能性单体通过聚合反应制备的一系列生物医用高分子相继被设计开发,部分已在生物医学领域获得临床应用。同时,高效的点击化学等有机合成反应也为生物医用高分子的修饰和改性提供了可能及充足的条件。除聚合反应、有机合成等化学方法之外,物理共混也是获得新型生物医用高分子的有效策略之一。

三、生物医用高分子的制备方法

生物医用高分子材料的构建过程可分为两个阶段:第一阶段为高分子化合物的合成,第二阶段为高分子材料的成型加工(本教材只重点介绍生物医用高分子材料构建的第一阶段)。第二阶段高分子材料的成型加工知识可参阅本章扩展阅读 4 和 5。

在高分子化合物的合成阶段,首先需要对聚合反应的原料进行准备和精制,常用的原料有聚合所需单体、引发剂、链转移剂、催化剂以及聚合所需的其他组分,如溶剂、分散剂、乳化剂等。精制过程则是指对单体、引发剂、溶剂等的纯化步骤,目的是去除阻聚剂和其他杂质,以免带来不可预见的副反应,影响聚合反应的顺利进行。通常来讲,液态原料可利用其沸点相对较低的特点,通过常压蒸馏或减压蒸馏的方法进行纯化,还可利用组分的极性差别,通过碱性氧化铝柱分离提纯;对于固态原料可利用组分在不同溶剂中的溶解性差异,通过重结晶的方法进行提纯。

聚合反应是将小分子的单体化合物通过共价键重复连接形成高分子的过程,最终产物即为聚合物。众所周知,高分子材料的结构决定性质,从而最终决定其用途和效果。因此,聚合物合成是高分子材料构建的基础和关键环节。根据聚合反应的不同原理,其可分为逐步聚合与连锁聚合两类,其中逐步聚合通常是指双官能团或多官能团单体,采用缩合聚合(简称缩聚)或加成聚合(简称加聚)的方式形成高分子链;连锁聚合又称链式聚合反应,是指含有碳碳双键等不饱和键的单体通过连锁聚合反应生成高分子链,在聚合反应过程中有活性中心(自由基或离子),主要包括链引发、链增长和链终止三个基元反应。依据不同的活性中心,连锁聚合又可细分为离子聚合(如阴离子聚合、阳离子聚合)、配位(定向)催化聚合以及自由基聚合。需要指出的是,引发链转移终止剂法、氮-氧稳定的自由基聚合(NMP)、原子转移自由基聚合(ATRP)、可逆加成-裂解-链转移聚合(RAFT)等都属于活性可控自由基聚合,是当今高分子合成领域的研究热点,已广泛应用于生物医用高分子材料的制备。图 3-4 为聚合反应分类图。

逐步聚合是单体官能团之间通过缩合或加成反应,生成二聚体、三聚体等低聚物,然后由低聚物逐步转化为高聚物,因而通常需要较长的反应时间才能达到高分子量,且逐步聚合反应大多为可逆反应,即一边聚合一边解聚,转化率及分子量随时间呈正比升高。

连锁聚合是以自由基、阴离子或阳离子为活性中心进行链增长的,由于活性中心异常活泼,连锁聚合瞬间就能达到高分子量,延长时间只是提高单体的转化率。常见连锁聚合的特征及对比如表 3-5 所示。

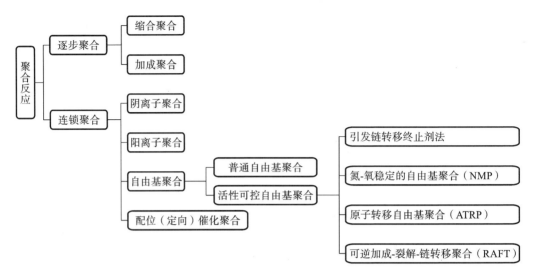

图 3-4　聚合反应分类图

Figure 3-4　Classification diagram of polymerization reactions

表 3-5　常见连锁聚合的特征

聚 合 反 应	自由基聚合	阴离子聚合	阳离子聚合	配位(定向)催化聚合
活性中心	自由基	碳负离子	碳正离子	阴离子性质
活性中心形成方式	共价键均裂	共价键异裂,富电子基团	共价键异裂,缺电子基团	单体 π 电子进入嗜电子金属空轨道,配位形成 π 络合物,进一步形成过渡态
引发剂	偶氮化合物、过氧化合物	Lewis 碱、碱金属、有机金属化合物、碳负离子、亲核试剂	Lewis 酸、质子酸、碳正离子、亲电试剂	Ziegler-Natta 引发剂、茂金属引发剂
引发速率	很慢,需热、光、电等引发	单体与引发剂配合得当时,聚合速率较快		与吸附过程及催化剂比表面积相关
单体	大多数乙烯基单体、共轭单体	带吸电子基团的共轭烯类单体	带供电子基团的共轭烯类单体	大多数烯烃、二烯烃单体
聚合机理特征	慢引发、快增长、快终止、有链转移	快引发、慢增长、无终止、无链转移	快引发、快增长、难终止、有链转移,主要向单体或溶剂转移或单分子自发终止	配位、四元环过渡态、单体插入、增长链末端为阴离子性

续表

聚 合 反 应	自由基聚合	阴离子聚合	阳离子聚合	配位(定向)催化聚合
聚合活化能	较大	小		
聚合温度	一般 50～120 ℃	低温,温度太高则聚合度下降		

自由基聚合反应是当今高分子合成领域研究最普遍、实验操作最简便、工业化程度最高的连锁聚合反应。然而,普通自由基聚合却存在缺陷或不足,如分子量分布较宽,聚合物分散性指数(PDI)常高于 2.0。同时,聚合物分子量及分子结构难以控制,经常出现支化和交联等问题。为克服上述问题,活性可控自由基聚合通过降低自由基(如活性中心)的浓度及反应活性,实现有效抑制双基终止和链转移反应,使其达到可忽略不计的目的,从而使链增长反应处于绝对主导地位。活性可控自由基聚合,如氮-氧稳定的自由基聚合(NMP)、原子转移自由基聚合(ATRP)、可逆加成-裂解-链转移聚合(RAFT)被广泛研究,已成为高分子科学领域具有学术意义和应用价值的重要方向之一。与普通自由基聚合相比,活性可控自由基聚合最显著的优点在于可控的聚合物分子量以及很窄的分子量分布(1.0＜PDI＜1.5),同时按照特定的单体投料顺序,能够设计合成指定链段结构的嵌段共聚物及拓扑结构(如星形、梳状、环状、接枝聚合物等)。

因聚合机理不同,聚合反应实施的方法也有所不同(图 3-5)。逐步聚合采用的聚合方法有熔融缩聚、界面缩聚、溶液缩聚及固相缩聚。连锁聚合采用的聚合方法有本体聚合、悬浮聚合、溶液聚合及乳液聚合。熔融缩聚是在单体和聚合物的熔点以上(一般高于生成聚合物的熔点

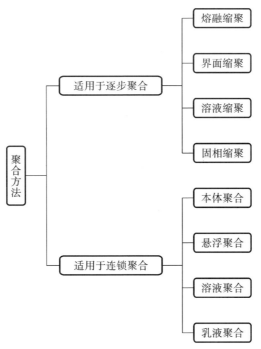

图 3-5 常见的聚合方法

Figure 3-5 Common polymerization methods

$10\sim25\ ℃$)进行的缩聚反应,其反应温度比连锁聚合高很多,一般在200 ℃以上。界面缩聚是指单体、催化剂等处于不同的相态中,单体在多相体系的相界面处发生的缩聚反应。溶液缩聚是指单体、催化剂完全溶解于溶剂中进行的缩聚反应。固相缩聚是指在单体、催化剂等原料的熔点或软化点以下进行的缩聚反应。缩聚反应的特点是不同官能团之间发生反应,形成目标聚合物的同时,还伴有水、氨等低分子副产物的生成。

通过聚合反应合成的粗产物体系一般为多组分混合体系,包含目标聚合物、未参与反应的剩余单体、残留引发剂、链转移剂、催化剂、反应溶剂等。为获得纯净的目标聚合物,需要对粗产物体系进行纯化,必须将聚合物与其他杂质分离,还需脱除溶剂。常见的实验室分离主要分为两个步骤,首先将目标聚合物从液体介质中分离,再脱除溶剂等残留的易挥发成分。从液体介质中分离目标聚合物的常用方法有化学破坏凝聚分离、离心分离、透析分离等。化学破坏凝聚分离的原理是目标聚合物和其余杂质组分及沉淀溶剂、酸、碱、盐发生相互作用,打破原有的混合状态,利用目标聚合物与杂质在沉淀溶剂中显著的溶解性差异,使固体聚合物以沉淀或结晶的形式析出,进而实现将聚合物分离的目的。离心分离的原理是通过离心力、重力的作用,利用聚合物等固体颗粒在液体介质中的沉降作用或利用非均相体系各组分的比重不同,将固液相分离。透析分离利用单体、催化剂、引发剂等小分子物质在溶液中可通过透析膜,而聚合物等大分子物质不能通过透析膜的性质,达到分离提纯目的。脱除溶剂等易挥发成分的方法是将易挥发组分从液态变为气态,进而通过挥发作用除掉气态组分,分离效率由气液相界面的浓度差及扩散系数共同决定,最终可实现的浓度则由气液相平衡决定。

当生物医用材料应用于人体时,人体组织细胞或血液最先与材料表面相互接触,并产生某种应答。而遗憾的是,大多数生物医用材料与细胞或血液之间不能相互适应、相互容纳,即不具备良好的组织相容性与血液相容性,最终引起严重的机体排斥反应,导致材料失去生物医用的价值。通常,为了使材料能够激发生物体恰当的应答能力、展现良好的生物相容性,需要对材料表面进行相应的修饰与改性,优化改善生物相容性已成为拓宽高分子材料在生物医用领域中的应用范围的核心问题,因此生物医用高分子材料的表面改性具有重要的研究意义和实用价值。常见的表面改性方法有物理改性、化学改性以及仿生化改性,如表3-6所示。

表3-6   生物医用高分子材料的表面改性方法

表面改性方法		改性目的
物理改性	物理共混	改善生物医用高分子材料表面的抗凝血性
	表面涂层	
化学改性	光/力化学改性	氧化、粗造化表面,引入不同基团或聚合物链等
	低温等离子体处理	
	紫外线/射线辐照	
	电晕放电处理	
	火焰处理	
仿生化改性	表面肝素化	交联、引入官能团等
	表面磷脂化	
	表面内皮化(内皮细胞固定法)	

物理改性通常是指通过层层自组装技术或物理吸附等包裹一层生物相容性薄膜或聚合物。例如,在生物医用高分子材料表面,通过增加抗凝血涂层来起到钝化高分子材料表面的作用,使血液不会直接接触高分子材料表面,这是改善生物医用高分子材料表面的抗凝血性的有效方法。多种高分子材料成型加工方法也是制备具有不同形态结构、物理化学特性及表界面性质等生物医用高分子材料的有效手段,其中物理共混是构建生物医用高分子材料的重要方法。例如,聚乳酸虽是具有良好生物相容性、生物可降解性、可加工性的生物医用高分子,但其较慢的体内降解速度、高疏水性、低抗冲击强度等,严重限制了其在生物医学领域的应用。为解决上述问题,研究者们将聚乳酸与其他种类的生物医用高分子,如壳聚糖、透明质酸、聚羟基乙酸、聚乙二醇、聚己内酯等通过物理共混的方法,构建了性能优异的复合生物医用高分子材料,这种材料已成功应用于药物载体、形状记忆材料及组织工程支架等。此外,为提高聚砜的血液相容性,研究者们将合成的两亲性抗凝血添加剂共聚物(2-甲基丙烯酰氧基乙基磷酰胆碱-甲基丙烯酸正十二烷基酯及 2-甲基丙烯酰氧基乙基磷酰胆碱-甲基丙烯酸正丁酯的共聚物)与聚砜物理共混,共混后的两亲性共聚物抗凝血添加剂会为了降低界面自由能而富集包裹在聚砜表面,因此提高了聚砜透析膜的血液相容性,最终构建了性能优良的抗凝血材料。

对生物医用高分子材料表面进行涂层处理(即表面涂层技术)也是对生物医用高分子材料进行表面改性的主要手段之一。通过在生物医用高分子材料表面增加抗凝血涂层,钝化敏感的生物材料表面,使血液不能直接与其接触,从而有效地提高材料的生物相容性。例如,通过涂抹抗凝血物质,使生物医用高分子材料表面产生血纤维蛋白质,减少血小板的聚集,使得生物医用高分子材料表面产生抗凝血性能。一般来说,常用抗凝血物质主要有苯乙烯及其转化物、环氧树脂、丙烯酸酯转化物等。这些物质有着很强的黏性,能够用于医疗器械表面,避免出现脱落。另一种方法就是将抗凝血物质和基础材料混合,使基础材料表面能够形成聚集,产生一定的抗凝血性。

物理改性具有操作简单、方便的优势,但如果仅通过物理吸附作用在生物医用高分子材料表面进行涂层,相互作用力较弱,导致稳定性较差,涂层物质有从基材表面脱落的可能。通过化学方法进行表面接枝改性是生物医用高分子材料改性的一个重要途径。通过该方法构建的改性生物医用高分子材料,其表面层与基材通过共价键键合,结合牢固,不会轻易脱落。常见的改性方法有通过高效的点击化学等反应引入功能性基团、键合高分子链、偶联生物活性大分子等。众所周知,许多生物医用高分子材料(如常见的聚硅氧烷、聚四氟乙烯、聚乳酸、聚己内酯等)虽具有良好的生物相容性,但由于高分子的长链式结构易与血液融合、产生吸附。为阻止高分子长链对血液的吸附,利用聚氧乙烯在溶血方面相对稳定的性能,将生物医用高分子与聚氧乙烯共同融合,使其形成水溶性的长链结构,从而尽可能降低生物医用高分子对血浆蛋白的影响,阻止其对血液的吸附。此外,多数生物医用高分子自身无法实现抗菌、自修复、药物缓释等功能。同时,这些聚合物本身不具有反应活性位点,不带有可反应的化学基团,往往难以实现期望的功能材料使用效果。因此,为构建多重响应性和功能性的生物医用高分子材料,对上述聚合物进行表面修饰与改性就显得尤其重要。目前,常见的表面修饰方法有化学溶液处理法(如氧化、磺化、浸渍、水解)、低温等离子体处理、紫外线/射线辐照、原子层沉积、电化学、原子力显微振荡等技术和策略。

等离子体是继固、液、气之后的物质第四态。当外加电压达到击穿电压时,气体分子被电离,产生大量活性粒子的混合体,包括电子、离子、原子、原子团和自由基等,从而为等离子体技术通过化学反应改性材料表面提供了条件。使用低温等离子体改性生物医用高分子材料是用等离子体对高分子材料表面进行处理,将其置于甲烷、氮气、氧气或稀有气体中,通过高压放电的原理产生等离子体,其中的能量粒子及活性物质与高分子材料表面发生反应,改善表面结构来实现表面改性的目的。此外,甲烷等聚合性气体可使生物医用高分子材料表面生成一层聚合物膜,从而提高材料的黏附性。紫外线/射线辐照方法是使用紫外线或射线照射生物医用高分子材料,使其表面发热及活性基团、活性物质能够附着于其表面,这种方法的优点是操作简单、成本低、抗凝血效果好。

表面仿生化改性是改善生物医用高分子材料血液相容性的理想方法之一。仿生化改性使高分子化合物不被血液视为异物,因此在机体内不会被清除、代谢。常见的仿生化改性途径有以下三种:表面肝素化、表面磷脂化、表面内皮化。

肝素因首先在肝脏中被发现而得名,是动物体内一种天然抗凝血物质,也是最早被人们认识和研究的天然抗凝血药物。将肝素分子固定在生物医用高分子材料的表面,是材料抗凝血性能改善的重要途径,采用的方法有物理吸附法和化学键合法。物理吸附法:虽然肝素结合不太牢固,但具有保持肝素构象不变的优势。化学键合法:肝素结构稳定,但不易保持原有构象,使其抗凝血性能降低。磷脂是组成生物膜外表面的主要成分。卵磷脂中的两亲性磷酸胆碱(phosphorylcholine,PC)基团具有很强的抗凝血活性,改善生物医用高分子材料血液相容性的有效方法是在材料中引入磷酸胆碱基团,使生物医用高分子材料表面磷脂化。

表面内皮化又称内皮细胞固定法。众所周知,生物医用高分子材料由于接触到的生物体系成分(如体液、酶、细胞、自由基等)复杂,且生物学环境极其复杂,仅仅依靠表面修饰很难使其血液相容性得到很大的改善。研究者发现,改善材料血液相容性的重要途径是通过应用组织工程技术在材料表面原位培养人体内皮细胞。血管内皮细胞是体内新陈代谢十分活跃的内分泌细胞。通过血管内皮细胞的物理屏障作用及调节维持凝血因子与抗凝血因子之间的动态平衡,可使血液正常流动,而不发生凝血。目前,改善材料血液相容性的理想方法是在生物医用高分子材料表面种植、培养血管内皮细胞。然而,直接将内皮细胞种植在基质材料表面不仅增殖速度慢,而且容易脱落分离。因此,通过共价键结合作用将内皮细胞固定在材料表面,然后在其上种植和培养内皮细胞,可产生更好的效果。

第四节　挑战与展望

一、皮肤疾病诊疗中的生物医用高分子临床开发方向

生物医用高分子材料已经发展成为现代生物医学领域不可或缺的重要材料之一。过去数十年中,生物医用高分子材料的研究和临床应用经历了从生物惰性材料到生物可降解活性材料、智能材料、电子信息材料等的跨越式转变与发展,其在皮肤美容、皮肤疾病诊疗领域的应用涉及多种疾病的生物成像、纳米药物递送系统、透皮给药技术、免疫治疗、皮肤修复与再生、可穿戴皮肤器件及电子皮肤等多个领域,并取得了十分显著的成效。但是,迄今生物医用高分子所涉及的材料种类偏少,不能适应和满足人体各器官所需的复杂的功能,距离通过生物医用高分子材料治病救人的理想目标还很远,亟须深入研究。因此,拓展高分子的结构与组成、设计

合成新型高分子材料、拓展新的适用领域是未来的发展方向。

在诸多慢性疾病及疑难杂症等的用药领域,中药等天然药物都能充分发挥其多靶点的治疗作用。此外,通过现代化技术系统地筛选天然物质,从中药中提取的药物有效组分(如喜树碱、紫杉醇等)已广泛用于肿瘤的临床化疗。前景光明的中药现代化以及从中提取的天然高分子等在皮肤美容、皮肤疾病诊疗行业会越来越受到重视,这也将是未来的发展方向。

此外,为满足生物医用高分子材料更广泛、更智能、更个性化的临床应用需求,同时适应和满足皮肤器官复杂的功能,生物医用高分子材料在皮肤领域的应用形式也更加多样化,发展适合皮肤美容、皮肤疾病诊疗领域特殊需求的复合功能材料,定时、定位、定量的精准智能药物释放,即发挥生物医用高分子材料所具备的优异性能,构建智慧医疗材料是未来生物医用高分子材料的另一个发展方向。

我国的高分子基础研究处于世界前列,但是有关生物医用高分子在皮肤美容及皮肤疾病诊疗领域的研究及应用起步较西方国家晚数十年。因此,目前开发的品种不够多、规格不完善、质量不稳定,导致研发与生产能力与国际仍有巨大差距。高端生物医用高分子材料及制品在很大程度上依赖进口,专业生物医用高分子企业存在规模小、品种少、研发投入少、技术水平相对较低等问题。但是,近年来我国生物医用高分子材料的发展日新月异,已展现出蓬勃的生命力和良好的发展前景,并且已拥有一批国际前沿产品(如植入性生物芯片、组织诱导性骨和软骨、组织工程制品等)。因此,进口生物医用高分子材料制品被国产化替代已成为趋势,是未来生物医用高分子材料发展的另一个重要方向。同时,伴随着人们生活水平的提高和医疗消费的升级,及医疗产品的不断升级换代,生物医用高分子材料制品的品牌效应也将持续提升和发挥重要作用。

二、皮肤美容、皮肤疾病诊疗中的生物医用高分子医疗经济和医疗产业

健康是人类的永恒梦想和毕生追求目标,医用材料及其制品是健康的物质基础。皮肤美容、皮肤疾病诊疗中的生物医用材料是极具潜力的"朝阳产业",未来生物医用高分子材料市场潜力巨大、充满机遇,被国家以及普通消费者寄予厚望。一方面,生物产业"十四五"发展规划强调要大幅提升生物医药及高性能医疗器械领域的新材料应用水平;另一方面,我国人均医疗器械费用远低于发达国家,叠加我国巨大的人口基数,城镇化、老龄化的趋势刺激,生物医用高分子材料将会迎来新一轮的高速发展。由于皮肤疾病发病率升高、患者自我诊疗意识提升、皮肤保健美容需求旺盛、消费升级、高端技术更新换代等,我国医院的就医人次和住院人数持续增长,尤其皮肤保健及皮肤美容已引起大众越来越多的重视,其增长幅度更为明显。持续增长的医疗需求促进了我国医疗服务市场的快速持续发展,预计未来5年复合增速将超过15%。

随着经济发展和受教育程度的提高,人们的皮肤保健及皮肤美容意识也逐步增强,这将极大地提升我国皮肤医疗服务行业的市场需求,为行业发展带来巨大的空间。此外,现代女性已不再满足于美容和抗衰老的基础护肤需求,在此背景下,近年来专业美容皮肤科进入普通民众生活。不同于整形外科的手术治疗,美容皮肤科的非手术项目具备安全、高效、便捷、时尚的特点,符合当今社会普遍价值观,有望成为继整形外科后医疗美容的又一大支柱产业,同时催生出各类医疗美容材料及其制品。生物医用高分子材料将在皮肤医疗市场展示巨大潜力,获得更加广泛的临床应用,同时为皮肤用生物医用高分子医疗经济和医疗产业的稳步发展提供契机,并不断开拓新的应用领域。

思 考 题

1. 简述自由基聚合、阴离子聚合、阳离子聚合和配位(定向)催化聚合的优缺点。
2. 简述生物医用高分子合成的几种常见方法。
3. 简述生物医用高分子表面修饰与改性的几种常见方法。
4. 生物医用高分子有哪些特殊性能要求?
5. 皮肤美容领域通常使用的生物医用高分子材料有哪几种?

扩 展 阅 读

[1] 陈学思,陈红.生物医用高分子[M].北京:科学出版社,2018.
[2] 赵长生,孙树东.生物医用高分子材料[M].2版.北京:化学工业出版社,2016.
[3] Sahana T G,Rekha P D. Biopolymers:applications in wound healing and skin tissue engineering[J]. Mol Biol Rep,2018,45(6):2857-2867.
[4] 王小妹,阮文红.高分子加工原理与技术[M].北京:化学工业出版社,2006.
[5] 温变英.高分子材料成型加工新技术[M].北京:化学工业出版社,2014.

参 考 文 献

[1] Teo A J T,Mishra A,Park I,et al. Polymeric biomaterials for medical implants and devices[J]. ACS Biomater Sci & Eng,2016,2:454-472.
[2] Brandrup J,Immergut E H,Grulke E A. Polymer handbook[M]. 4th ed. Toronto:John Wiley & Sons Inc. ,2013.
[3] 程宁新.注射用整形美容外科材料进展[J].中华医学美学美容杂志,2005,11(6):375-380.
[4] Böttcher-Haberzeth S,Biedermann T,Reichmann E. Tissue engineering of skin[J]. Burns,2010,36(4):450-460.
[5] Chen Y F,Yang P Y,Hu D N,et al. Treatment of vitiligo by transplantation of cultured pure melanocyte suspension:analysis of 120 cases[J]. J Am Acad Dermatol,2004,51(1):68-74.
[6] Yu B,Kang S Y,Akthakul A,et al. An elastic second skin[J]. Nat Mater,2016,15(8):911-918.
[7] 肖春生,田华雨,陈学思,等.智能性生物医用高分子研究进展[J].中国科学(B辑:化学),2008,38(10):867-880.
[8] Ishihara K,Fukumoto K,Iwasaki Y,et al. Modification of polysulfone with phospholipid polymer for improvement of the blood compatibility. Part 1. Surface characterization[J]. Biomaterials,1999,20(17):1545-1551.
[9] Hetemi D,Pinson J. Surface functionalisation of polymers[J]. Chem Soc Rev,2017,46(19):5701-5713.
[10] Fuoco T,Cuartero M,Parrilla M,et al. Capturing the real-time hydrolytic degradation of a library of biomedical polymers by combining traditional assessment and

electrochemical sensors[J]. Biomacromolecules,2021,22(2):949-960.

[11] Zhang Y,Qi Y,Ulrich S,et al. Dynamic covalent polymers for biomedical applications [J]. Mater Chem Front,2020,4(2):489-506.

[12] Seppälä J, van Bochove B, Lendlein A. Developing advanced functional polymers for biomedical applications[J]. Biomacromolecules,2020,21(2):273-275.

[13] Palza H,Zapata P A,Angulo-Pineda C. Electroactive smart polymers for biomedical applications[J]. Materials,2019,12(2):277.

[14] Alegret N, Dominguez-Alfaro A, Mecerreyes D. 3D scaffolds based on conductive polymers for biomedical applications[J]. Biomacromolecules,2019,20(1):73-89.

[15] Zhang H,Zhao T,Newland B,et al. Catechol functionalized hyperbranched polymers as biomedical materials[J]. Prog Polym Sci,2018,78:47-55.

[16] Nezakati T, Seifalian A, Tan A, et al. Conductive polymers: opportunities and challenges in biomedical applications[J]. Chem Rev,2018,118(14):6766-6843.

[17] Hu Y,Li Y,Xu F J. Versatile functionalization of polysaccharides via polymer grafts: from design to biomedical applications[J]. Acc Chem Res,2017,50(2):281-292.

[18] Bajpai A K, Bajpai J, Saini R K, et al. Smart biomaterial devices: polymers in biomedical sciences[M]. Boca Raton:CRC Press,2017.

[19] Yan Y,Zhang J,Ren L,et al. Metal-containing and related polymers for biomedical applications[J]. Chem Soc Rev,2016,45(19):5232-5263.

[20] Peterson G I,Dobrynin A V,Becker M L. α-amino acid-based poly(ester urea)s as multishape memory polymers for biomedical applications[J]. ACS Macro Lett,2016, 5:1176-1179.

[21] Green J J, Elisseeff J H. Mimicking biological functionality with polymers for biomedical applications[J]. Nature,2016,540(7633):386-394.

[22] Wu W,Wang W G,Li J. Star polymers:advances in biomedical applications[J]. Prog Polym Sci,2015,46:55-85.

[23] Fairbanks B D, Gunatillake P A, Meagher L. Biomedical applications of polymers derived by reversible addition—fragmentation chain-transfer (RAFT) [J]. Adv Drug Deliv Rev,2015,91:141-152.

[24] Dong R,Zhou Y,Huang X,et al. Functional supramolecular polymers for biomedical applications[J]. Adv Mater,2015,27(3):498-526.

[25] Delplace V,Nicolas J. Degradable vinyl polymers for biomedical applications[J]. Nat Chem,2015,7(10):771-784.

[26] Gu L,Faig A,Abdelhamid D,et al. Sugar-based amphiphilic polymers for biomedical applications:from nanocarriers to therapeutics[J]. Acc Chem Res, 2014, 47(10): 2867-2877.

[27] Hoffman A S. Stimuli-responsive polymers:biomedical applications and challenges for clinical translation[J]. Adv Drug Deliv Rev,2013,65(1):10-16.

[28] Lynge M E, van der Westen R, Postma A, et al. Polydopamine—a nature-inspired

polymer coating for biomedical science[J]. Nanoscale,2011,3:4916-4928.

[29] Zhou Y,Huang W,Liu J,et al. Self-assembly of hyperbranched polymers and its biomedical applications[J]. Adv Mater,2010,22(41):4567-4590.

[30] Lendlein A,Langer R. Biodegradable,elastic shape-memory polymers for potential biomedical applications[J]. Science,2002,296(5573):1673-1676.

[31] Zhang H. Molecularly imprinted nanoparticles for biomedical applications[J]. Adv Mater,2020,32(3):e1806328.

[32] Yang J,Yang Y W. Metal-organic frameworks for biomedical applications[J]. Small, 2020,16(10):1906846.

[33] Walia R,Akhavan B,Kosobrodova E,et al. Hydrogel—solid hybrid materials for biomedical applications enabled by surface-embedded radicals[J]. Adv Funct Mater, 2020,30(38):2004599.

[34] Nele V,Wojciechowski J P,Armstrong J P K,et al. Tailoring gelation mechanisms for advanced hydrogel applications[J]. Adv Funct Mater,2020,30(42):2002759.

[35] Tutar R,Motealleh A,Khademhosseini A,et al. Functional nanomaterials on 2D surfaces and in 3D nanocomposite hydrogels for biomedical applications[J]. Adv Funct Mater,2019,29(46):1904344.

[36] Fu Q,Zhu R,Song J,et al. Photoacoustic imaging:contrast agents and their biomedical applications[J]. Adv Mater,2019,31(6):e1805875.

[37] Yang G,Li X,He Y,et al. From nano to micro to macro:electrospun hierarchically structured polymeric fibers for biomedical applications[J]. Prog Polym Sci,2018,81: 80-113.

[38] Shabahang S,Kim S,Yun S H. Light-guiding biomaterials for biomedical applications [J]. Adv Funct Mater,2018,28(24):1706635.

[39] Li W,Zhang L,Ge X,et al. Microfluidic fabrication of microparticles for biomedical applications[J]. Chem Soc Rev,2018,47(15):5646-5683.

[40] Kim D,Shin K,Kwon S G,et al. Synthesis and biomedical applications of multifunctional nanoparticles[J]. Adv Mater,2018,30(49):e1802309.

[41] Ding X,Duan S,Ding X,et al. Versatile antibacterial materials:an emerging arsenal for combatting bacterial pathogens[J]. Adv Funct Mater,2018,28(40):1802140.

[42] Cho J H,Lee J S,Shin J,et al. Ascidian-inspired fast-forming hydrogel system for versatile biomedical applications:pyrogallol chemistry for dual modes of crosslinking mechanism[J]. Adv Funct Mater,2018,28(6):1705244.

[43] Becker G,Wurm F R. Functional biodegradable polymers via ring-opening polymerization of monomers without protective groups[J]. Chem Soc Rev,2018,47: 7739-7782.

[44] Song Z,Han Z,Lv S,et al. Synthetic polypeptides:from polymer design to supramolecular assembly and biomedical application[J]. Chem Soc Rev,2017,46(21):

6570-6599.

[45] Li J, Mo L, Lu C, et al. Functional nucleic acid-based hydrogels for bioanalytical and biomedical applications[J]. Chem Soc Rev, 2016, 45(5):1410-1431.

（陈森斌　朱锦涛）

Chapter 3
Introduction of Biomedical Polymers

3.1　A Brief History of Biomedical Polymers

Starting from the practical requirements of polymeric compounds in the fields of clinical medicine and medical treatment, biomedical polymers are the designed polymer materials and their corresponding products, extensively used in the fields of biology and medicine, reflecting a multidisciplinary research fields of life science, material science, medicine and polymer chemistry (see extended reading 1 & 2). Biomedical polymer materials generally refer to all polymer materials used in biomedical fields such as diagnosis, treatment, and organ repair and regeneration, committed to meeting the industrial needs for the biomedical field and serving people's higher pursuit of a healthy and beautiful life. Biomedical polymer materials holds an irreplaceable important position in biological materials. Its application will be helpful to improve human health, extend the life of patients, and improve the quality of human life.

3.1.1　The development history of biomedical polymers

Having been developed for about a century, biomedical polymer materials and related devices have become important auxiliary tools and functional materials in the various fields of diagnosis and treatment in modern medicine, hold an irreplaceable important position in modern medicine, and continue to promote the innovation and sustainable development of various diagnosis and treatment technologies. The composition basis of biomedical polymer materials is polymer compounds. Therefore, in order to explain the development history of biomedical polymer materials, we first briefly introduce the basic knowledge of polymer science.

Polymer science and synthetic polymer technology began to sprout in the 1920s and 1930s. So far, it has become an essential part of human daily life and industrial production.

Polymer materials, metallic materials, and ceramic materials are the three key materials of modern society. Polymer compounds are generally named as macromolecules, or polymers for short. It is made up of many repeated structural units linked by repeated covalent bonds. Its relative molecular weight can reach thousands or even millions, showing certain mechanical properties of macromolecular compounds.

Each repeated structural unit that makes up a polymer is known as the monomer of the polymer, i. e., the starting material of the synthetic polymer, capable of forming high molecular weight compounds through the polymerization reactions.

Compared to the small molecular compounds, polymer compounds have the following remarkable characteristics: ①The molecular weight is high and the molecule is like a "long chain". ②It has a certain aspect ratio. ③If there are branches on the molecular chain, it can form star-shaped, hyperbranched, network and other topological structures. ④ The molecular weight is not uniform and featured by heterogeneous, i. e., the polydispersity of polymers. ⑤Strong interchain interactions lead to liquid and solid-state polymers, and can't be vaporized. ⑥Solid polymers have certain mechanical strength, can be used as load-bearing materials, and can be used to form a clot, draw silk and make film. Among them, biomedical polymer materials are one type of polymer materials used in the fields of artificial organs, tissue engineering and regenerative medicine, physical therapy and rehabilitation, internal and external diagnosis, slow and controlled drug release, blood preparations, and medical devices.

In fact, before the concept of "polymer science" and the technology of "man-made polymers" appeared, some natural polymer materials (e. g., cotton fiber, horsehair) have been used by ancient humans to heal the wounds. Bamboo chips and wooden planks are used for fracture fixation, and these natural polymer products are recognized as the earliest biomedical polymer materials. It is well known that the most important substances in the composition of animal and plant bodies (e. g., protein, muscle, cellulose, starch, biological enzymes and pectin) are all belong to polymer compounds. Therefore, it is accepted that natural polymers are the basis of life, and the biological world is a huge resource of natural polymers. The ubiquity of polymer compounds in the biological world determines their special status in the medical field. Among various materials, the molecular structure, chemical composition, and physical and chemical properties of man-made polymer materials have important similarities with biological tissues, therefore they can be widely used as biomedical materials.

Modern biomedical polymer materials were born with the concept of "polymer science" and the technology of "man-made polymer". After that, there have been many significant evolutions in the polymer field, and polymer science and technology have been rapidly developed. As a consequence, new polymer synthetic materials continue to emerge, providing more options for the medical fields, leading to the continuous development of biomedical polymer materials for clinical application, as shown in Table 3-1.

Table 3-1　Development and progress of biomedical polymers

Years	Inventions in the field of polymers	Clinical applications
1930s	Poly(methyl methacrylate) (PMMA)	Dentures and fillings
1940s	Celluloid film	Hemodialysis
1950s	Organosilicon rubber	Artificial kidney
1950s	Polyurethane (PU)	Artificial heart
1950s	Polytetrafluoroethylene，PTFE，Teflon®	Artificial blood vessel
1960s	Poly (hydroxyethyl methacrylate) (PHEMA) cross-linked hydrogel (water swellable soft transparent elastic colloid)	Soft contact lens，arterial blood vessel，surgical repair material
1960s	Poly (glycolic acid) (PGA, Dexron®), poly (lactic acid) (PLA)	Absorbable suture
1970s	Poly(lactic-co-glycolic acid) (PLGA)	Absorbable suture
1980s	Sodium alginate/calcium ion cross-linked hydrogel to embed insulin	Artificial pancreas
1980s	Collagen-glycosaminoglycan cross-linked hydrogel used as a mimic extracellular matrix	Skin regeneration and repair
1990s	Functional, intelligent and responsive biomedical polymers	Artificial lens, wound dressing, tissue engineering, regenerative medicine, controlled drug release
21st century	Personalization, precision, bionic intelligence, function integration	Dynamic structure adjustable polymer scaffold, tissue engineering and implantable device/organ, responsive polymer nanomedicine precision diagnosis and treatment system

3.1.2　Advances in biomedical polymers and skin beauty，diagnosis and treatment of skin diseases

With the development of biomedical polymers，it has become an indispensable material in the field of modern medicine，especially in the past 30 years，which has experienced a rapid development globally. Biomedical polymers，as the model of interdisciplinary，integrate polymer chemistry and physics，biochemistry，synthetic material technology，pathology，pharmacology，anatomy，and clinical medicine. It also involves many engineering issues，including the design and manufacturing of various medical devices. The collaboration and penetration of the above disciplines has promoted more varieties of biomedical polymer materials being applied to clinical medical treatment and daily protection，showing outstanding performance and advanced functions. Biomedical polymer materials are related to where and how they are used. At the same time, different application fields require materials to have certain special functions. In the fields of skin beauty, skin health, skin disease diagnosis and treatment, and daily protection, biomedical polymer materials have been widely accepted and applied.

The skin covers the surface of the whole body and is the largest organ of the human body. The total area of adult skin is 1. 5-2 m^2, accounting for 5%-15% of the total weight. The skin is in direct contact with the external environment. The first chapter of this textbook "Structure and Function of the Skin" demonstrated that the skin has important functions, including protecting the human body from heat, microorganisms or pathogens, protecting the deep tissues and organs of the human body, excreting, regulating body temperature, and feeling external stimuli. As people get older, their skin will gradually loosen, sag, reduce elasticity, and appear wrinkles. Now, injecting the polymeric supporting materials or fillers into the dermis and/or subcutaneous tissue to fill and increase the volume of the tissue will help correct or increase the function of the soft tissue clinically, and finally achieve the effect and propose of skin beauty.

The ideal facial fillers must demonstrate the good biocompatibility, safety and excellent cosmetic effects. The facial fillers can be divided into two types: non-absorbable and absorbable fillers. Non-absorbable fillers are prepared from non-degradable polymer materials, including poly (methyl methacrylate) (PMMA), polyacrylamide (PAM), expanded polytetrafluoroethylene (PTFE) and silica gel, etc. Absorbable fillers are prepared from degradable biomedical polymer materials, including collagen, hyaluronic acid (HA) and poly(L-lactic acid) (PLLA), etc. Expanded PTFE is prepared from a biaxial stretching process of PTFE to form "fibrous nodules", showing the porous with the diameters less than 1 μm. As a result, cells can be easily grown in and demonstrate excellent biocompatibility, therefore considered as an excellent facial filling material. Expanded PTFE has the advantages of natural lifelike, safe and permanent, and strong plasticity, so it is usually used for rhinoplasty, soft tissue repair, facial filling, mandibular prosthesis, nasolabial filling, etc. In addition, absorbable injectable fillers are the future developing direction of a novel generation of medical implants, which can be spontaneously degraded after being injected into the body for a certain period of time. Moreover, the degradation products have good biocompatibility and can be eliminated by the body through metabolism. At present, in addition to the usage for skin wrinkle removal propose, absorbable plastic implants are also widely used for depression filling, scar repair, and facial plasticity. Its main polymer materials include sodium hyaluronate gel, collagen implants, creotoxin and 3D PLA microsphere materials, etc.

The skin is the human body's first line of physical defense, and it also participates in various functional activities of the body. Therefore, abnormal conditions and even lesions of the body can also be reflected through the skin. If the physiological function of the skin is affected or damaged, it will cause the skin disease. The common pathogenic factors in skin diseases are infection and allergy, but with the degenerative changes of aging, senile skin diseases and skin cancer appear as the vital skin diseases. In addition, damage or loss of skin integrity may affect the function of the skin, leading to severe disability or even death. Therefore, wound healing is very important to the human body and is a major challenge faced by scientific research and clinical medicine. For a detailed introduction to skin diseases, please refer to the chapter 2 "Skin Health and Representative Skin Diseases". Biomedical polymers also play a significant role in the diagnosis and treatment of skin diseases and have been widely used, including skin wound dressings, pharmaceutical excipients, and composite artificial skins.

Healing of the skin wounds is one of the basic, yet key issues encountered by the entire human and medical circles. The process of wound healing is complicated, and an ideal surgical dressing can protect the wound, prevent infection, and promote healing. In recent years, the treatment of skin wounds and the variety of products are increasing day by day (see extended reading 3). Traditional dressings such as cotton gauze only have simple functions of protection and reducing infection, and play a limited protective role in covering wounds and absorbing the exudate. New synthetic dressings constructed from biomedical polymer compounds, such as hydrogels, alginate dressings and foam dressings, are more effective for skin wound care, and can interact with the wound. In addition to absorbing the exudate, it also shows the effect of allowing gas exchange, preventing the invasion of external microorganisms and preventing wound infections, and creates an environment conducive to wound healing, which can alleviate the pain of patients and reduce scars and shrinkage. The dressing material itself can promote and accelerate wound healing. With the establishment and improvement of epidermal cell culture methods, active artificial skin, namely tissue engineered skin, is gradually born on the basis of the research of biological materials and synthetic materials. Biomedical polymer dressings and tissue engineered skins have significant advantages such as "wet" environment and good healing function that they provide for wounds, therefore leading to wide clinical applications.

Natural biomedical polymer materials, such as alginate and chitosan dressings, have been widely used in the repair of skin wounds. Dressing extracted from natural seaweed plants, contains calcium alginate ingredients. The calcium ions in the dressing exchange with the sodium salt secreted by the blood and wounds, forming gels with the effect of clotting and stopping bleeding and stabilizing biofilm, protect the wound surface and promote the growth of granulation tissue. Commercially available alginate dressing products include AlgiSite, Sorbsan and Kaltostat, etc., which are suitable for wounds with moderate to large amounts of exudation, mild bleeding wounds, and yellow rotting and necrotic tissue wounds, but cannot be used for dry and eschar wounds. Most products are not self-adhesive and require secondary dressings to be fixed, with relatively high cost. Many synthetic biomedical polymer materials, such as polyvinylon, polypropylene, polyamide (Nylon), polyurethane, poly(vinyl alcohol), polyacrylonitrile, polycaprolactone, poly (lactic acid), poly (amino acid), polytetrafluoroethylene, and silicone elastomer, can also be used as a dressing. The more important and widely used ones are polyurethane and silicone.

Membrane-like dressings (e. g. , OpSite and Tegaderm) which are made of polyurethane, have a certain degree of elasticity, and at the same time reflect good adhesion performance, and the water vapor can smoothly permeate. Yet, water and bacteria cannot permeate the membrane-like dressings made of polyurethane, and they do not interfere with the normal healing process of the wound. The prepared film has high transparency and is easy to observe. In addition, due to good biocompatibility, the film will not cause immune response, and can stay on the wound until the wound heals. Sometimes, it needs to be used in combination with other materials. For example, the melanocyte transplantation is used to treat vitiligo. After the cells are transplanted to the ground surface of the lesion, a layer of silica gel and a dressing impregnated with F12 medium are attached immediately, and then covered with Tegaderm. The FlexiGrid unidirectional breathable membrane produced by S & N in the UK, whose main components are polyurethane and polyacrylic, has the advantage of being a "molecular valve" function. The rancid gas decomposed by the necrotic tissue in the wound can outward penetrate the membrane smoothly, while the bacteria and air outside the membrane cannot penetrate the membrane to penetrate the skin wound, endowing the great permeability to the wound. In addition, polyether-based polyurethane has strong membrane permeability, so the moisture of the wound exudate can pass through and precipitate, and the protein and other components are transformed into gel under the dressing, which can relieve pain.

Generally, synthetic polymer dressings can be divided into film type, foam type, hydrogel, hydrocolloid and composite type according to the different status. The commercialized products are generally the composite materials. The advantages and disadvantages of the common dressings and the scope of applications are shown in Table 3-2.

Table 3-2　The advantages and disadvantages of the common dressings and the scope of applications

Dressing types	Advantages	Disadvantages	Scope of applications
Transparent dressing film	1. Gas and water vapor can permeate, while bacteria and liquid cannot permeate; 2. Provide a moist healing environment to promote autolytic debridement; 3. Transparent and easy to observe the wound; 4. Can be used as inner dressing or outer dressing; 5. Flexible and adaptable	1. Poor ability to absorb the exudate and may soak the surrounding skin; 2. Cannot be used on infected wound; 3. May tear the surrounding fragile skin when removing	1. Protect the wound from external contamination; 2. Wound with minor exudate or without exudation; 3. Also often used as a secondary dressing, such as in combination with hydrogel for wound with black necrosis or yellow carrion

Continued

Dressing types	Advantages	Disadvantages	Scope of applications
Hydrocolloid dressing (main component is sodium carboxymethyl cellulose)	1. Provide a moist healing environment to promote autolytic debridement; 2. Absorb a small amount of the exudate; 3. Waterproof, anti-bacterial, moisturizing, promote epithelial cells craw; 4. The granulation tissue is not easily damaged when removing; 5. The flake dressing is self-adhesive and does not require external fixation	1. Cannot be used on infected wound or wound with exposed bones or tendons; 2. Cannot be used for deep diving or excessively exuding wounds; 3. Easy to tear the fragile skin around the wound, prone to curl	1. Partially damaged wound; 2. Wound with a small amount of exudate; 3. Wound with yellow carrion or black necrosis; 4. Can be used as a topical dressing
Hydrogel dressing	1. Keep the wound moist, provide a moist healing environment to promote autolytic debridement; 2. Non-sticky, easy to remove; 3. Can fill sinus and cavities, protect exposed periosteum, tendons, etc. ; 4. Has a gentle movement and can relieve pain	1. Easy to cause wound maceration; 2. Cannot be applied to normal skin; 3. Need secondary dressing for fixation; 4. Not recommended to be used for wound with excessive exudate or infected wound	1. Dermal and full-thickness damaged wounds; 2. Wound with yellow carrion or black necrosis; 3. Burns and electrotherapy wounds
Alginate dressing	1. Provide a moist healing environment to promote autolytic debridement; 2. The exchange of calcium and sodium ions can stop bleeding; 3. Form a gel to protect the wound; 4. Promote the growth of granulation tissue, can be non-invasive removed; 5. The amount of absorbing exudate is 17-20 times of its own weight	1. Cannot be used on dry or eschar wound; 2. Need secondary dressing for fixation	1. Wounds with moderate to large amounts of exudate; 2. Mild bleeding wound; 3. Wound with yellow carrion or necrotic tissue

Continued

Dressing types	Advantages	Disadvantages	Scope of applications
Foam dressing	1. Gas and water vapor can freely permeate; 2. Provide a moist healing environment; 3. Protect the wound and relieve pain; 4. Promote the growth of granulation tissue; 5. Dissolve necrotic tissue; 6. Absorb a large amount of exudate to prevent edema of granulation tissue and not soak the surrounding skin; 7. Flatten over-long granulation; 8. Soft, can be used under pressure	1. Cannot be used on dry or scab wound; 2. It is a non-adhesive dressing and requires secondary dressing for fixation; 3. Opaque, inconvenient to observe wound; 4. Relatively poor compliance	1. Can be used on cavity wound in conjunction with debridement gel and alginate dressing; 2. For venous ulcer wound, preferably with elastic bandage
Silicone dressing	1. Non-invasive during replacement, protect the wound and surrounding skin; 2. Patented technology to achieve vertical absorption, effectively avoiding impregnation; 3. Provide a more suitable moist healing environment; 4. Rapid epithelialization; 5. The application is soft and fits the skin well; 6. Self-adhesive and can be cut freely; 7. Can be pasted repeatedly	1. Cannot be used on infected wound; 2. Not suitable for dry wound or wound with eschar; 3. If there is no exudate, it will cause dryness	1. Avulsion wound; 2. Vulnerable wound of the surrounding skin; 3. Prevention of pressure ulcers
Silicone foam	1. Super absorbent, 3D dendritic foam structure; 2. Soft and thin, good compliance, self-adhesive and self-fixing, can be pasted repeated	1. Disabled on damaged skin and open wound; 2. Disabled for wound that has not been removed; 3. Stop using it when you have dermatitis or eczema, or use it after the symptoms are relieved	1. Various exudative wounds; 2. Fragile wound of the surrounding skin, and elderly and children; 3. The thin type can be applied to patients and joint wounds that require more mobility

Continued

Dressing types	Advantages	Disadvantages	Scope of applications
Hypertonic salt dressing (Meisho, composed of polyester fiber and 28% NaCl)	1. Absorb a large amount of exudate and necrotic tissue, clean up for creation; 2. Reduce edema and promote wound healing; 3. Easy to operate, no foreign matter remains; 4. Arbitrary cutting, can fill the cavity and gap; 5. Hypertonic environment, inhibit the growth of bacteria	1. Cannot be used for dry wound; 2. Cannot be in contact with normal tissues, cannot be used on dry eschar wound or healthy granulation; 3. Requires additional outer dressing	1. Wound with a lot of exudate 2. Edematous granulation; 3. Debridement of yellow carrion; 4. Suppurative or foul-smelling infected wound
Hydrophilic cellulose dressing (main ingredient: sodium carboxymethyl cellulose)	1. Powerful exudate management ability, strong absorption, strong locking, anti-impregnation; 2. Unique softness and compliance; 3. No adhesion to the wound, painless	1. Cannot be used for dry wound; 2. Need external fixation dressing	A variety of exudative wounds

Scar is a general term for the appearance and histopathological changes of normal skin tissues caused by various kinds of wounds, including skin cutting injury, skin burn, skin infection, surgical operation, etc. Scar is an inevitable product in the process of human wound repair. When the growth of scar exceeds to a certain limit, all kinds of complications will occur, such as damage of appearance and dysfunction of function and activity, which will bring great physical and mental pain to the patients, especially scars left after burns, scalds and other severe trauma. The polymer material usually used to treat scar is cross-linked polydimethylsiloxane, commonly known as silicone, which forms a covering that is as soft and stretchable as human skin. Silicone used for scar treatment usually has three forms of ointment, film and gel, which can prevent the formation of new scars and relieve the symptoms and signs of existing hypertrophic scars, including erythema, hardness, size and pruritus. The use of polyurethane film alone or combined with pressure therapy can also reduce the color and hardness thickness of scar. The usage is similar to that of silicone products, 12 to 24 hours per day and last for 2 to 4 months. Advantages lie in transparent appearance, suitable for exposed parts such as the head, face and hands, and not easy to macerate.

The cross-linked polydimethylsiloxane films also help moisturize the skin well and can be used in skin care products or cosmetics, as well as medical skin applications. Robert Langer from the Massachusetts Institute of Technology, collaborating with Massachusetts

General Hospital, Living Proof and Olivo Laboratories, jointly developed the "second skin" elastic thin film materials. The material, a cross-linked polymer layer based on polydimethylsiloxane, is breathable, has "no feeling" against the skin and has not yet been found to have side effects on humans. Most importantly, it can effectively restore the mechanical properties of skin, eliminate the users' face bag and make the skin more moisture at the same time. If the product is successfully marketed, it is expected to be directly used to treat patients' skin or prevent UV exposure, for example, treating skin diseases such as eczema. When sunscreen is added, the "second skin" film also protects against damage from the sunlight.

Skin encapsulation therapy is a kind of therapy in which non-permeable films (e. g., plastic wrap, plastic bags, bandages, gloves and medical dressings) are enclosed and wrapped on the surface of the affected part coated with drugs, so as to achieve the therapeutic purpose. Topical application of glucocorticoid encapsulation is the traditional method for the treatment of chronic inflammatory dermatosis, including chronic hypertrophic dermatitis, keratosis dermatosis, verrucous hyperplastic dermatosis, etc. The materials of packets developed from the initial polyethylene plastic materials to the present water gel sticker, and glucocorticoids can be made into a composite preparation with the encapsulated material or used separately. Topical use of glucocorticoids combined with hydrocolloid coated DuoDerm is effective for the treatment of psoriasis, which is also used for the treatment of refractory atopic dermatitis and other chronic inflammatory skin diseases. Another hydrocolloidal film Actiderm plus medi-effect hormone was used for external treatment of metatarsal pustular disease, and the effect was far better than that of strong hormone alone. Hydrocolloidal 3M AcneDressing can significantly improve the condition of acne patients by reducing hand exposure and ultraviolet radiation. These methods which use the hydrocolloidal external materials with strong adhesion and closure, can promote drug absorption, and can reduce scratching. Scratching has the effect of promoting chronic local skin inflammation, thus reduction of scratching has the therapeutic effect.

3.1.3 Applications of biomedical polymers in skin beauty and diagnosis and treatment of skin diseases

Polymer material is one of the three major materials in today's society, and it is an indispensable material basis for human production and life. With the birth of polymer science and technology, the almost simultaneous development of biomedical polymers and their products have been widely recognized and clinically applied. Polymer materials and their products can be seen in every step of medical work. In recent years, the application of polymer materials in the field of skin, including the diagnosis and treatment of skin diseases, skin beauty, wearable skin devices and electronic skin, and skin repair and regeneration, etc., has achieved remarkable results and more complete cognition through scientific research and clinical practice.

Skin disease is a general term for a variety of diseases that occur in the skin and skin appendages. There are many types of skin diseases and currently more than 2000 skin diseases with different clinical characteristics can be named. They can be affected by all ages from birth to death, and any part of the body can be affected. From a medical point of view, there are almost no individuals who are not troubled by skin diseases in a person's life. Therefore, skin disease is the most common disease. At the same time, the lesions that occur in the internal organs often present on the skin. In addition, skin diseases caused by infectious factors (e. g., leprosy, scabies, skin bacteria, fungal diseases) are usually contagious, which not only affects physical health, but also leads to social discrimination and psychological problems, etc. The common skin diseases are infectious diseases and allergic dermatitis, but with the degenerative changes of aging, senile skin diseases and skin cancer are also important skin diseases. With people's pursuit of a healthy and beautiful life, the diagnosis and treatment of skin diseases have attracted more and more attention. The diagnosis and differential diagnosis of skin diseases include physical examination, laboratory examination, etc. At the same time, in order to clarify the tissue structure of the organism and clarify the various physiological functions of the organism, bioimaging technology has been widely used in the research and clinical diagnosis of skin diseases. For this content, please refer to chapter 5 "Imaging in Dermatology".

Traditional treatments of skin diseases mostly employ external use medicines, which have some disadvantages such as low drug utilization, and multidrug resistance. Recent studies have shown that the usage of polymer nanoparticles (NPs) as drug carriers can achieve targeted delivery and slow down the purpose of controlled-release drug delivery, which has gradually developed into an effective way to treat skin diseases. For details, please refer to chapter 6 "Polymer Nano-Drug Carriers and Their Applications in Skin Diseases Treatments". Melanoma is a tumor produced by melanocytes of the skin and other organs. It has early metastasis, high malignancy, and high mortality, and is a very important content in the treatment of skin diseases. For detailed introduction, please refer to chapter 7 "Applications of Biomedical Polymers in Immunotherapy of Melanoma". Compared with traditional drug delivery methods, new drug delivery technologies (e. g., transdermal drug delivery) refer to new technologies that administer drugs on the surface of the skin to allow drugs to pass through the skin into the body circulation at a controlled rate or procedure to achieve local or systemic treatment. Transdermal drug delivery technology has significant advantages in the treatment of skin diseases, including not being interfered by factors such as strong acidity in the digestive tract, food, and transit time. It can avoid the liver first-pass effect, and can overcome the adverse reactions resulted from the high blood concentration caused by the rapid drug absorption. The drug delivery speed can be controlled continuously, and the drug delivery can be personalized and flexible. For the latest research progress and clinical application of transdermal drug delivery, please refer to chapter 8 "Transdermal Drug Delivery".

The biomedical polymers in skin cosmetology can be classified into three types according to the duration of the filling material: short-acting (6-12 months), semi-permanent (18-30 months) and permanent (over 5 years). The important basic materials for skin filling are collagen, poly (lactic acid) and hyaluronic acid, as shown in Table 3-3. Regarding the biomedical polymer materials in skin cosmetology, please refer to chapter 9 "Applications of Biomedical Polymers in Cosmetic Dermatology" for details.

Table 3-3　Introduction to biomedical polymers in skin beauty

Biomedical polymers	The US FDA approval time	Duration	Representative products	Advantages	Disadvantages
Collagen	1981	Short-acting	Double Beauty I	Biosafety	Short validity
Hyaluronic acid	2003	Short-acting, semi-permanent	Ruilan, Joe Yadeng, Ewan, Evelyn, Ellivia, Haiwei	It widely exists in organisms, and is the main component of extracellular matrix, safe and reliable	Wrinkles deepen after injection, cross-linking agent remains
Poly(lactic acid)	2009	Semi-permanent	Sculptra, AestheFill, Derma Veil	High biosafety, long-acting time, mild and natural	Easy to form nodules after injection

In addition, wearable electronic skin is a detection technology that can measure human health physiological indicators, such as heart rate, pulse, blood pressure, body temperature, and muscle vibration. Its advantages lie in the timely sensing and feedback of changes in human health data, and even the early prevention and diagnosis of diseases. For this part of the content, please refer to chapter 10 "Wearable Electronic Skin Devices". Organisms have great ability to repair and restore tissue damage and defects, including the repair of different levels of skin tissue structure, and the reconstruction of its tissue and body function. For skin damage, epidermal damage can usually be regenerated. It is usually difficult to completely repair it once the damage reaches the dermis and subcutaneous tissue. Biomedical polymer materials for skin repair and regeneration include traditional wound dressings and artificial skins that have recently been developed. The characteristic of wound dressings is the pursuit of fast and good wound repair, while artificial skin is mainly dedicated to the complete restoration of the structure and function of the skin (e. g. , skin regeneration). The structure and function of natural skin are very complicated. Therefore, based on the knowledge of skin structure and function, research and thorough understanding of the mechanism of skin wound repair and healing are important for the design and construction of new facial fillers, wound dressings and artificial skin significance. For the physiological process of skin wound healing, complications and treatment of skin wound repair, and biomedical polymer materials for skin repair and regeneration, please refer to chapter 11 "Applications of Biomedical Polymers in Skin Wound Repair".

3.2 Basic Knowledge of Biomedical Polymers in Skin Cosmetology and the Diagnosis and Treatment of Skin Diseases

3.2.1 Necessary conditions and special performance requirements for biomedical polymers

When biomedical polymers are used for the skin beauty and the diagnosis and treatment of skin diseases, it is necessary to contact with human tissues, blood and body fluid. Due to the natural protective reaction of human body, when the material acts on human body or skin surface, rejection phenomenon is bound to occur, which will often produces very serious consequences, and even endanger life. Therefore, compared with general polymer materials, the requirements of biomedical polymer materials are very strict, and also have special specific requirements for properties. Before medical polymer materials are used in clinic, the physical and chemical properties, mechanical properties, and the mutual adaptability of the materials with organisms and human bodies must be evaluated in detail and comprehensively, and then they can be used in clinic only after being approved by the national administrative departments. Therefore, biomedical polymer materials must have the following properties.

1. Biosafety

Biomedical polymer materials must be non-toxic or have minimal side effects. Biomedical polymer materials, after contact with the body's tissues, will produce a series of complex biological, physical, and chemical reaction, and a variety of temporary or profound influences. On the one hand, the material requires high molecular compound purity, clean production and processing environment, less residual impurities, and no disease, sterile or non-toxic transmission. On the other hand, after contact with body fluid, the polymer materials must demonstrate no sensitization, irritation, genetic toxicity, or three causes (carcinogenic, teratogenic, and mutation), and reflects biological inertness. In other words, no changes in structure and composition occur in the body, or it can be degraded in the body, while no adverse reactions and no harmful by-products are produced. The first application of biodegradable biomedical polymer materials is absorbable suture, and the representative of which are poly(glycolic acid) (PGA), poly(lactic acid) (PLA), and poly (lactic-*co*-glycolic acid) (PLGA), as described in Table 3-1.

The influences of human environment on the polymer materials basically have the followings: body fluid can cause the degradation, cross-linking and phase change of polymers; free radicals in the body can cause materials oxidation and degradation; enzyme can cause polymers decomposition reaction. Under the action of body fluid, the additives in polymer materials may be dissolved out. In the meantime, the substance such as lipid, steroid and adipose in blood and body fluid also can seep into polymer materials, leading to falling mechanical strength. But for biomedical polymers, in some cases, the reactions of human environment to aging, decomposition and degradation of polymer materials are not always negative, and even have positive significance. The surgeon, for example, does not want the sutures to be chemically stable or biologically inert, but rather to be broken down, absorbed, or expelled by the tissue as soon as possible. In this case, the additional requirement for biomedical polymer materials is that no harmful by-products are produced during the decomposition process.

2. Physical, chemical and mechanical properties

It should meet the design and function requirements of skin beauty and the diagnosis and treatment of skin diseases. Differing from high mechanical strength for dentistry and orthopedics, the strength requirements of polymer materials used in skin beauty and fractured wound repair are not that high; however they must demonstrate a certain degree of flexibility, especially dermal fillers, which should reflect similar or even consistent mechanical properties such as elasticity and elasticity to normal skin, and should have a certain degree of adhesion and adaptability with the skin, in order to match and integrate with the skin. The repair materials at the damaged part of the skin are physically combined with human skin tissue. Such soft tissue repair materials should have certain activity, which can not only promote the repair of the injured part, but also degrade after repair, and finally be absorbed and metabolized by the body.

3. Low clinical application cost

The materials with non-expensive can be suitable for civilian consumption. And the materials should be relatively easy to prepare and obtain, so they can finally achieve the wide application.

3.2.2 Composition and classification of biomedical polymers

Biomedical polymer materials can be divided into natural and synthetic biomedical polymer materials according to their sources. These two kinds of materials have their own advantages and disadvantages. Usually, the natural polymers have good biocompatibility and the synthetic polymers have good mechanical properties. Among them, natural biomedical polymer materials are usually a kind of macromolecular materials extracted from living organisms or directly obtained in the natural environment, mainly including natural polysaccharides and natural protein materials, animals or human body's own acellular matrix materials, and natural polymer materials from microbial fermentation. Synthetic biomedical polymer materials can also be subdivided into non-degradable and degradable biomedical polymer materials.

The chemical structures of some common natural biomedical polymers are shown in Figure 3-1. Natural polysaccharides materials mainly include starch/cellulose/chitosan and their derivatives, alginate, hyaluronic acid, heparin and chondroitin sulfate, etc. Natural protein materials mainly include collagen, gelatin, silk fibroin, albumin and soybean protein. The acellular matrix materials of animal or human body can come from small intestine, bladder, skin, bone, heart, heart valve and others. The natural macromolecular materials derived from microbial fermentation include poly (3-hydroxybutyrate), poly (γ-glutamic acid) and poly (ε-lysine), etc. Natural biomedical polymer materials are abundant and easy to obtain, generally display good biocompatibility and biodegradability. They have been widely used in pharmaceutical excipients, absorbable sutures, medical isolation membranes, wound repair membranes, wound dressings, medical adhesives, artificial skin, degradable tissue engineering scaffolds, and nano-drug carriers. However, natural biomedical polymer materials also have some defects, such as potential immunogenicity, complex structure, difficult to chemical modification and poor mechanical properties of proteins and acellular matrix materials.

Among the synthetic polymer materials, non-degradable materials are the first polymer materials used in the field of biomedicine. They are characterized by long-term stability under the physiological environment, not prone to degradation, cross-linking reaction or physical wear, and have excellent mechanical properties. Simultaneously, they generally have poor adhesion to cells and tissues, poor matching of mechanical properties with surrounding tissues, and poor adaptability. They are mainly used in various medical devices and consumables, including packaging materials for medical products, *in vitro* diagnostic equipment, disposable medical products, medical protective equipment, interventional embolization materials, blood bags, ophthalmic lenses, artificial tissues, artificial organs, etc. The chemical structures of some common synthetic non-degradable biomedical polymers are shown in Figure 3-2.

Compared with non-degradable polymer materials, synthetic degradable materials are the new generation of medical materials and the hot-spot in the field of scientific research. Meanwhile, in recent years, synthetic degradable materials have been widely applied in the field of medicine and have achieved success in clinical practice, making them an important direction of future development. Degradable biomedical polymer materials refer to a kind of polymer materials that can be gradually degraded into low molecular weight compounds or monomers through hydrolysis and enzymolysis in biological environment, and the degradation products can be excreted from the body or participate in the normal metabolism in the body and disappear. Commonly-used degradable polymer materials include poly(lactic acid) (PLA), poly(glycolic acid) (PGA), poly(lactic-*co*-glycolic acid) (PLGA), polycarbonate (PC), poly (*p*-dioxanone) (PPDO), poly(ε-carprolactone) (PCL), poly(amino acid) (PA), polyphosphoester

(PPE), poly(ortho ester)(POE), polyanhydride, polyphophazene, etc. The corresponding chemical structures are shown in Figure 3-3.

In addition, biomedical polymers can also be divided into soft biomedical polymers, semi-crystalline biomedical polymers and other related biomedical polymers according to their structural characteristics, as shown in Table 3-4.

Table 3-4 Soft, semi-crystalline and other related biomedical polymers

Classification	Polymer name	Main applications
Soft biomedical polymers	Silicone rubber	Tissue substitutes, drug release devices, adhesives, tubular materials, contact lenses, etc.
	Poly(ether-urethane)	Blood pump, blood storage bag, artificial heart, tubular materials
	Poly(vinyl chloride)	Tubular materials, blood storage bag
	Rubber	Tubular materials
Semi-crystalline biomedical polymers	Polyester	Vascular grafts, sutures, heart valve suture rings
	Polytetrafluoroethylene	Vascular grafts, blood, oxygenator membranes
	Nylon 66	Sutures, dressings
	Polyethylene	Artificial joints, intrauterine devices, drug release devices
	Cellulose	Kidney dialysis membrane, drug release device, contact lenses
Other related biomedical polymers	Poly(alkyl methacrylate)	Hard and soft contact lenses, dental fillings, bone cement, endophthalmoscopes
	Poly(methacrylate β-hydroxyethyl ester)	Soft contact lenses, burns dressings, coated drug release matrix
	Poly(methacrylic acid)	Soft contact lenses, biological function fine beads
	Polyacrylamide	Soft contact lenses, biological function fine beads
	Poly(N-vinylpyrrolidone)	Soft contact lenses, pre-generation plasma expanders
	Poly cyanoacrylate	Tissue adhesive, vascular closure agent
	Zinc polyacrylate	Dental cement

3.3 Preparation and Modification of Biomedical Polymers

3.3.1 Purpose and significance of preparation and modification of biomedical polymers

In biological research and long-term clinical practice, scientists have gradually realized that direct use of a unitary polymer material is often difficult to achieve the desired results. For example, the mechanical strength of polymer materials is inconsistent with the mechanical strength of human tissues, and the adhesion between the polymer materials and the tissue interface is weak. The mechanical properties of materials are lost too quickly during the degradation process, and the degradation time is different from the working time *in vivo*. Non-specific adsorption of tissue or blood components, which in turn triggers intractable problems such as local inflammation. In addition, considering that nanodrug needs to overcome multiple physiological barriers in order to achieve the successful delivery of the drug in the body, it is required that the prepared polymer drug carrier exhibits a variety of functions and has multiple responsiveness. It is necessary to design new synthetic ideas, explore new synthetic methods, and modify and improve traditional polymer materials. Therefore, the prospect of synthesizing ideal medical polymer materials with biomedical functions through the approach of molecular design is very broad, and the final realization of biomedical polymer materials with outstanding performance is one of the important directions for future development.

3.3.2 Design of biomedical polymers

Differing from the general polymer materials, biomedical polymer materials will directly contact and interact with the living organisms. In addition to the aforementioned physical and chemical performance requirements of general materials, special performance demanding in biomedical fields must also be fulfilled. Therefore, the design scheme of biomedical polymer materials needs to be comprehensively considered in terms of raw material selection, synthesis strategy, material structure and physical morphology. At the same time, the goal of biomedical polymer synthesis is to bring new functions (e. g., intelligence, targeting, responsiveness, and visualization), and to optimize material properties (e. g., biocompatibility, hydrophilicity and hydrophobicity, and mechanical properties). At present, the design methods of biomedical polymers mainly include the synthesis of new biomedical polymers, and the modification of traditional polymers. Whether it is for the design and synthesis of new biomedical polymers, or for the modification and improvement of traditional polymers, the structure and composition of existing materials can be enriched, the vacancy of existing materials can be filled, and the biomedical polymer materials with new properties and special functions can be obtained.

To prepare biomedical polymers, the common design and synthesis methods mainly include polymerization, organic synthesis and physical blending. In recent years, benefiting from the rapid development of "living" controllable polymerization technology, a series of biomedical polymers prepared by functional monomers through polymerization have been successively designed and developed, and some of them have been clinically applied in the biomedical field. Meanwhile, the efficient organic synthesis reaction such as click-chemistry also provides sufficient possibility and conditions for the modification of biomedical polymers. In addition to polymerization, organic synthesis and other chemical methods, physical blending is also one of the effective strategies to obtain new medical polymer materials.

3.3.3 Preparation methods for biomedical polymers

The construction process of biomedical polymer materials can be divided into two stages: the first stage is the synthesis of polymer compounds, and the second stage is the molding of polymer materials. This textbook only focuses on the first stage of the construction of biomedical polymer materials. For the second stage of polymer material molding and processing knowledge, please refer to extended reading 4 & 5.

In the synthesis stage of polymer compounds, the raw materials for polymerization need to be prepared and refined first. Commonly-used raw materials include monomers, initiators, chain transfer agents, catalysts, and other components required for polymerization, such as solvents, dispersant, and emulsifier. The refining process refers to the purification steps of monomers, initiators, solvents, etc. The purpose is to remove polymerization inhibitors and other impurities, so as to avoid unforeseen side reactions and affect the smooth progress of the polymerization reaction. Generally speaking, liquid raw materials can take advantage of their relatively low boiling point and can be purified by atmospheric distillation or vacuum distillation, and can also be separated and purified by alkaline alumina column by using the polar difference of the components. For solid raw materials, the difference in solubility of components in different solvents can be used to purify by recrystallization.

The polymerization reaction is the process of repeatedly linking small molecules of monomeric compounds through covalent bonds to form polymers, and the final product is the polymer. It is well known that the structure of polymer materials determines the properties, which ultimately determine its usage and effects. Therefore, the synthesis of polymers is the basis and key link in the construction of polymer materials. According to the different principles of polymerization, it can be divided into two types: stepwise polymerization and chain polymerization, among which stepwise polymerization usually refers to bifunctional or multifunctional monomers, using condensation polymerization (e.g., polycondensation) or addition polymerization. Chain polymerization implies that monomers containing carbon-carbon double bonds and other unsaturated bonds generate polymer chains through chain polymerization. During the polymerization process, there are active centers (e. g. , radicals or ions), mainly including three elementary reactions of chain initiation, chain growth and chain termination. According to different active centers, chain polymerization can be subdivided into ionic polymerization (e. g. , anionic polymerization, cationic polymerization), coordination (directional) catalytic polymerization, and free radical polymerization. It should be pointed out that the initiation chain transfer terminator method, the nitroxide-mediated living free-radical polymerizations (NMP), atom transfer radical polymerization (ATRP), and reversible addition fragmentation chain transfer polymerization (RAFT), belong to living/controllable free radical polymerization. It is a research hotspot in the field of polymer synthesis and has been widely used in the preparation of biomedical polymer materials. Figure 3-4 shows the classification diagram of polymerization reactions.

Step polymerization is the formation of oligomers (e. g. , dimers and trimers) through condensation or addition reactions between monomer functional groups, and then the oligomers are gradually transformed into high polymers. Therefore, it usually takes a long reaction time to reach high molecular weight. In addition, most stepwise polymerization reactions are reversible, meaning the polymerization and depolymerization occurs at the same time, while the conversion rate and molecular weight increase proportionally with time.

Chain polymerization takes free radicals, anions, or cations as the active center for chain growth. Since the active center is extremely active, the chain polymerization can reach high molecular weight instantly, and the extension of the time only increases the conversion rate of the monomer. The characteristics and comparison of common chain polymerization are shown in Table 3-5.

Table 3-5 Characteristics of common chain polymerization

Polymerization	Radical polymerization	Anionic polymerization	Cationic polymerization	Coordination (directed) catalytic polymerization
Active center	Free radicals	Carbanion	Carbocation	Anionic properties
Active center formation method	Homolysis of covalent bond	Heterolysis of covalent bond, electron-donating group	Heterolysis of covalent bond, electron-deficient group	The monomer π electron enters the empty orbital of the electrophilic metal, coordinates to form a π complex, and further forms a transition state

Continued

Polymerization	Radical polymerization	Anionic polymerization	Cationic polymerization	Coordination (directed) catalytic polymerization
Initiator	Azo compounds, peroxides	Lewis base, alkali metal, organometallic compounds, carbanion, nucleophilic reagents	Lewis acid, protonic acid, carbocation, electrophilic reagents	Ziegler-Natta initiators, metallocene initiators
Initiation rate	Very slow, requires heat, light, electricity, etc.	When the monomer and initiator are matched properly, the polymerization rate is faster		Related to the adsorption process and catalyst specific surface area
monomer	Most vinyl monomers, conjugated monomers	Conjugated vinyl monomers with electron withdrawing groups	Conjugated vinyl monomers with electron-donating groups	Most olefin and diene monomers
Characteristics of polymerization mechanism	Slow initiation, fast growth, fast termination, chain transfer	Fast initiation, slow growth, no termination, no chain transfer	Fast initiation, fast growth, difficult to terminate, chain transfer, mainly to monomer or solvent transfer, or single molecule spontaneous termination	Coordination, four-membered ring transition state, monomer insertion, anionic growing chain end
Polymerization activation energy	High	Low			
Polymerization temperature	Generally 50-120 ℃	Low temperature, too high temperature will reduce the degree of polymerization		

Free radical polymerization reaction is a kind of chain polymerization reaction, which is the most common in the field of polymer synthesis, and the most convenient experimental operation and the highest degree of industrialization. However, common free radical polymerization has some defects or deficiencies. For example, the molecular weight distribution is relatively wide, and the polymer dispersibility index (PDI) is often higher than 2.0. The polymer molecular weight and molecular structure are difficult to control, and branching and cross-linking often occur. In order to overcome the above problems, active controllable free radical polymerization can effectively inhibit double radical termination and chain transfer reactions by reducing the concentration and reactivity of free radicals (e. g., active center), making it achieves negligible purpose, thus, the chain growth reaction is absolutely dominant. Living controllable free radical polymerization, such as NMP, ATRP, RAFT, has been widely studied, which has become one of the important directions of academic significance and application value in the field of polymer science. Compared with common free radical polymerization, the most significant advantage of active controllable free radical polymerization is that the molecular weight of the polymer is controllable and the molecular weight distribution is very narrow ($1.0 < PDI < 1.5$). At the same time, according to the specific monomer feeding order, it can design and synthesize block copolymers with specified segment structure and topological structures (e. g., star, comb, cyclic, graft polymer).

Because of the different polymerization mechanisms, the polymerization process is implemented in different ways (Figure 3-5). The polymerization methods of step polymerization include melt condensation polymerization, interfacial condensation polymerization, solution condensation polymerization and solid-phase condensation polymerization. The polymerization methods of chain polymerization include bulk polymerization, suspension polymerization, solution polymerization and emulsion polymerization. Melt condensation polymerization is a polycondensation reaction that is carried out above the melting point of monomer and polymer (generally 10-25 ℃ higher than the melting point of the resulting polymer). The reaction temperature is much higher than chain polymerization, generally above 200 ℃. Interfacial condensation polymerization refers to the polycondensation reaction of monomers and catalysts in different phases and the monomers at the phase interface of the multiphase system. Solution condensation polymerization is a polycondensation reaction in which monomers and catalysts are completely dissolved in the solvent. Solid-phase condensation polymerization refers to a polycondensation reaction in which raw materials (e. g., monomers and catalysts) are below their melting point or softening point. The polycondensation reaction is characterized by the reaction between different functional groups to form the target polymer, and the formation of low molecular by-products (e. g., water and ammonia).

The crude product system synthesized by the polymerization reaction is generally a multi-component mixed system, including the target polymer, the remaining monomers that have not participated in the reaction, residual initiators, chain transfer agents, catalysts, reaction solvents, etc. In order to obtain a pure target polymer, the crude product system needs to be purified, the polymer must be separated from other impurities, and the solvent must be removed. Common laboratory separation is mainly divided into two steps. Firstly, the target polymer is separated from the liquid medium, and then the residual volatile components (e. g. , solvent) are removed. The commonly-used methods of separating target polymer from liquid medium include chemical destruction coagulation separation, centrifugal separation, dialysis separation, etc. The principle of chemical destruction coagulation separation is that the target polymer and the remaining impurity components interact with the precipitation solvent, acid, alkali, and salt to break the original mixed state, utilizing the significant difference in solubility between the target polymer and the impurities in the precipitation solvent. The solid polymer is precipitated in the form of precipitation or crystallization, thereby achieving the goal of separating the polymer. The principle of the centrifugal separation is to use the effect of centrifugal force and gravity, use the sedimentation of polymer and other solid particles in the liquid medium, or use the different specific gravity of each component of the heterogeneous system to separate the solid and liquid phases. Dialysis separation utilizes that monomers, catalysts, initiators and other small molecules in solution can pass through the dialysis membrane, while polymers and other large molecules cannot pass through the dialysis membrane to achieve separation and purification. The method to remove volatile components such as solvents is to change the volatile components from liquid to gas, and then remove the gaseous components through volatilization. The separation efficiency is determined by the concentration difference of the gas-liquid interface and the diffusion coefficient. The achieved concentration is determined by the vapor-liquid equilibrium.

When biomedical materials are applied to the human body, human tissue cells or blood first come into contact with the surface of the material and produce a certain response. Unfortunately, most biomedical materials cannot adapt and accommodate each other with cells or blood. In other words, they do not have good histocompatibility and blood compatibility, which will eventually cause serious rejection of the body and lead to the loss of biomedical value of the materials. Therefore, in order to enable biological materials to stimulate appropriate response capabilities and exhibit good biocompatibility, the surface of the materials needs to be decorated and modified accordingly. Optimizing and improving biocompatibility has become a core issue in broadening the application of biomedical polymer materials in the biomedical field. Therefore, the surface modification of biomedical polymer materials has important research significance and practical value. Commonly-used modification methods include physical modification, chemical modification, and biomimetic modification, as shown in Table 3-6.

Table 3-6　The surface modification methods of biomedical polymer materials

Surface modification methods		Modification targets
Physical modification	Physical blending	Improve the anticoagulant properties of the surface of biomedical polymer materials
	Surface coating	
Chemical modification	Optical/mechanical chemical modification	Oxidation, surface roughening, introducing different groups or polymer chains, etc.
	The treatment of low temperature plasma	
	Ultraviolet/ray radiation	
	The treatment of corona discharge	
	Flame treatment	
Biomimetic modification	Surface heparinization	Cross-linking, introducing functional groups
	Surface phospholipidization	
	Surface endothelialization (endothelial cell fixation)	

Physical modification usually refers to wrapping a layer of biocompatible film or polymer through layer-by-layer self-assembly technology or physical adsorption. For example, on the surface of biomedical polymer material, the anticoagulant coating can passivate the surface of the polymer material so that the blood will not contact directly with the surface of the polymer material, which is an effective method to improve the anticoagulant blood on the surface of biomedical polymer material. A variety of polymer materials processing methods are also effective means to prepare biomedical polymer materials with different morphological structures, physicochemical properties and surface interface properties, among which physical blending is an important method to construct functional biomedical polymer materials. For example, poly (lactic acid) is a biomedical polymer material with good biocompatibility, biodegradability and machinability, but its application scope in biomedical field is severely limited due to its slow degradation rate *in vivo*, high hydrophobicity and low impact strength. In order to solve the above problems, scientists have combined poly(lactic acid) with other kinds of biomedical polymers (e. g. , chitosan, hyaluronic acid, poly (glycolic acid), poly (ethylene glycol), and polycaprolactone) to construct the composite biomedical polymer materials with excellent performance, which have been successfully applied to drug carriers, shape memory materials and tissue engineering scaffolds. In addition, in order to improve the blood compatibility of polysulfone, scientists have synthesized the amphiphilic anticoagulant additive copolymer (2-methacryloyloxyethyl phosphorylcholine-*n*-dodecyl methacrylate ester and 2-methacryloyloxyethyl phosphorylcholine-*n*-butyl methacrylate copolymer) physically blended with polysulfone. The blended amphiphilic copolymer anticoagulant additive can enrich and wrap on the polysulfone surface to reduce the free energy of the interface, which can improve the blood compatibility of the polysulfone dialysis membrane, and construct an anticoagulant material with excellent performance.

Coating the surface of biomedical polymer materials (e. g. , surface coating technology) is also one of the main methods for surface modification of biomedical polymer materials. By adding an anticoagulant coating on the surface of biomedical polymer materials, the surface of sensitive biomaterials is passivated. Thus, blood cannot directly contact with it, thereby effectively improving the biocompatibility of the material. For example, by applying anticoagulant substances, fibrin is produced on the outer surface of the biomedical polymer, which reduces the coagulation of platelets, so that the medical polymer material has anticoagulant properties on the surface. Generally speaking, commonly-used anticoagulant substances mainly include styrene and its conversion products, epoxy resin, acrylate conversion products, etc. These substances have strong viscosity and can be used on the surface of medical devices to avoid falling off. Another method is to mix the anticoagulant substance with the basic material to make it have anticoagulant properties. Generally, the base material can aggregate on the surface and has a certain degree of anticoagulation to mix the copolymer, which can effectively play a role in medical treatment.

The physical modification has the advantage of simple and convenient operation, but it only acts on the surface of the biomedical polymer material through physical adsorption. The weak interaction force results in poor stability, and it may fall off the surface of the substrate. Surface grafting modification by chemical methods is an important way for biomedical polymer modification. The surface layer constructed by the improved method is covalently bonded to the substrate through a covalent bond, and will not easily fall off. Commonly-used modification methods include introduction of functional groups through efficient click chemistry and other reactions, bonding polymer chains, coupling biologically active macromolecules, etc. In addition, it is well known that many biomedical polymer materials have good biocompatibility (e. g. , common polysiloxane, polytetrafluoroethylene, poly(lactic acid), polycaprolactone). Due to the long-chain structure of polymers, they are easily fused with blood. Utilizing the relatively stable performance of polyoxyethylene in hemolysis, the biomedical polymer and polyoxyethylene are fused together to form a water-soluble long-chain structure, so as to minimize the impact of the biomedical polymer on blood proteins and prevent the adsorption of blood. In addition, most biomedical polymers themselves cannot achieve antibacterial, self-repair, drug sustained release and other functions. At the same time, these polymers themselves do not have reactive sites or reactive chemical groups, which often makes it difficult to achieve the desired effect of using functional materials. Therefore, in order to construct biomedical polymer materials with multiple responsiveness and functionality, it is particularly important to modify the surface of the above-mentioned polymers. At present, commonly-used surface modification methods include chemical solution treatment (e. g. , oxidation, sulfonation, immersion, and hydrolysis), low-temperature plasma treatment, ultraviolet/ray radiation, atomic layer deposition, electrochemistry, atomic force microsurgery and other technologies and strategies.

Plasma is the fourth state of matter after solid, liquid, and gas. When the applied voltage reaches the breakdown voltage, gas molecules are ionized to produce a mixture of a large number of active particles, including electrons, ions, atoms, radicals, and free radicals, which can provide conditions for plasma technology to modify the surface of materials through chemical reactions. The use of low temperature plasma to modify biomedical polymer materials means treating the surface of polymer materials with plasma. Typically, place them in methane, nitrogen, oxygen or rare gases, and generate plasma through the principle of high-voltage discharge. The energic particles and the active substance react with the surface of the polymer material, to improve the surface structure and to achieve the purpose of surface modification. In addition, polymerizable gases (e. g. , methane) can form a polymer film on the surface of biomedical polymer materials and improve the adhesion of the materials. The ultraviolet/ray radiation method uses ultraviolet or ray to radiate biomedical polymer materials, so that the surface is heat and active groups and active substances can be attached to the surface. The advantages of this method are simple operation and low cost, and its anticoagulation effect is good.

Surface biomimetic modification is one of the ideal methods to improve the blood compatibility of biomedical polymer materials. Biomimetic modification prevents polymer compounds from being treated as foreign bodies by the blood, thus they will not be cleared and metabolized in the body. There are three common biomimetic approaches: surface heparinization, surface phospholipidization, and surface endothelialization.

Heparin was firstly discovered from the liver and got its name. It is a natural anticoagulant substance in animals and one of the first natural anticoagulant drugs to be recognized and studied. Fixing heparin molecules on the surface of biomedical polymer materials is an important way to improve the anticoagulant properties of the materials. The methods used include physical adsorption and chemical bonding. Although the physical adsorption method is not very strong, it has the advantage of keeping the conformation of heparin unchanged. The structure of the chemical bonding method is stable, but it is not easy to maintain the original conformation of heparin, which reduces the anticoagulant performance. Phospholipids are the main components that make up the outer surface of biological membranes. The amphiphilic phosphorylcholine (PC) group in lecithin has strong anticoagulant activity. An effective way to improve the blood compatibility of biomedical polymer materials is to introduce phosphorylcholine groups into medical materials, which can make the surface of biomedical polymer materials phospholipidization.

Surface endothelialization is also called endothelial cell fixation. As we all know, because of the complex biological system components (e. g. , body fluid, enzymes, cells, free radicals) that biomedical polymer materials come into contact with, and the extremely complex biological environment, it is difficult to achieve great blood compatibility only by surface modification. Researchers have found that an important way to improve blood compatibility of materials is to cultivate human endothelial cells *in situ* on the surface of the material through the application of tissue engineering technology. The blood can flow normally without clotting through the physical barrier function of vascular endothelial cells and the regulation and maintenance of the dynamic balance between coagulation factors and anticoagulation factors. At present, the ideal method to improve the blood compatibility of materials is to plant and culture vascular endothelial cells on the surface of biomedical polymer materials. However, directly planting endothelial cells on the surface of the matrix materials not only proliferates slowly, but also easily falls off and separates. Therefore, endothelial cells can be fixed on the surface of the materials by covalent bonding, and then endothelial cells can be planted and cultured on it.

3.4   Challenges and Perspectives

3.4.1   Clinical development direction of biomedical polymers in the diagnosis and treatment of skin diseases

Biomedical polymers have developed into one of the important materials indispensables in the field of modern biomedicine. In the past decades, the research and clinical application of biomedical polymer materials have undergone a leap-forward transformation and development from biologically inert materials to biodegradable active materials, smart materials, and electronic information materials. The application of biomedical polymers in the fields of skin cosmetology and the diagnosis and treatment of skin diseases involves various fields such as bioimaging, nanodrug delivery system, transdermal drug delivery technology, immunotherapy, skin repair and regeneration, wearable skin devices and electronic skin, and has obtained remarkable results. Yet, so far, the types of materials involved in biomedical polymers are few, and they cannot adapt to or meet the complex functions of various organs of humans. The ideal goal of curing diseases through biomedical polymer materials is still far away, and in-depth research and exploration are urgently needed. Therefore, expanding the structure and composition of polymers, designing and synthesizing new polymer materials, and expanding new applicable fields are the future development directions.

In the medication fields of many chronic diseases and intractable diseases, natural medicines such as traditional Chinese medicines can give full play to their multi-target therapeutic effects. In addition, through modern technologies that have the systematic screening of natural substances, the effective components of drugs extracted from traditional Chinese medicines (e. g., camptothecin, paclitaxel) have been widely used in clinical chemotherapy for tumors. The promising modernization of traditional Chinese medicines and the natural polymers extracted from it will receive more and more attention in the industries of the skin beauty and the diagnosis and treatment of skin diseases, and will also be the future development directions.

In addition, in order to meet the needs of more extensive, smarter and more personalized clinical applications of biomedical polymer materials, while adapting and satisfying the complex functions of skin organs, the application of biomedical polymer materials in the skin field is also more diverse. The development of composite functional materials suitable for the special needs of skin beauty and dermatological diagnosis and treatment fields, timing, positioning, and quantitative precise smart drug formulations, the excellent properties of biomedical polymer materials are used. The construction of smart medical materials is another development direction for biomedical polymer materials in the future.

In China, the basic polymer research is at the forefront of the world, but the research and application of biomedical polymers in the field of skin beauty and the diagnosis and treatment of skin diseases started decades later than western countries. Therefore, there are not enough varieties, incomplete specifications, and unstable quality that are currently being developed, resulting in a big gap of R & D and production capabilities between China and the international levels. High-end biomedical polymer materials and products are largely dependent on imports. Professional biomedical polymer companies have problems such as small scale, few varieties, low R & D investment, and relatively low technical level. However, in recent years, the development of biomedical materials in China has been changing rapidly. It has demonstrated vigorous vitality and good development prospects, and has a number of international cutting-edge products, such as implantable biochips, tissue-inducing bone and cartilage, and tissue engineering products. Therefore, it has become a general trend that imported biomedical polymer material products are replaced by localization, which is another important direction for the development of biomedical polymer materials in the future. At the same time, with the improvement of people's living standards, the upgrading of medical consumption, and the continuous upgrading of medical products, the brand effect of biomedical polymer products will continue to improve and play an important role.

3.4.2 Medical economy and medical industries of biomedical polymer in skin cosmetology and the diagnosis and treatment of skin diseases

Health is the eternal dream of mankind and the goal of lifelong pursuit. Medical materials and related products are the material basis of health. Biomedical material in skin cosmetology and dermatological diagnosis and treatment is a "sunrise industry" with great potential. The future market of biomedical polymer materials has huge potential and full of opportunities, and is highly expected by the country and ordinary consumers. On the one hand, "The 14th Five-Year Development Plan" of the biological industry emphasizes the need to greatly improve the application level of new materials in the fields of biomedicine and high-performance medical devices. On the other hand, the average medical device cost in China is much lower than developed countries. Stimulated by huge population base, urbanization, and aging trends, biomedical materials will trigger a new round of rapid development in China. Due to the increase in the incidence of skin diseases, the increase in patients' self-diagnosis and treatment awareness, the strong demand for skin health and skin beauty, consumption upgrades, and the upgrading of high technology, the number of medical visits and hospitalizations in our country's hospitals continues to increase. In particular, skin health and skin beauty have attracted more and more attention from the public, and the growth rate is even more obvious. The continuous growth of medical demand has promoted the rapid and sustainable development of our country's medical service market, and the compound growth rate is expected to exceed 15% in the next five years.

With economic development and improved education levels, people's awareness of skin health and skin beauty has gradually increased, which will greatly enhance the market demand of China's dermatology medical service industry and bring huge space for industry development. In addition, modern women are no longer satisfied with basic skin care products for aesthetics and anti-aging needs. In this context, professional cosmetic dermatology has entered the lives of ordinary people recently. Different from the surgical treatment of plastic surgery, the non-surgical items of cosmetic dermatology are safe, efficient, convenient and fashionable. They are in line with the universal values of today's society and are expected to become another pillar industry of medical cosmetology after plastic surgery, and at the same time give birth to various medical cosmetology materials and products. Biomedical polymer materials will play a huge potential in the dermatological medical market and obtain more extensive clinical applications. At the same time, they will provide opportunities for the steady development of medical economy and medical industry of dermatological biomedical polymers, and will continue to explore new applicable fields.

Questions

1. Briefly describe the advantages and disadvantages of free radical polymerization, anionic polymerization, cationic polymerization and coordination (directed) catalytic polymerization.

2. Briefly describe several common methods of the synthesis of biomedical polymers.

3. Briefly describe several common methods of the surface modification of biomedical polymers.

4. What are the special performance requirements of biomedical polymers?

5. What kinds of biomedical polymers are commonly-used in the field of skin cosmetology?

Extended Reading

[1] 陈学思,陈红. 生物医用高分子[M]. 北京:科学出版社,2018.

〔2〕 赵长生,孙树东.生物医用高分子材料[M].2版.北京:化学工业出版社,2016.

〔3〕 Sahana T G,Rekha P D. Biopolymers:applications in wound healing and skin tissue engineering[J]. Mol Biol Rep,2018,45(6):2857-2867.

〔4〕 王小妹,阮文红.高分子加工原理与技术[M].北京:化学工业出版社,2006.

〔5〕 温变英.高分子材料成型加工新技术[M].北京:化学工业出版社,2014.

(Chen Senbin　Zhu Jintao)

第四章
皮肤防护、清洁与消毒

第一节　皮肤防护

（一）皮肤防护的概念

随着人类社会的发展和科学技术的进步，环境中能对皮肤造成伤害的因素越来越多，主要分为三种：物理因素，如放射性辐射、电、光、热、机械摩擦等；化学因素，如石油分馏产品、强酸、强碱、重金属、石棉等；生物因素，如细菌、真菌、病毒、昆虫叮咬、花粉等。因此，针对生产生活中这些危害皮肤健康的因素进行个人皮肤防护显得十分重要。

（二）皮肤防护用品分类

皮肤防护用品包括个人防护装备（personal protective equipment，PPE）和皮肤保护剂。

1. 个人防护装备（PPE）

PPE 是指作业者在工作中为免遭或减轻事故伤害和职业危害，个人随身穿（佩）戴的用品，如防护服、防护面罩和防护手套等（图 4-1）。

按使用对象不同，PPE 可分为以下几类：为军人配备的单兵防护装备，如防弹头盔、防弹衣、防毒面具、作战靴等；为警察配备的警员防护装备，如防爆服、防刺衣、防眩光眼镜等；为各行各业劳动者（如工农业生产人员、医务人员、科技工作者等）配备的劳动防护装备，涉及范围广泛。

按防护对象不同，PPE 可分为以下几类：物理防护装备，如绝缘手套、安全帽、耳罩等；化学防护装备，如防毒面具、防酸服、防碱服等；生物防护装备，如医用口罩、护目镜、医用防护服等；为公共场所配备的公共安全防护装备，如宾馆、民航客机等场所准备的逃生面具、救生衣等；个人生活中的防护装备，如防霾、防紫外线护目镜等。

按防护部位不同，PPE 可分为呼吸防护器、防护眼罩、防护面罩、护耳器、防护帽盔、防护服、防护手套和防护鞋套等。

总之，个人防护装备就是结合具体工作环境对工作人员的口、鼻、眼、耳、裸露皮肤等吸入、吸收部位及头部等易受伤部位实施相应保护的用品。

2. 皮肤保护剂

皮肤保护剂主要包括防护膏、皮肤清洁剂、皮肤防护膜、护肤霜及滋润性防护膏等。

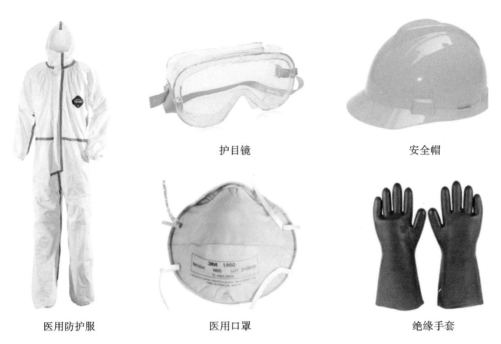

护目镜 安全帽

医用防护服 医用口罩 绝缘手套

图 4-1 常见的个人防护装备

Figure 4-1 Common personal protective equipment

（1）防护膏：防止职业性皮肤疾病的护肤制剂，可用于预防生产中有害物质作用于暴露的皮肤。防护膏的性质分为易溶于水和不溶于水两类。将防护膏涂在皮肤上可形成一种黏性的被覆体或韧曲性的保护膜，从而对皮肤起机械保护作用或特殊保护作用，如氧化、还原、中和、络合或吸收有害物质等。常见的防护膏包括亲水性防护膏、疏水性防护膏和遮光性护肤膏等。

①亲水性防护膏：含油脂量少，涂于皮肤表面能够起到耐油作用，于接触矿物油、有机酸等作业时使用。

②疏水性防护膏：含油脂量多，涂于皮肤表面可以堵塞毛孔，起到防止水溶性物质（如低浓度酸、碱、盐类液体）的滴溅伤害的作用。

③遮光性防护膏：涂抹后有避光作用，主要用于预防沥青、焦油等光敏性物质对皮肤的刺激作用，于接触焦油、接触沥青、电焊及雪中作业时使用。人们日常使用的防晒霜也属于其中一种。

（2）皮肤清洗剂：主要用于洗涤皮肤表面的各种污染，特别是对于毒、尘接触作业人员，需要及时清理、去除附着在皮肤和工作服上的毒物。最常用的皮肤清洗剂是肥皂，但许多作业中接触到的化学物品不易被肥皂洗净，而且肥皂洗涤时会损伤一部分皮肤脂肪。难去除的油污可以使用有机溶剂（如汽油、煤油、松节油等）洗去，但这些溶剂本身会引起或者加剧皮肤的损害。

（3）皮肤防护膜：又称隐形手套，通常是将纤维素、干酪素、松香等溶于酒精等中制成；涂抹后可在皮肤表面形成耐油、耐水、耐刺激的薄膜，适用于电镀、刷油漆、印染等工作场所。

（4）护肤霜及滋润性防护膏：含油脂多，通常加入高蛋白、蜂王浆、珍珠粉等容易被人体吸收的物质，具有滋润、保护皮肤的作用。其适合在长期接触水分、碱性溶液和有机溶剂后，皮肤出现脱脂时使用。

相较个人防护装备存在的不严密、不舒适、易渗漏以及影响工作等缺陷,皮肤保护剂更为轻便,能直接在皮肤表面发挥防护作用,但防护效果可能不如个人防护装备。

（三）日常皮肤防晒

1. 紫外线对皮肤的影响

日常生活中,太阳光辐射中的紫外线是最常见的造成皮肤损伤的原因。根据波长的不同,紫外线可分为长波紫外线(ultraviolet A,UVA)、中波紫外线(ultraviolet B,UVB)和短波紫外线(ultraviolet C,UVC)三个区段,其中到达地面的成分为 95% 左右的 UVA 和 5% 左右的UVB,而 UVC 基本被臭氧层吸收而无法到达地面。长时间暴露于阳光下而未采取任何保护措施时,阳光中的紫外线会对皮肤产生不同程度的伤害。紫外线照射皮肤的过程中会产生自由基及氧化副产物,对皮肤细胞的 DNA、脂质及蛋白质造成破坏,造成皮肤红斑、黑化、光老化、免疫功能异常和皮肤肿瘤等。

紫外线造成的皮肤损伤主要包括以下几种。

①红斑反应:即日晒红斑,为急性炎症反应。晒后 2~7 h 出现,12~24 h 达高峰,主要表现为日晒部位出现红斑、肿胀,重者发生水疱,自觉灼痛。数日后红斑消退,出现脱屑。浅肤色的人更易发生,作用光谱主要为 UVB。

②皮肤黑化:即皮肤晒黑。表现为光照部位边界清晰的灰黑色斑,无自觉症状。根据色素出现的时间,皮肤黑化可分为以下几种。

a. 即刻性黑化(immediate pigment darkening):照射过程中或照射后立即发生的灰黑色色素沉着,一般仅持续数分钟至 2 h。

b. 持续性黑化(persistent pigment darkening):随着 UV 剂量加大,可与红斑反应重叠发生,皮肤变为灰黑色或深棕色,高峰期在 2~24 h,可持续数小时至数天。

c. 延迟性黑化(delayed tanning):照射后数日内发生,可持续数周至数月。即刻性黑化和持续性黑化是通过氧化黑素颗粒并输送到角质形成细胞而产生的,作用光谱是 UVA 和可见光。延迟性黑化则是由黑素细胞功能活跃,合成更多的黑素引起的,作用光谱包括 UVB、UVA、可见光。

③皮肤光老化:长期日光照射会加速皮肤衰老,这一变化主要由 UVA 引起。表现为光暴露部位皮肤粗糙、皱纹增多和色素加深,皮肤弹性降低,毛细血管扩张或增生、红斑形成。

④免疫功能异常:皮肤受到紫外线照射后,不但会导致照射部位发生皮肤光变态反应,还会导致局部皮肤和全身免疫系统的功能异常。光线引起的免疫改变涉及免疫活性细胞、细胞因子、补体以及这些物质之间的相互作用,多种光线性疾病、光加剧皮肤疾病均与之有关。

⑤皮肤肿瘤:UVB 照射导致细胞核碱基结构改变,UVA 诱导细胞产生活性氧簇,引起细胞膜结构异常,DNA 变性,破坏脂质、蛋白质,导致光线性角化病、基底细胞癌、鳞状细胞癌、黑素瘤等。

2. 常见防晒措施及用品

2002 年世界卫生组织(World Health Organization,WHO)提出紫外线指数(ultraviolet index,UVI),用以表示日光紫外线强度。通常,UVI 越高,日光对皮肤和眼睛的伤害越大。一般中午时分为 UVI 最高的时段,而春末和夏季是 UVI 较高的季节;UVI 随海拔升高而增高。另外,海边沙滩、雪地、城市高层建筑的墙面或幕墙玻璃、汽车窗玻璃以及沥青或水泥硬化的地面都会反射紫外线,从而增高 UVI。日常防晒措施主要包括遮挡性防晒及使用防晒剂。

(1) 遮挡性防晒:利用防晒伞、遮阳镜、防晒帽、防晒衣或防晒口罩等遮挡物遮挡身体裸露部位。遮挡物通过阻挡紫外线以达到防晒效果。遮挡物的织纱密度越高、颜色越深或遮挡物加有防晒涂层,则其遮挡能力越强,防晒效果越好。如使用防晒帽,则帽檐的边长最好在 7.5 cm 以上,这样才有较好的防晒效果。同时,建议选购紫外线防护系数(UPF)大于 25,UVA 透过率小于 5% 标识的织物产品(表 4-1)。如使用遮阳镜,应选购覆盖全部 UV 的遮阳镜,并尽量减少蓝光和紫光透过。

表 4-1   织物防紫外线照射指标(《皮肤防晒专家共识(2017)》)

紫外线防护系数	防护分级	UVA 透过率/(%)	紫外线防护系数等级
15～25	较好	6.7～4.2	15,20
25～39	非常好	4.1～2.6	25,30,35
40～50,50＋	非常优异	≤2.5	40,45,50,50＋

(2) 使用防晒剂:防晒剂是利用对光的吸收、反射或散射作用,以保护皮肤免受特定 UV 伤害的物质。目前,市场上的防晒产品主要分为以紫外线吸收剂为主的有机防晒剂、以紫外线屏蔽剂为主的无机防晒剂以及间接起到防晒作用的抗氧化剂。

①有机防晒剂:又称化学性 UV 吸收剂。绝大部分有机防晒剂含有芳香基团类化合物,苯环上特殊基团的改变可影响防晒剂的光谱特性。一般而言,这类物质可选择性吸收 UV,从而发挥防晒作用。吸收 UVA 的防晒剂主要是丁基甲氧基二苯甲酰基甲烷等;吸收 UVB 的防晒剂主要有水杨酸盐及其衍生物和肉桂酸酯类等;对两者兼可吸收的有二苯甲酮及其衍生物等。有机防晒剂具有质地轻薄、透明感好的优点,但也有一些缺点,如光稳定性较差、易透皮吸收、致敏等。近年来,大量新型有机防晒剂不断上市,这些防晒剂通过异构化、微粒化等方式显著提高了溶解性和光稳定性,并且不易透皮吸收,安全有效,因此备受市场青睐。

②无机防晒剂:又称物理 UV 屏蔽剂。这类防晒剂主要通过反射或散射日光从而发挥防晒作用,如二氧化钛(TiO_2)、氧化锌(ZnO)。主要作用原理是在皮肤表面形成一层均匀的保护层,该保护层可对紫外线进行反射、折射和散射,从而减少紫外线对皮肤的伤害。近年来的研究发现,无机防晒颗粒具有类半导体性能,其内电子跃迁过程可选择性吸收 UV 而发挥防晒作用。无机防晒剂防晒谱宽、相对光稳定。同时这类防晒剂不易致敏,因而适用于皮肤敏感的人群。然而,这类防晒剂存在不易涂抹、不透明、容易有白色残留物影响美观等缺点,并且过多使用易堵塞毛孔,会造成新的皮肤疾病。

③抗氧化剂:这类防晒剂对日光没有直接吸收或反射作用,但将其加入化妆品后可提高皮肤抗氧化能力,从而间接地发挥防晒作用。这类化合物主要是一些植物提取物如维生素 C 或维生素 E、β 胡萝卜素、金属硫蛋白、超氧化物歧化酶(superoxide dismutase,SOD)、花青素、四氢甲基嘧啶羧酸(Ectoin)。甘草、芦荟、绿茶、三七、葡萄籽等中也含有抗氧化剂。

综上,目前各类防晒剂各有利弊。但为了同时覆盖 UVB 和 UVA,兼顾安全性和适用性,多数防晒化妆品是用不同作用机制的原料复配,从而获得更好的防晒效果。

(四)防护用品带来的皮肤损伤

尽管使用皮肤防护用品的目的是保护皮肤,但是反复或长时间的接触防护用品可能会引起皮肤伤害。通常,个人防护装备透气性不强并且会摩擦和压迫皮肤,而皮肤保护剂具有一定程度的可吸收性和致敏性。尽管防护的目标和用品的材质可能不同,但用于人体同一部位的防护用品可能会引起类似的皮肤问题。

1. 皮肤压力性损伤

包括呼吸防护器(如头盔、各类口罩、防毒面具)以及护目镜在内的防护用具常常会造成面部和耳部皮肤的损伤。由于密闭性的要求,此类防护用具需要紧贴于皮肤表面。这会使固定部位皮肤长期处于受压状态,容易出现器械相关压力性损伤。受压部位局部血液循环不佳,组织缺血缺氧。皮肤蒸发及口鼻呼出的大量水汽聚集在口罩和面具内侧,从而使面部皮肤长期处于潮湿的环境中。皮肤在潮湿的环境中软化浸渍,进而导致角质层对抗外界压力和剪切力的能力下降,皮肤更容易出现压痕(图4-2)。与此同时,由于活动过程中防护用具常常在皮肤受压点附近来回摩擦,这更易使皮肤发红,严重者有水疱形成和破溃,继而引发疼痛甚至继发感染。

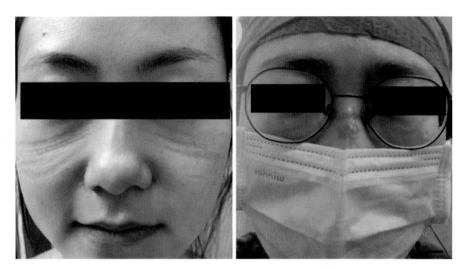

图 4-2 防护用品带来的皮肤压力性损伤照片

Figure 4-2 Photos of skin pressure injuries caused by protective products

2. 毛囊炎

长时间戴头盔或帽子可能会导致毛囊炎。头皮的毛囊、皮脂腺及汗腺丰富,因而油脂、汗液分泌较多。由于头发、帽子、头盔等透气性差,头皮分泌的汗液和油脂混合后停留在头部皮肤表面会堵塞毛孔。同时,由于细菌在头皮定植,容易引起毛囊炎,炎症加重则会出现脓疱、疖、脂溢性皮炎,继发真菌感染等皮损。

3. 皮肤真菌、细菌感染

为了彻底隔绝环境中有害物质的接触,手套和防护服多以橡胶、塑料等透气性极差的防水材料制成。在长时间不透气的环境中,皮肤的汗液蒸发受阻。此时,皮肤容易出现浸渍、湿疹、汗疱疹等症状;同时,湿热环境也利于细菌、真菌繁殖。特别是外阴、股内侧及肛周部位,由于存在排泄物的刺激,且行走时常常被反复摩擦,更易出现皮肤炎症及继发细菌、真菌感染。

4. 湿疹

在化学和生物防护中,手部保护除了戴手套外,还需要保持手卫生。然而,反复的清洗会导致皮肤表面油脂减少,从而破坏正常的皮肤屏障,使皮肤出现干燥和瘙痒等症状以及手足部湿疹。

5. 接触性皮炎

反复接触手消毒剂、手套等刺激性的物质后,部分人会出现接触性皮炎,伴有红斑、丘疹、丘疱疹、渗出或糜烂。研究发现,患手部湿疹的医务人员中有 52% 的人既往洗手频率大于 10 次/天。另外,长期接触消毒剂里的一些消毒成分会抑制皮肤表面寄生的正常菌群,使得皮肤表面的免疫微环境发生改变,进而可能导致接触性皮炎。汗液的刺激、使用防晒剂等也可能导致皮肤过敏反应。

6. 痤疮

防爆服、防刺衣等防护用品的材质硬度较大,可能会因为防护服边缘部位与皮肤的摩擦而引起器械相关压力性损伤。工业防护服、医用防护服密闭性高,会使全身皮肤处于湿润环境中,容易出现浸渍。而部分皮脂腺分泌旺盛的人,由于汗液和皮脂堵塞毛孔,容易在皮脂腺丰富的部位如胸背部出现痤疮。同时,无机防晒剂也容易堵塞毛孔从而引发痤疮。

(五)新型高分子材料在皮肤防护中的应用

随着工业的发展和科技的进步,人们对皮肤防护用品有了更高的要求。对于个人防护装备,不仅要实现防护功能,更要求穿戴舒适、简单、轻便。同时,皮肤防护剂如日常的防晒霜等,也需要更加安全有效。新型高分子材料的发展及其在皮肤防护领域的应用使人们的这些需求得以部分实现。

1. 新型高分子材料用于防护用品制造

(1)高性能防护服材料。

①聚对苯撑苯并双噁唑(poly (p-phenylene benzobisthiazole),PBO)纤维:PBO 纤维是经液晶纺丝技术,由 PBO 制得的高性能纤维。这种纤维的强度和模量是目前最高的,被认为是超级纤维。通常,PBO 纤维有 4 大优越性能:耐热和阻燃性能好;高强度、高模量、耐冲击和耐磨性强;化学稳定性强;表面粘接性能、耐光色牢度和染色性佳。PBO 纤维可用于制作耐热、阻燃以及高强度和高拉力的防护服,如消防服、炉前工作服、焊接工作服、防切割工作服和安全手套等。

②聚苯并咪唑(PBI)纤维:PBI 纤维的密度为 1.43 g/cm³,强度和伸长与粘胶纤维相似。该材料的特点如下:a. 优良的耐热性能,甚至可以在 350 ℃ 左右的温度下长期使用;b. 优良的纺织加工性能,其因具有较高的回潮率(约 15%),在加工过程中不会产生静电;c. 舒适性与天然纤维相似。PBI 纤维可用来制作高温炉前工、焊接工、翻砂工的防护服,还可用于制作赛车服、飞行服、救生服等。

③聚四氟乙烯(PTFE)纤维:PTFE 纤维的密度为 2.2 g/cm³,其拉伸强度不高,约为 13 cN/tex。该材料的特点如下:化学稳定性优异,其化学稳定性超过其他所有天然纤维和化学纤维;耐气候性最好,PTFE 纤维既能在高温条件下使用,也能在低温条件下使用;具有抗辐射性能且无毒性。PTFE 纤维在航空航天和医疗卫生领域有着重要用途,常被用于制作宇航服、屏蔽服和医疗防护服。

(2)防毒面罩材料:随着合成橡胶工业的发展,各国目前采用越来越多种类的综合性能优良的合成橡胶作为罩体材料,如丁基橡胶、氯化丁基橡胶、溴化丁基橡胶、硅橡胶、三元乙丙橡胶、聚氨酯等。其中,溴化丁基橡胶和硅橡胶是两大罩体材料。溴化丁基橡胶在硫化速度、耐老化性、黏合性、耐气候性、耐疲劳性方面比其他丁基类橡胶优异,因而更适合用于罩体材料。

而硅橡胶无味、无毒,具有优良的生理惰性和抗生理老化性,生物相容性优异,制成面罩后,其佩戴舒适性、适配性和面部密封性均非常好。

(3)口罩材料:医用口罩由口罩面体和拉紧带组成,其中口罩面体分为内、中、外三层,内层为亲肤材质(普通卫生纱布或无纺布)制成,中层为隔离过滤层(超细聚丙烯纤维熔喷材料层),外层为特殊材料抑菌层(无纺布或超薄聚丙烯熔喷材料层)。

口罩的防护性指标主要包括防护阻隔异物的过滤效率、防止外部液体侵入的防溅射性能和防止口罩形状不同而引起的异物吸入的密闭性。

长时间佩戴医用非织造口罩后,口罩的鼻梁条容易损伤鼻梁及颊部皮肤。同时,由于较差的吸湿性,这类口罩变湿后滤过性能会下降。此外,医用非织造口罩的原材料为热塑性聚合物,会加重后期处理的环保压力。

(4)防晒剂:新型防晒剂多应用纳米技术,主要分为两种:一种是将化妆品制成具有纳米级粒径的纳米粉体;另一种是使用纳米载体搭载紫外线吸收剂,常用的纳米载体主要包括脂质体、固体脂质纳米粒、纳米乳液、微球等。

物理性紫外线屏蔽剂中,氧化铁、二氧化钛、氧化锌、高岭土和滑石粉是常用的物质。通常纳米级粒子的粒径为几纳米或几十纳米,这种规格的二氧化钛、氧化锌、氧化铝或氧化铁等对紫外线具有良好的屏蔽作用。

不同的载体直接影响着防晒剂的性能。目前,在防晒剂领域使用的纳米系统包括聚合物和中孔二氧化硅纳米颗粒、脂质纳米颗粒、纳米乳剂,而非纳米系统包括微粒/微球、脂质体和环糊精。将这些载体应用于化妆品中可以起到提高活性组分的稳定性、促进渗透和降低刺激性等作用:①减少活性物质与皮肤的直接接触,从而降低潜在的毒理学风险;②减少活性物质的光降解,稳定防晒剂;③增强紫外线活性物质的作用或者减少紫外线吸收剂的使用,提高防晒效果;④消除配方中各种成分之间可能发生的不良相互作用。

根据不同防晒剂的性质,可以将不同的防晒剂进行复配以加强防晒效果。UVA防晒剂与UVB防晒剂的复配、有机防晒剂与无机防晒剂的复配等都可以提高防晒产品的性能,这也是目前改进防晒产品的一个重要研究方向。

2. 新型高分子材料用于解决防护用品使用中存在的问题

(1)高分子敷料预防PPE带来的面部压力性损伤:预防器械相关压力性损伤的关键是减轻皮肤局部压力和缩短压迫时间。在保证防护效果的前提下,材质柔软、可塑性强的PPE对皮肤的顺应性强,压力分布更为均匀,局部压强相对较小。在受压集中部位及反复摩擦部位,如额部护目镜上缘压迫处,可通过使用敷料来重新分布压力、减小压强及避免相对位移产生的摩擦从而预防压力性损伤。临床医疗中使用较多的水凝胶敷料、水胶体敷料及泡沫敷料等均可以起到预防压力性损伤的作用。

水凝胶是一类含水量丰富、具有三维网络结构的材料,有利于伤口愈合。水凝胶敷料具有良好的生物相容性和顺应性,多孔结构保障其透气性,并可通过吸收和释放水分来保证皮肤含水量适宜,还可以起到冷却和镇痛的效果(图4-3)。

水胶体敷料主要由包裹在弹/黏性合成基质中的吸水性羧甲基纤维素钠(carboxymethyl cellulose,CMC)颗粒构成,其外层是一种聚氨酯半透性薄膜,不仅可以阻隔微生物,还具有良好的顺应性,吸收水分后会形成一层凝胶,有利于减小皮肤组织直接受到的压力或剪切力。有研究表明,在使用水胶体敷料后,气管切开处器械相关性压力性损伤明显减轻。水胶体敷料在

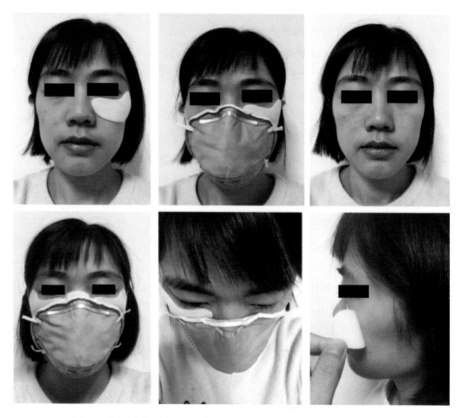

图 4-3　水凝胶敷料用于预防防护用品带来的皮肤压力性损伤照片

Figure 4-3　Photos of hydrogel dressings for the prevention of skin pressure injuries from protective products

头面部防护中的使用可以减轻护目镜等防护设备对面部的压力。

　　泡沫敷料厚度一般为 0.5 cm。该敷料中间垫有泡沫垫,因此能够有效地缓冲和分散局部压力。此外,该敷料柔滑、防水又透气,因此牢固粘贴后便可在局部形成保护膜,减小皮肤所受的压力和摩擦力。不仅如此,该敷料还可以吸收大量渗液,从而有效地预防浸渍,全面阻断潮湿对皮肤造成的侵蚀和刺激。然而,泡沫敷料的厚度及材质特点决定了其顺应性不如水凝胶敷料和水胶体敷料,使用过程中需注意不能影响护目镜和口罩的密闭性。

　　此外,各种新型伤口敷料对防护用品带来的皮肤损伤,尤其是压力性损伤有重要的治疗作用,其在保护创面的同时可加速伤口的愈合。

　　(2) 防雾涂层减少护目镜起雾:护目镜镜片材质主要为聚碳酸酯(polycarbonate, PC),耐冲击性强,且折射率高、镜片薄。针对这种透明塑料材料的防雾方法主要如下:①通过电、辐射等加热方式改变基材表面与空气的温差,防止雾化;②使用防雾剂来改变基材表面的润湿性,通过使基材表面亲水,水膜铺展,从而提高材料的透光率。第一种方法工艺复杂,使用的限制条件比较苛刻;第二种方法在日常生活中更为实用。根据防雾剂主要成分的不同,其可以分为表面活性剂型防雾剂、高分子型防雾剂、有机-无机杂化型防雾剂、光催化型超亲水防雾剂及特殊纳米结构超亲水防雾剂等。目前,国内外的研究人员在有机-无机杂化型以及纳米光催化型等新型防雾剂方面进行了很多研究,并取得了一定的进展。随着防护用品的应用日益广泛,用于透明塑料材料的防雾剂需要具备更加优异的性能来满足生产生活中的需求。

第二节　皮肤的清洁

（一）皮肤的类型及皮肤清洁的意义

1. 皮肤的类型

不同种族和个体的皮肤存在很大的差异，对皮肤的分类方法也有很多种。根据皮肤 pH、皮肤含水量、皮脂分泌情况和皮肤对外界刺激的反应性进行分类，是目前最方便且常用的方法。一般生理状态下，皮肤可分为以下四种类型（图 4-4）。

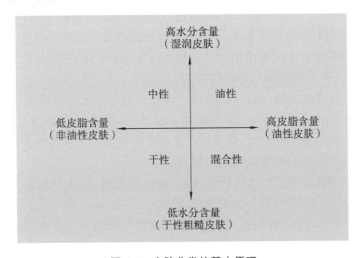

图 4-4　皮肤分类的基本原理

Figure 4-4　The basic principle of skin typing

（1）中性皮肤：即普通型皮肤，这是相对理想的皮肤类型。pH 为 4.5～6.5，角质层含水量在 20% 左右。皮脂分泌量适中，皮肤表面较为光滑、细腻、有弹性，无明显干燥感，对外界刺激有较强的适应能力。

（2）干性皮肤：又称干燥型皮肤。pH 大于 6.5，而角质层含水量低于 10%，皮脂分泌量较少而易感干燥，洗脸后常有紧绷感。此外，皮肤温度较低，毛孔不明显。对外界刺激较为敏感，易出现皱纹、脱屑甚至发生皲裂。干性皮肤除了与先天性因素有关，还与生活习惯密切相关，如经常风吹日晒或过多使用碱性洗涤剂等。

（3）油性皮肤：也称多脂性皮肤，多见于肥胖者及中青年人群。pH 常小于 4.5，角质层含水量为 20% 左右，皮脂分泌较为旺盛，皮肤外观常油腻发亮，从而易黏附灰尘。皮肤毛孔常常粗大，肤色往往较深，但弹性好且不容易出现皱纹，对外界刺激一般不敏感。雄激素分泌旺盛、喜好高脂食物者多为油性皮肤，且易发痤疮、脂溢性皮炎等皮肤疾病。

（4）混合性皮肤：中性、干性或油性混合存在的皮肤类型。多表现为面中央部位（即前额、鼻部、鼻唇沟及下颌部）呈油性，而双面颊、颞部等则为中性或干性皮肤。躯干部皮肤和毛发性状常与头面部一致，即干性皮肤者毛发亦显干燥，而油性皮肤者毛发亦多油。

2. 皮肤清洁的意义

皮肤表面常有生理性污垢和外源性污垢黏附，前者包括人体产生、分泌或排泄的各种代谢产物,如老化脱落的细胞、皮脂、汗液、黏膜和腔道的排泄物,后者包括微生物、环境污染物、各类化妆品和外用药物的残留。同时,皮肤疾病患者皮肤表面还有病理性污垢,如汗液、鳞屑、脓液和痂等。这些皮肤污垢会影响毛孔通畅,妨碍皮肤和黏膜正常生理功能的发挥。因此,正确地清洁皮肤尤为重要,也是保持皮肤健康的基本方法。此外,清洁皮肤还可促进皮肤血液循环、增进皮肤健康。

(二)皮肤清洁剂的分类及选用

1. 皮肤清洁剂的分类

尘土、金属或非金属的氧化物常以颗粒状物沉积在皮肤表面,通过清水即可以除掉。然而,呈膜状的油脂、脓液或污垢中的分子可以通过静电引力或分子间作用力与皮肤紧密贴合,则需要清洁剂才能清除。清洁剂通过润湿、渗透、乳化和分散等多种作用,使污垢脱离皮肤进入水中,经充分乳化增溶后分散于水中,再经清水反复漂洗即可去除。理想的皮肤清洁剂应尽量不损害皮肤,并保持皮肤表面的清洁和湿润感。其按化学性质,主要分为皂类清洁剂和合成型清洁剂。

(1)皂类清洁剂:常由脂肪、油脂、盐组成。通过形成皂盐乳化皮肤表面污物而发挥清洁作用。由于皂盐成分 pH 为 9.0~10.0,呈碱性,其去污力较强,皮脂膜容易被清除,但会使皮肤 pH 增高,导致皮肤的耐受性降低,对皮肤产生一定的刺激。含甘油的手工皂或添加了保湿成分的改良皂类性质较温和,对皮肤的刺激较低。

(2)合成型清洁剂:一种非皂化表面活性剂,加上保湿剂、防腐剂和黏合剂等而由人工合成的清洁剂。其根据化学特性,可分为阴离子、阳离子、两性离子、非离子及硅酮等合成型清洁剂。阴离子表面活性剂的清洁作用强,但对皮肤的刺激性也较大。合成型清洁剂主要通过表面活性剂的乳化和包裹等作用来清洁皮肤;配方中常添加具有湿润皮肤和降低皮肤敏感性等作用的保湿剂及润肤剂,使用后可在皮肤表面形成一层薄的保湿膜,由此减轻由表面活性剂造成的皮肤屏障受损。研究表明,与皂类清洁剂相比,使用合成型清洁剂可更好地保护皮肤脂质和蛋白质结构,减轻由表面活性剂导致的皮肤屏障破坏。为了进一步提高液体皮肤清洁剂的适度取出性及低温稳定性,也常添加水溶性高分子成分,包括丙烯酸-(甲基)丙烯酸烷基酯的共聚物、羟乙(丙)基纤维素等,可单独使用一种或两种及以上组合使用。

2. 皮肤清洁剂的选用

可根据不同的皮肤类型、不同清洁部位和不同季节选择合适的清洁剂与适宜的使用频次。如油性皮肤可根据皮脂量的多少来调节清洁剂使用量和清洁频率,一般以皮肤不油腻、不干燥为度。油性皮肤者可选择控油洁面产品,如香皂、浴盐、富含泡沫的洗面奶等,但同时需要避免过度清洁。过度清洁会破坏皮脂膜,导致经皮失水率增高,反馈性地刺激皮脂腺分泌皮脂而出现所谓的"外油内干"现象。反之,干性皮肤者应尽量避免使用皂类清洁剂,碱性皂盐成分会导致经皮水分丢失加重、皮肤 pH 升高,对皮肤屏障功能破坏较大。皮肤敏感的人应仅用清水洗浴,或使用非常温和的清洁剂,同时考虑选用对皮肤无刺激性的自来水、河水、湖水等软质水。

面部清洁:每天早晚均应清洗 1 次,水温随季节而调节。

全身沐浴:应根据体力活动的强度、环境和季节不同,以及是否出汗和个人习惯做适当调整。一般情况下,2~3 天沐浴 1 次,炎热的夏季或运动爱好者可以每天 1 次。水温以皮肤温度为准,夏季可低于体温,而冬季可略高于体温,一般以 35~38 ℃为宜。清洗过多反而会使皮脂含量降低,促进皮肤老化。

（三）过度清洁的危害及皮肤保湿剂的分类与选用

1. 过度清洁的危害

清洁的目的是清除多余的皮肤代谢产物、沾染的灰尘及化妆品等。但是，过于频繁地清洗、过度使用去污及去角质能力强的清洁产品，均会造成皮肤屏障的损伤，严重影响皮肤正常pH，破坏皮肤微生态平衡；严重者可诱发或加重一些皮肤疾病如皮肤干燥、瘙痒症、皮肤过敏及湿疹等。

2. 皮肤保湿剂的分类与选用

在皮肤清洁后使用保湿剂是减少清洁剂对皮肤屏障产生的不利影响、维护皮肤屏障稳态的重要措施。保湿剂又称湿润剂，能够保持并补充皮肤角质层中的水分，防止皮肤干燥，或使已干燥、失去弹性并干裂的皮肤恢复光滑、柔软和富有弹性的状态。按其来源，保湿剂可分为天然保湿剂和合成保湿剂，按保湿的作用机制又分为封闭性保湿剂和湿润性或吸湿性保湿剂。

（1）封闭性保湿剂：一类不溶性的脂类物质，通过对皮肤角质层脂类物质的补充，形成表面润滑膜层，其能将角质层包裹从而不仅阻挡皮肤内的水分丢失，而且促进了水分不断向角质层内部扩散，使之保持一定含水量。这类保湿剂的特点：有较好的吸湿、保湿能力且不易受环境条件的影响；黏度适宜、使用感好，对皮肤较为亲和；挥发性低、凝固点低；无色、无臭且无味，与其他成分相容性强。封闭性保湿剂主要有以下6类：①矿物油和蜡类，如凡士林、矿物油等；②植物与动物脂肪，如羊毛脂等；③硅油类，如环甲聚硅氧烷等；④脂肪酸和酯类，如硬脂酸、亚麻酸等；⑤磷脂、胆固醇类，如卵磷脂、胆固醇硫酸盐等；⑥植物与动物蜡，如巴西棕榈、蜂蜡等。

（2）湿润性或吸湿性保湿剂：该类保湿剂的成分是与表皮中天然保湿因子和人体多糖、蛋白质等相似的物质，主要包括透明质酸和甘油等，是水分补充体。当皮肤水分丢失时，保湿因子通过毛孔进入皮肤内部，或携带水分，或包裹皮肤内尚未丢失的水分使其不再丢失，从而保留皮肤内的水分。这类保湿剂有以下特点：①涂抹后使皮肤含水量上升，变得饱满；②使表皮深层和真皮组织的水分进入角质层，使角质层细胞再给水；③防止水分蒸发和经表皮水分丢失，使皮肤角质层细胞柔韧、软化。

保湿剂的选用可根据自身皮肤情况而定，如油性皮肤者可以多选择水溶性的保湿剂；而干性皮肤者用油脂成分更多的保湿剂则能在皮肤表面形成更好的保护层。对于眼、唇以及颈部等皮脂腺较少、角质层比较薄的部位，尤其需要保湿。

（四）高分子材料在皮肤清洁和保湿中的应用前景

近年来，高分子纳米材料蓬勃发展。其因具有可增强的皮肤渗透性、可控而持续的药物释放能力、更高的稳定性、一定的靶向性、较高的包封效率和良好的感官特征等众多优点，被广泛应用于皮肤美容领域，如防脱发、促生发的洗发水和护发素产品，以及新型保湿剂等。在药妆领域，多种类型的纳米载体如脂质体、囊泡、固体脂质纳米粒、纳米脂质载体、纳米乳等已被用于皮肤保湿和清洁成分的递送，包括迪奥、兰蔻、黛珂等在内的多个知名化妆品品牌已有多种纳米药妆产品。纳米载体可以实现对活性物质的可控释放，并可改变药物的透皮效率。高分子纳米材料还可通过可变的聚合物与添加剂的比例和组分之间的物理或化学相互作用来组合具有不同生化性质的药物，因此其在皮肤疾病治疗及美容领域具有广阔的应用前景。

第三节　皮肤的消毒

(一)皮肤消毒的概念及意义

皮肤消毒是预防皮肤微生物感染的重要措施之一。皮肤消毒剂是指为达到预防和控制病菌感染的目的,用于皮肤、黏膜的伤口、烧伤创面等部位的消毒产品。此类消毒剂可通过改变病原体中酶系统、蛋白质的生理活性,破坏其生理功能,使其死亡。

(二)皮肤消毒剂的分类及使用

1. 常见的皮肤消毒剂

消毒剂的主要分类方式包括两种。

按照作用机制,消毒剂通常可分为化学消毒剂和生物消毒剂(如酶、噬菌体等)。其中,化学消毒剂应用较为广泛,种类也较多,按照反应类型可进一步分成氧化型和非氧化型。氧化型主要包括卤素类(氯、溴、碘)和过氧化物类(过氧化氢、过氧乙酸、二氧化氯等);非氧化型常见的有醇类(如乙醇)、酚类(如对氯间二甲苯酚)、季铵盐类(如苯扎氯铵)、胍类(如盐酸聚六亚甲基双胍、氯己定)、醛类(如戊二醛)和金属类(如银)。

按照杀灭微生物效果的强弱,消毒剂一般可分为高效、中效和低效消毒剂。通常认为高效消毒剂能杀灭包括细菌芽孢、真菌孢子、病毒在内的各种微生物,这类成分主要有氯类、过氧化物类、醛类等。中效消毒剂不能杀灭细菌芽孢,通常包括碘类、醇类等。低效消毒剂只能杀灭一般细菌繁殖体、部分真菌和亲脂性病毒,不能杀灭结核分枝杆菌、亲水性病毒和细菌芽孢。

常用化学消毒剂主要包括碘类、醇类、酚类、过氧化物类、胍类、季铵盐类等。

(1)碘类:碘是被临床广泛应用的皮肤消毒剂,碘分子能快速渗透细胞壁,通过与氨基酸和不饱和脂肪酸结合,导致蛋白质合成困难和细胞膜改变。临床常用的含碘制剂主要是碘酊(碘酒)、碘伏和聚维酮碘溶液。聚维酮碘是当前最主要的含碘皮肤消毒剂,也是皮肤黏膜消毒剂,是碘与表面活性剂结合而成的不定形络合物。其所含表面活性成分能改变溶液对物体的湿润性,可在皮肤表面形成一层极薄的杀菌薄膜,从而协助碘穿透细胞壁,并且可以乳化脂肪,缓慢、持久地释放有效碘来加强碘的杀菌作用。

(2)醇类:乙醇属于中效消毒剂,最佳作用浓度为75%~85%。60%~90%的乙醇水溶液浸泡或擦拭可杀灭细菌繁殖体、分枝杆菌、酵母菌、真菌以及部分病毒,但不能杀灭细菌芽孢。乙醇通过脱水作用使菌体蛋白质凝固、变性,其渗透作用可以使其穿透细胞壁进入菌体内发挥消毒作用。乙醇能够迅速杀灭细菌繁殖体,但具有活性不持久、易挥发、刺激性大等缺点,不宜应用于黏膜或较大创面上。乙醇还可与其他化学抗菌剂协同抗菌,如多种醇溶液进行复配可以提高杀菌能力,延长有效作用时间,尤其是对病毒杀灭效果更佳。

异丙醇的杀菌作用和机制与乙醇相似,常用浓度为70%~80%。70%异丙醇可以在10 min内杀灭乙型、丙型肝炎病毒和人类免疫缺陷病毒。异丙醇杀菌能力、毒性均比乙醇稍强,能完全杀灭脂质病毒,但对非脂质肠道病毒无灭活作用。

(3)酚类:酚类皮肤消毒剂主要为三氯羟基二苯醚。三氯羟基二苯醚属于广谱、高效抗菌剂,又名三氯生。抗菌浓度为0.2%~2.0%。三氯生的抗菌机制是进入细菌细胞膜来影响胞膜、RNA、脂肪酸和蛋白质的合成。三氯生主要发挥抑菌的作用。三氯生对革兰阳性菌(包括

MRSA)的作用强于革兰阴性菌,特别是铜绿假单胞菌。三氯生对分枝杆菌属和假丝酵母菌属有一定的活性,但对丝状真菌的活性较弱。然而,有研究显示,三氯生有轻度的致畸作用。

（4）过氧化物类:过氧化物类皮肤消毒剂主要有过氧化氢和过氧乙酸。其可以杀灭细菌、真菌、细菌芽孢和病毒等所有微生物,其中过氧乙酸杀菌能力最强,过氧化氢次之。过氧化物类消毒剂属于高效、速效、低毒消毒剂,需现用现配,高浓度时可刺激、损害皮肤黏膜。过氧化氢溶液浓度达 1000 mg/L 时具有杀菌作用。临床上,过氧化氢溶液常被用于口腔炎症者漱口和清洗创伤。过氧乙酸溶液用于皮肤消毒时浓度应低于 2000 mg/L,用于黏膜消毒时浓度应低至 200 mg/L。

（5）胍类:氯己定又名洗必泰,属于双胍类抗菌剂,具有毒性低、刺激性小、抗菌谱广等特点,主要用于皮肤及黏膜的抗菌处理,属于低效消毒剂。其易吸附于菌体细胞膜上,致使细胞膜破裂损伤,抑制细菌系统酶的作用,造成细菌的代谢障碍。高浓度可使菌体细胞质聚集成块、浓缩变性,达到杀菌目的。氯己定能有效杀灭细菌繁殖体,但对细菌芽孢、结核分枝杆菌及真菌仅有抑制作用,对乙型和丙型肝炎病毒、真菌菌株黑曲霉菌杀灭能力较弱。

（6）季铵盐类:季铵盐类皮肤消毒剂属于低效消毒剂,包括单链季铵盐和双链季铵盐,主要有十二烷基二甲基苄基溴化铵(苯扎溴铵)、十二烷基二甲基苯氧乙基溴化铵(度米芬)和十四烷基二甲基吡啶溴化铵(消毒净)等。其杀菌机制是吸附于菌体表面,改变细胞膜通透性,造成胞内物质外漏和蛋白质的变性,从而达到杀菌的效果。季铵盐类皮肤消毒剂具有杀菌浓度低、水溶性好、毒性小、刺激性小、性质稳定等特点,但价格较贵,对某些病毒杀灭效果较差,配伍禁忌多。苯扎溴铵的抑菌作用强,但不能杀灭真菌、结核分枝杆菌、细菌芽孢和非包层病毒。临床常用浓度为 1000 mg/L,可应用于患者皮肤清洁、医务人员手部清洁等,通常与醇类消毒剂联合应用。

2. 皮肤消毒的步骤及注意事项

（1）彻底清洁是保证消毒效果的前提。皮肤消毒前要视皮肤的污染情况对皮肤进行不同的清洁,清洁或去污不彻底会影响消毒效果。

（2）正确选择消毒剂的类型及使用浓度。以乙醇为例,乙醇在 70%～80% 的浓度时消毒效果最佳。

（3）消毒剂要有足够的作用时间。不同的皮肤消毒剂所需的作用时间不同,通常为 1～5 min,或者以所用消毒剂彻底自然干燥为准。

（三）消毒剂对皮肤的损伤及相应护理措施

与过度清洁引起的损伤类似,频繁接触消毒剂也会破坏皮肤屏障的正常结构。消毒剂中的一些物质(如乙醇等)长期使用会造成皮肤干燥粗糙、失去弹性、油脂分泌过多等问题,并使得皮肤表面的免疫微环境发生改变,可能会导致湿疹、过敏性皮炎等一系列疾病。另外,消毒剂中的刺激性成分接触皮肤后可能引发接触性皮炎等不良反应。

1. 过敏反应

过敏反应主要见于对所含消毒成分过敏的特殊体质人群,常见表现是过敏性接触性皮炎。常在接触部位出现,与皮肤接触的范围大体一致。症状较轻时,多在局部皮肤出现红、肿、瘙痒等症状;严重者可出现丘疹、水疱,甚至糜烂破溃,可在破溃后继发感染。

处置原则:①首先停止使用可疑消毒剂,更换为其他非过敏产品;②若皮疹较轻,可在停用

3~5天后自行改善,无须特殊处理;③若皮疹严重,瘙痒明显,可口服第二代抗组胺药,外用中强效糖皮质激素如糠酸莫米松、卤米松乳膏等,有系统症状者可以给予系统糖皮质激素治疗;④当有继发感染时,应局部或系统性地使用抗生素。

2. 皮肤屏障破坏与刺激反应

由于脂溶性消毒剂可以溶解皮肤表面皮脂膜,反复使用这类消毒剂容易导致皮肤屏障功能破坏,出现皮肤皲裂。如继续使用,消毒剂渗入皮肤产生刺激性皮炎。表现为反复使用该消毒剂后,接触部位瘙痒,皮疹可为红斑、丘疹、水疱、皲裂。

处置原则:加强润肤剂的使用,其他措施同过敏反应的处理。

此外,随着具有抗菌、抑菌功效的皮肤护理和洗消用品长期、大量使用,皮肤菌群中的常见致病菌和定植的条件致病菌对消毒产品有效成分的抗性不断增强,耐药谱增加,影响了皮肤消毒的效果。

(四)部分新型消毒剂

1. 酸性氧化电位水

酸性氧化电位水是指将低浓度的氯化钠溶液加入水中,通过电化学方法电解而制成的一种消毒剂,分为微酸性电解水、弱酸性电解水和强酸性电解水。目前普遍认为,酸性氧化电位水的杀菌作用与其 pH、氧化还原电位(oxidation-reduction potential,ORP)、有效氯、活性氧等有关。酸性氧化电位水的低 pH 和高 ORP 可以改变微生物的细胞膜电位,增强细胞膜的通透性,使细菌肿胀,破坏细胞代谢酶,导致细胞内物质溢出、溶解,达到杀菌效果。酸性氧化电位水杀菌谱广、高效、无毒性、无刺激性、不产生耐药性,但稳定性较差,易受有机物和金属离子的影响。

2. 生物消毒剂

生物消毒剂是指用于杀灭或消除病原微生物的天然的或应用基因工程方法获得的生物酶、噬菌体、蛭弧菌、抗菌肽等。相比化学消毒剂,其杀菌速度快、特异性强、毒性小、温和无刺激、不易产生耐药性并且无有害物质残留。生物消毒剂主要有植物消毒剂和微生物制剂。某些植物精油具有自身特定的杀菌谱(包括防己科、樟科、芸香科、茜草科的植物),可制备成植物消毒剂。微生物制剂分为两类:一类是直接用微生物作为杀菌剂;另一类是由微生物的代谢产物分离而得或人工合成。微生物制剂主要有蛭弧菌、生物酶和噬菌体。生物酶包括溶菌酶和溶葡萄球菌酶,对革兰阳性菌杀灭能力强。目前溶菌酶已用于烧伤创面的消毒清创。

3. 含银消毒剂

含银消毒剂发挥杀菌作用的主要成分是银离子,其杀菌机制包括以下几点:与细胞膜结合,改变原有结构和功能;作用于质子泵,影响物质传输,干扰代谢;与胞内蛋白质的巯基、氨基和羧基等结合,破坏可分解葡萄糖、蔗糖、尿素等的酶的结构和功能;与 DNA 结合,导致化学键断裂,破坏分子结构并阻断繁殖。与离子形式存在的银相比,银纳米材料由于具有量子效应、小尺寸效应和较大的比表面积等优势,容易与病原微生物密切接触,从而发挥更大的生物效应。因此,银纳米材料的抗菌效果更强,且安全性高、效力持久。银纳米材料杀菌机制复杂多样,属非抗生素类杀菌剂,故不易发生耐药。但银纳米材料在不加保护剂的常规条件下容易发生颗粒聚集而失去纳米特性,或被氧化为棕色的氧化银,从而影响其杀菌效果。

第四节 挑战与展望

本章主要介绍了皮肤防护、清洁和消毒用品的发展近况,包括个人防护装备、皮肤保护剂、防晒剂和各种皮肤清洁、保湿、消毒剂,以及高分子材料用于解决防护用品使用中存在的问题。在人们的生产生活中,皮肤的防护、清洁和消毒对维持皮肤健康以及保护机体不受外界理化、生物等因素的侵害十分重要。

随着高分子材料在生物医药等领域的飞速发展,各种新型防护用品、皮肤清洁保湿剂及皮肤消毒剂的出现给人们生产生活中的皮肤健康带来了更多保障。例如在材料方面,新型的防护服纤维材料、口罩聚合物材料以及纳米防晒剂,还有高分子皮肤清洁保湿剂和消毒剂等,均能很好地发挥相应功能。然而,由于皮肤特定的生物学特点,皮肤屏障也容易受到环境、防护用品和清洁剂、消毒剂的损伤。生物医用高分子材料的开发需在注重防护、清洁、消毒等效果的同时,更多地关注材料的人体安全性、使用舒适度以及对皮肤屏障的长期保护,真正突出生物医用高分子材料的优势。新型水凝胶、水胶体等敷料用于预防防护用品带来的压力性损伤就是很好的例子。

思 考 题

1. 请指出当前主要的皮肤防护用品、皮肤清洁剂、皮肤消毒剂的分类。
2. 高分子材料在皮肤防护中主要有哪些应用?在材料方面还可以如何优化?
3. 皮肤清洁剂、保湿剂中的高分子材料需要具备什么样的特点?
4. 皮肤防护、清洁与消毒领域还有哪些主要的问题和需求需要解决?
5. 在皮肤防护、清洁与消毒领域,未来还能如何应用高分子材料?

扩 展 阅 读

[1] Rook A,Burns T F. Rook's textbook of dermatology[M]. 8th ed. Oxford:Blackwell Science,2010.
[2] 李航,陶娟. 重大疫情中皮肤黏膜屏障防护手册[M]. 北京:北京大学医学出版社,2020.
[3] Bucci P,Prieto M J,Milla L,et al. Skin penetration and UV-damage prevention by nanoberries[J]. J Cosmet Dermatol,2018,17(5):889-899.
[4] Zhao Z,Fang R,Rong Q,et al. Bioinspired nanocomposite hydrogels with highly ordered structures[J]. Adv Mater,2017,29(45):e1703045.
[5] Rutala W A,Weber D J. Disinfection and sterilization in health care facilities:an overview and current issues[J]. Infect Dis Clin North Am,2016,30(3):609-637.

参 考 文 献

[1] Honda H,Iwata K. Personal protective equipment and improving compliance among healthcare workers in high-risk settings[J]. Curr Opin Infect Dis,2016,29(4):400-406.
[2] Holland M G,Cawthon D. Personal protective equipment and decontamination of adults

and children[J]. Emerg Med Clin North Am,2015,33(1):51-68.

[3] Villano J S,Follo J M,Chappell M G,et al. Personal protective equipment in animal research[J]. Comp Med,2017,67(3):203-214.

[4] Black J M,Cuddigan J E,Walko M A,et al. Medical device related pressure ulcers in hospitalized patients[J]. Int Wound J,2010,7(5):358-365.

[5] Arnold-Long M,Ayer M,Borchert K. Medical device-related pressure injuries in long-term acute care hospital setting[J]. J Wound Ostomy Continence Nurs,2017,44(4):325-330.

[6] Pailler-Mattei C,Pavan S,Vargiolu R,et al. Contribution of stratum corneum in determining bio-tribological properties of the human skin[J]. Wear,2007,263(7):1038-1043.

[7] Ham W H,Schoonhoven L,Schuurmans M J,et al. Pressure ulcers,indentation marks and pain from cervical spine immobilization with extrication collars and headblocks:an observational study[J]. Injury,2016,47(9):1924-1931.

[8] Lazzarini R,Duarte I A,Sumita J M,et al. Allergic contact dermatitis among construction workers detected in a clinic that did not specialize in occupational dermatitis[J]. An Bras Dermatol,2012,87(4):567-571.

[9] Ibler K S,Jemec G B E,Agner T. Exposures related to hand eczema:a study of healthcare workers[J]. Contact Dermatitis,2012,66(5):247-253.

[10] Rosenthal M,Goldberg D,Aiello A,et al. Skin microbiota:microbial community structure and its potential association with health and disease[J]. Infect Genet Evol,2011,11(5):839-848.

[11] Apold J,Rydrych D. Preventing device-related pressure ulcers:using data to guide statewide change[J]. J Nurs Care Qual,2012,27(1):28-34.

[12] Wyatt D,McGowan D N,Najarian M P. Comparison of a hydrocolloid dressing and silver sulfadiazine cream in the outpatient management of second-degree burns[J]. J Trauma,1990,30(7):857-865.

[13] Whittle H,Fletcher C,Hoskin A,et al. Nursing management of pressure ulcers using a hydrogel dressing protocol:four case studies [J]. Rehabil Nurs,1996,21(5):239-242.

[14] Han L,Lu X,Liu K,et al. Mussel-inspired adhesive and tough hydrogel based on nanoclay confined dopamine polymerization[J]. ACS Nano,2017,11(3):2561-2574.

[15] Lan J,Song Z,Miao X,et al. Skin damage among health care workers managing coronavirus disease-2019[J]. J Am Acad Dermatol,2020,82(5):1215-1216.

[16] Dong L,Yang L,Li Y,et al. Efficacy of hydrogel patches in preventing facial skin damage caused by mask compression in fighting against coronavirus disease-2019:a short-term,self-controlled study[J]. J Eur Acad Dermatol Venereol,2020,34(9):e441-e443.

[17] Zhou N,Yang L,Li Y,et al. Hydrogel patches alleviate skin injuries to the cheeks and nasal bridge caused by continuous N95 mask use[J]. Dermatol Ther,2020,33(6):e14177.

[18] Zhou N, Suo H, Alamgir M, et al. Application of hydrogel patches to the upper margins of N95 respirators as a novel anti-fog measure for goggles: a prospective, self-controlled study[J]. J Am Acad Dermatol, 2020, 83(5): 1539-1541.

[19] Zhou N, Yang L, Dong L, et al. Prevention and treatment of skin damage caused by personal protective equipment: experience of the first-line clinicians treating 2019-nCoV infection[J]. Int J Dermatol Venereol, 2020, 3(2): 70-75.

[20] Walker R M, Gillespie B M, Thalib L, et al. Foam dressings for treating pressure ulcers[J]. Cochrane Database Syst Rev, 2017, 10: CD011332.

[21] Chambers E S, Vukmanovic-Stejic M. Skin barrier immunity and ageing[J]. Immunology, 2020, 160(2): 116-125.

[22] Draelos Z D. The science behind skin care: moisturizers[J]. J Cosmet Dermatol, 2018, 17(2): 138-144.

[23] Draelos Z D. The science behind skin care: cleansers[J]. J Cosmet Dermatol, 2018, 17(1): 8-14.

[24] Treffel P, Gabard B. Stratum corneum dynamic function measurements after moisturizer or irritant application[J]. Arch Dermatol Res, 1995, 287(5): 474-479.

[25] Rawlings A V, Harding C R. Moisturization and skin barrier function[J]. Dermatol Ther, 2004, 17: 43-48.

[26] Graninger M, Grassberger M, Galehr E, et al. Comments, opinions, and brief case reports: biosurgical debridement facilitates healing of chronic skin ulcers[J]. Arch Intern Med, 2002, 162(16): 1906-1907.

[27] Kaul S, Gulati N, Verma D, et al. Role of nanotechnology in cosmeceuticals: a review of recent advances[J]. J Pharm(Cairo), 2018, 2018: 3420204.

[28] 赵辨. 临床皮肤病学[M]. 南京: 江苏科学技术出版社, 2001.

[29] 张星, 刘金鑫, 张海峰, 等. 防护口罩用非织造滤料的制备技术与研究现状[J]. 纺织学报, 2020, 41(3): 168-174.

[30] 王然, 冯瑞娟, 刘佳. 皮肤保护剂对老年失禁相关性皮炎防治的研究进展[J]. 实用临床护理学电子杂志, 2019, 4(26): 193, 198.

[31] 周晶, 张溢. 纳米技术在防晒化妆品中的应用[J]. 广东化工, 2017, 44(15): 175-176, 185.

[32] 吴薇, 陈思, 郭虹. 空气过滤用静电纺PAN纳米纤维膜的制备及性能研究[J]. 国际纺织导报, 2019, 47(5): 1-4, 6-8, 10.

[33] 中国医师协会皮肤科医师分会皮肤美容事业发展工作委员会. 皮肤防晒专家共识(2017)[J]. 中华皮肤科杂志, 2017, 50(5): 316-320.

[34] 阎迪, 郝爱萍. 功能性防护服及新材料应用[J]. 棉纺织技术, 2012, 40(2): 65-68.

[35] 韩玲, 马英博, 胡梦缘, 等. 国内外医用口罩防护指标及标准对比[J]. 西安工程大学学报, 2020, 34(2): 13-19.

[36] 张婷婷, 李佳星, 张紫君, 等. 预防院内压力性损伤敷料的应用现状[J]. 职业与健康, 2018, 34(14): 2010-2013.

［37］ 高宁,刘太奇.塑料防雾剂的研究进展[J].新技术新工艺,2014(4):98-101.

［38］ 崔兵彦,姚俊,刘红,等.美军单兵用防护眼镜防雾性能的现状及发展[J].中国新技术新产品,2019(7):60-62.

［39］ 王敏,郭亮.皮肤清洁剂及其在各种皮肤病中的应用[J].中华医学美学美容杂志,2019,25(5):443-445.

［40］ 李利,何黎.中国皮肤清洁指南[J].中华皮肤科杂志,2016,49(8):537-540.

［41］ 郑志忠,李利,刘玮,等.正确的皮肤清洁与皮肤屏障保护[J].临床皮肤科杂志,2017,46(11):824-826.

［42］ 邹祖鹏,朱磊.保湿剂的临床应用实践[J].中国临床医生杂志,2020,48(4):398-401.

［43］ 陈亚飞,余汉谋,姜兴涛,等.皮肤保湿剂的功效评价方法[J].日用化学品科学,2015,38(12):27-30.

［44］ 何黎.皮肤屏障与保湿[J].实用医院临床杂志,2009,6(2):25-27.

［45］ 虞瑞尧.皮肤屏障功能与润肤保湿霜[J].皮肤性病诊疗学杂志,2003,10(3):222-224.

［46］ 杨娜,杨彬,孙文魁,等.皮肤消毒剂开发应用研究进展[J].中国消毒学杂志,2018,35(4):297-300.

［47］ 王冬梅,莫遗盛,江晓筠.纳米银临床应用研究进展[J].中国药房,2007,18(5):386-387.

［48］ 李阳友.生物消毒剂及其前景[J].畜牧兽医科技信息,2012(4):117.

(周诺娅　陶娟)

Chapter 4
Skin Protection, Cleaning and Disinfection

4.1　Skin Protection

4.1.1　The concept of skin protection

With the development of human society and the advancement of science and technology, the environment that we face is becoming more and more complex. In the process of production, there are many factors that can cause harm to the skin, which can be summarized as physical factors, such as radiation, electricity, light, heat, and mechanical friction; chemical factors, such as petroleum fractionation products, strong acids, strong bases, heavy metals, and asbestos; biological factors, such as bacteria, fungi, viruses, insect bites, and pollen. Therefore, it is very important to carry out personal skin protection against these physical, chemical and biological factors that endanger skin health in production and life.

4.1.2　Classification of skin protective products

Skin protective products includes personal protective equipment (PPE) and skin protective agents.

1. PPE

PPE refers to the items that operators wear at work, e. g. , protective masks, work clothes and gloves (Figure 4-1), in order to avoid or reduce accidental injuries and occupational hazards.

When classified by the use objectives, PPE includes: individual protective equipments for military personnel, such as bullet-proof helmets, bullet-proof clothing, gas masks, and combat boots; protective equipments for police, such as explosion-proof clothing, anti-stab clothing, and anti-glare glasses; protective equipments for diverse types of workers, mainly industrial and agricultural production staff, medical staff, and scientific and technological workers.

When classified by the protection objectives, PPE includes: physical protective equipments such as insulating gloves, hardhats, and earmuffs; chemical protective equipments such as gas masks, acid-proof clothing, and alkali-proof clothing; biological protective equipments such as medical masks, goggles, and medical protective clothing; public safety protective equipments for public places, such as escape masks and life jackets in civil aviation passenger planes; protective equipments used in personal life, such as anti-haze and anti-UV goggles.

When classified by the protected body parts, PPE includes respiratory protectors, eye shields, face shields, ear protectors, helmets, protective clothing, gloves, and shoe covers.

In short, personal protective equipment is combined with the specific working environment to protect workers' mouth, nose, eyes, ears, exposed skin and other vulnerable parts such as inhalation, absorption and head.

2. Skin protective agents

Skin protective agents mainly include protective ointment, skin cleanser, skin protective films, skin cream and moisturizing protective ointment.

(1) Protective ointment: Protective ointment is a kind of skin care preparation to prevent harmful substances from acting on exposed skin and occupational skin diseases. The protective ointment is soluble or insoluble in water, and its function is to apply to the skin and become a viscous coating or a flexible film, thus playing a mechanical or special protective role on the skin. For example, protective ointment can play the roles in redox, neutralization, complexation and absorption of harmful substances. Long-term use of protective ointment can play a certain role of isolation, so that the skin can be protected. Common protective ointment includes hydrophilic protective ointment, hydrophobic protective ointment and sunshade protective ointment, and others.

①Hydrophilic protective ointment: It contains less oil and is applied to the surface of the skin when it is used. This kind of ointment can play the role of oil resistance and is used in contact with mineral oil, organic acid and other operations.

②Hydrophobic protective ointment: It contains a lot of oil and is applied to the surface of the skin and can plug pores. This kind of ointment prevent individuals from the splashing injuries of water-soluble substances, such as low concentration of acid, alkali and salt liquid.

③Sunshade protective ointment: It can help to avoid light after smearing. It is mainly used to prevent the irritation of photosensitive substances such as asphalt and tar to the skin. It is suitable for tar, asphalt, electric welding and snow operation. Sunscreen that people use daily is also one of them.

(2) Skin cleanser: Skin cleanser is mainly used to wash all kinds of pollution on the surface of the skin, especially for workers exposed to poison and dust, when it is necessary to clean up and remove the poison on the attached skin and overalls in time. The most commonly used skin cleanser is soap, but many chemicals exposed to work are not easily

washed by soap, and soap will damage part of the skin fat when washed. Organic solvents can be used to wash away stubborn stains such as gasoline, kerosene and turpentine, but these cleansers themselves can cause or aggravate skin damage.

(3) Skin protective films: Skin protective films are also known as invisible gloves, which are usually made of cellulose, casein or rosin dissolved in alcohol. The skin protective films can be applied to the surface of the skin to form an oil-resistant, water-resistant and irritant film, which is suitable for irritating work such as electroplating, paint, printing, dyeing and dust.

(4) Skin cream and moisturizing protective ointment: This kind of ointment contains a lot of oil, and it is usually added with substances such as high protein, royal jelly and pearl powder that are easily absorbed by the human body to increase the effects of moisturizing and protecting the skin. It is suitable for preventing defatting of skin caused by long-term contact with water, alkaline solution and organic solvent.

Compared with the defects of PPE(e. g. , lack of tightness, leakage, affecting work and discomfort), skin protective agents are lighter and can come into close contact with the skin. Yet, the protection by skin protective agents may not be as good as PPE.

4. 1. 3　Daily skin sunscreen

1. Effect of ultraviolet radiation on skin

In daily life, ultraviolet radiation is the most common cause of skin damage. According to the different wavelengths, ultraviolet can be divided into three sections: long-wave ultraviolet (ultraviolet A, UVA), medium-wave ultraviolet (ultraviolet B, UVB) and short-wave ultraviolet (ultraviolet C, UVC). Among them, the ultraviolet reaching the ground are about 95% of UVA and 5% of UVB, while UVC is basically absorbed by the ozone layer and cannot reach the ground. When exposed to the sun for a long time without taking any protective measures, the ultraviolet rays in the sun will cause varied degrees of damage to the skin. In the process of ultraviolet irradiation, free radicals and oxidation will be produced, which will damage the DNA, lipids and proteins of skin cells, resulting in skin erythema, skin blackening, skin photoaging, abnormal immune function and skin tumors.

The skin damage caused by ultraviolet radiation mainly includes the followings.

① Erythema reaction: Also called sun erythema, which is an acute inflammatory reaction. Erythema appears at 2-7 hours after sun exposure and reached the peak at 12-24 hours, which was mainly manifested as erythema and swelling in the sun site, and blisters occurred in severe cases, which could cause burning pain consciously. After a few days, the erythema disappeared and desquamation appeared. Patients with light skin are more likely to have erythema. The main light causing erythema reaction is UVB.

②Skin blackening: Also called skin tanning. It is characterized by clear gray-black spots with clear boundaries on the light site, and there are no self-conscious symptoms. According to the appearance time of pigment, it can be divided into immediate pigment darkening, persistent pigment darkening and delayed tanning.

a. Immediate pigment darkening is gray-black pigmentation that occurs during or immediately after irradiation and usually lasts only a few minutes to two hours.

b. With the increase of UV dose, persistent pigment darkening can overlap with erythema reaction, and then shows gray-black or dark brown. The peak is reached at 2-24 hours, which can last from several hours to several days.

c. Delayed tanning usually occurs within a few days after radiation and can last from weeks to months. Immediate pigment darkening and persistent pigment darkening are produced by oxidizing melanin particles and transporting them to keratinocytes, which are affected by UVA and visible light. Delayed tanning is caused by the active function of melanocytes and the synthesis of more melanin, which are affected by UVB, UVA and visible light.

③Skin photoaging: Long-term sunlight exposure will accelerate skin aging, which is mainly caused by UVA. It is characterized by rough skin, decreased elasticity, increased wrinkles and deepened pigmentation, accompanied by telangiectasia or hyperplasia and erythema formation.

④ Abnormal immune function: The skin exposed to the ultraviolet can occur photoallergy, and abnormal function of local skin and systemic immune system can occur at the same time. Immune changes caused by light involve immunoreactive cells, cytokines, complements and the interaction between these substances, which can cause a variety of photolinear diseases and light-exacerbated skin diseases.

⑤Skin tumors: UVB irradiation can cause nuclear base structure changes. UVA induces cells to produce reactive oxygen clusters, which leads to abnormal structure of cell membrane, DNA degeneration and destruction of lipids and proteins. As a result, malignant skin diseases occur, including photolinear keratosis, basal cell carcinoma, squamous cell carcinoma and melanoma.

2. Common sunscreen measures and products

In 2002, ultraviolet index (UVI) was put forward by the World Health Organization (WHO), which is used to indicate the ultraviolet intensity of sunlight. And the higher UVI induces the greater damage of sunlight to the skin and eyes. Generally, noon is the highest period for UVI, and late spring and summer are the higher seasons for UVI. UVI increased with the increase of altitude. In addition, seaside beaches, snow, wall or curtain glass of urban high-rise buildings, car windowpanes and hardened floors by the asphalt or cement all reflect ultraviolet and increase UVI. Daily sunscreen measures mainly include shielding sunscreen and the use of sunscreen agents.

(1) Shielding sunscreen: Shielding sunscreen refers to the use of sunscreen umbrellas, sunscreen mirrors, sunscreen caps, sunscreen clothing or masks and other shielding objects to block the exposed parts of the body. The shield can block ultraviolet rays to achieve sunscreen. High-density weaving, darker colors and sunscreen coatings can enhance the

shielding ability of the shielding to ultraviolet rays, which means better sunscreen. If a sunscreen hat is used, the edge length of the brim should be above 7.5 cm for requiring a better sunscreen. It is recommended to buy fabric products marked with UFP>25 dyn and UVA transmittance<5% (Table 4-1). Sunshades that cover all UV and minimize the penetration of blue and purple light are recommended.

Table 4-1　Ultraviolet radiation protection index of fabric (*Skin Sun Protection Expert Consensus 2017*)

Ultraviolet protection factor	Protection grade	UVA transmittance/(%)	Ultraviolet protection factor grade
15-25	Good	6.7-4.2	15, 20
25-39	Great	4.1-2.6	25, 30, 35
40-50, 50+	Excellent	≤2.5	40, 45, 50, 50+

(2) The use of sunscreen agents: Sunscreen is a substance that absorbs, reflects or scatters light to protect the skin from specific UV damage. At present, the sunscreen products on the market are mainly divided into three categories: organic sunscreen based on ultraviolet absorbers, inorganic sunscreen based on ultraviolet shielding agents and antioxidants that indirectly play a role in sunscreen.

①Organic sunscreen: It is also called chemical UV absorbent. Most organic sunscreen agents contain aromatic compounds, where the special groups on the benzene ring can affect the spectral properties of sunscreen agents. Generally, this kind of substance can selectively absorb UV and result in sunscreen. The sunscreen agents that absorb UVB mainly include salicylates and their derivatives and cinnamates; butyl methoxydibenzoylmethane is the main absorbent of UVA; benzophenone and its derivatives are both absorbable. Organic sunscreen is favorable for the light and thin texture and excellent sense of transparency. However, the photostability of traditional organic sunscreen is not as stable as that of inorganic sunscreen. Moreover, organic sunscreen is easy to be absorbed through the skin and has a certain degree of sensitization, which may lead to contact sensitization and photosensitization. In recent years, a large number of new organic sunscreen agents have been put on the market, which not only overcome the shortcomings of traditional organic sunscreen agents, but also significantly improve the solubility and photostability of sunscreen agents through isomerization and micronization, and these are not easy to be absorbed through the skin. The new organic sunscreen agents have been becoming favored by the market for their safety and effectiveness.

②Inorganic sunscreen: It is also called physical UV shielding agent. This kind of sunscreen reflect and scatter sunlight, such as titanium dioxide (TiO_2), and zinc oxide (ZnO). The main principle is to form a uniform protective layer, which can reflect, refract and scatter ultraviolet, thus reducing the damage of ultraviolet to the skin. In recent years, it has been found that inorganic sunscreen particles have semiconductor-like properties, and electron transition process in the atoms can selectively absorb ultraviolet, resulting in sunscreen.

Inorganic sunscreen is favored for wide sunscreen spectrum and relatively light stability. Meanwhile, this kind of sunscreen is not sensitized. Thus, it is suitable for people with sensitive skin. However, the disadvantage of this kind of sunscreen is that it is not easy to apply, and excessive use is easy to clog pores and cause new skin diseases.

③Antioxidants: This kind of sunscreen has no direct absorption or reflection effect on sunlight. Yet, addition of it to cosmetics can improve the antioxidant capacity of the skin, thus indirectly play the role of sunscreen. These compounds mainly include plant extracts such as vitamin C/E, β-carotene, metallothionein, superoxide dismutase (SOD), anthocyanin, and tetrahydromethyl pyrimidine carboxylic acid (Ectoin). Licorice, aloe, green tea, panax notoginseng and grape seeds also have antioxidants.

Generally speaking, all kinds of sunscreen agents at present have their own advantages and disadvantages. In order to cover both UVB and UVA, and take into account both safety and applicability, most sunscreen cosmetics are compounded of raw materials with different mechanisms of action.

4.1.4 Skin damages caused by protective products

Although the purpose of skin protective products is to protect the skin, repeated or prolonged contact with the protective products may cause skin damages at the same time. Overall, the PPE is short in poor air permeability and will rub and oppress the skin, and the protective agent has a certain degree of absorbability and sensitization. Although the protective products used in different industries are made from various materials, the skin problems caused by protective products used for the same part of the body are basically similar.

1. Skin pressure injuries

PPE (e.g., helmets, masks, gas masks, and goggles) often cause skin damage to the face and ears. Such equipment needs to be tightly attached to the skin surface, which compresses the skin at the fixed site for many hours and may result in device-related pressure injuries. The factors contributing to device-related pressure injuries include poor local blood circulation, and ischemia and hypoxia of tissue. The accumulation on the inside of the mask of a large amount of water vapor exhaled from the mouth and nose and skin evaporation, keep the facial skin in a moist environment for a long period. This softens and impregnates the skin, and reduces the ability of the stratum corneum to resist external pressure and shear forces. Thus, the skin is prone to indentations(Figure 4-2). In addition, the friction between the PPE and the skin enhances the development of erythema, blisters, or ulcers, along with pain and even secondary infection.

2. Folliculitis

Wearing a helmet or hat for a long time may lead to folliculitis. The scalp is rich in hair follicles, sebaceous glands, and sweat glands, and therefore secretes large amounts of oil and sweat. Due to the poor permeability of hair, hats, and helmets, the sweat and oil secreted by the scalp mix together and remain on the skin surface of the head, consequently blocking the pores and making it easier for folliculitis to develop when bacteria colonize. Aggravation of this inflammation may lead to skin lesions such as pustules, boils, seborrheic dermatitis, and secondary fungal infection.

3. Skin fungal and bacterial infections

To completely isolate the wearer from harmful substances in the environment, gloves and protective clothing are mostly made of waterproof materials with poor air permeability, such as rubber and plastic. If the skin is left in an air-impermeable environment for long periods, the sweat evaporation is decreased, and the skin is prone to impregnation, eczema, and sweat herpes. Furthermore, the hot and humid environment is conducive to fungal reproduction. In particular, the vulval, medial thigh, and perianal areas are predilection sites for skin inflammation and secondary bacterial and fungal infections due to excretion irritation and repeated friction during walking.

4. Eczema

In addition to wearing gloves, hand hygiene is also essential for chemical and biological protection. However, repeated cleaning can lead to a reduction of grease on the skin surface, thus damaging the normal skin barrier. As a result, the skin shows symptoms such as dryness and itching, as well as hand and foot eczema.

5. Contact dermatitis

Repeated contact with irritants such as disinfectants and gloves can cause contact dermatitis with erythema, pimples, exudation, or erosion. One study found that 52% of medical staff with hand eczema wash their hands more than 10 times per day. Long-term disinfectant use also influences the microbiota and changes the immune microenvironment on the skin surface, resulting in conditions such as eczema, fungal infection, bacterial infection, and allergic dermatitis. Irritation of sweat and sunscreen may also cause an allergic skin reaction.

6. Acne

The materials used to make explosion-proof clothing, stab-resistant clothing, and other protective clothing are relatively hard, which may cause device-related pressure injuries due to friction between the clothing edge and the skin. Industrial and medical protective clothing have requirements for tightness, which keeps the skin over the whole body in a humid environment and makes it prone to impregnation. People with large amounts of sebaceous gland secretions are likely to develop acne in areas rich in sebaceous glands (e. g. , chest and back), due to the pores being blocked by sweat and sebum. At the same time, inorganic sunscreen is also easy to clog pores and cause acne.

4.1.5 Applications of new polymer materials in skin protection

With the development of industry and the progress of science and technology, people have put forward higher requirements for skin protective products. PPE should not only achieve the protective function, but also should be comfortable, simple and light to wear. At the same time, skin protective agents (e. g. , daily sunscreen) also need to be more safe and effective. With the development of new polymer materials and its application in the field of skin protection, these requirements can be partially realized.

1. New polymer materials used in the manufacture of protective products

(1) High performance fiber for protective clothing

①Poly (*p*-phenylene benzobisoxazole) (PBO) fiber: PBO fiber is a high performance fiber prepared by liquid crystal spinning of PBO polymer. This kind of fiber has the highest strength and modulus at present and is considered to be a super fiber of the century. At present, this fiber in our country is still under research and development. PBO fiber has four special properties: a. good heat resistance and flame retardancy; b. high strength, modulus, impact resistance and wear resistance; c. excellent chemical stability; d. excellent surface adhesion, color fastness to light and dyeing. PBO fiber can be used as heat-resistant and flame-retardant materials, as well as high-strength and high-tension protective clothing, such as fire clothes, furnace overalls, welding overalls, cutting-proof overalls, and safety gloves.

②Polybenzimidazole (PBI) fiber: PBI fiber is non-flammable in the air with excellent heat resistance, and can even be used for a long time at 350 ℃. The fiber is excellent in stability to chemicals and good tolerance to carbonic acid, hydrochloric acid and nitric acid. The density is 1. 43 g/cm³, and the strength and elongation are similar to those of viscose fiber. The high moisture regain (about 15%) of PBI fiber prevents static electricity generation in the production process; thus, it is excellent in textile processing performance. Moreover, the wearing comfort of protective clothing made of PBI fiber is similar to that of natural fiber and much better than that of other synthetic fibers. Since the PBI fiber is smoke-free and non-toxic at high temperature, it can be used to make protective clothing for high-temperature furnace workers, welders and sand workers, as well as racing suits, flight suits and life suits.

③Polytetrafluoroethylene (PTFE) fiber: The density of PTFE fiber is 2. 2 g/cm³. The tensile strength is not high (about 13 cN/tex), but the PTFE fiber is excellent in chemical stability, and its chemical stability is higher than that of all other natural fibers and chemical fibers. At the same time, PTFE fiber can be used not only at high temperature, but also at low temperature. Therefore, it is the best weather-resistant fiber among all kinds of chemical fibers. PTFE fiber also has good heat resistance and radiation resistance, and PTFE fiber itself does not have any toxicity. As a kind of high-tech fiber, PTFE fiber has important applications in aerospace and medical and health fields, and is often used to make spacesuits, shielding clothing and medical protective clothing.

(2) Gas mask material: With the development of synthetic rubber industry, more and more kinds of synthetic rubber with excellent comprehensive properties are being used as cover materials, such as butyl rubber, chlorinated butyl rubber, brominated butyl rubber,

silicone rubber, EPDM rubber and polyurethane. Brominated butyl rubber is better than other butyl rubber in curing speed, aging resistance, adhesion, weather resistance and fatigue resistance; thus, it is more suitable for cover material. Silicone rubber is tasteless and non-toxic, and has no adverse effect on human body. Meanwhile, silicone rubber has excellent physiological inertia, and it reacts slightly with human tissue. Therefore, the cover materials using silicone rubber are more popular in the wearing comfort, adaptability and facial leakproofness.

(3) Mask material: The medical mask is composed of a mask face and a tension band, in which the mask face is divided into three layers: inner, middle and outer. The inner layer is made of skin-friendly material (e. g. , ordinary sanitary gauze or non-woven); the middle layer is isolation filter layer (e. g. , ultra-fine polypropylene fiber melt-blown material layer), and the outer layer is a special material bacteriostatic layer (e. g. , non-woven or ultra-thin polypropylene melt-blown material layer). The protective indexes of the mask mainly include the filtration efficiency of the foreign body, the anti-splashing performance of preventing the invasion of external liquid, and the tightness of preventing the inhalation of the foreign body caused by the different shape of the mask. The main raw materials of medical non-woven masks are anti-adhesive cloth and melt-blown cloth made of thermoplastic polymer; yet, with the sharp increase in the use of disposable masks, such masks will increase the environmental pressure of post-treatment. In addition, this kind of mask also needs to be improved in terms of comfort and hygroscopicity. For example, after wearing a medical non-woven mask for a long time, the plastic strip of the mask is easy to damage the skin around the nasal bridge and cheek. At the same time, due to poor hygroscopicity, the filtration performance of this kind of mask will decrease after getting wet.

(4) Sunscreen agents: The application of nanotechnology in the field of sunscreen cosmetics can be divided into two kinds: one is to make cosmetics into nano-sized powders, and the other is to use nanocarriers to carry ultraviolet absorbents. Commonly-used nanocarriers mainly include liposomes, solid lipid nanoparticles (NPs), nano-emulsions, microspheres and others.

Among the physical ultraviolet shielding agents, iron oxide, titanium dioxide, zinc oxide, kaolin and talc powder are commonly-used substances. Usually, the size of NPs is less than tens of nanometers, and titanium dioxide (TiO_2), zinc oxide (ZnO), alumina or iron oxide of this specification have a good shielding effect on ultraviolet. Zinc oxide and titanium dioxide NPs are broad-spectrum inorganic ultraviolet shielding agents, which have been widely used in sunscreen cosmetics in recent years because of their good shielding performance, safety, stability, heat resistance and certain antibacterial properties. According to the properties of different sunscreen agents, different sunscreen agents can be compounded to enhance the effect of sunscreen. The composite of UVA sunscreen and UVB sunscreen, organic absorbent and inorganic scattering agent can improve the performance of sunscreen products, which is also an important research direction to improve sunscreen products. For example, the absorption performance of titanium dioxide NPs is better at the wavelength of 280-350 nm and weaker at other wavelengths. Zinc oxide NPs is a broad-spectrum sunscreen, while its absorption property at short wavelength is worse than that of titanium dioxide NPs. However, it can provide broad-spectrum UV protection. Some researchers have prepared a broad-spectrum sunscreen with ZnO/TiO_2 composite NPs, which combines the advantages of TiO_2 NPs and ZnO NPs. This composite particle has a strong ability to shield against ultraviolet and has a broad-spectrum sunscreen effect. In addition, organic sunscreen and inorganic sunscreen can be compounded to improve the safety of products and reduce the cost of sunscreen development.

Different delivery systems directly affect the performance of sunscreen. At present, the nano-systems used in sunscreen include mesoporous silica NPs, lipid NPs, nano-emulsions, while non-nano-systems include particles or microspheres, liposomes and cyclodextrins. The application of these delivery systems in cosmetics can improve the stability of active components, promote penetration and reduce irritation by the following ways: ① There is no direct contact between active substances and skin components, and these systems can reduce potential toxicological risks. ② These systems can reduce the photodegradation of active substances. ③ These systems can promote the effect of UV-active substances and improves the effect of sunscreen. ④ Since some nanocarriers themselves can scatter or reflect UV, it can reduce the use of UV absorbers and achieve a synergistic UV blocking effect. ⑤ The adverse interactions that may occur between various components in sunscreen formulations can be eliminated. Although the materials and structures of carrier systems vary widely, biodegradable materials (e. g., lipids or biodegradable polymers) should be preferred since they play key roles in improving chemical and physical stability.

2. New polymer materials for solving problems accompanying the use of protective products

(1) Polymer dressings for preventing skin damage caused by PPE: The key to preventing device-related pressure injuries is to reduce local skin pressure and shorten the compression time. Under the premise to ensure the protective effect, soft plastic PPE has strong compliance with the skin, relatively uniform pressure distribution, and relatively little local pressure. In areas where pressure is concentrated and there is repeated rubbing (e. g., the upper edge of goggles, the upper edge of the bridge of the nose, and the ear-closing parts of facemasks), the application of a dressing can help prevent pressure injuries by redistributing and reducing the pressure and avoiding the friction caused by relative displacement. Many types of hydrogel dressings, hydrocolloid dressings, and foam dressings are used in clinical practice to prevent pressure injuries.

Hydrogel has a rich water content and three-dimensional network structure, and has many characteristics that are beneficial for wound healing. Hydrogel dressings have good biocompatibility and compliance, as the porous structure guarantees breathability and absorbs and releases moisture to ensure that the skin moisture content is appropriate. Hydrogel also has cooling and analgesic effects (Figure 4-3).

Hydrocolloid dressings are fabricated from colloidal, gel-forming materials carboxymethyl cellulose, mixed with elastomers and adhesives. Hydrocolloid dressings consist of two main layers. The outer layer generally consists of polyurethane, and it protects the wound from bacteria, foreign debris, and shear forces. The inner layer is a self-adhesive layer mainly composed of a hydrophilic polymer matrix. After water absorption, a modification in the physical state occurs because of the gel formation, which could help to reduce the pressure or shear force directly on the skin tissue. Previous studies reported that the application of hydrocolloid dressings could significantly reduce the device-related pressure injuries of tracheotomy. Using hydrocolloid dressings can reduce the pressure by PPE (e. g. , goggles).

Foam dressing is a decompression dressing with the thickness of 0. 5 cm. Since the dressing is covered with a foam pad, it can effectively buffer and disperse the local pressure. The dressing is soft, smooth, waterproof and breathable. A protective film can be formed locally to reduce the pressure and friction on the skin after the dressing being firmly pasted. In addition, the dressing can also absorb a large amount of exudate, thereby effectively preventing impregnation, and comprehensively reducing the erosion and irritation caused by moisture on the skin. However, its compliance is not as good as hydrogel dressing and hydrocolloid dressing because of the thickness and material characteristics. Care should be taken during use to not affect the tightness of goggles and masks.

In summary, wound dressings have important therapeutic effects on treating skin damage caused by protective products, especially pressure injuries. These dressings could accelerate wound healing while protecting wounds.

(2) Anti-fogging coating reduces fogging of goggles: The material of the goggles is mainly polycarbonate (PC), which has strong impact resistance, high refractive index and thin lenses. The anti-fogging methods for this transparent plastic material mainly include: ① variation of the temperature difference between the substrate and the air through heating methods (e. g. , electricity and radiation); ② using an anti-fogging agent to change the wettability of the substrate surface. By making the surface hydrophilic, a water film is formed to spread on the substrate, and finally the light transmittance of the substrate is increased. The first method is complicated in process and the conditions used are harsh while the second method is more practical in daily life. According to the main components of anti-fogging agent, it can be divided into surfactant-type anti-fogging agent, polymer type anti-fogging agent, organic-inorganic hybrid anti-fogging agent, photocatalytic super-hydrophilic anti-fogging agent and new nano-structure hydrophilic anti-fogging agent, etc. Scientists also have conducted a lot of research on organic-inorganic hybrid type, nano-photocatalytic type and other new anti-fogging agents, and have made certain progress. With the increasing application of protective products, anti-fogging agents used in plastic materials need to have more excellent performance to meet the demand.

4.2　Skin Cleaning

4.2.1　Skin type and significance of skin cleaning

1. Skin type

The skin varies greatly between races and individuals. And there are many methods to classify skin types, most of which are based on skin hydration, sebum secretion, skin pH value and skin reactivity to external stimuli. Under physiological conditions, the skin can be divided into the following four types (Figure 4-4).

(1) Neutral skin: Also known as ordinary skin, and it is the ideal skin type. The water content of the stratum corneum is about 20% and the pH value ranges from 4.5 to 6.5. The skin is soft, delicate and elastic, with moderate sebum secretion. This type of skin has strong adaptability to external stimuli.

(2) Dry skin: The water content of stratum corneum is less than 10% and the pH value is greater than 6.5. The skin of this type is dry and lack of oil because of less sebum secretion. The skin lines are fine and pores are not obvious. People with dry skin tend to feel tight after washing face, and are sensitive to external stimuli (e.g., climate and temperature changes). The skin is also prone to chapping, scaling and wrinkles. The development of dry skin is related to genetic factors, as well as environmental factors and inappropriate habits, including overexposure of wind and sunlight and excessive use of alkaline detergents.

(3) Oily skin: Also known as fatty skin, and it is more common in young and middle-aged people and obese people. The water content of stratum corneum is about 20% and the pH value is less than 4.5. A distinctive feature of this skin type is the strong sebum secretion resulting in greasy and shiny appearance, easy to adhere to dust and large pores. The color of oily skin is often darker, while skin elasticity is great and not easy to wrinkle. And it's generally not sensitive to external stimuli. Oily skin is mostly related to hyperleydigism, high-fat diets and fragrant condiments, and is prone to skin diseases (e.g., acne and seborrheic dermatitis).

(4) Combination skin: It is a skin type in which neutral skin, dry skin or oily skin coexist. This skin type is mostly characterized by oily skin in the central part of the face (i.e., forehead, nose, nasolabial fold, and chin), while neutral or dry skin in the bilateral cheeks and temples, etc. The skin and hair characteristics of the trunk are generally consistent with that of the head and face. The hair of oily skin is always oily, while the hair of dry skin is always dry.

2. Significance of skin cleaning

The surface of the skin is often adhered by physiological dirt and exogenous dirt. The former case includes metabolites produced, secreted or excreted by the human body, including aging and shed cells, sebum, sweat, mucous membranes and excretions of the lumen. The latter case includes microorganisms, environmental pollutants, residues of various cosmetics and topical drugs. In addition, there are pathological dirt on the skin surface of patients with dermatosis, such as scales, pus, scab, and increased sweat. These skin dirt block pores and hinder the normal physiological functions of the skin and mucous membranes. Therefore, it is of great significance to clean the skin regularly, which is the basic method to maintain skin health. Moreover, skin cleaning can also stimulate blood circulation to improve skin health.

4.2.2　Classification and selection of skin cleansers

1. Classification of skin cleansers

Particles of dust, metal or non-metal oxides deposited on the skin can be removed by water. However, oil, pus, or dirt in a film form are tightly bound to the skin by electrostatic or even chemical interactions, and often require the use of cleansers to remove them. Through wetting, permeating, emulsifying and dispersing, the cleansers make the dirt escape from the skin and enter the water. After fully emulsifying and solubilizing, the dirt is dispersed in the water, and then it can be removed by repeated rinsing with clean water. The ideal skin cleansers should be harmless to the skin and can keep the surface of the skin clean and moist. According to its chemical properties, skin cleansers are often divided into soap cleanser and synthetic cleanser.

(1) Soap cleanser: It consists of fat, grease and salt, which exerts the cleaning effect by forming soap salts to emulsify the dirt on the skin surface. Because the soap salt component is alkaline (pH 9.0-10.0), it has strong detergency and the sebum film of the skin can be easily removed, which may cause skin irritation by increasing the skin pH and reducing skin tolerance. Modified soaps with added moisturizing ingredients and handmade soaps containing glycerin are gentle in nature and have low skin irritation.

(2) Synthetic cleanser: It is a non-saponified artificial surfactant with some added ingredients including moisturizers, adhesives, and preservatives. According to the chemical characteristics of surfactants, they can be divided into anionic surfactant, cationic surfactant, zwitterionic surfactant, nonionic surfactant, silicone surfactant, etc., among which the anionic surfactant has the strongest cleaning ability and is also more irritating to the skin. Synthetic cleanser can clean the skin by emulsification and wrapping effect of the surfactants. Moisturizers and emollients added in the formula can form a thin moisturizing film on the surface of the skin to reduce skin sensitivity and alleviate the skin barrier damage caused by surfactants. Transmission electron microscopy investigation shows that the skin lipid and protein structures are superbly protected after the use of synthetic cleansers. Compared with soap cleansers, synthetic cleansers are more gentle in nature and significantly less irritating to the skin. In order to further improve the moderate extractability and low temperature stability of the cleansers, water-soluble polymer components are often added to the cleansers, including acrylate-(methyl) alkyl acrylate copolymer, hydroxyethyl (propyl)

cellulose and others. These water-soluble polymer components can be used alone or in combination of two or more.

2. Selection of skin cleansers

The selection of cleansers and the frequency of use depend on the skin type, different part of skin and the seasons to use. For example, for oily skin, the amount of cleansers and the frequency of cleaning can be adjusted according to the amount of sebum to make the skin neither greasy nor dry. Oily skin is recommended to choose mild nature oil-control cleansers to avoid excessive cleaning. Excessive cleaning may damage the sebum film and increase the rate of transdermal water loss, which will then stimulate the skin sebaceous glands to secrete more sebum by negative feedback mechanism and cause "oil outside while dry inside" phenomenon. However, those with dry skin should avoid the use of soap-based cleansers. The further increase in transdermal water loss and in skin pH caused by alkalinity of the soap salt will lead to greater damage to barrier function of skin. Skin cleaning for those with sensitive skin only requires bathing with clean water or using very mild cleansers. And using tap water, river water, lake water and other soft water are relatively not irritating to the skin, so become a better choice for them.

Face should be washed once every morning and evening. The water temperature should be adjusted with seasons' change.

Bathing frequency varies with the intensity of physical activity, seasons, environment, sweating and one's personal habits. Take a bath every 2 to 3 days under normal circumstances and the frequency can be increased to once a day in hot summer or for those who love sports. The water temperature is based on the skin temperature, which can be lower than the body temperature in summer and slightly higher than the body temperature in winter, generally 35-38 ℃. Excessive washing will reduce the sebum film content, which means less protection and moisturization of the skin, and the skin aging will be promoted.

4.2.3 The hazards of excessive cleaning and the classification and selection of skin moisturizers

1. The hazards of excessive cleaning

The purpose of cleaning is to remove excess skin metabolites, contaminated dust and cosmetics. However, too frequent cleaning and excessive use of cleaning products with strong decontamination and exfoliation capabilities will cause damage to the skin barrier, affect normal pH and destroy the micro-ecological balance of the skin. In severe cases, it can induce or aggravate some skin diseases such as dry skin, itching, skin allergies, and eczema.

2. The classification and selection of skin moisturizers

The use of moisturizers after cleaning is an important measure to reduce the adverse effects of the cleansers on the skin barrier and maintain the steady state of the skin barrier. Moisturizers, also known as humectant, can maintain and replenish moisture in the stratum corneum of the skin to prevent skin dryness, or rescue skin that has dried, loss of elasticity and chapped, to make it smooth, soft and elastic again. Moisturizers are divided into natural moisturizers and synthetic moisturizers according to their sources. According to the mechanism of moisturizing, they can be divided into sealing moisturizers and wetting or hygroscopic moisturizers.

(1) Sealing moisturizers: They are a type of insoluble lipid substance. By supplementing the stratum corneum with lipid substance, it forms an additional lubricating film layer on the surface of the skin, wraps the stratum corneum, and blocks the loss of moisture from the skin. And the water can continuously diffuse from the inner layer of the skin into the stratum corneum to help maintain a certain water content in it. There are many characteristics of this type of moisturizers, including good moisture absorption and moisturizing capacity which is rarely affected by environmental conditions (e. g. , temperature and humidity), low volatility and low freezing point, suitable viscosity and good affinity to skin, colorless, odorless, tasteless, and good compatibility with other ingredients. Sealing moisturizers mainly have the following 6 categories: ① Mineral oils and waxes, such as petrolatum and mineral oil. ② Plant and animal fats, such as lanolin. ③ Silicone oils, such as cyclomethicone. ④ Fatty acids and esters categories, such as stearic acid and linolenic acid. ⑤ Phospholipids, cholesterol, such as lecithin and cholesterol sulfate. ⑥ Plant and animal waxes, such as carnauba and beeswax.

(2) Wetting or hygroscopic moisturizers: The substances of this kind of moisturizers is similar to natural moisturizing factors, and human polysaccharides and proteins in the epidermis, including glycerin, hyaluronic acid, etc. It is a water supplement and enters the inside of skin through pores, or carries moisture into skin when skin moisture is lost, or wraps the unlost moisture to preserve it in the skin. The characteristics of this type of moisturizers are that they can increase the skin water content and reduce the transepidermal water loss to make stratum corneum flexible and softening, as well as attract moisture from the skin deep and dermis tissue into stratum corneum to be easily acquired by cell.

The selection of moisturizers should be based on skin conditions. People with oily skin are recommended to choose more water-soluble moisturizers, while people with dry skin can form a better protective layer on the skin surface with more oil composition moisturizers. It is necessary to apply moisturizers in areas where sebum glands are small and the stratum corneum are thinner, such as eyes, lips and neck.

4. 2. 4 Application prospects of polymer materials in skin cleaning and moisturizing

In recent years, polymer nanomaterials have been popular in areas of cosmetic dermatology because of their advantages of enhancing skin permeability, controlling and sustaining drug release capability, higher stability, certain targeting ability, higher encapsulation efficiency and good sensory characteristics. There are many polymer products such as in the areas of shampoos for preventing hair loss or promoting hair growth, as well as new moisturizers. In the field of cosmeceuticals, various types of nanocarriers, such as liposomes, niosomes, solid lipid nanoparticles, nanostructured lipid carriers and nanoemulsion have been used in the delivery of skin moisturizing and cleaning ingredients. Many well-known cosmetic brands, including Dior, Lancome and Decorte, have developed a variety of nano-cosmeceuticals. Nanocarriers can achieve controlled release of active substances and change the transdermal efficiency of drugs. Polymer nanomaterials can also be used to synthesize drugs with different biochemical properties through physical or chemical interactions between components and variable ratios of polymers and additives, which has broad prospects in the field of cosmetics and skin disease treatment.

4.3　Skin Disinfection

4.3.1　Concept and significance of skin disinfection

Skin disinfection is one of the important measures to prevent microbial infections on the skin. Skin disinfectants refer to a group of disinfection products for wounds, burned area and other parts of skin and mucous membranes for the purpose of preventing and controlling bacterial infections. They can destroy the physiological function of pathogens and consequently kill them by changing the physiological activities of their inner enzyme system and protein.

4.3.2　Classification and use of skin disinfectants

1. Common skin disinfectants

Disinfectants are classified by mechanisms, effect, objects, etc. According to the mechanisms, they can be ambiguously classified into chemical disinfectants and biological disinfectants (e.g., enzymes and bacteriophages). Of which, chemical disinfectants are the most widely used and most diverse disinfectants which can be further classified into oxidized and non-oxidized disinfectants according to the types of chemical reaction. Oxidized disinfectants mainly include halogens (e.g., chlorine, bromine, and iodine) and peroxides (e.g., hydrogen peroxide, peroxyacetic acid, and chlorine dioxide); non-oxidized disinfectants mainly include alcohols (e.g., ethanol), phenols (e.g., para-chlorometa xylenol), quaternary ammonium salts (e.g., benzalkonium chloride), guanidines (e.g., polyhexamethylene biguanide hydrochloride, chlorhexidine), aldehydes (e.g., glutaraldehyde) and metals (e.g., silver).

According to the ability of killing microorganisms, disinfectants can be classified into high-efficiency, medium-efficiency and low-efficiency. It is believed that high-efficiency disinfectants, which in general contain chlorine, peroxides, or aldehydes, can kill all microorganisms including bacterial spores, fungal spores, and viruses. Medium-efficiency disinfectants which in general contain iodine or alcohol, can not kill bacterial spores. Low-efficiency disinfectants (e.g., certain guanidines and certain quaternary ammonium salts), can only kill general bacterial propagules, some fungi and lipophilic viruses, without ability of killing *Mycobacterium tuberculosis*, hydrophilic viruses and bacterial spores.

Common categories of skin disinfectants include iodine, alcohols, phenols, peroxides, guanidines, and quaternary ammonium salts, etc.

(1) Iodine-containing disinfectants: Iodine is a widely used ingredient of skin disinfectants. Iodine molecules can quickly penetrate the cell wall to combine with amino acids and unsaturated fatty acids, resulting in difficulty in protein synthesis and changes in cell membranes. The iodine-containing disinfectants commonly used in clinical practice are iodine tincture (e. g. , iodine wine), iodophor and povidone-iodine solution. Povidone iodine, an amorphous complex formed by the combination of iodine and surfactant, is currently the most important iodine-containing skin disinfectant, as well as mucous membrane disinfectant. The surface active ingredients contained in it can change the wettability of the solution to the object and form an extremely thin sterilization film on the skin surface which is able to assist iodine to penetrate organics, emulsify fat, release effective iodine slowly and permanently to strengthen the sterilization ability of iodine.

(2) Alcohol-containing disinfectants: Ethanol belongs to the medium-efficiency disinfectants, with an optimal effective concentration of 75% to 85%. Soaking or wiping with 60% to 90% ethanol aqueous solution can kill bacterial propagules, mycobacteria, yeasts, fungi and some viruses, except bacterial spores. The dehydration of ethanol can make the bacterial protein coagulate and denature, and its penetration can make it penetrate the cell wall and enter the bacterial body to play the disinfecting role. Although ethanol can quickly kill bacterial propagules, it is not lasting. In addition, it is volatile and irritating, which can not be applied to mucosa or large wounds. The combination of ethanol and other chemical antibacterial agents produces a synergistic antibacterial effect. For example, the compounding of multiple alcohol solutions can shorten the effective action time and improve the sterilization ability, especially to virus.

Isopropyl alcohol belongs to the medium-efficiency disinfectants as well, with similar sterilization mechanism to that of ethanol. Isopropyl alcohol has a slightly stronger sterilizing ability and toxicity than ethanol. Currently, ethanol is extensively used in China, while isopropyl alcohol is widely used abroad. Isopropyl alcohol can completely kill lipid viruses, but it has no inactivating effect on non-lipid enteroviruses. Its commonly-used concentration is 70%-80%, and 70% isopropanol can kill hepatitis B virus, hepatitis C virus and human immunodeficiency virus within 10 min.

(3) Phenol-containing disinfectants: Trichloro hydroxyl diphenyl ether, a broad-spectrum, high-efficiency antibacterial agent, also known as triclosan, is an important phenol-containing disinfectant. Its effective antibacterial concentration is 0. 2%-2. 0%. Triclosan penetrates into the bacterial cell and affects the cell plasma membrane and synthesis of RNA, fatty acid and protein. Triclosan has a certain degree of antibacterial effect, but tends to show more bacteriostatic effect. In addition, it has a stronger effect on

Gram-positive bacteria (including MRSA) than Gram-negative bacteria, especially *Pseudomonas aeruginosa* and a certain activity against *Mycobacterium* and *Candida*, but has a weak activity against filamentous fungi. Studies have shown that triclosan is mildly teratogenic.

(4) Peroxide-containing disinfectants: Peroxide-containing disinfectants mainly include hydrogen peroxide and peracetic acid, and can kill all microorganisms such as bacteria, fungi, spores and viruses. Of which, peracetic acid has the strongest sterilization ability, followed by hydrogen peroxide. Peroxide-containing disinfectants are high-efficiency, quick-acting, and low-toxic disinfectants, which need to be used and prepared instantly. At high concentrations, they can irritate and damage skin and mucous membranes. The concentration of hydrogen peroxide solution up to 1000 mg/L has a bactericidal effect. Clinically, hydrogen peroxide solution is often used to gargle and clean wounds in patients with oral inflammation. The concentration of peroxyacetic acid solution should be less than 2000 mg/L when it is used for skin disinfection, and be reduced to 200 mg/L when it is used for mucosa disinfection.

(5) Guanidine-containing disinfectants: Chlorhexidine, a low-efficiency disinfectant, also known as chlorhexidine, is a biguanide antibacterial agent with low toxicity, low irritation, and broad antibacterial spectrum. The chlorhexidine is easily adsorbed on the bacterial body to damage the cell membrane and inhibit the action of bacterial system enzymes to hinder the bacterial metabolism, through which it is mainly used as an antibacterial treatment for skin and mucous membranes. Moreover, high concentration of chlorhexidine can make the cell cytoplasm aggregated, concentrated and denatured to achieve the purpose of sterilization. Chlorhexidine can effectively kill bacterial propagules, but has only an inhibitory effect on spores, tuberculosis and fungi, and a weak ability to kill hepatitis B and C viruses and fungal strains of *Aspergillus niger*.

(6) Quaternary ammonium salt-containing disinfectants: Quaternary ammonium salt-containing disinfectants are low-efficiency disinfectants, including single-chain quaternary ammonium salts and double-chain quaternary ammonium salts, such as dodecyl dimethylbenzyl ammonium bromide (e. g. , benzalkonium bromide), dodecyl dimethylphenoxyethyl ammonium bromide (e. g. , domiphen) and myristyl dimethylpyridine ammonium bromide. It can adsorb on the surface of the bacteria to change the permeability of the bacteria, along with leakage of intracellular substances and denaturation of proteins, consequently obstructing the process of cell metabolism to achieve the effect of sterilization. The disinfectants have the characteristics of low bactericidal concentration, good water solubility, low toxicity, low irritation, stable properties, etc. , but the price is comparatively expensive, the effect of killing certain viruses is poor, and there are many compatibility taboos. The presentative product, benzalkonium bromide, has a strong antibacterial effect, but it cannot kill fungi, *Mycobacterium tuberculosis*, bacterial spores, and non-cladding viruses. The clinically used concentration of benzalkonium bromide is 1000 mg/L, which can be used to clean the skin of

patients, and clean the hands of medical staff, etc. It is usually used in the combination with alcohol disinfectants.

2. Disinfection procedures and attention points

(1) Thorough cleaning is the prerequisite to ensure the disinfection effect. Prior to skin disinfection, the skin should be cleaned specifically in accordance with the pollution types of the skin. Incomplete cleaning or decontamination will affect the disinfection effect.

(2) Correctly select the type and concentration of disinfectant. Take ethanol as an example, it has the best disinfection effect at a concentration of 70%-80%.

(3) Sufficient action time is required. The action time of different skin disinfectants varies. Generally, it takes 1-5 min or is subjected to thorough natural drying to reach the disinfection standard.

4.3.3　Damages of disinfectant to skin and corresponding nursing measures

Similar to the damages caused by excessive cleaning, frequent exposure to disinfectants will destroy the normal structure of the skin barrier, and change the pH of the sebum membrane, making the skin presented with dryness, redness, itch, and even molting. Long-term exposure to some compositions in the disinfectants (e.g., ethanol) can render the skin dry and rough, loss of elasticity, excessive oil secretion, and changes in the immune microenvironment on the skin surface, which can lead to eczema, allergic dermatitis, etc. In addition, the irritant components in the disinfectant may cause adverse reactions such as contact dermatitis.

1. Allergic reaction

It is usually seen in people with special physical condition who are allergic to the disinfectant ingredient. The common manifestation is allergic contact dermatitis which often appears at the contact site, and the range of which is roughly the same with that of the contact area. Mild symptoms are presented with redness, swelling, itch and other symptoms appearing on the local skin. While in severe cases, papules, blisters, and even erosion and ulceration may occur, posing great risk of secondary infections. Treatment principles: ① Stop using suspicious disinfectants at once and replace with other non-allergenic products. ② If the rash is light, it can be mitigated on its own within 3-5 days without special treatment after discontinuing contact with allergen. ③ If the rash is severe and itching is obvious, the second-generation antihistamine can be administrated orally plus topical application of moderate to strong glucocorticoids such as mometasone furoate and halometasone cream. Oral glucocorticoids are needed only when systematic symptoms show. ④ When there is a secondary infection, antibiotics should be used topically or systematically.

2. Damage and irritation of skin barrier

As fat-soluble disinfectant dissolves the sebum film on the skin surface, repeated use of such disinfectant can easily lead to the destruction of the skin barrier function and the appearance of cracked skin. If fat-soluble disinfectant continues to be used, it will penetrate into the skin and cause irritation, manifested with itch, erythema, papules, blisters, chap, etc. on the contact skin area. Treatment principles: strengthen the use of emollients; other measures are consistent with the treatment of allergic contact dermatitis.

Of note, with the long-term and large-scale use of skin care and disinfection products with antibacterial effects, the common pathogenic bacteria in the skin flora and the colonizing conditioned pathogen are increasing their resistance to the disinfectant ingredient, as well as the drug resistance spectrum, which reduces the effect of skin disinfection.

4.3.4 Other novel disinfectants

1. Acidic oxidation potential water

Acidic oxidation potential water refers to a disinfectant made by adding a low concentration of sodium chloride solution to water and electrolyzed by electrochemical methods which includes slightly acidic electrolyzed water, weakly acidic electrolyzed water and strong acidic electrolyzed water. At present, it is generally believed that the bactericidal effect of acidic oxidation potential water is determined by its pH value, oxidation-reduction potential (ORP), available chlorine, and active oxygen. The low pH value and high ORP value of acidic oxidation potential water can change the cell membrane potential of microorganisms to enhance their cell permeability, making bacteria swell, destroying inner cell metabolic enzymes, and causing intracellular substances to overflow and dissolve to achieve the bactericidal effect. Acidic oxidation potential water has characteristics of broad-spectrum, high-efficiency, non-toxic, non-irritating, non-drug-resistant, but has poor stability and is easily affected by organics and metal ions.

2. Biological disinfectants

Biological disinfectants mainly include plant disinfectants and microbial preparations. Compared with chemical disinfectants, biological disinfectants have characteristics of fast sterilization speed, strong specificity, low toxicity, mild, non-irritating, non-drug-resistant, and no harmful substances remain. The active ingredient is mainly essential oil. Several kinds of botanical extracts (e. g., vegetable oil, sophora flavescens, chrysanthemum and dried ginger) can be formulated into bactericidal preparations. Microbial preparations have two categories: one is the direct use of microorganisms as bactericides; the other is the separation or synthesis of microbial metabolites. Microbial preparations mainly include bdellovibrio, biological enzymes and bacteriophage. Biological enzymes include lysozyme and staphylococcal enzyme, which have a strong ability to kill Gram-positive bacteria. Lysozyme has been used for disinfection and debridement of burn wounds. The bacteriophage is highly specific and can infect specific bacteria.

3. Silver disinfectants

It is Ag^+ that finally plays the role of sterilization effect in all silver-containing disinfectants. The sterilization mechanisms of Ag^+ include: combine with the cell membrane to change the original structure and function; act on the proton pump to affect the material transmission and metabolism; combine with thiol, amino and carboxyl groups of intracellular proteins to destroy the structure and function of enzymes that can decompose glucose, sucrose, urea, etc.; combine with DNA to block reproduction and break chemical bonds to destroy the molecular structure. Compared with silver in the form of ions, silver NP is easily contacted with pathogenic microorganisms due to quantum effect, small size effect and a large specific surface area, thereby exerting a greater biological effect. Therefore, silver NP is more secure and durable with stronger antibacterial effect. The sterilization mechanism of silver NP is complex and diverse. As it belongs to non-antibiotic fungicides, it is not easy to develop drug resistance. However, in the setting of lacking protective agents, silver NP materials are prone to aggregate particles and lose nano-characteristics, or are oxidized into brown silver oxide, both affecting its sterilization effect.

4.4　Challenges and Perspectives

This chapter mainly introduces the development of skin protection, cleaning and disinfection products, including personal protective equipment, skin protective agents, sunscreen and a variety of skin cleansers, moisturizers, disinfectants, as well as polymer materials used to solve the problems in the use of protective products. In people's production and daily life, the protection, cleaning and disinfection of skin are very important for maintaining skin health and protecting the body from external physical, chemical, biological and other factors.

With the rapid development of polymer materials in biomedicine and other fields, the emergence of various new protective products, skin cleaning and moisturizing agents and skin disinfectants has brought more guarantees to the skin health in production and life. For example, in terms of materials, new protective clothing fiber materials, masks polymer materials and nano-sunscreen, as well as polymer skin cleansers, moisturizers and disinfectants, all can play good roles. However, due to the specific biological characteristics of skin, the skin barrier is also susceptible to damage caused by environment and the protective equipment, cleansers and disinfectants. The development of medical polymer materials should pay attention to the human safety, comfort of use and long-term protection of skin barrier, so as to truly highlight the advantages of biomedical polymer materials. A good example is the use of new hydrogels, hydrocolloid and other dressings for the prevention of pressure injuries caused by protective equipment.

Questions

1. What's the main classification of skin protective products, skin cleansers and skin disinfectants at present?

2. What applications do polymer materials basically have in skin protection? How can we optimize the materials?

3. What are the characteristics of polymer materials in skin cleansers and moisturizers?

4. What are the main issues and needs in the field of skin protection, cleaning and disinfection?

5. How can polymer materials be used in the future for skin protection, cleaning and disinfection?

Extended Reading

[1] Rook A, Burns T F. Rook's textbook of dermatology[M]. 8th ed. Oxford: Blackwell Science, 2010.

[2] 李航,陶娟. 重大疫情中皮肤黏膜屏障防护手册[M]. 北京:北京大学医学出版社,2020.

[3] Bucci P, Prieto M J, Milla L, et al. Skin penetration and UV-damage prevention by nanoberries[J]. J Cosmet Dermatol, 2018, 17(5):889-899.

[4] Zhao Z, Fang R, Rong Q, et al. Bioinspired nanocomposite hydrogels with highly ordered structures[J]. Adv Mater, 2017, 29(45):e1703045.

[5] Rutala W A, Weber D J. Disinfection and sterilization in health care facilities: an overview and current issues[J]. Infect Dis Clin North Am, 2016, 30(3):609-637.

(Zhou Nuoya　Tao Juan)

第五章
皮肤影像学诊断技术

皮肤疾病是指发生于人体皮肤、黏膜及皮肤附属器的疾病。皮肤疾病种类繁多、治疗时间长且易反复，是临床上的常见病、多发病。随着大气污染日益严重，皮肤疾病发病率不断提高，皮肤疾病的致病因素也在不断增多。世界卫生组织曾宣布，皮肤疾病将是 21 世纪人类历史上发病率最高、致残率最高、传染性最强的一种疾病。受生活条件和环境的影响，皮肤疾病多发于经济发展落后、贫困的地区，且皮肤疾病患者年龄日趋低龄化，数量逐年递增。特别是我国患者对皮肤疾病的认识不足，导致病情拖延；且皮肤疾病容易反复，治疗费用高等，给人民的健康生活和经济社会发展带来了困扰。鉴于皮肤疾病类型繁多、病情复杂，发展无创性、原位、实时、动态的皮肤疾病影像学诊断技术，对可疑皮损进行早期检查、定期复查，提供客观、量化的评价指标，成为目前皮肤科临床的重要需求。

皮肤疾病诊断以皮损形态和视诊为基础。在专业的皮肤影像学诊断技术出现之前，皮肤科医生只能利用裸眼直接辨识诊断，但这种诊断方法基于主观判断，需要皮肤科医生在长期临床实践中积淀深厚的临床经验，而且由于传统病历通常只有文字描述，无法留存图像资料，不利于后续进行诊疗随访和疗效比较。后来，虽然通过手工绘图和蜡型制模的方式在一定程度上改善了病历缺乏图像资料的问题，但绘图和制模过程烦琐，且需要专业人才，缺乏普适性。随着科学技术的不断发展，涌现出了电子计算机断层扫描（CT）、磁共振成像（MRI）、正电子发射断层扫描（PET）、超声成像以及皮肤镜、皮肤共聚焦技术、多光子成像、光学相干断层成像和光声成像等多种光学成像技术。上述光学成像技术可对可疑皮损进行可视化检查，能不同程度地实现皮下组织的无创性、原位、实时成像，为临床诊断提供了客观的评价依据。不断发展的皮肤影像学与皮肤组织病理学相互促进、相互补充，势必将带动现代皮肤病学的飞跃发展。

第一节　皮　肤　镜

皮肤镜，又称皮表透光显微镜、入射光显微镜等，是一种可以放大数十倍的皮肤显微镜，能够无创性观察活体皮肤表面以下微细结构。它可以观察到表皮下部、真皮乳头层和真皮深层等肉眼不可见的组织结构与特征，这些特征与皮肤组织病理学的变化有着特殊和相对明确的对应关系，根据这些对应关系确定了皮肤镜诊断的灵敏度、特异性。皮肤镜被称为"皮肤科医生的听诊器"，在皮肤影像学技术中应用最为广泛，发展也较为成熟。

早在 1663 年，Kohlhaus 首次利用显微镜观察到甲床血管。1893 年，Unna 首次利用浸油和玻片在显微镜下观察寻常狼疮患者的皮损，并在德语中使用"diaskopie"（透照法）表示。

1916年,Zeiss制成首个双目皮肤血管镜。1920年,德国皮肤科医生Saphier首次使用术语"dermatoskopie",并对皮肤镜进行了升级改造,首次将传统的外置光源用内置光源来替代,从而能够清晰地观察皮肤病变部位的毛细血管。现代皮肤镜的雏形出现在1951年,美国皮肤科医生Goldman首次用单目放大镜观察、评估各种色素性皮肤疾病(包括色素痣和黑素瘤等)的镜下特征。1970年以后,皮肤镜在皮肤科临床上得到了广泛的推广和应用。1971年,Mackie研究并总结了皮肤镜对色素性皮肤疾病术前诊断的意义及其在鉴别良性色素痣和黑素瘤中的作用。1981年,Fritsch等根据皮肤镜下不同色素结构特征区别黑素瘤和色素痣。1987年,Pehamberger等发表论文,详细记载了各种色素性皮肤疾病在皮肤镜下的特征,建立了模式分析法,用于诊断色素性皮肤疾病,促进了皮肤镜诊断方法的形成。1991年,Kreusch和Rassner出版了第一本皮肤镜图谱,强调皮肤镜下观察结构与组织病理学的联系。时至今日,皮肤镜在皮肤科临床上的应用越来越广泛,不论是在色素性或非色素性皮损、血管形态,还是毛发生长方面都可以进行观察,皮肤镜诊断标准也在不断完善。

一般情况下,由于皮肤表面的角质层光密度和折射率与空气不同,照射到皮肤表面的大部分光在皮肤表面被直接反射,一部分光被皮肤吸收,而仅有少量光通过散射进入皮肤,因此皮肤表皮下的结构用肉眼很难观察到。皮肤镜(图5-1)的具体使用方法:首先在皮肤表面滴加浸润液(如水、矿物油、乙醇和凝胶等)以增加皮肤角质层的透光性和减少反射光;然后在浸润液上面覆盖玻片,压平局部皮肤;光源从适当的角度射入,在光学放大设备的协助下,能够观察到表皮下部、真皮乳头层和真皮深层等肉眼不可见的影像结构与特征。最新研究表明,医用乙醇作为浸润液产生的气泡较少,从而能获得更为清晰的图像,并且具有不油腻、不染色、自然挥发而无须擦拭、可有效减少细菌污染等优点。此外,水凝胶(例如超声用耦合剂)具有非流动性和无刺激性的优势,在眼睛或者黏膜区域应用较为广泛。

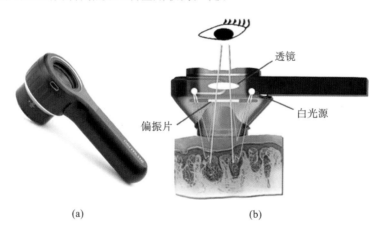

图5-1 手持式皮肤镜实物图(a)和示意图(b)

Figure 5-1 Photograph (a) and schematic diagram (b) of handheld dermatoscope

在早期皮肤科临床工作中,皮肤疾病的诊断主要依靠临床医生的经验和组织病理学检查。虽然组织病理学是行业的金标准,正确诊断率高,是目前临床最为可靠的诊断依据,但它是一种创伤性的检查方法,对于多发色素性皮损很难进行逐一检查。而皮肤镜在多发色素性皮损的早期排查和随访观察方面有着得天独厚的优势,可以判定需要做活组织检查的皮损病灶,还可对大面积皮损部位进行病情定位,保证了切除范围的准确性,以及对皮损进行定期的随访观察。作为临床上诸多疾病的筛选和诊断工具,皮肤镜具有无创、无痛、诊断迅速等优点,有良好

的发展前景。目前,关于皮肤镜的诊断方法有很多,如模式分析法、ABCD 规则法、Menzies
法、7 点分类法、TADA 法等。其中,模式分析法在各种色素性皮损鉴别诊断方面,尤其是良恶
性黑素性皮损的鉴别方面展现了极大的优势。

　　黑素瘤是一种多发生于皮肤的恶性肿瘤,其因持续增高的发病率和死亡率而引起了人们
越来越高的重视。降低黑素瘤患者死亡率最有效的方法是早期诊断。尚未发展成侵袭性黑素
瘤以前,治愈率是 98%。一旦黑素瘤突破真皮层甚至发生转移,治愈率将降低至 15%。模式
分析法被认为是评估色素沉着性皮肤疾病的经典皮肤镜方法,即"提炼整体模式,结合局部标
准"。此方法包括评估病变的对称性、一种或多种颜色、基本模式以及局部特征。整体模式是
指占大面积病变的主要特征,由一个(通常)或两个(较少见)主要特征组成。而局部特征可以
被识别为单个特征或分组特征,并且它们中的几个可以共存于同一病变中。常见的基本模式
有四种:网状模式(对应色素网络)、球状模式(对应多个点、球)、星爆状模式(对应外周条纹或
伪足)和均质模式(对应无结构色素区)。此外,还存在组合模式,即源自两种以上模式的组合。
这四种模式在痣和黑素瘤中均可见,而组合模式则多在黑素瘤中出现(图 5-2)。如果病变表现

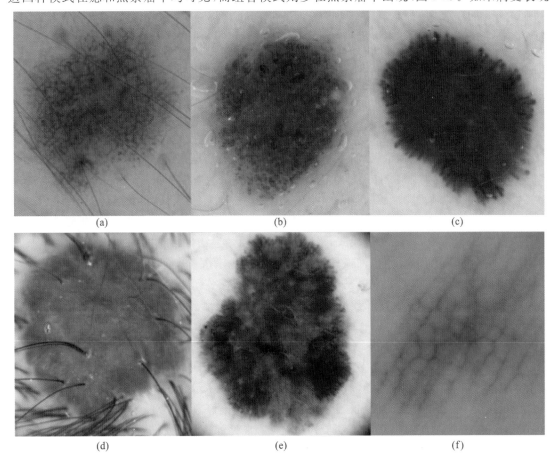

图 5-2　代表性皮肤痣与黑素瘤的皮肤镜图片

(a)网状痣;(b)球状痣;(c)星爆状 Spitz 痣;(d)均质蓝色痣;(e)组合模式黑素瘤;(f)平行沟肢端痣

Figure 5-2　Global dermoscopic patterns of representative nevus and melanoma

(a) Reticular (nevus);(b) Globular (nevus);(c) Starburst (Spitz nevus);(d) Homogeneous (blue nevus);
(e)Multicomponent (melanoma);(f)Parallel furrow pattern (acral nevus)

出这四种模式中的一种,则将根据整体对称性、颜色和局部特征进行进一步评估,即所谓的"黑素瘤特异性标准"。通常,痣的特征是结构对称,并显示一种或两种颜色。相比之下,黑素瘤结构紊乱,通常具有两种以上的颜色。

一、黑素瘤特异性标准

非典型色素网络:棕黑色网络,具有不规则的网孔和不规则分布的不同厚度的线(对黑素瘤的诊断具有很高的特异性)。

不规则的点和(或)小球:棕黑色或灰色,大小不同的点和(或)小球,不规则地分布在病变区域内。

不规则斑点:黑色,棕色或灰色区域,形状和(或)分布不规则。

不规则条纹和(或)伪足:呈放射状不规则地分布在病变区域周围(条纹),有时在其周围末端呈球状突起(伪足)。

退化结构:见于病变的平坦区域,可能表现为与纤维化相对应的白色瘢痕样区域或与黑素细胞相对应的蓝灰色区域(胡椒粉)。

蓝白色面纱:见于病变的隆起部分。呈蓝灰色或蓝白色,弥漫性,有不规则色素沉着。

血管结构不规则:多形血管,在同一病变中并存点状、线状或发夹状血管等。

由于特定的皮肤解剖结构,在某些位置(如面部、手掌、足掌和指甲等)上色素性黑素细胞病变表现出独特的皮肤镜特征。

二、肢端黑素瘤

肢端黑素瘤见于手掌、足底、甲下等肢端部位,是我国乃至亚洲发生率较高的黑素瘤亚型(约占 50%),因此鉴别肢端的良、恶性色素沉着性肿瘤尤为重要。肢端黑素瘤早期常常表现为褐色斑疹,临床上通过肉眼观察很难与肢端黑素痣区分开,皮肤科医生在面对肢端色素性皮损时难以明确诊断,而皮肤镜能极大地提高皮肤科医生对肢端黑素瘤的临床诊断能力。肢端黑素痣皮肤镜下主要表现为三种模式:平行沟,是肢端黑素痣最常见的模式,表现为沿着皮肤表面纹路走形的褐色色素沉着;网格样,表现为平行的色素沉着中间连接着桥梁样的色素沉着线,形似网状格子;纤维状,表现为密集的纤维样色素沉着平行排列。

肢端黑素瘤与肢端黑素痣在皮肤镜下的表现形式有显著差异。平行嵴模式是肢端黑素瘤最常见且最具特异性的表现,该模式由平行于皮嵴的带状色素构成,灵敏度和特异性分别高达86%和99%,从而大大提高了肢端黑素瘤诊断的准确率。与肢端黑素痣的平行沟模式中色素位于皮沟处不同,肢端黑素瘤的平行嵴模式中色素平行线位于皮嵴处。除了平行嵴模式之外,肢端黑素瘤还存在不规则的弥漫色素沉着模式,表现为弥漫、无结构的黑褐色色素沉着同时带有颜色的渐变,多见于晚期的皮损。其他表现诸如不规则斑点或小球、不规则条纹、蓝白色面纱、溃疡形成、非典型血管形态,甚至是肢端黑素痣常见的三种模式都可见于肢端黑素瘤中。对于位于肢端的后天黑素瘤皮损,Saida 等建议在临床上面对疑似肢端黑素瘤患者时,首先利用皮肤镜诊断是否为平行嵴模式,阳性患者立刻做组织病理学检查,阴性患者则需进一步确认是否具有典型的肢端黑素痣模式(如平行沟、网格样、纤维样)。如有,则可进行长期的临床随访观察;如没有,且皮损直径大于 7 mm,则需做组织病理学检查进行确认。

三、恶性雀斑样黑素瘤

恶性雀斑样黑素瘤多发于阳光暴晒区域,从恶性雀斑样痣发展而来。通常是在恶性雀斑样痣多年以后,皮疹扩大,出现蓝黑色结节和溃疡,在老年人面部最为常见。组织病理学表现为表皮基底层异形黑素细胞增生,且皮肤镜观察的位于面部的黑素细胞皮损表现不同于其他部位。Stolz等率先用皮肤镜观察面部恶性雀斑样黑素瘤,并总结了四个发展阶段的特征性表现模式:阶段Ⅰ,出现色素沉着过度的不对称毛囊开口,表明黑素瘤细胞向单个毛囊不均匀浸润;阶段Ⅱ,在毛囊口周围出现短而细的条纹、点和小球,表现为环形颗粒状图案;阶段Ⅲ,随着毛囊口周围的条纹变长、相交,逐渐形成菱形色素结构;阶段Ⅳ,随着毛囊内部黑素瘤细胞的浸润,色素沉着区域融合,直至毛囊口消失。此模式诊断恶性雀斑样黑素瘤的灵敏度和特异性分别是89%和93%,可用于临床上诊断和随访观察恶性雀斑样黑素瘤。

总之,除了黑素瘤以外,皮肤镜在非黑素细胞来源的肿瘤中应用也非常广泛,包括基底细胞癌、鳞状细胞癌等。皮肤镜在评估皮肤肿瘤方面具有不可替代的作用,它显著提高了临床医生诊断的准确性,降低了误诊率。此外,随着皮肤疾病在皮肤镜下表现形态及模式的不断完善,皮肤镜逐渐扮演着类似于皮肤科医生听诊器的角色。

第二节 光学相干断层成像

光学相干断层成像(optical coherence tomography,OCT)技术是一种以光反射为基础的非侵入性二维成像技术,具有高分辨率(分辨率可达微米级)、非接触性、非侵入性和实时性等优势,在生物组织活体检测和在体成像方面具有极高的应用前景。1991年,美国麻省理工学院的Huang和哈佛医学院的Schuman等用半导体激光器(中心波长为830 nm)研制出首台OCT仪器,用于测量离体的冠状动脉和视网膜。随着技术的进步,OCT逐渐发展成为一种实用的临床检测工具,并于1993年率先在眼科临床进行活体成像。从1997年开始,OCT逐渐被应用于皮肤病学、胃肠病学、泌尿科、妇科和神经外科等,并出现了多款用于皮肤病学的商用OCT系统。通过应用OCT技术,可以从皮肤组织的OCT图像中获取其结构上的变化,而这种结构变化可以用来表征不同类型的皮肤肿瘤。OCT的局限性在于,其最大成像深度仅为2 mm,这常使其无法评估网状真皮之外的皮肤变化。

一、OCT的原理

OCT利用光学干涉原理成像,整个系统包括一个光源、一个分束器和一个探测器,也被称为迈克尔逊干涉仪。OCT集半导体激光技术、光学技术、超灵敏探测技术和计算机图像处理技术于一身,能够提供分辨率达$1\sim15\ \mu m$的生物组织轴向断层图像。OCT将近红外光源发出的光线分为两束,一束射向被测物质,称为样品臂;另一束射向参照反光镜,称为参考臂。从被测物质和参照反光镜反射回来的两束光在探测器上进行信号叠加。当样品臂与参考臂的长度一致时,两束光发生干涉。对从组织中反射回来的光信号来说,组织的性状不同,反射光信号强弱不同。样品臂的反射光与参考臂的反射光信号叠加,光波顶点一致时信号增强(增加干涉),光波顶点方向相反时信号减弱(削减干涉)。形成干涉的条件是频率相同,相位差恒定。利用干涉原理,OCT通过比较标准光源信号与反射光源信号,增强单一光线反射,减弱散射光线反射。由于干涉只发生在样品臂与参考臂长度一致时,通过调节反光镜的位置,可以改变参考臂的长度,继而得到不同深度的组织信号。这些光信号经过计算机处理便可得到组织断层图像。

与以往的成像技术相比,OCT具备以下优势:①采用对人体无害的近红外光源;②采用干涉技术实现断层成像,分辨率极高,可达微米级;③采用直径约100 μm的光纤传输信号,可以连接各种仪器,包括导管、内镜、腹腔镜和手术探针,这可以实现身体内的器官系统成像;④可以在原位进行成像,无须像常规的活组织检查和组织病理学那样处理标本,并且图像为实时传输图像,无需复杂的数学计算和图像重建,可实现实时诊断,并将此信息与手术联系起来,可实现手术指导;⑤设备紧凑且便携,这是临床上可行设备的重要考虑因素。

根据成像工作原理,OCT可以分为两大类,即时域OCT(time domain OCT,TD-OCT)和频域OCT(frequency domain OCT,FD-OCT)(图5-3)。TD-OCT是将在同一时间从组织中反射回来的光信号与参照反光镜反射回来的光信号叠加、干涉,然后成像。TD-OCT采用机械移动反光镜的方法,速度有限。FD-OCT为第二代OCT技术,使得更有效的低相干干涉测量原理得以实现。FD-OCT的参考反光镜固定不动,通过改变光源光波的频率实现信号的干涉。由于取消了机械移动部件,利用电子扫描方式,FD-OCT的扫描成像速度大大提高,信噪比也得到改善,特点是无需纵向扫描,信号灵敏度大幅度提高,动态范围大。

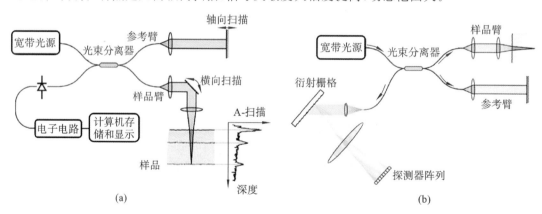

图 5-3　时域 OCT(TD-OCT)(a)和频域 OCT(FD-OCT)(b)系统图

Figure 5-3　Schematic diagram of time domain OCT (a) and frequency domain OCT (b)

二、OCT 的应用

随着OCT的不断完善,OCT因无创性、非侵入性、高分辨率、结构简单、设备简单便携等优势在皮肤检查、眼科检查、胃肠道检查等多方面有着广泛的应用,特别是在皮肤疾病的检测和诊断上。目前医学上皮肤癌诊断的金标准是组织病理学活检,但组织病理学活检具有创伤性,会遗留瘢痕,无法定量检测,而通过应用OCT技术,可以从皮肤组织的OCT图像中获取其结构上的变化,这种结构变化可以用来表征不同类型的皮肤肿瘤。迄今为止,OCT的最大潜力在于皮肤病学中非黑素瘤皮肤癌（NMSCs）的诊断和治疗检测，尤其是基底细胞癌。此外，OCT在色素性病变中的应用仍面临巨大挑战，而在黑素瘤的诊断中，OCT的准确率低于皮肤镜或反射式共聚焦显微镜（RCM）。其原因在于，黑素是光的强散射体，像黑素瘤和色素痣这样的色素性病变的图像已经被证明很难通过基于光线穿透的技术获得。

（一）基底细胞癌（BCC）

BCC是OCT适用的主要皮肤疾病之一。OCT图像在描述这些肿瘤方面已经显示出良好的结果，并且已经建立了BCC的诊断标准。对正常皮肤来说，OCT可以有效地识别不同的皮肤层，能够深入深层网状真皮（取决于成像的皮肤区域和所用的OCT系统），真表皮交界处呈现为一条完整的窄的低反射线（图5-4（a））。而对BCC来说，整体的变化表现为正常皮肤结

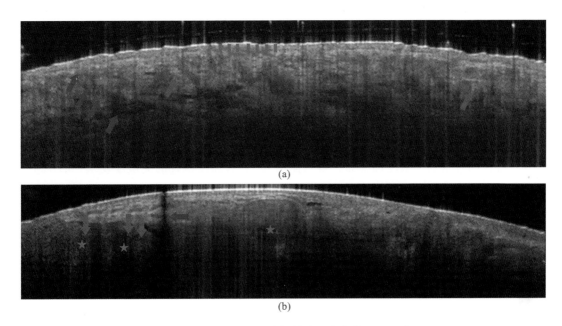

(a)

(b)

图 5-4　正常皮肤和结节性基底细胞癌的 OCT 图像

（a）下巴处正常皮肤的OCT图像。该层是完整的，并且在表皮（蓝色竖线）与真皮之间的界面处（真表皮交界处）呈现为一条完整、细密、高反射的线条。低反射对角线对应于毛囊和发干穿过表皮突出（红色箭头），血管用蓝色箭头标记。（b）脸颊处结节性基底细胞癌的OCT图像。表现出正常的分层破坏和与肿瘤岛相对应的低反射椭圆形结构（蓝色星号）。在肿瘤岛（蓝色箭头）的边缘观察到一条不反射的线，与组织学切片中观察到的溃疡性裂口/周围性麻痹相对应。红色箭头标记毛发投射阴影

Figure 5-4　Conventional cross-sectional OCT images of normal skin and nodular basal cell carcinoma

(a) Conventional cross-sectional OCT image of normal skin located on the chin. The layering is intact and the dermal-epidermal junction (DEJ) is seen as an unbroken, fine, and hyperreflective line at the interface between the epidermis (blue bars) and dermis. The hyporeflective diagonal line corresponds to a hair follicle and the hair shaft protruding through the epidermis (red arrows). Vessels are marked by blue arrows. (b) Conventional cross-sectional OCT image of nodular basal cell carcinoma located on the cheek showing disruption of normal layering and hyporeflective oval structures (blue asterisks) corresponding to tumor islands. An unreflective line is seen bordering the tumor islands (blue arrows) corresponding to mucinous clefting/peripheral palisading often recognized in histology sections. The red arrow marks a hair casting shadow

构的缺失(图 5-4(b))。在 OCT 观察下,BCC 表现为真表皮交界处的变化和真皮(基底细胞巢)中暗卵圆形区域周围出现白色的晕(基质)。在细胞巢的外围,基底细胞巢边缘的细胞栅栏/瘤周裂陷通常显示为低强度 OCT 信号。

次要特征包括正常毛囊和腺体的缺失,以及真皮毛细血管向基底细胞岛方向生长。虽然早期的研究发现很难区分 BCC 亚型,但已有研究显示了皮肤肿瘤的 OCT 特征与组织学的相关性。高清 OCT(HD-OCT)具有更高的横向分辨率(以穿透深度为代价),可以区分 BCC 亚型。HD-OCT 中描述的特征只表现在病变的表面,包括明显的小叶组织,乳头丛中占优势的血管模式以及是否存在对基质的拉伸作用。

如上所述,OCT 在区分病变与正常皮肤方面具有较高的准确性,在识别肿瘤边界方面也有重要意义。在区分正常皮肤和非黑素瘤皮肤癌方面,OCT 的灵敏度为 79%~94%,特异性为 85%~96%。OCT 在鉴别 BCC 中具有较高的诊断准确性,受到了广泛关注。Wahrlich 等通过使用基于五个预定的 OCT 诊断标准的特定评分系统(Berlin 评分)发现,经熟悉 OCT 的皮肤病学专家评估,多光束 OCT 的灵敏度和特异性分别为 96.6% 和 75.2%。其中,基于 OCT 的 BCC 诊断的病例中有 88% 最终被病理组织学证实是正确的。Ulrich 等的研究评估了 OCT 对典型临床环境中 BCC 的诊断价值。对 155 例可疑 BCC 患者的 235 处无色素性粉红色皮损进行了临床评估,并分别使用皮肤镜检查、OCT 和活检/组织学检查进行了诊断。结果表明,这三种诊断技术的灵敏度都很高。虽然使用 OCT 后临床检查的灵敏度仅从 90.0% 升高到 95.7%,但特异性从 28.6% 显著升高到 75.3%,具有统计学意义。OCT 的阳性预测值和阴性预测值最大,对 BCC 的总体诊断准确度从 65.8%(仅临床检查)提高到 87.4%。该研究强调,虽然 OCT 不能代替临床检查和皮肤镜检查,但可以作为一种辅助的非侵入性诊断工具使用。

(二)色素痣和黑素瘤

迄今为止,只有少数研究探讨了色素痣和黑素瘤的 OCT,原因是黑素是光的强散射体,通过光透过技术很难获得色素性病变(如黑素瘤和色素痣)的图像。常规 OCT 的成像分辨率为 5~7 mm,无法可视化细胞特征,因此病变黑素细胞的图像分析必须依赖于组织中明显的形态变化。良性痣的 OCT 图像中经常看到完整的真表皮交界处和皮肤棘层松解。相比之下,由于浸润性肿瘤的生长,黑素瘤常常表现出明显的结构紊乱,很少显示出清晰的表皮边界。黑素瘤在常规 OCT 观察下,最典型的特征是大的、垂直冰柱状结构,这在良性痣中是看不到的。但是,这并不足以证明常规 OCT 能够有效区分恶性和良性色素性病变,不能用作黑素瘤的诊断工具。

与常规 OCT 相比,HD-OCT 具有较高的细胞水平组织成像分辨率。HD-OCT 的高分辨率有助于对病变黑素细胞的病理学变化进行详细成像,研究表明,HD-OCT 可以提供形态学成像,可以区分表皮和真皮浅层色素性病变和细胞的结构模式和细胞学特征。关于 HD-OCT 在黑素瘤中的诊断准确性,最近的一项研究评估了 HD-OCT 在良性黑素细胞性皮肤病变和黑素瘤鉴别中的诊断性能。该研究包括 93 个经组织病理学证实的黑素细胞性皮肤病变,其中 27 个是黑素瘤。HD-OCT 的灵敏度为 74.1%,特异性为 92.4%。阳性预测值为 80%,阴性预测值为 89.7%。HD-OCT 的诊断准确性取决于肿瘤的厚度和边界病变的存在,在极薄的黑素瘤中假阴性率高,在增生性痣中假阳性率高。总之,尽管最近的研究提供了新的视角,但 OCT 在诊断黑素瘤方面的表现仍不如其他竞争技术(如 RCM)。为了优化黑素瘤的早期诊断,OCT 可能会发展成为一个有价值的辅助诊断工具。但在此之前,需要对 OCT 进行进一步的技术开发和更广泛的研究。

第三节　激光扫描共聚焦显微镜

荧光成像是一种近年来在生物医学领域中逐渐发展起来的成像模式。荧光是自然界常见的一种发光现象,当分子受到光激发后,电子从稳定的基态跃迁到不稳定的激发态,电子在吸收光子后,可能到达第一激发态的高振动能级或第二激发态,然后经历内转换或弛豫振荡过程到达第一激发态的最低振动能级。由于激发态是不稳定状态,电子从第一激发态的最低振动能级回到基态,同时产生荧光。荧光成像具有实时图像采集、高灵敏度、无毒性和荧光造影剂丰富等优点,广泛应用于基础科学研究和临床实践。随着现代科技的不断进步,荧光显微镜技术也有了长足的发展,涌现出一系列荧光显微镜技术,如激光扫描共聚焦显微镜、双光子激光扫描共聚焦显微镜等,它们在生物医学研究和临床诊断方面发挥着重要的作用。

一、双光子激光扫描共聚焦显微镜

鉴于单光子共聚焦荧光成像技术在活体组织光学成像中的局限性,Denk 等于 1990 年开创性地提出了双光子荧光显微概念,为活体组织光学成像提供了新的思路,后来又发展出多光子荧光成像技术,进一步拓展了荧光成像技术在临床医学上的应用。相比于传统的单光子共聚焦荧光成像技术,双光子或多光子荧光成像技术的优势在于:对生物样品的光损伤小,延长了有效观测时间,便于长时间活体观测和研究;使用长波长激光,在活体组织中散射系数较小,提高了组织穿透深度,从而可获取深层组织的清晰荧光图像;荧光收集率高,增强了图像对比度;对光路收集系统的要求低,光学系统相对简单(图 5-5);可以利用单一波长的激发光同时激发多种染料,从而得到同一生命现象中的不同信息,便于相互对照、补充。因此,多光子荧光成像技术在活体组织成像,尤其是皮肤组织的成像中得到了广泛的应用。近年来,该技术在临床诊断方面也取得了突破,基于多光子层析成像的皮肤检测系统在早期皮肤癌诊断、皮肤衰老检测等方面均有应用。

二、双光子荧光成像原理

双光子荧光指在飞秒脉冲激光器产生的强激光辐照下,荧光分子吸收两个光子,从基态跃迁到两倍光子能量的激发态,然后恢复到基态并发出荧光的过程。当被合适波长的激光辐照时,一些活体组织内的物质分子能够发射出稳定荧光,它们也因此被称为内源性荧光团。内源性荧光团广泛分布于活体组织中,例如还原型烟酰胺腺嘌呤二核苷酸磷酸(NADPH)、卟啉类化合物、黑素等。通常,有黑素瘤的皮肤部位的黑素细胞形态与边界将发生改变,可用于黑素

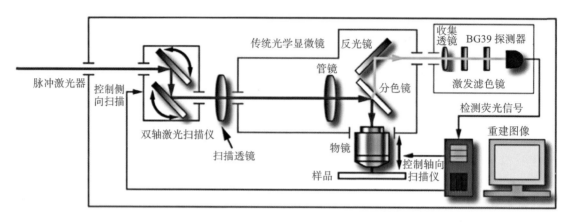

图 5-5　双光子激光扫描共聚焦显微镜示意图

Figure 5-5　Schematic diagram of two-photo excitation confocal laser scanning fluorescence microscope

瘤的早期诊断；皮肤组织中 NADPH 的含量与细胞内氧化还原和新陈代谢水平相关，可作为皮肤衰老检测的分子标志物。因此，双光子荧光成像技术在皮肤疾病的早期诊断和皮肤衰老检测方面有着广泛的应用。

三、双光子激光扫描共聚焦显微镜在皮肤肿瘤诊断方面的应用

　　临床上皮肤肿瘤微创诊断的需求极大地促进了双光子激光扫描共聚焦荧光成像技术的发展。按照发生率由高到低排列，皮肤肿瘤的类别如下：基底细胞癌（起源于构成表皮基底层的细胞）、鳞状细胞癌（起源于鳞状细胞，构成表皮的主要部分）和黑素瘤（起源于黑素细胞）。尽管黑素瘤病例的比例相对较低，但它的死亡率却最高。Teuchner 等最早于 1999 年利用双光子荧光共聚焦显微镜观察了皮肤组织切片中黑素的双光子荧光。随后，Skala 等研究了仓鼠颊囊癌（一种鳞状细胞癌）模型，并对肿瘤进行活检和三维成像。从这些图像中，鉴定出五个特征来区分正常、癌变前和癌变组织。随后，这项工作扩展到包括基于 NADPH 和黄素腺嘌呤二核苷酸(FAD)的荧光寿命代谢成像，并指出肿瘤中的代谢与正常组织不同。

　　人体组织的研究是朝着最终临床应用迈出的重要一步，这些研究大多数基于内源性荧光团的双光子荧光。Cicchi 等在基底细胞癌的概念验证研究中，观察到患者癌变组织中荧光强度增高的现象。Riemann 等利用 NADPH 和弹性蛋白的荧光以及胶原蛋白的 SHG 信号对黑素瘤进行了荧光成像，观察到黑素瘤细胞发射的荧光强度大大高于周围的正常细胞。另外，Koenig 等通过对 250 例黑素瘤患者癌变组织的荧光成像观察，进一步证实了癌变黑素细胞发射的荧光强度增高，并且还观察到细胞形态的差异。癌变黑素细胞相比正常细胞拉长，而且倾向于一起迁移。一项招募了 115 例患者的大型研究，评估了双光子荧光成像诊断黑素瘤的灵敏度和特异性，其灵敏度高达 95%，特异性高达 97%（图 5-6）。因此，双光子荧光成像是一种有前途的无创诊断方法，其提供的形态学和分子信息与切除活检类似，具有诊断意义。

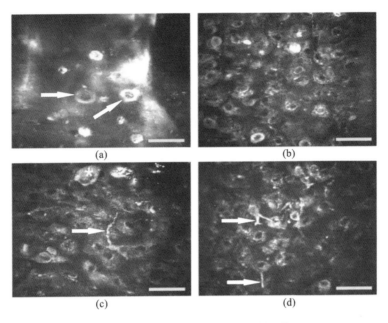

图 5-6 黑素瘤的原位光学显微镜图像

(a)上表皮角质层内出现荧光强度增高的黑素细胞(白色箭头);颗粒层(b)和棘突层(c 和 d)的特征表现为具有较大的细胞间距离和轮廓不清晰的角质化细胞边界;棘突层(c 和 d)多观察到细胞碎片、多形细胞(星号)和树枝状结构(白色箭头)。标尺:40 μm

Figure 5-6　Optical sectioning of melanoma

Ascending highly fluorescent melanocytes (white arrows) appear within the upper epidermal layers, for example, stratum corneum (a). Large intercellular distance and poorly defined keratinocyte cell borders characterize the stratum granulosum (b) and stratum spinosum (c and d). Cell fragments, pleomorphic cells (asterisk) and dendritic structures (white arrows) were frequently found in the stratum spinosum (c and d). *In vivo*, scale bar: 40 μm

第四节　反射式共聚焦显微镜

反射式共聚焦显微镜(RCM)是一种常用的皮肤科临床影像学检查手段,其特点是利用光在皮肤组织结构中的折射或者散射成像,可以实时、原位地观察皮肤组织和细胞,在非侵入性的方式下诊断皮肤病灶。它具有实时性、非侵入性、可重复性和高分辨率等特点,在临床上广泛应用于大部分皮肤疾病(包括炎症性皮肤疾病、感染性皮肤疾病、色素性皮肤疾病、皮肤良恶性肿瘤)的诊断以及皮肤美容等,尤其是其在皮肤良恶性肿瘤的诊断和应用方面受到了研究人员的广泛关注。相比于普通光学显微镜,RCM 具有以下特点:①超高分辨率(最高可达 1 μm);②可对样品进行无损伤性连续光学切片,实现三维重构成像,获取样品内部精细结构;③可对样品进行厚度小于 1 μm 的光学切片,避免机械切片造成的损伤;④聚焦针孔可有效地抑制杂散背景散射光,大大提高了图像对比度,成像质量好。RCM 已经逐渐成为国内外大型医疗中心诊断、治疗、随访皮肤肿瘤患者的重要辅助仪器。

一、RCM 成像原理

RCM 系统主要由点光源、分束器、聚焦透镜和探测器组成(图 5-7)。点光源发射的光聚焦到样品上,样品的散射光经过一个放置在焦平面共轭处的针孔抵达探测器。针孔只允许来自焦点的光通过,而阻挡来自其他方向的光。因此,探测器只接收照射到焦点处组织结构的散射光,而对其他位置的散射光不敏感。该系统的激光光源在扫描样品的过程中经历两次聚焦,因此称为共聚焦显微镜。点光源在 X 轴和 Y 轴的移动,实现对样品的二维扫描来获得样品不同层面的图像;在 Z 轴的不断移动,可实现对皮肤组织的无损伤性连续光学切片。由于与 CT 类似,RCM 也被称为皮肤 CT。获得的图像经计算机三维重构,有助于实现对皮肤组织三维剖面或整体结构的多角度观察。RCM 基于皮肤的细胞器和其他组织结构自身的折射率不同而得以实现高分辨率。皮肤组织中的黑素、角蛋白和纤维组织具有较高的折射率,是自然对照物。折射率高的结构较明亮,折射率低的结构则显灰暗。

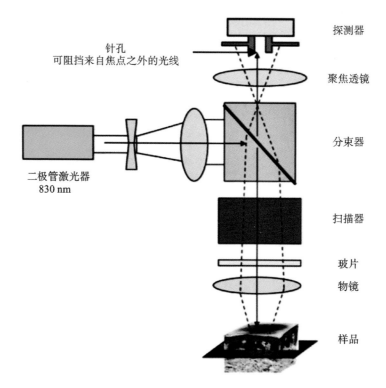

图 5-7　在体反射式共聚焦显微镜示意图

Figure 5-7　Schematic diagram of *in vivo* reflectance confocal microscope (RCM)

目前,临床检测用 RCM 系统使用波长为 830 nm 的二极管激光器,其组织水平的输出功率低于 35 mW。系统最大成像范围为 500 μm×500 μm,最大成像深度为 500 μm,放大倍数为 40~100 倍,横向分辨率为 0.5 μm,最小光学切片厚度为 1.7 μm。数值孔径为 0.9 的 30 倍物镜与浸没介质水(折射率为 1.33)或凝胶(折射率 1.3335)一起使用,以横向尺寸为 0.5~1.0 μm、轴向尺寸为 4~5 μm 捕获图像。RCM 系统的优点:无创性,可实时动态地监测细胞组织形态和生理功能,可对同一皮损进行多次成像,以对其发展变化、治疗后的改善状态进行随访观察;能观察皮肤血管中血流的动态变化;当常规组织病理学检查难以确定取材部位时,可以在一次检查中观察许多可疑病灶,无须取材及组织病理学复杂烦琐的处理过程;成像迅速,数据易于存储和输出。

二、RCM 在黑素瘤诊断方面的应用

黑素瘤是早期或预防性检测的挑战之一。在肿瘤发展的早期阶段,手术切除可以提高治愈率,而延迟识别会增加肿瘤生长和转移导致死亡的风险。RCM 的出现对黑素瘤诊断和黑素细胞病变生物学研究起到了显著的推动作用。由于黑素体和黑素是内源性对比的重要来源,因此黑素细胞在 RCM 图像中呈现更为明亮的结构。经过长期的研究,黑素细胞病变的 RCM 特征逐渐建立和完善,这大大提高了黑素瘤的诊断准确性,而且 RCM 和皮肤镜检查结合使用,将进一步提高诊断准确性。

(一)浅表扩散型黑素瘤

Pellacani 等评估了 RCM 特征在良性和恶性黑素细胞病变中的频率及其对黑素瘤鉴别的诊断意义。他们研究了 102 例黑素细胞病变的病例,包括 37 例黑素瘤,49 例获得性痣(21 例交界痣、27 例复合痣和 1 例皮内痣),以及 16 例上皮样和(或)梭形细胞(3 例交界性 Spitz 痣、8 例复合性 Spitz 痣和 5 例 Reed 痣)。通过详细描述每种类型病变的 RCM 特征,确定与黑素瘤诊断独立相关的六个标准。两个主要标准:在基底层存在细胞学上的非典型性(轻度或明显)和无边缘的乳头。四个次要标准:浅层中存在圆形细胞,呈 Paget 样扩散;Paget 样细胞遍布整个病变;真皮乳头处的脑回结构;真皮乳头内出现有核细胞。因此,在临床和皮肤镜评估中,RCM 可用于在体明确黑素细胞病变的特征。

2007 年,Pellacani 等开发了一种算法,利用标准统计方法定义 RCM 特征,来区分黑素瘤和痣。用于诊断黑素瘤的 RCM 特征如下。

(1)表皮(颗粒层/棘层):在黑素瘤中经常观察到明显的表皮细胞排列紊乱,但是并不能将其作为黑素瘤诊断的依据,因为这种现象也存在于三分之一的痣中。相反,以规则的蜂窝状或鹅卵石图案为特征的表皮只表现于良性病变中。据报道,在 78% 的黑素瘤和 19% 的痣中,可观察到圆形细胞 Paget 样浸润,而树突状的 Paget 样细胞(尽管非常明显)在黑素瘤中出现率则相对较低。对黑素瘤来说,每个 RCM 图像中能观察到超过三个大于 20 μm 的细胞。多形性和遍及整层的 Paget 样细胞广泛扩散是特异性特征,但并不是特别敏感的特征。

(2)皮肤真表皮交界处:在 90% 的黑素瘤和 41% 的痣中能够观察到无边缘的乳头,而有边缘的乳头主要存在于痣中。在 73% 的黑素瘤和 27% 的痣中观察到轻度至明显的非典型性。细胞呈片状结构分布,破坏了基底层的乳头状结构,具有高度特异性,但对诊断黑素瘤的灵敏度较低。此外,真表皮交界处的细胞巢,无论是簇状分布还是增厚都是良性病变的特征。

(3)真皮上层:在真表皮交界处的下方,一半以上的病灶中可见痣细胞成巢分布。规则致密的细胞巢多出现在痣中,而非典型细胞巢(如不均一的巢,稀疏的细胞巢和脑形巢)多出现在恶性肿瘤(53% 的黑素瘤)中,需要指出的是,非典型细胞巢也会在 26% 的痣中出现。在真皮乳头中,几乎一半的黑素瘤表现为大的有核细胞,而只有 13% 的痣中表现出这一特征。在恶性肿瘤和痣中,未观察到丰富的明亮细胞(明亮的小细胞和高折光点)以及增宽的网状胶原束的差异。在对不同厚度黑素瘤(≤1 mm 和 >1 mm)进行比较时,表皮排列紊乱、片状结构细胞、脑形巢和真皮乳头内的有核细胞等现象多出现于较厚的黑素瘤中。

(二)恶性雀斑样痣

恶性雀斑样痣是黑素瘤的一种早期形式,在过去的 20 年中发病率有所增高。多项研究表明,RCM 可用于区分恶性雀斑样痣和面部其他色素沉着。RCM 可以帮助确定恶性雀斑的边缘,同样,RCM 也可以用于确定恶性雀斑样痣的边缘,甚至无色素性的黑素瘤。2010 年,Guitera 等通过判别分析确定了与恶性雀斑样痣诊断独立相关的六个特征,按相关性顺序依次如下:无边缘的乳头;尺寸较大的圆形 Paget 样细胞;真皮乳头中出现有核细胞;在五个 0.5 mm×0.5 mm 的真表皮交界图像中出现三个或更多非典型细胞;毛囊周围出现 Paget 样细胞和非典型细胞;单个阴性(良性)特征——表皮增宽的蜂窝状结构(图 5-8)。

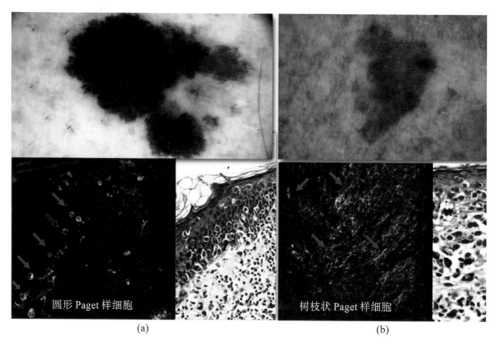

圆形 Paget 样细胞   树枝状 Paget 样细胞

(a)   (b)

图 5-8 不同类型黑素瘤的 RCM 图像

(a)浅表扩散型黑素瘤,带有多个棕点、假足、放射状流、瘢痕样色素沉着和不规则且宽阔的色素网,能够观察到表皮紊乱和圆形 Paget 样细胞(红色箭头);(b)黑素瘤出现在长期遭受太阳照射的皮肤表面,能够观察到在组织学上也可见的树枝状 Paget 样细胞(红色箭头)

Figure 5-8 Reflectance confocal microscopy(RCM) images for distinct melanoma types

(a) A superficial spreading melanoma with multiple brown dots, pseudopods, radial streaming, scar-like depigmentation, and irregular and broad network. Under RCM, we can observe epidermal disarray and roundish pagetoid cells (red arrows) corresponding to the pagetoid spread under histopathology. (b) A melanoma appearing on chronically sun-damaged skin. Under RCM, we can observe dendritic pagetoid cells (red arrows) that are also visible on histology

(三)结节性黑素瘤

在 RCM 观察下,结节性黑素瘤与浅表扩散型黑素瘤表现出多种差异。这些差异通常与皮肤镜检查和组织病理学特征相关。在表皮内,结节性黑素瘤缺乏黑素瘤的特征,如表皮结构紊乱和 Paget 样扩散。取而代之的是它们通常表现出蜂窝状图案,或是由具有黑色核和明亮的、厚边界的多形细胞组成的特殊加宽图案。在真表皮交界处,由于真皮中恶性细胞大量增殖引起表皮变平,典型的乳头状结构在结节中不可见。在结节性黑素瘤中能够观察到称为"脑回样巢"的低分形巢,其出现与深部肿瘤浸润相关。另外,出现胞质丰富的细胞与病灶处存在中等程度的炎症有关。

第五节 光声成像

一、光声成像的原理

光声成像(PAI)是一种新型非侵入性生物成像技术。当脉冲激光或连续调制激光辐照生物组织时,生物组织内的肿瘤、黑素、血红蛋白等物质吸收光子,导致组织局部温度瞬间升高,周围的介质产生周期性的热胀冷缩而激发超声波(图 5-9)。利用位于生物体表的超声探测器接收这些超声波信号,并对采集到的信号进行适当的处理和采用相应的图像重建算法,反演组织内吸光物质的光学特性,并据此重建光照射区域的光声图像。

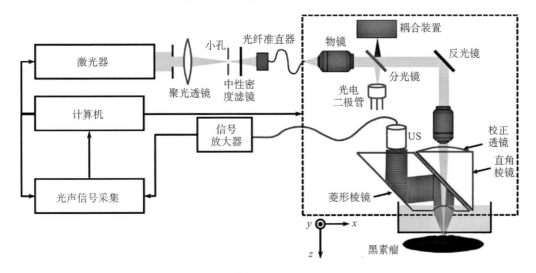

图 5-9 光声成像系统示意图
Figure 5-9 Schematic diagram of photoacoustic imaging (PAI) system

光声成像兼具光学成像高分辨率和超声成像深穿透性的优势。一方面,光声成像基于生物组织内部物质的光学吸收差异,与光学成像类似,具有高分辨率和高对比度;另一方面,光声成像探测的是超声波信号而不是光学信号,克服了光学成像因组织高度光散射而导致的成像深度浅的不足。因此,光声成像是近年来发展最迅速的一种成像技术,可以为深层组织(50~70 mm)提供高分辨率和高对比度的组织图像。对于像皮肤这样的浅表器官,光声成像几乎可以实现在整个皮肤深度范围内的成像。

皮肤疾病的发生和发展,往往伴随着皮肤组织理化性质的变化,如组织形态结构和成分、新陈代谢、血氧含量和色素变化等。组织病理学分析作为临床上的金标准,虽然可以精确检测上述理化性质的变化,但耗时长、侵入性强等缺点限制了其广泛应用。而光声成像能够快速、无损地展示活体组织中血氧饱和度和血流量、生物组织的化学成分和功能等信息(如脂肪、肿瘤、血红蛋白、胶原、黑素和水的含量以及所处组织层等)。此外,皮肤作为浅表器官,能够充分吸收光能量,受声衍射和声衰减影响较小。因此,光声成像在皮肤疾病诊断领域中得到了飞速发展。

二、光声成像在皮肤疾病诊断中的应用

光声成像在皮肤疾病的诊断中应用广泛,涉及黑素瘤、鲜红斑痣、血管瘤、基底细胞癌、鳞状细胞癌及硬皮病等诸多皮肤疾病。其中,鉴于光声对血管的高度敏感性,对人体皮肤血管的结构与功能和血管增生进行成像是近年来光声成像在皮肤疾病影像学诊断中较为热门的应用,例如,利用光声成像成功实现了对手掌中血管结构和功能的成像。Viator 等对鲜红斑痣进行了光声成像,发现采集到的图像可清晰地呈现鲜红斑痣的血管深度和皮损厚度。也有研究者通过光声成像与光学相干断层扫描技术的联合,实现了对基底细胞癌的检测,并得到了其血管模式和胶原基质。由于血管模式和胶原基质是基底细胞癌分类的两个关键参数,所以通过对比血管模式和胶原基质有望实现基底细胞癌的早期诊断。

光声成像在皮肤疾病诊断方面的另一个重要应用是黑素瘤的诊断和评估。由于具有较强的吸光特性,黑素在组织光声成像中与周围其他组织呈现极高的对比度,而黑素瘤是非常典型的色素相关皮肤癌。研究结果表明,基于光声成像,通过检测肿瘤内源性黑素可实现皮肤黑素瘤的诊断和监测黑素瘤的生长及其转移。目前,光声成像在黑素瘤中的应用主要表现在以下几个方面。

1. 测量黑素瘤厚度

厚度测量在黑素瘤的诊断中至关重要,肿瘤厚度在很大程度上决定了将采取何种治疗手段及预后。Oh 等将光声成像技术用于体内皮肤黑素瘤的成像。结果表明,该技术可以对黑素瘤顶部和底部边界进行清晰成像(图 5-10),且测量得到的黑素瘤的厚度与实际值是高度一致的。此外,方便的手持设计使得光声成像系统在黑素瘤厚度的研究中有很好的应用前景。

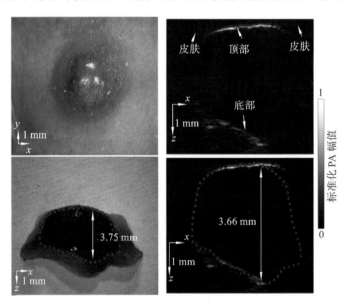

图 5-10　裸鼠体内黑素瘤的光声成像结果(测量黑素瘤厚度)

Figure 5-10　Photoacoustic image of melanoma *in vivo* in a nude mouse (detection of melanoma depth)

2. 检测黑素瘤增长率

有研究表明,与肿瘤厚度相比,黑素瘤的增长率特征可能是更为可靠的诊断指标。黑素瘤

可能有不规则的形状,为了准确量化其体积,需要可视化整个边界。最近,基于光声计算机断层成像的线性传感器阵列系统可以用来测量黑素瘤体积和增长率,该系统可以成像体内的整个黑素瘤,成功地测量黑素瘤的厚度和体积,并且可以直接计算出黑素瘤的增长率,这在很大程度上促进了黑素瘤的精准检测(图 5-11)。

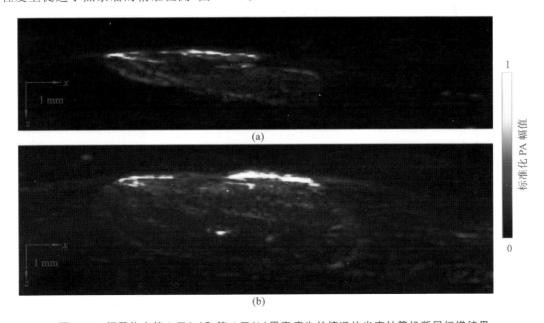

图 5-11　裸鼠体内第 3 天(a)和第 6 天(b)黑素瘤生长情况的光声计算机断层扫描结果

Figure 5-11　Photoacoustic computed tomography of melanoma *in vivo* in a nude mouse at day 3 (a) and day 6 (b)

3. 前哨淋巴结的定位

光声层析成像可以实现对前哨淋巴结的定位和活检,并可以实现较高的对比度和分辨率,使更精确的前哨淋巴结活检和转移性黑素瘤诊断成为可能。例如,有研究者将从美国临床阵列系统改进而来的手持探针用于前哨淋巴结检测。结果表明,光声成像可用于高精度的前哨淋巴结活检的图像引导,且具有较高的临床可行性。

4. 前哨淋巴结的筛查

继血氧素和肌素染色后的活检是评估转移性黑素瘤在前哨淋巴结中的护理标准。然而,对前哨淋巴结的不完全检查可能会错过黑素瘤细胞,从而导致转移性黑素瘤的误诊。光声层析成像在黑素瘤成像中具有较高的灵敏度,可以实现对前哨淋巴结的完整评估和筛查。已有研究发现,光声层析成像可以检测人类前哨淋巴结黑素瘤转移的能力,如非侵入性多光谱光声成像可检测出被切除的人类淋巴结中的黑素瘤转移(图 5-12)。

5. 监测循环肿瘤细胞

黑素瘤的高死亡率主要归因于其高转移倾向,而循环肿瘤细胞的出现可作为早期黑素瘤转移的预测因素。因此,有研究人员利用近红外高脉冲激光器辅助的超高速光声流式细胞术实现了对人类黑素瘤细胞的信号监测。此外,随着光声流式细胞术的进一步发展和成熟,其对循环肿瘤细胞监测的灵敏度将大幅提高,这将极大地促进光声成像在转移性黑素瘤诊断中的应用。

此外,光声成像在移植皮肤、热烧伤等方面也有较多的应用。随着光声成像的深入研究和

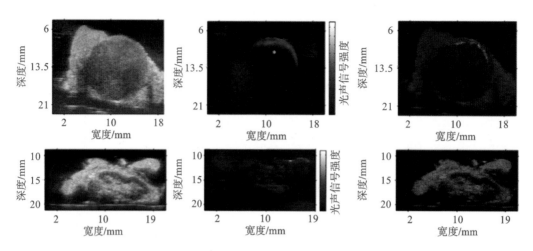

图 5-12　恶性(上)和良性(下)前哨淋巴结的光声计算机断层扫描结果

Figure 5-12　Photoacoustic computed tomography of malignant
(upper) and benign (bottom) human sentinel lymph node

技术的进一步发展,光声成像在皮肤疾病中的应用从单纯的成像诊断拓展至治疗领域。Kim等将光声成像应用在黑素瘤切除手术中,发现其可以更加精准地确定黑素瘤的边缘,这有利于黑素瘤的完全切除,大大降低了术后复发率。此外,He 等利用双波长光声流式细胞术对黑素瘤细胞进行体内的无标记成像,并进一步结合纳秒脉冲激光技术产生精确定位的热效应,实现对黑素瘤细胞的特异性杀伤,这对监控和预防黑素瘤的早期转移具有极为重要的意义。目前,光声成像在皮肤疾病中的应用还存在着分辨率不够、成像速度较慢等不足,但随着光声成像技术的不断发展和成熟以及联合其他成像技术,其在皮肤疾病领域的研究将不断拓展和完善,并将逐渐从单纯的诊断成像升级到诊疗一体化。

第六节　光 热 成 像

光热成像技术是一个发展前景广阔的新兴高科技产业,在国民生活的许多部门都发挥着重要作用。1956 年,美国外科医生 Lawson 用红外扫描技术证实乳腺癌皮肤的温度高于正常部位,由此拉开了光热成像技术临床应用的序幕。光热成像技术是一种以红外成像为基础,与X 线、CT、MRI、超声等形态学影像学技术完全不同,以锁定细胞相对新陈代谢强度为途径的医用功能学影像学技术。光热成像技术是一种反映人体生理和病理状况的全新热显像技术。其工作原理是利用红外扫描采集系统来接收人体辐射的红外能量,经计算机智能分析和图像处理形成红外热图,以不同的色彩显示人体表面的温度分布,定量地分析温度变化,从而判断出某些病灶的性质、位置,达到诊断疾病的目的。随着光电技术和计算机技术的迅猛发展,光热成像技术在医学领域也得到了更广泛、更深入的发展。此外,光热成像技术具有简便、快速、无创、直观、全面、灵敏度高等优势,在疾病的早期探查、动态观测以及诊断、疗效评价等方面均有重要作用。

一、光热成像技术原理

任何温度高于绝对零度(−273.15 ℃)的物体均向外辐射能量,人体就是一个天然生物红外辐射体,不断地向外散发红外辐射能。研究表明,人体红外辐射与机体的能量代谢、体热平衡、体温调节及组织结构有着密切的联系。而人是恒温动物,皮肤是人体的主要散热器官。在室温略低于体温的条件下,根据人体峰值辐射波长,通常选用敏感波长为 8~14 μm 的红外探测器,通过遥感技术收集人体发出的红外线信号,并转化为电信号;利用模数转换将电信号转换为数字信号,经计算机以伪彩色显示温度分布场,从而形成可视性的和可定量的红外热图像(图 5-13)。因生理结构以及体表各处温度不等,当人体某处发生病变或生理状况发生变化时,必将因其血流和代谢变化而产生高于或低于正常温度的偏离。由此,红外辐射能发生改变。基于这一原理的热成像仪,可以精确测量人体温度的变化,甚至在病变尚未出现临床症状或组织结构学改变时就出现阳性扫描结果。

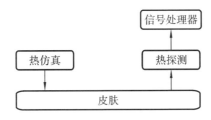

图 5-13 光热成像系统示意图

Figure 5-13 Schematic diagram of photothermal imaging system

二、光热成像在皮肤疾病诊断中的应用

早在 20 世纪 60 年代初,光热成像技术就被认为在皮肤癌检测,尤其是早期黑素瘤诊断中具有很好的发展前景。不幸的是,早期的热成像仪的研究并不尽如人意,假阴性结果的百分比很高,极大地降低了医学界的热情。具体原因在于:早期病变中涉及的潜在热信号变化很小,并且当时还没有高灵敏度的红外成像设备;这种小的热信号变化通常被掩盖在源自皮下组织的较大的热信号变化中。在这种情况下,即使使用当前最灵敏的红外摄像头,也很难检测到小的热点或冷点。

1995 年,Di Carlo 提出通过主动热成像测量来克服以上困难。他利用脉冲热成像装置,通过接触装有恒温乙醇溶液的气球来刺激皮肤。与周围健康皮肤相比,去除刺激后,黑素瘤和色素沉着的基底细胞癌在几秒内表现出明显的温度差异。几年后,Buzug 等用冷凝胶袋和高灵敏度的红外热成像仪重复了 Di Carlo 的实验。约翰斯・霍普金斯大学的 Çetingül 和 Herman 研究了黑素瘤病变的瞬时热信号,通过建立多层热传递皮肤模型,可以从瞬态热信号中提取定量信息。图 5-14 展示了用脉冲热成像仪检查的位于肩部的色素沉着病变,然而稳态热分析图无法提供任何诊断信息。在去除冷刺激后,所拍摄的红外图像能清晰地展示黑素瘤病变区域。Çetingül 和 Herman 认为此方法能够检测 Clark Ⅰ级(原位黑素瘤)病变。

Bonmarin 和 Le Gal 开发了一种基于锁相热成像的装置,专门用于皮肤癌的相关研究。该装置利用气流周期性调节皮肤表面温度,而红外摄像机则记录皮肤所发射的热辐射。与以前基于脉冲刺激的设置相比,锁相热成像具有抑制横向热扩散的能力,从而获得更清晰的温度记录图。图 5-15 展示了锁相热成像准确检测皮肤癌病灶边缘的能力。

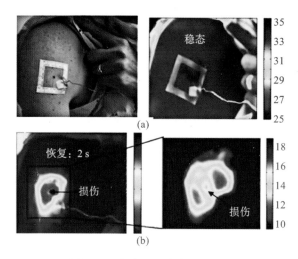

图 5-14　色素沉着病变的热成像

(a)用脉冲热成像仪检查的位于肩部的色素沉着病变(左:光学照片。右:红外照片);(b)去除冷刺激后(2 s 后),相同区域红外图像

Figure 5-14　Thermal imaging of pigmented lesions

(a) Photograph (left) and infrared image (right) of the shoulder area with a cluster of pigmented lesions and the adhesive window;(b) Infrared images of the same area after cooling (2 s after the removal of the thermal stimulation)

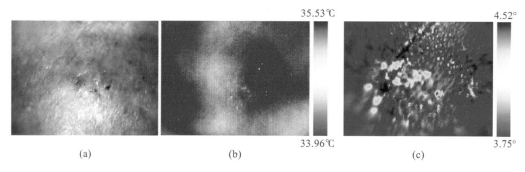

图 5-15　前额处基底细胞癌(BCC)的光学照片(a)、热成像(b)和相位图像(c)

Figure 5-15　Photograph (a), thermal image (b), and phase image (c) of basal cell carcinoma (BCC) located on the forehead

第七节　拉 曼 成 像

　　拉曼光谱技术基于印度物理学家 Raman 于 1928 年发现的拉曼散射效应,是一种常用的振动光谱技术。由于拉曼谱图中特征峰的位置、强度和宽度等能够有效地提供物质分子的指纹信息,而且特征峰的强度具有浓度依赖性,因此拉曼光谱也是一种定量分析方法。相比于其他光谱技术,拉曼光谱有其独特的优势:可以通过改变激发波长来选择性地激发分子的所需部分;不需要任何样品预处理,测量过程中样品也不会被破坏;由于水的拉曼光谱带小到可以忽略不计,因此在测量含水样品或水溶液的拉曼信号时也比较容易。拉曼光谱在长波方向上有

较宽的测量范围,能够提供一些重原子的振动情况。在拥有诸多优势的拉曼光谱基础上衍生出了各种各样的新型分析技术,如表面增强拉曼光谱技术(SERS)、傅里叶变换拉曼光谱技术(FT-Raman)、共振拉曼光谱技术(RRS)、显微共聚焦拉曼光谱成像技术(CRMI)和相干拉曼散射显微术(CRSM)等。

CRMI 是在显微共聚焦光路的基础上结合拉曼分析发展起来的一种检测技术。共聚焦技术使得只有聚焦平面的信号被共聚焦针孔接收,而聚焦平面以外的信号将被滤除,因此大大提高了信号质量,增高了信噪比。这项技术可对微小样品甚至单细胞水平的样品进行探测,配置高倍率光学显微镜及多种类型的激发光源,具有高空间分辨率、高信噪比、高准确率等优点,可进行逐点扫描并获得样品的显微拉曼图像。这些年来,CRMI 在肿瘤检测、文物考古、公安法学等领域得到了大力发展。在用拉曼光谱对生物组织进行成分分析时,一些不确定性因素如生物组织结构不均匀和化学组成复杂会对结果造成影响。融合了拉曼光谱和显微成像两种分析方法的优点的 CRMI,能够有效弥补这些不确定性因素所导致的认知局限,它是一种研究生物组织的生化成分与组织结构特点的分子量级光学成像方法。图 5-16(a)所示为 CRMI 系统的简化示意图。由于弱的拉曼散射(斯托克斯和反斯托克斯位移),CRMI 系统的激光光源比普通吸收光谱弱,约为其的百万分之一。分束器将光分开,光束路径通过物镜聚焦到样品上。光束可以分别在相机和光谱仪上进行观察或测量,并且在通过带阻滤波器去除瑞利散射之后,斯托克斯(和反斯托克斯)波长的光经过光栅衍射到检测器(或 CCD 或 InGaAs 阵列)上。CRMI 凭借不需要样品预处理的独特优势以及与常规显微镜相比能够提供更高的轴向和空间分辨率的能力,可以对细胞或生物组织的自然状态进行非常详细的分析。在细胞生命周期、细胞受损或癌变时及时观察到生化成分含量及分布的改变情况对研究人员来说是非常有价值的。使用 CRMI,不仅可以随时监测各种组织或细胞的变化,而且能够进行健康组织与癌变组织间的差异分析。

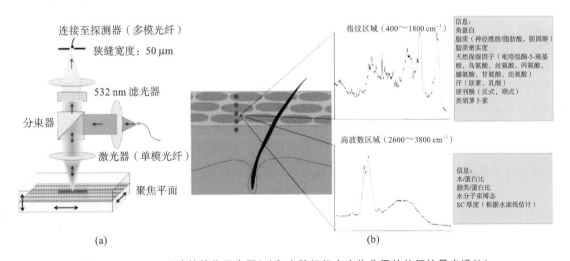

图 5-16 CRMI 系统的简化示意图(a)和皮肤组织内生物分子的特征拉曼光谱(b)

Figure 5-16 Schematic diagram of confocal Raman microspectral imaging (CRMI) (a) and characteristic Raman spectra of biomolecules in skin tissue(b)

皮肤由蛋白质、核酸、糖、辅酶等成分组成,是人体最大的器官,主要作用是保护体内器官和组织不受外界物理化学刺激以及病原体等的影响。皮肤组织由表皮、真皮、皮下组织组成,还包括一些附属器(如汗腺、皮脂腺、指甲)、血管、淋巴管、肌肉等。各层组织、细胞形态和生物功能各不相同,但其含有相同类型、不同拉曼光谱特征的生物分子。在实验中,通过研究各层皮肤组织的拉曼光谱特征,能够描述不同皮肤层中所具有的化学组分差异。例如,角质层和表皮层之间主要的光谱差异表现在 1062 cm^{-1}、1126 cm^{-1}、1296 cm^{-1} 处,表明了大量神经酰胺分布于角质层中。相比于拉曼光谱分析技术,CRMI 研究离体皮肤组织的拉曼光谱特性,将含有大量化学成分组成信息的拉曼光谱浓缩为高信息内涵的光谱图像,能够更为直观地呈现皮肤组织内部不同的化学成分以及其相对含量差异,更有利于归纳分析皮肤组织内部的生化组成特性。

第八节　挑战与展望

随着医学和生命科学的不断进步,人们对自身健康状态的关注程度越来越高。先进的医学影像学技术是人们利用医学诊断技术认识人类健康状态的核心技术手段之一,它可以利用荧光成像、光声成像、光热成像、超声成像、磁共振成像、拉曼成像等多种生物成像模式来获取人体的医学影像信息。与传统疾病诊断方法相比,医学影像学技术具有更直观、准确、灵敏的优势。鉴于每种成像模式的特点,其成像对象、成像空间分辨率和深度、成像灵敏度均存在差异。随着成像技术的不断发展,单一模式的成像方法逐渐显示出许多不足,如:荧光成像空间分辨率低,由于穿透深度的限制很难获得深层组织的成像信息;光声成像深度仍显不足,图像对比度和探测灵敏度需进一步提高,缺少既对成像对象无害又能提供足够对比度的分子对比剂;超声成像分辨率低,具有对操作经验的依赖性;磁共振成像时间较长,成本高,灵敏度相对较低等。

近几年发展的多模态成像是医学成像发展的一个新的趋势,它将两种或者多种成像模式合并在一起从而避免了单一模式成像的缺陷。不同成像模式获得的医学影像信息存在互补性,因而对受诊者进行多种成像模式的检查,有利于实现对健康或疾病状态的准确诊断,但是这将增加受诊者的经济负担,增强造影多次用药对受诊者产生毒副作用的风险也将增加,多模态成像技术应运而生。多模态成像技术是选择临床成像技术中互补性强的有利于疾病诊断的技术加以融合,进而在同一仪器上实现多种成像方式的检查,它的应用前景已为广大科研和临床工作者所认同。多模态成像系统的开发对成像探针的性能提出了新的要求,开发与多模态成像系统相匹配的多模态活体成像探针成为医学影像学技术的发展前沿与热点。

思　考　题

1. 除皮肤科之外,光学相干断层成像技术还可以在哪些科室得到广泛的临床应用?

2. 试分析各种影像学诊断技术在黑素瘤早期诊断方面的优缺点。

3. 请查阅资料,对比各种影像学诊断技术在对比度来源、穿透深度、轴向分辨率、侧向分辨率、成像速率方面的异同。

4. 试分析人工智能在皮肤影像学领域中的机遇与挑战。

5. 相比于 CT、MRI、PET 等成像技术,光学成像技术在皮肤疾病诊断中应用更为广泛,请列出本章中各种光学成像技术的优缺点。

扩 展 阅 读

[1] Wilhelm K P, Elsner P, Berardesca E, et al. Bioengineering of the skin: skin imaging & analysis[M]. 2nd ed. Los Angeles: CRC Press, 2006.

[2] Hamblin M R, Avci P, Gupta G K. Imaging in dermatology[M]. Pittsburgh: Academic Press, 2016.

[3] Berardesca E, Maibach H, Wilhelm K P. Non invasive diagnostic techniques in clinical dermatology[M]. Heidelberg: Springer-Verlag, 2014.

[4] 孟如松,崔勇. 多模态皮肤病医学影像诊断图谱[M]. 北京: 人民卫生出版社, 2021.

[5] 孙秋宁,刘洁. 协和皮肤镜图谱[M]. 北京: 人民卫生出版社, 2015.

参 考 文 献

[1] Schneider S L, Kohli I, Hamzavi I H, et al. Emerging imaging technologies in dermatology Part Ⅰ: basic principles [J]. J Am Acad Dermatol, 2019, 80 (4): 1114-1120.

[2] Schneider S L, Kohli I, Hamzavi I H, et al. Emerging imaging technologies in dermatology Part Ⅱ: applications and limitations [J]. J Am Acad Dermatol, 2019, 80 (4): 1121-1131.

[3] Saida T, Koga H, Uhara H. Key points in dermoscopic differentiation between early acral melanoma and acral nevus[J]. J Dermatol, 2011, 38(1): 25-34.

[4] Kutzner H, Metzler G, Argenyi Z, et al. Histological and genetic evidence for a variant of superficial spreading melanoma composed predominantly of large nests[J]. Modern Pathol, 2012, 25(6): 838-845.

[5] Coleman A J, Richardson T J, Orchard G, et al. Histological correlates of optical coherence tomography in non-melanoma skin cancer[J]. Skin Res Technol, 2013, 19 (1): 10-19.

[6] Wahrlich C, Alawi S A, Batz S, et al. Assessment of a scoring system for basal cell carcinoma with multi-beam optical coherence tomography[J]. J Eur Acad Dermatol, 2015, 29(8): 1562-1569.

[7] Ulrich M, von Braunmuehl T, Kurzen H, et al. The sensitivity and specificity of optical coherence tomography for the assisted diagnosis of nonpigmented basal cell carcinoma: an observational study[J]. Brit J Dermatol, 2015, 173(2): 428-435.

[8] Boone M A, Norrenberg S, Jemec G B, et al. High-definition optical coherence tomography imaging of melanocytic lesions: a pilot study[J]. Arch Dermatol Res, 2014, 306(1): 11-26.

[9] Gambichler T, Schmid-Wendtner M H, Plura I, et al. A multicentre pilot study investigating high-definition optical coherence tomography in the differentiation of cutaneous melanoma and melanocytic naevi[J]. J Eur Acad Dermatol, 2015, 29(3): 537-541.

［10］ Skala M C,Squirrell J M,Vrotsos K M,et al. Multiphoton microscopy of endogenous fluorescence differentiates normal,precancerous,and cancerous squamous epithelial tissues［J］. Cancer Res,2005,65(4):1180-1186.

［11］ Conchello J A,Cogswell C J,Wilson T,et al. Three-dimensional and multidimensional microscopy:image acquisition and processing［M］. 13th ed. Bellingham:Proceedings of SPIE,2006.

［12］ Bartels K E,Bass L A,DeRiese W T W,et al. Photonic therapeutics and diagnostics ［M］. Bellingham:Proceedings of SPIE,2005.

［13］ Periasamy A,So P T C,König Karsten,et al. Multiphoton microscopy in the biomedical sciences［M］. 6th ed. Bellingham:Proceedings of SPIE,2006.

［14］ Ruini C,Schuh S,Sattler E,et al. Line-field confocal optical coherence tomography— practical applications in dermatology and comparison with established imaging methods［J］. Skin Res Technol,2021,27(3):340-352.

［15］ Pellicani G,Cesinaro A M,Seidenari S. Reflectance-mode confocal microscopy of pigmented skin lesions-improvement in melanoma diagnostic specificity［J］. J Am Acad Dermatol,2005,53(6):979-985.

［16］ Pellacani G,Guitera P,Longo C,et al. The impact of *in vivo* reflectance confocal microscopy for the diagnostic accuracy of melanoma and equivocal melanocytic lesions ［J］. J Invest Dermatol,2007,127(12):2759-2765.

［17］ Guitera P,Pellacani G,Crotty K A,et al. The impact of *in vivo* reflectance confocal microscopy on the diagnostic accuracy of lentigo maligna and equivocal pigmented and nonpigmented macules of the face［J］. J Invest Dermatol,2010,130(8):2080-2091.

［18］ Kim J,Kim Y H,Park B,et al. Multispectral *ex vivo* photoacoustic imaging of cutaneous melanoma for better selection of the excision margin［J］. Brit J Dermatol, 2018,179(3):780-782.

［19］ Hindelang B,Aguirre J,Schwarz M,et al. Non-invasive imaging in dermatology and the unique potential of raster-scan optoacoustic mesoscopy［J］. J Eur Acad Dermatol, 2019,33(6):1051-1061.

［20］ He Y,Wang L,Shi J,et al. *In vivo* label-free photoacoustic flow cytography and on-the-spot laser killing of single circulating melanoma cells［J］. Sci Rep,2016,6:39616.

［21］ Di Carlo A. Thermography and the possibilities for its applications in clinical and experimental dermatology［J］. Clin Dermatol,1995,13(4):329-336.

［22］ Cetinguel M P,Herman C. Quantification of the thermal signature of a melanoma lesion［J］. Int J Therm Sci,2011,50(4):421-431.

［23］ Bonmarin M,Le G F. A lock-in thermal imaging setup for dermatological applications ［J］. Skin Res Technol,2015,21(3):284-290.

［24］ Ida T,Iwazaki H,Omuro T,et al. Lensless high-resolution photoacoustic imaging scanner for *in vivo* skin imaging［J］. Opt Rev,2018,25(1):33-39.

［25］ Chen Z,Rank E,Meiburger K M,et al. Non-invasive multimodal optical coherence and photoacoustic tomography for human skin imaging[J]. Sci Rep,2017,7(1):17975.

[26] Hoogedoorn L,Gerritsen M J P,Wolberink E A W,et al. A four-phase strategy for the implementation of reflectance confocal microscopy in dermatology[J]. J Eur Acad Dermatol,2016,30(8):1308-1314.

[27] Franceschini C,Persechino F,Ardigo M. *In vivo* reflectance confocal microscopy in general dermatology:how to choose the right indication[J]. Dermatol Pract Concept, 2020,10(2):e2020032.

[28] Aksu A E K, Gurel M S. Application of reflectance confocal microscopy in dermatology practice[J]. Turk Dermatoloji Dergisi,2015,9(1):45-52.

[29] Wan B,Ganier C,Du-Harpur X,et al. Applications and future directions for optical coherence tomography in dermatology[J]. Brit J Dermatol,2020,184(6):1014-1022.

[30] Ring H C,Israelsen N M,Bang O,et al. Potential of contrast agents to enhance *in vivo* confocal microscopy and optical coherence tomography in dermatology:a review[J]. J Biophotonics,2019,12(6):e201800462.

[31] Olsen J, Holmes J, Jemec G B E. Advances in optical coherence tomography in dermatology—a review[J]. J Biomed Opt,2018,23(4):1-10.

[32] Hibler B P, Qi Q,Rossi A M,Current state of imaging in dermatology[J]. Semin Cutan Med Surg,2016,35(1):2-8.

[33] Liu M,Drexler W. Optical coherence tomography angiography and photoacoustic imaging in dermatology[J]. Photoch Photobio Sci,2019,18(5):945-962.

[34] Srivastava R,Manfredini M,Rao B K. Noninvasive imaging tools in dermatology[J]. Cutis,2019,104(2):108-113.

[35] Huang D,Swanson E A,Lin C P,et al. Optical coherence tomography[J]. Science, 1991,254(5035):1178-1181.

[36] Lallas A,Zalaudek I,Apalla Z,et al. Management rules to detect melanoma[J]. Dermatology,2013,226(1):52-60.

[37] Zalaudek I,Giacomel J,Schmid K,et al. Dermatoscopy of facial actinic keratosis, intraepidermal carcinoma and invasive squamous cell carcinoma:a progression model [J]. J Am Acad Dermatol,2012,66(4):589-597.

[38] Dalimier E,Salomon D. Full-field optical coherence tomography:a new technology for 3D high-resolution skin imaging[J]. Dermatology,2012,224(1):84-92.

[39] Bakos R M,Blumetti T P,Roldan-Marin R,et al. Noninvasive imaging tools in the diagnosis and treatment of skin cancers[J]. Am J Clin Dermatol,2018,19(1s):3-14.

[40] 中国医疗保健国际交流促进会皮肤科分会,中国医疗保健国际交流促进会华夏皮肤影像人工智能协作组.黑素细胞肿瘤皮肤镜特征及组织病理特征相关性专家共识(2020)[J].中华皮肤科杂志,2020,53(11):859-868.

[41] 何黎.皮肤影像技术概况、应用现状及前景[J].中国医学文摘(皮肤科学),2016,33(1):29-37.

[42] 孟雅丹,金京,徐琦,等.基于光学相干断层成像技术量化评估皮肤癌的二维傅里叶分形

维数[J].生物医学工程研究,2017,36(4):327-330,345.

[43] 詹庆霞,张峻岭.共聚焦激光扫描显微镜在皮肤科的应用[J].继续医学教育,2016,30(5):85-86.

[44] 吴冬梅,李青,戴耕武.反射式共聚焦显微镜在皮肤恶性黑素瘤中的应用进展[J].实用皮肤病学杂志,2015,8(2):122-125.

[45] 周楚,文龙,王佩茹,等.光声成像在皮肤肿瘤中的应用进展[J].中华皮肤科杂志,2021,54(3):256-259.

(蒋皓)

Chapter 5
Imaging in Dermatology

Dermatosis is a term that refers to diseases of the integumentary system, which includes everything on the surface of the body: skin, nails, and hair. Dermatosis is a common and frequently-occurring disease in the clinic. There is a wide variety of dermatosis with the feature of easy recurrence and long term treatment. Nowadays, the serious air pollution increases the incidence of dermatosis, and the pathogenic factors are constantly escalating. The World Health Organization (WHO) has announced that dermatosis will be the most infectious disease with the highest incidence and disability rate in the 21st century. Owing to the living conditions and environment, dermatosis is more common in areas of poor economic development and poverty, and the age of patients with pathological dermatosis is getting younger and the number is increasing. In particular, due to inadequate understanding of the condition of patients, the condition is always delayed. Besides, the easy recurrence and high cost of dermatosis have sounded the alarm for the people's healthy life, as well as for economic and social development. In view of the wide variety of dermatosis and complex conditions, non-invasive, *in-situ*, real-time and dynamic dermatological imaging diagnostic technology has been developed to characterize suspicious skin lesions and provide objective and quantitative evaluation indicators, which has become a clinical requirement for dermatology.

The diagnosis of dermatosis relies heavily on visual observation of the skin. Before the emergence of professional dermatological imaging technology, dermatologists could only use the naked eyes to directly identify the diagnosis, which is based on subjective judgment and professional background and clinical experience in long-term clinical practice of dermatologists. Cases were only described in text, and the image data could not be retained, which was not conducive to follow-up diagnosis and follow-up and comparison of efficacy. Later, although manual drawing and wax model making improved the condition to a certain extent, the drawing and model making process was cumbersome and required professional talents, which lacked universality. With the continuous development of science and technology, computer tomography (CT), magnetic resonance imaging (MRI), positron emission tomography (PET), ultrasound imaging, and various optical imaging technologies such as dermoscopy, skin confocal technology, multiphoton imaging, optical coherent tomography and photoacoustic imaging have emerged. The optical imaging technologies can visualize suspicious skin lesions, and achieve non-invasive, *in -situ*, real-time imaging of subcutaneous tissue to varying degrees, providing an objective evaluation basis for clinical diagnosis. The promotion and complementation between imaging technologies in dermatology and skin histopathology will inevitably lead to the rapid development of modern dermatology.

5.1　Dermoscope

Dermoscope, also known as skin surface microscope, incident light microscope, etc. , is a non-invasive microscopic imaging technique that can magnify tens of times and enables the visualization of submacroscopical structures invisible to the naked eyes, such as the lower epidermis, dermal papilla layer, and deep dermis. These features have special and clear correspondences with skin histopathological changes. Based on these correspondences, the dermoscopic diagnosis exhibits sensitivity and specificity. Thus, dermoscope is also called "dermatologist's stethoscope". It is the most widely used imaging technique in dermatology.

As early as 1663, Kohlhaus used a microscope to observe the blood vessels in the nail bed. In 1893, Unna used immersion oil and glass slides to observe the skin lesions of patients with lupus vulgaris under a microscope, and called this method as "diaskopie" in German. In 1916, Zeiss invented a binocular skin angioscopy. In 1920, a German dermatologist Saphier used the phrase "dermatoskopie" and upgraded the dermoscope. The traditional external light source was replaced with a built-in light source, so that the capillaries of the skin lesions could be clearly observed. The prototype of modern dermoscope appeared in 1951. An American dermatologist Goldman observed and evaluated the microscopic characteristics of various skin pigmented patients (including pigmented moles and melanoma) with monocular magnifying glass. After 1970, dermoscope has been widely developed and used in clinical dermatology. In 1971, Mackie studied and summarized the significance of dermoscope for the preoperative diagnosis of pigmented dermatosis and its role in distinguishing benign pigmented nevus and melanoma. In 1981, Fritsch et al. distinguished melanoma and pigmented nevus based on the characteristics of different pigment networks upon dermoscope. In 1987, Pehamberger et al. published a paper describing the characteristics of various pigmented dermatosis upon dermoscope, established a model analysis method for the diagnosis of pigmented dermatosis, and promoted the formation of dermoscope diagnostic methods. In 1991, Kreusch and Rassner published the first atlas of dermoscopy, emphasizing the relationship between characteristics upon dermoscope and histopathology of dermatosis. Till now, dermoscope has been more and more widely used in clinical dermatology, whether it is in pigmented or non-pigmented skin lesions, vascular morphology, or even hair growth can be observed, and the diagnostic criteria of dermoscopy is constantly improved.

In general, since the optical density and refractive index of the stratum corneum are different from those of air, most of the light irradiated on the skin is directly reflected, part of which is absorbed by skin. Only a small amount of light enters the skin through scattering. Therefore, the structure under the epidermis is difficult to observe with the naked eyes. The specific operation of dermoscope is as follows (Figure 5-1). Add an infiltrating fluid (e. g. , water, mineral oil, ethanol, and gel) on the skin to increase the light transmission of the stratum corneum and reduce the reflected light; cover the glass slide on it, flat the local skin, and the light source enters from an appropriate angle. With the assistance of optical magnification equipment, invisible structures and features such as the lower epidermis, dermal papilla layer and deep dermis can be observed. As shown in the latest research, medical alcohol as an infiltrating liquid produces fewer bubbles, thereby obtaining clearer images, with the characteristics of non-greasy, non-staining, natural volatilization without wiping, and effectively reducing bacterial contamination. In addition, in the eye or mucosal area, hydrogels (e. g. , ultrasonic coupling agents) are widely used due to their non-fluidity and non-irritating advantages.

In the early dermatological clinic, the diagnosis of dermatosis mainly relied on the experience of dermatologists and histopathological examination. Although histopathology is the gold standard and currently the most reliable clinical diagnosis technique in dermatology, it is a traumatic inspection method and is difficult to inspect one by one for multiple pigmented skin lesions. Dermoscope has a unique advantage to diagnose multiple pigmented skin lesions in the early stage. It can determine the lesions that need biopsy, and diagnose the features of skin lesions in a large area to ensure the accuracy of the resection site. As a screening and diagnosis tool for many clinical diseases, dermoscope has the advantages of non-invasive, *in vivo* and rapid diagnosis with a good prospect. At present, there are many types of diagnostic methods for dermoscope: pattern analysis, ABCD rule, Menzies' method, 7-point checklist, TADA method, etc. Among them, pattern analysis has shown great advantages in the differential diagnosis of various pigmented skin lesions, especially in the differentiation of benign and malignant melanocytic skin lesions.

Melanoma is a malignant tumor that usually occurs in skin. It has attracted more and more attention due to its increasing morbidity and mortality. Early diagnosis of melanoma is the most effective way to reduce its mortality. Before it goes into aggressive melanoma, the cure rate is 98%. Once melanoma breaks through the dermis or even metastasizes, the cure rate will be greatly reduced to 15%. Pattern analysis is regarded as the classic dermoscopic method for evaluating pigmented skin lesions. This method includes the assessment of the symmetry of the lesion, the presence of one or more colors, the global dermoscopic appearance of the lesion according to predefined patterns, and the presence of local features. The global pattern results from predominant features occupying large areas of the lesion. A global pattern usually consists of one (usually) or two (less often) predominant features. In the presence of more than two predominant features, the pattern is classified as multicomponent. Instead, local features can be recognized as single or grouped characteristics, and several of them can coexist in the same lesion. There are five basic global patterns, including reticular (resulting from pigment network), globular (resulting from multiple globules), starburst (resulting from peripheral streaks or pseudopods), homogenous (resulting from structureless pigmentation), and multicomponent (resulting from the combination of more than two of the above patterns). The first four patterns can be seen in both nevi and melanoma, whereas the multicomponent pattern is directly suggestive of melanoma (Figure 5-2). If a lesion exhibits one of the first four patterns, further assessment will be based on the overall symmetry, colors, and the presence of local features, so-called "melanomaspecific criteria". In general, nevi are characterized by symmetry of structures and display one or two colors. In contrast, melanoma exhibits architectural disorder and often display more than two colors.

5.1.1 Melanoma-specific criteria

Atypical pigment network: Brown-black network with irregular meshes and irregularly distributed lines of different thickness (high specificity for the diagnosis of melanoma).

Irregular dots and/or globules: Brown-black or gray, dots and globules of different size, irregularly distributed within the lesion.

Irregular blotches: Black, brown, or gray areas with irregular shape and/or distribution.

Irregular streaks and/or pseudopods: Radial lines irregularly distributed at the periphery of the lesion (streaks), sometimes with a bulbous projection at their peripheral ending (pseudopods).

Regression structures: Melanoma with regression structures appears in the flat area of the lesion and may exhibit as either white scarlike areas corresponding to fibrosis or blue-gray areas (peppering) corresponding to melanophages.

Blue-white veil: Melanoma with blue-white veil appears in the elevated part of the lesion, which is blue-gray or blue-white, diffuse and irregular pigmentation.

Irregular vascular structures: Polymorphous vessels, coexistence of dotted, linear, or hairpin vessels in the same lesion.

Due to the specific skin anatomy, pigmented melanocytic lesions on the certain locations (face, palms, soles, and nails) show unique dermoscopic features.

5.1.2 Acral melanoma

Acral melanoma is found in extremities (e. g. , palms, soles, nails). It is a subtype of melanoma with a high morbidity (about 50%) in China and even in Asia. Therefore, it is particularly important to distinguish between benign and malignant pigmented tumors in extremities. Acral melanoma often manifests as brown spotted rash in the early stage, and it is difficult to differentiate between early acral melanoma and acral melanocytic nevi through naked eyes observation. It is difficult for dermatologists to diagnose when facing acral pigmented skin lesions, and dermoscope is extremely powerful to help dermatologists to improve accuracy rate of diagnosis. Acral melanocytic nevi has three main patterns upon dermoscope: parallel furrow pattern, pigmentation along the furrows of the skin markings (the most common dermoscopic pattern in acral melanocytic nevi); lattice-like pattern, pigmentation along and across the furrows; fibrillar pattern, fine fibrillar pigmentation perpendicular to the furrows.

There is a significant difference between the features of acral melanoma and acral melanocytic nevi upon dermoscope. Parallel ridge pattern is the most common and specific manifestation of acral melanoma. This pattern is composed of pigmentation located on the ridges of the skin markings. The sensitivity and specificity are as high as 86% and 99%, respectively, which greatly improve the diagnosis accuracy of acral melanoma. Unlike the parallel furrow pattern of acral melanocytic nevi where the pigment is located along the furrows of the skin markings, the parallel ridge pattern of acral melanoma is where the pigment parallel line is located at the ridge. Besides, acral melanoma also has an irregular diffuse pigmentation pattern, which is more common in late skin lesions. The diffuse pigmentation pattern is manifested as a diffuse and unstructured dark brown pigmentation with color gradation. Other manifestations, such as irregular spots or globules, irregular stripes, blue-white veils, ulcer formation, atypical vascular morphology, and even the three common patterns of acral melanocytic nevi can be found in acral melanoma. In the case of melanoma skin lesions located on the extremities, Saida et al. suggested that when facing patients with suspected extremity melanoma in clinical practice, dermoscope should be firstly used to diagnose the parallel ridge pattern, and the positive patients should immediately undergo histopathology. For negative patients, it is necessary to further confirm whether they have a typical acral melanocytic nevi pattern (e. g., parallel furrow, lattice-like, fibrillar). If so, long-term clinical follow-up observation should be performed. If not, and the diameter of the skin lesion is larger than 7 mm, a histopathological examination is required.

5.1.3 Lentigo maligna melanoma

Lentigo maligna melanoma is a type of invasive skin cancer. It develops from lentigo maligna, which is sometimes called Hutchinson's melanotic freckle. Lentigo maligna stays on the outer surface of the skin. When it starts growing beneath the skin's surface, it becomes lentigo maligna melanoma. It's the least common type of melanoma. Lentigo maligna grows slowly and is usually harmless, but lentigo maligna melanoma can spread aggressively. It is important to recognize the symptoms of lentigo maligna melanoma in the early stage. Histopathological manifestations are the proliferation of heterotypic melanocytes in the basal layer of the epidermis, and the appearance of melanocyte lesions on the face observed by dermoscope is different from other parts. Stolz et al. took the lead in observing lentigo maligna melanoma on face with dermoscope, and summarized the characteristic manifestations at four stages: stage Ⅰ, the appearance of asymmetric follicular openings with hyperpigmentation indicates that the melanoma cells descend unevenly toward a single hair follicle; stage Ⅱ, short and thin stripes, dots and globules appear around the follicular opening, exhibiting a circular granular pattern; stage Ⅲ, as the stripes around the follicular opening become longer and intersect, a diamond-shaped pigmentation is gradually formed; stage Ⅳ, as the melanoma cells inside the follicle expand, the pigmentation begins to merge until the follicular opening disappears. The sensitivity and specificity of this model for the diagnosis of lentigo maligna melanoma are 89% and 93%, respectively. This model can be used for clinical diagnosis and follow-up to observe the progress of lentigo maligna melanoma.

Overall, dermoscope has an irreplaceable role in assessing skin tumors because it has significantly improved the performance of dermatologists. In addition, with the continuous improvement of the appearance and mode of dermatosis upon dermoscope, dermoscope has gradually played a role similar to a pathologist's stethoscope.

5.2 Optical Coherence Tomography

Optical coherence tomography (OCT) technique is a biological tissue imaging technique with many advantages, such as high resolution (up to micrometer), non-contact, non-invasive, and real-time. The potential of OCT for *in vivo* visualization of microstructural morphology *in situ* has attracted many attentions. In 1991, Huang from Massachusetts Institute of Technology and Schuman from Harvard Medical School developed the first OCT instrument with a semiconductor laser ($\lambda = 830$ nm) to measure isolated coronary arteries and retinas. OCT was then introduced in the clinical field of ophthalmology and the first *in vivo* OCT image was presented in 1993. Since 1997, OCT had been introduced in dermatology, gastroenterology, urology, gynecology and neurosurgery, etc., and several manufactures of OCT systems have made OCT imaging for dermatological purposes commercially available. During the last decade, OCT has advanced from being an interesting scientific tool in the laboratory to being a useful bedside tool for supplementing the clinical diagnosis and also for treatment monitoring of different types of skin tumors. One limitation of OCT is the restricted imaging depth of maximum 2 mm that usually makes it inadequate in the evaluation of skin changes stretching beyond the reticular dermis.

5.2.1 Principles of OCT system

OCT is a macro-optical imaging modality using light-tissue interaction for generating images. The OCT system is composed of a light source, a beam splitter and a detector, also known as Michelson interferometer. OCT integrates semiconductor laser technique, optical technique, ultra-sensitive detection technique and computer image processing technique, and can create *in vivo* cross-sectional images of skin with a resolution of 1-15 μm. The beam splitter of OCT divides the light emitted by the near-infrared light source into two beams: one beam is directed to the measured substance, called the sample arm; the other beam is directed to the reference reflector, called the reference arm. The two beams of light reflected from the measured substance and the reference mirror are superimposed on the detector. Under certain conditions, interference can be observed: coherent waves superimpose and their electromagnetic field amplitudes add constructively (i. e. , they reinforce each other) or destructively (i. e. , they cancel out each other) or meet any condition in between. The associated light intensity can be measured as an electrical signal using a photo detector. This signal is a function of the difference in optical path length between both arms. For a low coherent light source (like a superluminescent diode or a pulsed laser source), interference is only possible if the optical paths are matched to be equal in length within the short coherence length of the source, which usually is in the order of micrometers.

OCT is a non-invasive and two-dimensional imaging technique through measuring reflected or backscattered light from tissue by correlating it with light. Compared with other imaging techniques, OCT has the following advantages: ① a near-infrared light source that is harmless to human body; ② interference technology to achieve tomographic imaging with extremely high resolution (micrometer); ③ the optical fiber with a diameter of 100 μm transmits signals and can be connected to a variety of instruments, including catheters, endoscopes, laparoscopes and surgical probes, which allows imaging of organ systems in the body; ④ *in situ* imaging and real-time transmission image, without complicated mathematical calculations and image reconstruction, surgical guidance; ⑤ portability, an important factor for clinically viable devices.

According to the working principle, there are two OCT systems, time domain OCT (TD-OCT) and frequency domain OCT (FD-OCT) (Figure 5-3). In the case of TD-OCT, light from the light source is split into the reference beam and the sample beam. Back reflected light from both arms is combined again and recorded by the detector. To record one depth profile of the sample (A-scan), the reference arm needs to be scanned. This has to be repeated for each lateral scan position. FD-OCT is the second generation of OCT technology and provides a more efficient implementation of the principle of low-coherence interferometry. In contrast to TD-OCT, FD-OCT uses spectral information to generate A-scans without the need for mechanical scanning of the optical path length. Thus, the scanning imaging speed and the signal-to-noise ratio of FD-OCT are greatly improved. The advantages are no longitudinal scanning, great improvement of signal sensitivity, and large dynamic range.

5.2.2 Applications of OCT

Recently, OCT has been widely used in dermatology, gastroenterology, urology, gynecology and neurosurgery, etc. , especially in the detection and diagnosis of dermatosis, due to its advantages such as non-injury, non-invasive, high resolution, simple structure, and simple portability. Although histopathology is the gold standard and currently the most reliable clinical diagnosis technique in dermatology, it is a traumatic inspection method and is difficult to inspect one by one for multiple pigmented skin lesions. It is benefit that OCT is able to help diagnose and delineate lesions, identify subclinical lesions, and accurately assess their thickness. This structural change can be used to diagnose different types of skin tumors. So far, the greatest potential of OCT lies in the diagnosis and treatment of non-melanoma skin cancers (NMSCs) in dermatology, especially basal cell carcinoma. Besides, pigmented skin lesions still face great challenges in OCT. In the diagnosis of melanoma, OCT is not as accurate as dermoscope or reflectance confocal microscopy (RCM). The reason is that melanin is a strong scatterer of light, and images of pigmented skin lesions such as melanoma and pigmented moles have been proven difficult to obtain through light penetration-based techniques.

5.2.2.1 Basal cell carcinoma (BCC)

The BCC is one of the prime examples of indications for OCT. Promising results have already been demonstrated in delineating these tumors, and also the diagnostic criteria for BCC have been established. For normal skin, OCT can reliably identify the distinct layers of the skin usually down to the deep reticular dermis (depending on the imaged skin region and the OCT system used) and the dermal-epidermal junction (DEJ) appears as an intact narrow hyporeflective line (Figure 5-4(a)). In BCC lesions, loss of normal skin architecture is an overall finding (Figure 5-4(b)). The specific OCT characteristics of BCC include alteration of the DEJ and dark ovoid areas in the dermis (basal cell nests) surrounded by a white halo (e. g., stroma), sometimes referred to as a honeycomb pattern. Cellular palisading/ peritumoral clefting at the margins of basal cell nests is often seen as a low-intensity OCT signal at the periphery of the cell nests.

Secondary features include absence of normal hair follicles and glands and altered dermal capillaries directed toward the basaloid cell islands. Several studies have shown the correlation of OCT morphology with histology for several types of skin tumors, although earlier studies found it difficult to differentiate between BCC subtypes. HD-OCT has an increased lateral resolution (at the cost of penetration depth) and may permit differentiation of BCC subtypes. The features described in HD-OCT can be visualized only superficially in the lesion and include the combination of distinct lobular organization, a dominant vascular pattern in the papillary plexus, and the presence/absence of a stretching effect on the stroma.

As mentioned above, OCT provides relatively high accuracy in distinguishing lesions from normal skin, which is of great importance in identifying tumor borders. In differentiating normal skin from non-melanoma skin cancers (NMSCs) lesions, sensitivity of 79%-94% and specificity of 85%-96% were found for OCT. Looking specifically at the diagnostic accuracy of OCT in identifying BCC, recent extensive studies have investigated this aspect. By using a specific scoring system (e. g., Berlin score) based on five predetermined diagnostic OCT criteria, Wahrlich et al. found that the sensitivity and specificity for multibeam OCT amounted to 96. 6％ and 75. 2％, respectively, when evaluated by a dermatology specialist familiar with OCT. Specifically, 88％ of all BCC diagnoses based on OCT were correctly classified, confirmed by histopathology. In a multicenter study by Ulrich and Mayer et al. , the diagnostic value of OCT for BCC in a typical clinical setting was investigated. 235 non-pigmented pink lesions of 155 patients suspicious for BCC underwent clinical assessment, dermatoscope, OCT, and biopsy/histological examination, with the diagnosis recorded at each stage. The results showed that sensitivities are high for all three techniques, increasing from 90. 0％ by clinical examination only to 95. 7％ with the addition of OCT. However, there was a marked and statistically significant increase in specificity from 28. 6％ by clinical assessment to 75. 3％ with the addition of OCT. The positive predictive value and negative predictive value were the greatest for OCT, and the overall accuracy of diagnosis for BCC increased from 65. 8％ (clinical examination alone) to 87. 4％ with the addition of OCT. The authors of this study emphasized that OCT should not be used as a replacement for clinical examination or dermatoscope, but that OCT is best utilized as an adjunct non-invasive tool especially in difficult cases and in the management of patients with field cancerization or a large number of suspicious skin tumors.

5. 2. 2. 2   Pigmented nevi and melanomas

So far, only few studies have investigated OCT imaging of pigmented nevi and melanomas. The reason is that melanin is a strong scatterer of light; images of pigmented lesions like melanomas and nevi have been proven more difficult to obtain by techniques based on the penetration of light. Conventional OCT with an imaging resolution of 5-7 mm cannot visualize cellular features and therefore the image analysis of melanocytic lesions must rely on distinct morphological changes in the tissue. In benign nevi, an intact DEJ and acantholysis is often seen in OCT images. In comparison, melanoma often shows marked architectural disarray and rarely displays a clear dermoepidermal border because of the infiltrative tumor growth. The most characteristic feature seen in melanoma with conventional OCT is large, vertical, and icicle-shaped structures that are not observed in the benign nevi; however, despite this finding, conventional OCT cannot demonstrate enough clear-cut differences between malignant and benign pigmented lesions to be used as a diagnostic tool for melanoma.

Compared with conventional OCT, HD-OCT has a high enough resolution to image the tissue on a cellular level but with a limited penetration depth complementary to that of RCM. The high resolution of HD-OCT allows detailed imaging of pathological changes in melanocytic lesions, and studies have suggested that HD-OCT can provide morphological imaging that can discriminate architectural patterns and cytological features of pigmented lesions and cells in the epidermis and superficial dermis. With regard to diagnostic accuracy of HD-OCT in melanoma, a recent multicenter study employing one blinded investigator assessed the diagnostic performance of HD-OCT in the differentiation of benign melanocytic skin lesions and melanoma. The study included 93 histopathologically proven melanocytic skin lesions, of which 27 were melanoma. The sensitivity of HD-OCT was found to be 74.1% and the specificity was 92.4%. The positive predictive value was 80% and the negative predictive value was 89.7%. The performance of HD-OCT was dependent on tumor thickness and the presence of borderline lesions, indicated by high false negative rates in very thin melanomas and high false positive rates in dysplastic nevi. In conclusion, the performance in diagnosing melanoma by OCT is still inferior to other competing techniques such as RCM, although recent studies have provided some encouragement. To optimize early diagnosis of melanoma, OCT may develop into a valuable adjunct tool; however, further technical development and more extensive studies of OCT are required before this can be achieved.

5.3　Confocal Laser Scanning Microscope

Fluorescence imaging is an imaging mode that has gradually developed in the biomedical field in recent years. Fluorescence is the process whereby a molecule in the lower and stable of two electronic states (generally the ground state) is excited to a higher and unstable electronic state by radiation whose energy corresponds to an allowed absorption transition. After absorbing photon, electrons may reach the high vibrational energy level or the first excited state. The second excited state then undergoes internal conversion or relaxation oscillation process to reach the lowest vibrational energy level of the first excited state. Since the excited state is an unstable state, the electron returns to the ground state from the lowest vibrational energy level of the first excited singlet state, followed by the emission at the same time. Fluorescence imaging has the advantages of real-time image acquisition, high sensitivity, non-toxicity, and abundant fluorescent contrast agents. It is widely used in basic scientific research and clinical practice. With the development of science and technology, fluorescence microscopy has also made significant progress, and a series of technologies such as confocal laser scanning microscopy, and two-photon confocal laser scanning microscopy, have emerged, which play key roles in biomedical research and clinical diagnosis.

5.3.1　Two-photon confocal laser scanning microscope

In view of the limitations of single-photon confocal fluorescence imaging technique in the optical imaging of intravital tissues, Denk et al. proposed the concept of two-photon fluorescence microscopy in 1990, which provided open ideas for optical imaging of intravital tissues. Then, the development of multiphoton fluorescence microscopy had further expanded the application of fluorescence imaging technique in clinical medicine. Compared with traditional single-photon confocal fluorescence imaging technique, the advantages of two-photon or multiphoton fluorescence imaging are as follows: ① Negligible damage to biological samples prolongs effective observation time, which is convenient for long-term *in vivo observation*. ② The long-wavelength lasers exhibits the small scattering coefficient in living tissues, deep tissue penetration, clear and high resolution fluorescence image. ③ The high fluorescence collection rate enhances image contrast. ④ The requirement for the optical path collection system is lower than that of the single-photon confocal microscope (Figure 5-5). ⑤ A single wavelength of excitation light can simultaneously excite multiple dyes, so that different information in the same life activity can be obtained for mutual comparison and supplement. Therefore, multiphoton fluorescence imaging technique has been widely used in intravital tissue imaging, especially skin tissue imaging. Recently, this technique has also made breakthroughs in clinical diagnosis. The detection system based on multiphoton tomography has been applied in early skin cancer diagnosis and skin aging detection.

5.3.2 Principles of two-photon fluorescence imaging

Two-photon fluorescence is the process in which a fluorophore is excited via near simultaneous absorption of two photons, each having half the energy (twice the wavelength) required for the transition from the ground to the first singlet excited state. The prerequisite for near-simultaneous absorption and the timescale of molecular light absorption (10-16 s) dictates the use of specialized excitation sources. In current instruments, a mode-locked Ti-sapphire laser delivers infrared light pulses of femtosecond duration at high repetition rates. Two-photon excited fluorescence has a characteristic dependence on the square of the excitation light intensity. Namely, doubling the excitation intensity quadruples the fluorescence signal. In contrast, fluorescence derived from conventional one-photon absorption exhibits linear dependence on excitation light intensity. When irradiated by a laser of a suitable wavelength, some molecules in intravital tissues can emit stable fluorescence, and they are therefore called endogenous fluorophores. Endogenous fluorophores are widely distributed in intravital tissues, such as reduced nicotinamide adenine dinucleotide phosphate (NADPH), porphyrin derivatives, and melanin. Usually, the morphology and boundary of melanocytes in the area of melanoma will change, which can be used for early diagnosis of melanoma. Besides, the percentage of NADPH in skin tissue is related to the level of intracellular redox and metabolism, which can serve as molecular markers for skin aging detection. Therefore, two-photon fluorescence imaging technique has a wide range of applications in the early diagnosis of dermatosis and detection of skin aging.

5.3.3 Applications of two-photon confocal laser scanning fluorescence microscope in the diagnosis of skin tumors

Minimally invasive diagnosis of skin tumors is a major reason for developing multiphoton skin imaging. Ranked by levels of incidence from the highest to the lowest the major types of skin are as follows: basal cell carcinoma (originating from cells that make up the stratum basale of the epidermis), squamous cell carcinoma (originating from squamous cells that make up the major part of the epidermis), and melanoma (originating from melanocytes). Despite the comparatively low proportion of melanoma cases, it has the highest mortality rate. Early examples of multiphoton imaging for skin tumors include Teuchner et al., who measured the two-photon fluorescence of melanin in excised skin tissue. Subsequently, Skala et al. studied a hamster cheek pouch cancer model where tumors were biopsied and imaged in 3D. From these images, five features were identified for distinguishing normal, precancerous, and cancerous (squamous cell carcinoma) tissues. Skala and coworkers extended this work to include fluorescence lifetime metabolic imaging based on NADPH and flavin adenine dinucleotide (FAD) emission, noting that metabolism was different in tumors when compared with normal tissue.

Although the use of animal models is helpful, the study of human tissues is an important step towards eventual clinical applications. Most of these studies are based on two-photon fluorescence of endogenous fluorophores. In a proof-of-concept study on basal cell carcinoma by Cicchi et al., an increase in fluorescence intensity was observed in cancerous tissue taken from a single patient. In another early study, melanoma was imaged based on fluorescence emissions from NADPH and elastin, and SHG signal from collagen. Melanoma cells were observed to fluoresce much brighter than the surrounding cells. A much larger trial, with 250 patients, was also performed for imaging melanoma. The increased fluorescence from cancerous melanocytes was confirmed, and morphological differences could also be seen. In another large study, 115 patients were recruited to study the sensitivity and specificity of two-photon fluorescence for the diagnosis of melanoma; values of up to 95% sensitivity and up to 97% specificity were reported (Figure 5-6). The overarching message of these reports seems to be that multiphoton fluorescence imaging may be a promising non-invasive approach providing morphological and molecular information that appears to be diagnostic and provides similar information as excisional biopsy.

5.4　Reflectance Confocal Microscope

Reflectance confocal microscope (RCM) is a commonly used dermatology clinical imaging technique. It relies on reflectance (back-scattering) of light from structures with endogenous contrast, such as melanin, haemoglobin and some organelles. Reflectance occurs at the boundaries of two structures with different refractive indices, such as membranes, keratohyaline granules and melanosomes. RCM is a non-invasive imaging technique that enables *in vivo* visualisation of the epidermis down to the papillary dermis in real-time. Resolution is almost comparable to conventional histology. It has the advantage of allowing the clinician to do a "virtual biopsy" of the skin and obtain diagnostic clues while minimizing unnecessary skin biopsies. RCM is widely used in clinical diagnosis of most dermatosis, including inflammatory lesions, infestations and infections, pigmented tumors, epithelial tumors, etc, and cosmetics. Specifically, RCM has received extensive attention from researchers in the diagnosis and application of benign and malignant skin tumors. Compared with regular optical microscopes, RCM has the following features: ① ultra-high resolution (up to 1 μm); ② non-invasive continuous optical section of the sample to achieve three-dimensional reconstruction imaging and obtain the fine structure inside the sample; ③ optical section of samples with a thickness of less than 1 μm to avoid damage caused by biopsy; ④ the pinhole placed in front of the detector can effectively decrease stray background scattered light, and greatly improve image contrast and quality. RCM has gradually become an important auxiliary instrument for diagnosis, treatment and follow-up of skin tumor patients in large medical centers.

5.4.1　Principles of RCM

The RCM system is mainly composed of diode laser, beam splitter, focusing lens and detectors (Figure 5-7). The light passes through a beam splitter, a scanning and focusing optical lens and a skin contact device. It penetrates the skin and illuminates a small tissue spot. Light reflected from the focal point reflects back through the lens, which focuses it into a small pinhole and forms an image on a photodetector. The pinhole only allows light from a focal point to pass through (i. e. , confocal), and prevents light from another tissue point or out-of-focus plane from getting through. When the beam is moved in one direction (scanning), a line of reflected signals is generated (X-axis) and when the beam is moved in the other direction (Y-axis), a complete area can be scanned leading to an en face image of the tissue comparable to an "optical slice". By moving that plane into or out of the tissue (Z-axis, parallel to the beam direction), a stack of images can be generated representing the optical image of a tissue volume, enabling the confocal microscope to visualize at a slice in the sample, similar to CT. Therefore, RCM is also called skin CT. The obtained images are three-dimensionally reconstructed by computer, which is beneficial for the multi-angle observation of the three-dimensional section or overall structure of skin tissue. RCM images are based on the difference in refractive index of organelles and skin tissues to achieve high resolution; melanin, keratin and fibrous tissue in skin tissue have high refractive index, serving as a natural control. The tissue with high refractive index is bright, and the one with low refractive index is dark.

The device uses a diode laser at 830 nm with a power lower than 35 mW at tissue level. The maximum imaging range of RCM is 500 μm × 500 μm, with the maximum imaging depth of 500 μm. The magnification is up to 100 times, with the lateral resolution of 0.5 μm, and the minimum optical section thickness is 1.7 μm. A 30× objective lens with a numerical aperture of 0.9 is used with either water (refractive index, 1.33) or gel (refractive index, 1.3335) as an immersion medium. It captures images with a spatial resolution of 0.5-1.0 mm in the lateral dimension and 4-5 mm in the axial dimension. The advantages of RCM are as follows: ① Non-invasive, real-time and dynamic monitor of cell/tissue morphology and physiological functions in the same skin lesion, which is favorable for follow-up observation of its development, changes, and improvement after treatment. ② Dynamic changes of blood flow inside skin blood vessels can be observed. ③ When it is difficult to determine the location for routine histopathological examinations, multiple suspicious lesions can be simply observed with RCM measurement without complicated and tedious processing. ④ Imaging is rapid, and the data is easy to store and output.

5. 4. 2　Applications of RCM in the diagnosis of melanoma

Cutaneous melanoma represents the challenges in early or preventive detection. In early stages of tumor development, surgical excision is almost always curative, whereas delayed recognition increases the risk of tumor growth and death from metastatic disease. RCM represents a breakthrough in melanoma diagnosis and biology of melanocytic lesions. Because melanosomes and melanin are strong sources of endogenous contrast, melanocytes are particularly evident by means of this technique. Several studies have identified RCM features of melanocytic lesions, suggesting that further improvement in diagnostic accuracy for melanoma could be achieved, especially when this technique is used in the combination with dermoscope.

5. 4. 2. 1　Superficial spreading melanoma

A study by Pellacani et al. aimed to evaluate the frequency of confocal features in benign and malignant melanocytic lesions and their diagnostic significance for melanoma identification where a second end point was to identify the most relevant features for melanoma diagnosis. The study included 102 consecutive melanocytic lesions (37 melanomas, 49 acquired nevi (21 junctional, 27 compound, and 1 intradermal), and 16 epithelioid and/or spindle cell nevi (3 junctional Spitz, 8 compound Spitz, and 5 Reed)). After describing the RCM features of every type of lesion included, six criteria were identified as independently correlated with a diagnosis of melanoma. The two major criteria were the presence of cytological atypia (mild or marked) and nonedged papillae at the basal layer, and the four minor criteria included the presence of roundish cells in superficial layers spreading upward in a pagetoid fashion, pagetoid cells widespread throughout the lesion, cerebriform clusters in the papillary dermis, and nucleated cells within dermal papilla. The study concluded that RCM was useful for characterizing the equivocal melanocytic lesions *in vivo* at clinical and dermoscopic evaluation.

In 2007, Pellacani et al. developed an algorithm aimed to define the impact of RCM features that distinguish melanomas and nevi with standard statistical methods. They defined the following RCM features for the diagnosis of melanoma.

(1) Epidermis (stratum granulosum/stratum spinosum): The presence of a marked epidermal disarray was more frequently observed in melanomas, although it was also present in one-third of nevi. Conversely, a homogeneous epidermis characterized by regular honeycombed and/or cobblestone pattern was strongly related to benign lesions. Pagetoid

infiltration of roundish cells was reported in 78% of melanomas and 19% of nevi, whereas the observation of dendritic pagetoid cells, although significant, had a relatively lower odds ratio for melanomas. More than three cells per image and the presence of cells larger than 20 mm were predominantly observed in melanomas. Pleomorphism and widespread diffusion throughout the lesion of pagetoid cells were specific but not sensitive markers of malignancy.

(2) Dermal-epidermal junction: The presence of nonedged papillae was observed in 90% of melanomas and 41% of nevi, whereas edged papillae were predominantly present in nevi. Mild to marked atypia was observed in 73% of melanomas and 27% of nevi, respectively. Cells distributed in sheet-like structures, disrupting the papillary architecture of the basal layer, were highly specific, but with low sensitivity for melanoma. Besides, junctional nests, both clusters and thickenings, were characteristics of benign lesions.

(3) Upper dermis: Immediately below the dermal-epidermal junction, nested cell aggregates were visible in more than half of the lesions. Regular dense nests were significantly more represented in nevi, whereas the presence of atypical nests (e. g., the nonhomogeneous nests, sparse cell nests, and/or cerebriform nests) were correlated with malignancy (53% of melanomas), although they were also observed in 26% of nevi. Within the dermal papilla, almost half of the melanomas showed large nucleated cells, compared with 13% of nevi. No difference in the frequency of plump bright cells (bright small cells, and/or hyper-reflecting spots), and broadened reticulated and/or large bundles of fibers was reported within the two groups. When comparing melanomas equal or thinner than 1 mm with thicker ones, epidermal disarray, cells in sheet-like structures, cerebriform nests, and nucleated cells within dermal papilla were significantly associated with thick melanomas.

5.4.2.2　Lentigo maligna

Lentigo maligna (LM) is an early form of melanoma with an incidence that has increased during the past two decades. Several studies demonstrated that RCM can be used to differentiate LM from other pigmentations of the face. It can also assist in defining the peripheral margins of LM, even on amelanotic tumors. In 2010, Guitera et al. identified six features that were independently correlated with the diagnosis of LM by means of discriminant analysis, corresponding to, in order of relevance, nonedged papillae, large pagetoid round cells, nucleated cells in a dermal papilla, three or more atypical cells at the DEJ in five 0.5 mm×0.5 mm images, follicular localization of pagetoid cells and/or atypical junctional cells, and the single negative (benign) feature of a broadened honeycomb pattern of the epidermis (Figure 5-8).

5.4.2.3　Nodular melanoma

Under RCM, nodular melanoma (NM) exhibits several differential features compared with superficial spreading melanoma. These differences are often correlated with dermoscopic and histopathological findings. Within the epidermis, NM lacks characteristics of melanoma such as epidermal disarrangement and pagetoid spreading. Instead, they usually show a honeycomb pattern or a peculiar broadened pattern consisting of polygonal cells with black nuclei and bright and thick borders. At the DEJ, the typical papillary architecture is not visible in the nodules, corresponding to the epidermal flattening caused by massive proliferation of malignant cells in the dermis. Hyporefractive nests, called "cerebriform nests", are observed in NM, correlating with deep tumor infiltration. Plump cells are present and correlated with dermal macrophages, usually associated with a moderate degree of inflammation.

5.5　Photoacoustic Imaging

5.5.1　Principles of photoacoustic imaging

Photoacoustic imaging (PAI) is a new non-invasive biological imaging technique. When pulsed or intensity-modulated continuous-wave laser irradiates biological tissue, tumor, melanin, hemoglobin and other substances in the biological tissue absorb photon energy. After the absorption of the light, an initial temperature rise leads to a pressure rise, which propagates as a photoacoustic wave (Figure 5-9). The ultrasonic detector located on the surface of targets is utilized to receive these ultrasonic signals. The collected signals are processed and the corresponding image is reconstructed by computer, through inversion of the optical features of the light-absorbing substances in the tissue.

Photoacoustic imaging has the advantages of high resolution optical imaging and deep penetration of ultrasound imaging. On the one hand, photoacoustic imaging is based on the difference in optical absorption of substances inside tissues with the features of high resolution and high contrast, similar with optical imaging. On the other hand, photoacoustic imaging detects ultrasonic signals instead of optical signals, which overcomes the penetrating depth limitation of optical imaging due to the high light scattering of tissues. Therefore, photoacoustic imaging is the most promising imaging technique in recent years, which can provide high-resolution and high-contrast tissue images for deep tissues (50-70 mm). For superficial organs like skin, photoacoustic imaging can almost achieve imaging in the entire depth of skin.

The occurrence and development of dermatosis are often accompanied by changes in the physicochemical properties of skin tissue, such as morphology and composition, metabolism, blood oxygen content and pigment changes. Although histopathological analysis is the clinical gold standard, which can accurately detect above physicochemical properties, the drawbacks of long time consumption and invasion limit its wide application. Photoacoustic imaging can quickly and non-invasively display information such as blood oxygen saturation and blood flow in intravital tissues, chemical composition and functions of tissues (e. g. , fat, tumor, hemoglobin, collagen, melanin and water content, and their locations). In addition, as a superficial organ, skin can fully absorb light and the effects by sound diffraction and attenuation can be negligible. Therefore, photoacoustic imaging has developed rapidly in dermatology.

5.5.2 Applications of photoacoustic imaging in the diagnosis of dermatosis

Photoacoustic imaging is widely used in the diagnosis of dermatosis, including melanoma, nevus flammeus, hemangioma, basal cell carcinoma, squamous cell carcinoma, scleroderma, and others. Due to the high sensitivity of photoacoustic to blood vessels, photoacoustic imaging of blood vessel structure and function in skin and vascular proliferation has become popular in dermatological imaging diagnosis in recent years. One of the representative applications is to achieve the photoacoustic imaging of blood vessel structure and function in palm. Viator et al. performed photoacoustic imaging of nevus flammeus and the obtained images clearly showed the depth of blood vessels and the thickness of skin lesions. Some researchers have successfully diagnosed basal cell carcinoma through the combination of photoacoustic imaging and optical coherence tomography, and obtained its vascular pattern and collagen matrix. Since the vascular pattern and collagen matrix are two key parameters for the classification of basal cell carcinoma, early diagnosis of basal cell carcinoma can be expected.

Another important application of photoacoustic imaging in the diagnosis of dermatosis is the diagnosis and evaluation of melanin. Due to its strong light absorption, melanin presents extremely high contrast with other substances in tissues. Melanoma is a typical pigment-related and the most malignant skin tumor, which is prone to metastasis. It is demonstrated that photoacoustic imaging can be utilized to diagnose melanoma and monitor its growth and metastasis by detecting endogenous melanin in tumors. At present, the applications of photoacoustic imaging in melanoma diagnosis are mainly as follows.

5.5.2.1 Measuring melanoma thicknesses

Thickness measurement is critical in the diagnosis of melanoma. Besides, tumor thicknesses are associated with different prognoses and treatment procedures. In 2006, Oh et al. imaged skin melanomas *in vivo* by using a table-top photoacoustic microscopy system. The results showed that both the top and bottom boundaries of the melanoma phantoms could be detected (Figure 5-10). In addition, the measured thicknesses of the melanoma phantoms agreed well with the known values. To broaden the applicability to various anatomical sites, Oh et al. developed a hand-held photoacoustic microscopy system that could image melanomas in all tumor classifications, which is highly promising for clinical studies.

5.5.2.2 Detecting the rate of growth

The rate of growth has been proposed as an important feature and reliable diagnostic indicator of melanoma, compared with melanoma thickness. However, all these measurements are indirect, and there is still little direct information on the ROG of the melanomas. One roadblock is the lack of a method for noninvasive melanoma volume quantification. Because melanoma may have irregular shapes, in order to accurately quantify its volume, the whole boundary needs to be visualized. Recently, a linear transducer array-based photoacoustic computed tomography system was applied to measure melanoma volume and the rate of growth, and nearly the entire melanoma boundary could be detected in three dimensions. With the ability to image entire melanomas *in vivo*, photoacoustic imaging has successfully measured both the thickness and volume of melanoma. Thus, as a significant feature of melanoma, the rate of growth can be directly calculated, which may prove to be superior to tumor thickness as a diagnostic feature (Figure 5-11).

5.5.2.3　Locating sentinel lymph nodes

Photoacoustic imaging can be used for the localization and biopsy of sentinel lymph nodes, and achieve higher contrast and resolution, making it possible for more accurate sentinel lymph node biopsy and metastatic melanoma diagnosis. A hand-held photoacoustic microscopy system modified from a clinical ultrasound array system was applied for sentinel lymph node detection. Image-guided needle biopsies were successfully performed by using this hand-held photoacoustic microscopy system. The results indicated that photoacoustic imaging could be used for image-guided sentinel lymph node biopsy with high accuracy.

5.5.2.4　Screening of sentinel lymph nodes

Biopsy followed by hematoxylin and eosin staining is the standard of care in assessing metastatic melanomas in sentinel lymph nodes. However, incomplete examination of the sentinel lymph nodes may miss melanoma cells and thus leads to misdiagnosis of metastasis. For complete sentinel lymph node assessment, photoacoustic tomography, with its high sensitivity for melanoma imaging, is a promising modality. Specifically, melanoma cells hidden in a pig lymph node and melanoma metastasis in human sentinel lymph nodes can be effectively identified with a typical photoacoustic computed tomography system. Thus, it is believed that photoacoustic tomography could potentially be applied for detecting melanoma metastasis in SLNs *in vivo* (Figure 5-12).

5.5.2.5　Monitoring circulating tumor cells

The high mortality rate of melanoma is attributed mainly to its high propensity for metastasis. The presence of circulating tumor cells has been suggested as an early predictor for metastatic development, motivating intensive studies for detection and isolation of circulating tumor cells in recent years. Based on photoacoustic sensing, *in vivo* photoacoustic flow cytometry excites selected blood vessels with short laser pulses, followed by time-resolved photoacoustic measurements by an ultrasonic transducer placed on the skin. Based on the difference in the corresponding photoacoustic signals, pure blood and blood containing melanoma cells can be distinguished. However, the detection voxel is large and the fractional photoacoustic signal changes caused by circulating tumor cells is small, which restricts the clinical application of *in vivo* photoacoustic flow cytometry. One solution is to tag circulating tumor cells with a magnetosensitive contrast agent and then magnetically concentrate them in the detection voxel, thus increasing the photoacoustic signal changes. However, the potential toxicity of such an exogenous contrast agent hinders its applications in humans. Thus further improvement of *in vivo* photoacoustic flow cytometry is most likely to focus on increasing the sensitivity of label-free photoacoustic tomography to circulating tumor cells.

In addition, applications of photoacoustic imaging in skin grafts and thermal burns have also attracted much attention. With the development of photoacoustic imaging technique, the application of photoacoustic imaging in dermatosis has expanded from simple diagnostics to theranostics. Recently, photoacoustic imaging has been utilized for melanoma resection. It is found that photoacoustic imaging can more accurately determine the edge of melanoma, which is beneficial for the complete resection of melanoma and greatly reduces the recurrence rate after surgery. In addition, dual-wavelength photoacoustic flow cytometry with nanosecond pulsed laser has been used to perform label-free imaging of melanoma cells *in vivo*. The imaging-guided nanosecond pulsed laser can generate thermal effect at the specific position to achieve specific killing of the melanoma cells, which is extremely important for monitoring and preventing early metastasis of melanoma. At present, the drawbacks of photoacoustic imaging in dermatosis, such as insufficient resolution and slow imaging speed, restrict the wide clinical applications. However, it is believed that photoacoustic imaging will be gradually improved and upgrade from simple diagnostics to theranostics.

5.6 Photothermal Imaging

Photothermal imaging is a new and promising technique, which plays an important role in many fields. In 1956, American surgeon Lawson used infrared scanning technology to confirm that the temperature of breast cancer skin was higher than normal, which opened the prelude to the clinical application of photothermal imaging. Photothermal imaging is a medical functional imaging technique based on infrared imaging, which is totally different with other morphological imaging techniques such as X-ray, CT, MRI and ultrasound. Photothermal imaging can monitor the relative intensity of cell metabolism. The infrared scanning and collection system can receive infrared light radiated by human body. Because this radiation is temperature-dependent, the infrared images recorded can be converted into temperature maps, or thermograms, allowing retrieving valuable information about the object under investigation. The temperature changes are quantitatively analyzed to diagnose the location of lesions, which reflects the physiological and pathological conditions of human body. With the rapid development of optoelectronic technology and computer technology, photothermal imaging technique in the medical field has also been developed quickly and extensively. Besides, due to the advantages of simplicity, rapid, non-invasion, convenience and high sensitivity, it plays important roles in early detection, dynamic observation, diagnosis and efficacy evaluation of diseases.

5. 6. 1   Principles of photothermal imaging

Every object above the absolute zero temperature (-273.15 ℃) emits an electromagnetic radiation. Human body is a natural biological infrared radiator, which continuously emits infrared radiation. Besides, infrared radiation from human body is closely related with metabolism, body heat balance, body temperature regulation and tissue structures. Human is warm-blooded animal, and skin is the main infrared radiator of human body. When room temperature slightly lower than body temperature, according to the radiation wavelength of human body, an infrared detector with a sensitive wavelength of 8-14 μm is usually selected. The infrared signal emitted by human body is collected through remote sensing technique and is converted into an electrical signal, followed by converting to digital signals with analogs. The computer displays a visible and quantitative infrared thermal image via the pseudo-color temperature distribution field (Figure 5-13). When physiological condition changes somewhere in human body, inevitably deviation of lesion temperature appears due to changes in blood flow and metabolism. As a result, the infrared radiation changes. Therefore, based on this principle, photothermal imaging can accurately monitor changes in human body temperature, and even exhibits positive scan results before clinical symptoms or histological changes appear in the lesion.

5. 6. 2   Applications of photothermal imaging in the diagnosis of dermatosis

The potential of photothermal imaging for skin cancer detection and, in particular, as an early-stage melanoma diagnostic tool, was already noticed in the early 1960s. Unfortunately, pioneer thermographic studies devoted to the subject showed disappointing results with a high percentage of false-negative outcomes. Those poor results drastically reduced the enthusiasm of the medical community. Nevertheless, they can be explained by several factors. First, potential thermal signals involved in early-stage lesions are small, and highly sensitive infrared imaging devices were not available at the time of the first study. Second, such small temperature differences are usually buried in larger thermal signals originating from the subcutaneous tissue. In such circumstances, small hot or cold spots would be hardly detectable even using current highly sensitive infrared cameras.

In 1995, Di Carlo proposed to overcome those difficulties by performing active thermography measurements. He implemented a photothermal set-up where the skin is stimulated by the contact with a balloon filled with a thermostatic alcohol solution. A few seconds after the removal of the stimulation, melanoma and hyperpigmented basal cell carcinomas exhibited drastic temperature differences compared with the surrounding healthy skin. Several years later, Buzug and his coworkers reproduced Di Carlo's experiment using cold gel packs and a more recent infrared camera. Very recently, Çetingül and Herman at Johns Hopkins University investigated transient thermal signals of melanoma lesions. Using a multilayer heat transfer skin model, they could extract quantitative information from the

transient thermal signals. As an example, Figure 5-14 shows a cluster of pigmented lesions located on a shoulder and investigated with photothermal. Whereas the steady state thermogram can not provide any diagnostic information, the melanoma lesion is clearly distinguishable on the infrared image taken few seconds after the removal of the cold stimulation. Çetingül and Hermann claimed that the method was able to detect Clark level Ⅰ (melanoma *in-situ*) lesions.

Bonmarin and Le Gal developed a lock-in thermography-based set-up specifically dedicated to the investigation of skin cancer. In such apparatus, the skin surface temperature is periodically modulated using an airflow, while an infrared camera records the emitted thermal radiation. Compared with the previous set-ups based on pulsed stimulation, lock-in thermography has the ability to suppress lateral heat spreading, leading to sharper thermograms. Figure 5-15 demonstrates the capabilities of lock-in thermography for the accurate detection of skin cancer lesion margins.

5.7　Raman Imaging

Raman spectroscopy is a commonly used vibrational spectroscopy based on Raman scattering effect discovered by Indian physicist Raman in 1928. In Raman spectrum, wavenumber, intensity and width of the characteristic peaks effectively reveal fingerprint information of substances, and the intensity is concentration-dependent. Thus, Raman spectroscopy is a quantitative analysis method. Compared with other spectroscopy techniques, Raman spectroscopy has its unique advantages: ① It can selectively excites the required chemical bonds of molecules by changing the excitation wavelength. ② There is no requirement of any sample pretreatment. ③ The sample will not be destroyed during the measurement. ④ The Raman absorbance of water can be ignored, so it is easier to measure Raman spectra of samples in aqueous solution. ⑤ Raman spectroscopy has a wide measurement range, so that heavy atom vibrations can be detected. Based on the advantages of Raman spectroscopy, various new analytical techniques are derived, such as surface enhanced Raman spectroscopy (SERS), Fourier transform Raman spectroscopy (FT-Raman), resonance Raman spectroscopy (RRS), confocal Raman microspectral imaging (CRMI) and coherent Raman scattering microscopy (CRSM).

CRMI is a relatively novel technique for the construction of label-free images of biological entities, such as cells or tissue sections. This method utilizes thousands of spatially resolved Raman spectra, and sophisticated image analysis algorithms, to construct images which are strictly based on the inherent biochemical abundance contrast afforded by Raman microscopy. Since only the signal from the focal plane is collected through the confocal pinhole, the signal-to-noise ratio and the signal quality is greatly improved. CRMI can detect tiny samples or even single-cell level samples. Equipped with a high-magnification optical microscope and various types of excitation light sources, CRMI can scan and obtain a Raman microscopic image of the sample point by point, which exhibits high spatial resolution, high signal-to-noise ratio and high accuracy. In the past few years, CRMI has vigorously developed in the fields of tumor detection, cultural relics and archaeology, and public security law. When the composition of biological tissues is analyzed with Raman spectroscopy, some uncertain factors, such as the inhomogeneity of biological tissues and the complexity of chemical composition, will affect the results. CRMI with the advantages of Raman spectroscopy and confocal microscopic imaging, can effectively compensate for the cognitive limitations caused by these uncertain factors. It is a molecular level optical imaging method to study biochemical components and structure of biological tissues. Figure 5-16(a) shows a simplified schematic of CRMI system. Due to weak Raman scattering (Stokes and anti-Stokes shifts), the laser of CRMI system is about one millionth weaker than typical absorption spectroscopy. A beamsplitter splits the light, with the beam path focused onto the sample through an objective lens. The beam can be split between a camera and the spectrograph for observation or measurement, respectively, and after passing through a rejection filter to remove the Rayleigh scatter, the Stokes (and anti-Stokes) wavelengths are diffracted by a grating onto a detector, either a CCD or an InGaAs array. Thus, the spatial distribution of the chemical components within the sample are imaged. High-resolution confocal Raman microscopes acquire the information of a complete Raman spectrum at every image pixel and achieve a lateral resolution at the diffraction limit (circa $\lambda/2$ of the excitation wavelength). CRMI can perform analysis of cells or biological tissues at molecular level. It is valuable for researchers to observe the changes of the composition and distribution of biochemical components in the cell life cycle, cell damage or cancer. CRMI not only can monitor the changes of various cells or tissues at any time, but also can analyze the difference between healthy tissues and cancerous tissues.

Skin is composed of proteins, nucleic acids, sugars, coenzymes and other components. It is the largest organ in human body, whose function is to protect internal organs and tissues from external physical and chemical stimuli and pathogens, etc. Skin consists of epidermis, dermis, and subcutaneous tissue, as well as some accessory organs (e. g. , sweat glands, sebaceous glands, and nails), blood vessels, lymphatic vessels, muscles, and others. Because different molecules contain chemical structures that have unique vibrational frequencies, vibrational spectroscopy and microscopy techniques can provide intrinsic and specific chemical contrast. Among these vibrational techniques, Raman spectroscopy has been extensively utilized in biomedical applications (e. g. , disease diagnosis). In the experiment, Raman spectra of skin can provide the changes of the composition and distribution of biochemical components in different skin layers. For example, the difference of Raman spectra between stratum corneum and epidermis is the peaks located at 1062 cm^{-1}, 1126 cm^{-1}, and 1296 cm^{-1}, indicating that a large amount of ceramide is present in the stratum corneum. Compared with Raman spectroscopy, Raman spectral properties of isolated skin tissues are studied in CRMI. Raman spectra of chemical composition in skin tissues constitute a spectral image, exhibiting the changes of composition and distribution of biochemical components in different skin layers for visualized diagnosis.

5.8　Challenges and Perspectives

With the development of medicine and life science, health has been paid much attention. Advanced medical imaging technique is one of the core techniques, which serves as an effectively medical diagnostic technique, including fluorescence imaging, photoacoustic imaging, photothermal imaging, ultrasound imaging, magnetic resonance imaging, Raman imaging, etc. Compared with traditional disease diagnosis methods, medical imaging technique is visualized, more accurate and sensitive. In view of the features of each imaging technique, imaging objects, spatial resolution and depth, sensitivity, are different. Thus, a single imaging technique exhibits unavoidable drawbacks: ① The spatial resolution of fluorescence imaging is too low to image deep tissue, due to the limitation of penetration depth. ② Penetration depth of photoacoustic imaging is still insufficient, and image contrast and detection sensitivity should be further improved. ③ The molecular contrast agents, which are low cytotoxicity and provide sufficient contrast, are lack. ④ Ultrasound imaging has low resolution and is dependent on operating experience. ⑤ MRI is time-consuming, high cost, and relatively low sensitivity, etc.

The development of multimodal imaging in recent years has attracted much attention in the field of medical imaging, which combines two or more imaging techniques to avoid the defects of a single imaging technique. The medical information obtained by different imaging techniques is complementary. Therefore, it is beneficial for the accurate diagnosis of patients to examine them with multiple imaging techniques. However, it will increase the patients' financial burden and the risk of toxic and side effects of angiography, which promotes the presence of multimodal imaging technique. By incorporating anatomical and functional imaging in a common hybrid imaging platform, a synergism in the imaging capabilities can be achieved, thus making it possible to precisely visualize and delineate structural and functional information. Multimodal imaging thereby ensures better elucidation of physiological mechanisms at molecular and cellular levels. Therefore, multimodal imaging has an immensely beneficial role for improved diagnosis and therapeutic planning of a disease. The field of multimodal imaging has seen rapid progress in the last decade, with its value having been demonstrated in numerous studies.

Questions

1. In which department does optical coherence tomography have widely clinical applications except dermatology?

2. What are the advantages and disadvantages of the imaging techniques in the early diagnosis of melanoma?

3. Please indicate the contrast source, penetration depth, axial resolution, lateral resolution, and imaging rate of the imaging techniques.

4. Please indicate the opportunities and challenges of artificial intelligence in the field of skin imaging.

5. Compared to CT, MRI and PET, optical imaging technology is widely used in the diagnosis of dermatosis. Please list the advantages and disadvantages of various optical imaging technologies in this chapter.

Extended reading

[1] Wilhelm K P, Elsner P, Berardesca E, et al. Bioengineering of the skin: skin imaging & analysis[M]. 2nd ed. Los Angeles: CRC Press, 2006.

[2] Hamblin M R, Avci P, Gupta G K. Imaging in dermatology[M]. Pittsburgh: Academic Press, 2016.

[3] Berardesca E, Maibach H, Wilhelm K P. Non invasive diagnostic techniques in clinical dermatology[M]. Heidelberg: Springer-Verlag, 2014.

[4] 孟如松,崔勇. 多模态皮肤病医学影像诊断图谱[M]. 北京:人民卫生出版社,2021.

[5] 孙秋宁,刘洁. 协和皮肤镜图谱[M]. 北京:人民卫生出版社,2015.

(**Jiang Hao**)

第六章
高分子纳米药物载体及其在皮肤疾病治疗中的应用

第一节　纳米药物载体概述

一、纳米药物载体简介

纳米药物载体是一类尺寸为纳米尺度的药物载体,它们可通过物理吸附、包裹或者化学键合等方式将药物分子负载于其内部、基体或表面,从而构成纳米载药系统。纳米载药系统适用于静脉、肌内、皮下、黏膜给药及口服等多种给药途径,通过对其载体的设计,可达到调控药物释放速率、增加生物膜的透过性、改变体内分布、提高生物利用度等目的。自20世纪90年代起,伴随着纳米科技的兴起和发展,纳米载药技术应运而生并迅速发展。它是一种将药剂学与纳米技术相结合的新型药物制剂技术。纳米药物载体的诞生与药物的溶解性有关,这是因为约半数的药物分子难溶于水,难以制成常规的水性溶液制剂;而纳米粒子由于具有特定的尺寸,在水中具有良好的分散性,因此利用其负载难溶性药物分子可有效地解决药物的溶解性难题。同时,载体材料对活性药物分子具有一定的保护作用,从而实现提高药物稳定性的目的。更重要的是,纳米载药系统具有缓释功能,可延长药物的作用时间,减少给药次数。此外,纳米载药系统可通过多种内吞途径进入靶细胞,从而提高药物的利用率。

自1995年第一个纳米载药系统问世以来,现已有50余种纳米载药系统进入临床研究阶段,且随着这一领域的快速发展,越来越多的纳米载药系统将进入临床研究。由于临床应用不断对药物制剂提出更高的要求(如在提高药效的同时降低副作用),研发具有靶向递送和控制释放功能的纳米药物载体成为近年来生物医药领域的热点之一。随着纳米载药技术的不断进步,研究者们发现经特定物质或功能性基团修饰的纳米药物载体具有靶向性,可将药物传输至指定病灶;随后通过一系列的物理、化学及生物作用,将药物在合适的时间以适当的速率释放出来,可有效地改善药物的代谢动力学参数,达到定向、定时、定量发挥药效的目的。此外,纳米载药系统也可集成诊断、检测试剂和治疗药物,是一种颇有前景的诊疗剂。

二、高分子纳米药物载体

高分子纳米药物载体即以天然或合成高分子为原料的纳米药物载体。早期的高分子载药系统可以追溯到 1962 年研制的青霉素与聚乙烯胺的结合物。1975 年,Ringsdorf 提出了高分子药物载体的设想,即通过共价键将小分子药物结合到高分子载体上。相比于无机材料,高分子材料具备诸多优点:具有 pH、温度、光等多种刺激响应性,易制备成具有不同形状、尺寸的纳米颗粒。此外,高分子材料种类繁多,来源广泛,其中生物医用高分子材料具有生物相容性好、可生物降解、毒性较低或无毒等特点,在纳米药物载体领域应用最为广泛。

三、皮肤疾病治疗和皮肤美容对高分子纳米药物载体的需求

皮肤疾病、皮肤美容等领域都涉及药物递送。例如,黑素瘤是死亡率极高的一种疾病,因此开发具有更好疗效且更低毒副作用的纳米载药系统对黑素瘤的治疗具有重要意义。另外,纳米载药系统也可用于银屑病等皮肤疾病的治疗和皮肤美容(皮肤美容方面见第九章)等方面。与传统的外用药物制剂(膏、霜)相比,纳米载药系统具有诸多优势:能够有效地改善难溶活性成分的水分散性,提高活性成分的稳定性,促进活性成分透过角质层屏障,实现活性成分的皮肤靶向输送和持续释放,并显著延长活性成分在皮肤中的滞留时间,避免发炎、过敏反应。同时,负载、释放多种活性成分,实现不同活性成分的协同增效。近年来,以高分子纳米材料为载体的抗癌药物和新型外用制剂越来越多地被应用到皮肤疾病的治疗产品中。

第二节　高分子纳米药物载体的类型

一、按化学组成分类

用作纳米药物载体的具有生物相容性且可生物降解的高分子材料包括天然高分子与合成高分子,其中较常用的有三类:多糖类、聚氨基酸类和聚酯类。

(一) 多糖类

多糖含有大量羟基、羧基、氨基等高活性亲水基团,易修饰改性,且一些多糖自身具有免疫调节、抗肿瘤、抗病毒等功效,已被广泛用于纳米药物载体的研究。目前用于纳米药物载体的多糖主要有葡聚糖、透明质酸、肝素、海藻酸盐、壳聚糖和香菇多糖等,其中应用较广泛的为透明质酸和壳聚糖。透明质酸由于具有良好的肿瘤靶向性而受到了广泛关注,然而其吸水性极强、稳定性较差、生物半衰期短,这些特点使其在纳米药物载体方面的应用也受到了一定限制。例如,被用于负载水溶性药物时载药量低、药物泄漏快。壳聚糖具有良好的生物黏附性,对许多细菌、真菌等微生物有不同程度的抑制作用,具有止血、提高人体免疫力和抗肿瘤的作用,且在人体内能被溶菌酶等分解,因此被广泛应用于生物医用材料。透明质酸和壳聚糖的亲水性强,通常被制备成纳米凝胶用作药物载体,还常与功能性无机纳米粒子如纳米金、量子点、磁性纳米粒子等制备成复合纳米凝胶,以提高药物的功能性。此外,它们还常被用作疏水性高分子或无机纳米药物载体的外层,以提高这些纳米药物载体的亲水性、稳定性及靶向性。

(二) 聚氨基酸类

聚氨基酸具有很强的结构可设计性,其分子链上具有多个反应活性位点,便于通过进一步修饰来调控其亲水疏水性能、电荷性质及靶向特性等。目前常用作纳米药物载体的聚氨基酸有聚谷氨酸、聚赖氨酸、聚苯丙氨酸和聚天冬氨酸等。在用作纳米药物载体时,疏水性聚氨基

酸通常与亲水性聚合物链段如聚乙二醇(PEG)等结合来形成两亲性嵌段共聚物,再经溶液自组装形成球形胶束。由于具有羧基和氨基等活性基团,聚氨基酸能够与药物分子通过化学键合的方式结合,也可通过物理包埋、静电吸附等方式结合,从而将药物负载于胶束的不同部位。此外,两种或多种氨基酸通过共聚的方式可合成氨基酸共聚物。氨基酸种类丰富,因此可以根据不同药物的需求,选择结构、性能符合要求的氨基酸制备共聚物。

(三) 聚酯类

脂肪族聚酯类高分子由于生理毒性小、相容性好而被用作纳米药物载体材料。这些聚酯通常不溶于水,常被制备成球形纳米颗粒或微胶囊用作药物载体。目前已被美国食品药品监督管理局(FDA)批准用作药物载体的脂肪族聚酯包括聚乳酸(PLA)、聚乳酸-羟基乙酸(PLGA)、聚己内酯(PCL)等。Pitt 和 Schindler 早在 20 世纪 70 年代就提出 PCL 可用作药物控释载体,目前,PCL 在生物医药领域已有广泛应用。

PLA 无毒、无刺激性、无免疫原性,且具有良好的生物相容性,因此也常用作纳米药物载体。但是,PLA 亲水性差,降解速率较慢;与之相反,聚羟基乙酸(PGA)极性较高,降解速率更快,但结晶度较高。因此二者在临床应用中均受到一定的限制。PLGA 为乳酸和羟基乙酸的共聚物,通过调节两种结构单元的比例,可以调控 PLGA 的溶解性、机械性能和降解速率,从而获得符合要求的载体材料。Yoo 等将抗癌药物阿霉素键合到 PLGA 上,随后制备了球形纳米粒子。研究结果表明,PLGA 纳米粒子的药物包封率高达 96.6%,载药量为 3.45%(质量分数),药物可在 25 天内缓慢释放。

此外,疏水性聚酯类高分子也常与亲水性高分子相结合,制备成两亲性嵌段共聚物,用于制备胶束型纳米药物载体,由此可以增加纳米药物载体的水溶性及稳定性。纳米药物载体的表面亲水性与亲脂性将影响巨噬细胞对其的吞噬速率。一般而言,表面亲脂性越强,巨噬细胞的吞噬速率越快。因此,增加纳米药物载体的表面亲水性,还可延长药物在体内的循环时间。

二、按载体的形貌分类

高分子纳米药物载体根据其形貌可以分为三维大分子(树状高分子、蛋白质等)、高分子纳米球/胶囊、高分子胶束/囊泡、高分子纳米凝胶和纳米乳等不同类型,如图 6-1 所示。

(一) 三维大分子

用作纳米药物载体的三维大分子主要指树状高分子和蛋白质。树状高分子是指从核心分子出发,不断地向外重复支化生长而得到的结构类似树枝的具有多级分支结构的三维立体高分子,其尺寸均匀性好、精确可调,一般介于 5~50 nm 之间。树状高分子的内部及表面均可设计丰富的、不同类型的官能团,它们可通过物理或化学作用与药物分子结合。通过物理作用结合的药物释放过快且易泄漏;通过化学作用结合的药物稳定性好但难以释放。为了解决上述问题,可设计内部疏水而外部亲水的树状高分子载体,例如在其表面接枝 PEG 链段,可提高通过物理作用结合的药物的载药量和稳定性,并延长药物的体内循环时间。Bhadra 等研究发现,在聚酰胺-胺(PAMAM)表面接枝 PEG 后,其对抗癌药物 5-氟尿嘧啶(5-FU)的载药量提高了 12 倍,药物释放速率降低至原来的 1/6,血液循环时间延长至原来的 3 倍,药效是5-FU裸药的 10 倍。通过调控表面接枝 PEG 的聚合度和接枝率,可对 PAMAM 的载药量和释放速率进行精细调控。另外,为了改善通过化学作用结合的药物的释放性能,可选用易在体内断裂的化学作用,例如通过酯键连接的药物比通过酰胺键连接的药物更易释放。更重要的是,利用肿

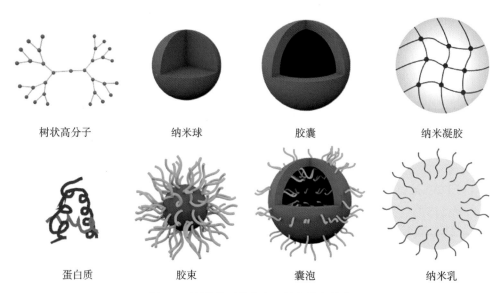

树状高分子　　　　纳米球　　　　胶囊　　　　纳米凝胶

蛋白质　　　　胶束　　　　囊泡　　　　纳米乳

图 6-1　不同类型的高分子纳米药物载体

Figure 6-1　Morphologies of polymer nano-drug carriers

瘤的弱酸性环境,通过酸敏感的化学作用(如腙键)将药物分子与树状高分子相结合,可实现刺激响应性释药,提高药物的细胞毒性并尽量避免对正常细胞的杀伤。Kono 等将阿霉素通过腙键键合到 PAMAM 表面,其细胞毒性比通过酰胺键连接的药物高 10 倍。此外,蛋白质也属于三维大分子,也被广泛用作纳米药物载体材料。

(二)高分子纳米球/胶囊

高分子纳米球(或纳米胶囊)一般是指由疏水性高分子聚集所形成的实心(或空心)零维纳米粒子,尺寸大多介于数十与数百纳米之间。例如,PLA、PLGA 常被用于制备纳米球/胶囊,以包覆抗癌药物。制备时,疏水性药物在纳米球形成的过程中可通过疏水作用被包裹到高分子基体中;在体内,药物随着高分子基体的逐渐降解而缓慢释放。纳米胶囊的空腔可包覆水溶性药物的水性溶液,也可包覆脂溶性药物的油性溶液,药物随着囊壁的溶解/破裂而释放。

(三)高分子胶束/囊泡

高分子胶束是指由两亲性嵌段共聚物自组装所形成的以疏水链为核、以亲水链为壳的球形聚集体,其尺寸一般介于 10~100 nm 之间,且非常均匀,是目前得到较多临床研究的高分子纳米药物载体。常用的疏水链段有 PLA、PLGA、PCL 及聚氨基酸等,常用的亲水链段为 PEG。药物可通过物理作用负载于胶束的疏水内核中,亲水壳层则可以维持胶束的稳定性,延长其体内循环时间。此外,也可通过化学作用先将药物分子键合到嵌段共聚物的疏水链上,再通过自组装形成胶束。高分子胶束疏水核的尺寸及其与药物之间的相互作用对其载药量具有重要的影响。

高分子囊泡则是两亲性嵌段共聚物自组装所形成的具有双分子层结构的胶囊状聚集体。与球形胶束不同的是,囊泡具有中空结构,内部空腔填充了水。用于制备囊泡的两嵌段共聚物的疏水链段的嵌段比则一般较大。囊泡的尺寸一般大于胶束,且均匀性不如胶束。类似于高分子纳米胶囊,囊泡也是一种纳米尺度的液体胶囊,既可包载传统的小分子药物,也可用于递送纳米颗粒以及蛋白质、核酸等生物大分子。与纳米胶囊不同的是,囊泡的囊壁内、外侧均有亲水高分子链,适用于装载亲水药物;但由于受到制备方法的制约,亲水药物在囊泡中的包封率一般较低。与球形胶束/纳米球不同的是,包覆在囊泡/纳米胶囊内的药物既可穿透囊壁缓释也可随着囊壁的破裂而暴释,得到较高的局部药物浓度。基于此,可以根据不同的需求来调控释药的速率。

（四）高分子纳米凝胶

高分子纳米凝胶是一种包含大量液体的纳米尺度分散体系,其中高分子通过物理交联或化学交联构成了连续的网络结构。常见的高分子纳米凝胶大多为水凝胶,其内部水含量可达90%左右。为了提高高分子纳米凝胶的性能,通常可将功能性无机纳米粒子,如纳米金、磁性纳米粒子、量子点等掺杂到纳米凝胶中。例如,杂化纳米凝胶中的非球形纳米金粒子可以作为光热传感器,应用于光动力疗法和光热疗法;含磁性纳米粒子的纳米凝胶可通过外部磁场实现药物体内靶向输送;此外,复合有量子点的纳米凝胶则可用于成像,构建诊疗一体化平台。

（五）纳米乳

纳米乳是指油相在表面活性剂的作用下以纳米液滴的形式分散于水中的一种稳定分散体系。类似于纳米液体胶囊,药物包覆在油滴中,其载药量取决于药物在油相中的溶解度。油滴直径一般为 $1\sim100$ nm,其均匀性因制备方法而异,但大多不如球形胶束。其中,油滴可选用食用油,而表面活性剂可选用生物相容性好、可生物降解的两亲性高分子。纳米乳中表面活性剂的疏水链段朝向油滴,而亲水链段则伸展在水相中,但高分子链的堆积密集度不如高分子纳米球/胶囊、高分子胶束/囊泡,因此药物的释放速率较快。

第三节　高分子纳米药物载体的制备技术

高分子纳米药物载体的制备方法因其结构类型和载药方式不同而异。高分子纳米药物载体负载药物的方式主要有三种:与高分子键合/吸附、嵌入高分子纳米载体的基体中、包裹在高分子纳米胶囊/高分子囊泡/纳米乳的内部。树状高分子、白蛋白等具有三维结构的大分子通过物理或化学作用与药物分子结合形成纳米载药系统。其中物理作用主要包括分子间作用力、氢键、静电作用、疏水作用,化学作用主要包括酯键、酰胺键、腙键等。其他类型的高分子纳米药物载体,如球形胶束、囊泡、纳米球/胶囊等都属于高分子聚集体,它们由许多高分子链在一定条件下聚集而成,根据聚集体的形貌,主要有以下制备方法。

一、单体聚合法

单体聚合法是指通过聚合反应直接制备高分子纳米粒子,并在纳米粒子形成的同时将药物分子包覆于其中的制备方法。其中,最主要的方法是乳液聚合。在乳液聚合过程中,首先将药物分子与疏水性单体混溶,之后在表面活性剂的作用下使之乳化,最后进行聚合反应即可获得包覆药物分子的高分子纳米球。该方法适用于疏水性高分子和药物,通常用于制备球形纳米药物载体。聚合反应过程中使用的高温条件可能影响药物的活性,且残留的单体、催化剂、表面活性剂、引发剂等可能会带来生物毒副作用。

二、溶液自组装

在选择性溶剂中,当两亲性嵌段共聚物的浓度高于其临界胶束浓度时,它们会自发聚集形成以疏水链段为核、亲水链段为壳的组装体,这个过程被称为溶液自组装(图 6-2)。根据嵌段共聚物亲水、疏水链段的嵌段比差异,自组装所得聚集体可以是球形胶束、囊泡或其他形状的胶束。疏水药物在自组装过程中被包覆到球形胶束的核中或囊泡的壁中;而亲水药物被包覆到囊泡的空腔中或连接到载体表面。溶液自组装法简单有效,所得胶束表面为亲水聚合物链段,有利于纳米药物载体的稳定性、靶向性和体内循环。因此,溶液自组装法成为目前临床研究中使用的主要方法。然而,该方法的药物包封率往往较低。此外,由于多数共聚物临界胶束浓度极低,因此制备过程中需消耗大量溶剂。近年发展起来的聚合诱导自组装法可实现高浓度制备不同形状的组装体,因此备受关注(见扩展阅读 1)。

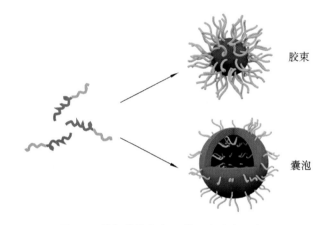

胶束

囊泡

图 6-2　嵌段共聚物自组装形成胶束和囊泡

Figure 6-2　Solution self-assembly of block copolymer into micelle and vesicle

三、纳米沉淀法

纳米沉淀法主要有两种,用于制备纳米球的自组织纳米沉淀法和用于制备纳米凝胶的交联沉淀法。

(一) 自组织纳米沉淀法

自组织纳米沉淀法是利用高分子和药物分子在良溶剂与不良溶剂中的溶解度差异而使高分子沉淀形成纳米颗粒并将药物包覆在其中的一种技术(图 6-3)。首先,将高分子和药物溶解于能与水互溶的有机溶剂中,再向其中缓慢加入水(此时确保无沉淀),然后使有机溶剂缓慢挥发而使高分子和药物共同沉淀形成纳米载药系统。该方法主要针对疏水性高分子,如 PLA、PLGA、PCL 等,所得颗粒大多为球形。自组织纳米沉淀法制备条件温和(常温、常压),无需其他助剂,产物易纯化,所得纳米颗粒的尺寸与聚合物及药物浓度密切相关。随着浓度的增加,纳米颗粒尺寸增大,而尺寸均匀性往往会降低。该方法的药物包封率也较低,若使药物分子先与高分子通过一定的相互作用连接,随后进行纳米沉淀反应可大大提高包封率。

(二) 交联沉淀法

交联沉淀法是指在溶液中对高分子进行交联,从而制备纳米凝胶的方法,主要针对多官能

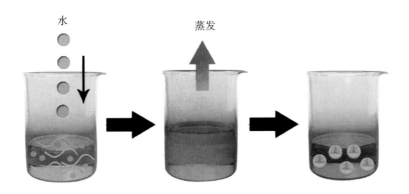

图 6-3 自组织纳米沉淀法制备高分子纳米药物载体的示意图

Figure 6-3 Scheme of self-organizing nano-precipitation method for
the preparation of polymer nano-drug carriers

团高分子,如多糖类、聚氨基酸类等。其中,通过该方法制备壳聚糖纳米药物载体的研究较多。根据交联的机理不同,交联沉淀法可细分为物理交联法和化学交联法。

离子交联法是一种较常用的物理交联法,当壳聚糖溶解在酸性溶液中时,其氨基($-NH_2$)被质子化形成带正电荷的阳离子($-NH_3^+$)。此时,加入带负电荷的阴离子交联剂即可通过静电作用使壳聚糖分子交联并聚集形成纳米凝胶。常用的阴离子交联剂有三聚磷酸钠、偏磷酸钠、十二烷基硫酸钠。其中,三聚磷酸钠因具有交联速度快、反应条件温和、所得纳米凝胶大小均匀、表面电荷可调控、安全无毒性等特点而被广泛应用。

化学交联法(如共价交联法)是较早用于制备壳聚糖纳米凝胶的方法之一,其原理是利用壳聚糖上的羟基、氨基等官能团以共价键的形式与交联剂结合,进而聚集形成纳米凝胶。Sadighian 等以戊二醛为交联剂,制备了具有 pH 响应性的磁性壳聚糖纳米凝胶,同时探讨了物理和化学两种交联方式对磁性壳聚糖纳米凝胶用作阿霉素靶向药物载体时性能的影响。此外,化学交联的纳米粒子稳定性好、控释性强,但残留的交联剂毒副作用较大,后处理工作量大。

四、乳液法

乳液法是指以乳液液滴为模板制备纳米药物载体的方法,主要包括乳液-溶剂挥发法、自乳化/溶剂扩散法和乳液交联法等。其中,前两种主要用于制备纳米球/胶囊,后一种则用于制备纳米凝胶。

(一)乳液-溶剂挥发法

乳液-溶剂挥发法是指将疏水性高分子和药物一起溶于与水不互溶的低沸点有机溶剂中作为油相,随后将其加入含有表面活性剂的水相体系中进行乳化,形成水包油(O/W)型乳液,然后使有机溶剂完全蒸发,从而获得纳米药物载体的水分散体系的方法(图 6-4)。油相中有机溶剂需具有比水更强的挥发性,常用的有二氯甲烷、氯仿、甲苯或乙酸乙酯等,其中乙酸乙酯毒性极低。药物分子在载体中的分布取决于二者疏水性及相互作用的强弱。若相互作用极弱,则疏水性弱的药物倾向于分布在载体的近表面处;反之,疏水性强的药物分布于载体的内部。如需制备亲水性纳米药物载体,则需采用反相(W/O)乳液,即高分子和药物均溶解在水中,而表面活性剂溶解在有机溶剂中,再使水挥发。反相乳液则要求有机溶剂难以挥发。

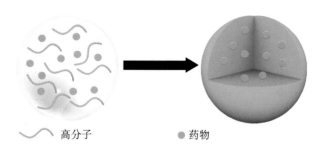

高分子　　　　　　　　●药物

图 6-4　基于膜乳化的乳液-溶剂挥发法制备高分子纳米药物载体

Figure 6-4　Emulsion-solvent evaporation method for the preparation of polymer nano-drug carriers based on membrane emulsify

乳液-溶剂挥发法的优点在于包封率高、载药量可控性强,且可同时包覆多种药物或检测试剂。疏水性可生物降解高分子如 PLA、PLGA 等可通过该方法制备纳米药物载体。所得纳米药物载体的尺寸易于调控,取决于乳液液滴的尺寸及高分子的浓度。尺寸均匀性依赖于乳化方法,一般不如球形胶束均匀,但优于自组织纳米沉淀法。所得产物中的大部分表面活性剂可通过离心或透析等方式去除,但难免有少量残余。为降低表面活性剂的毒副作用,可选用非离子型表面活性剂,如聚乙烯醇(PVA)等。

在乳液-溶剂挥发法的基础上,研究者们又发展了复乳液-溶剂挥发法,该法可用于制备纳米胶囊。复乳液是由普通乳液(即单乳液)进行二次乳化而形成的复杂乳液,又称多层乳液,若油包水(W/O)型单乳液被二次乳化在水相中,则可形成 W/O/W 型复乳液;反之,若 O/W 型单乳液被二次乳化在油相中,则可形成 O/W/O 型复乳液。复乳液中各相依次被称为内相、中间相和外相。目前研究得较多的是 W/O/W 型复乳液,将水溶性药物溶解在内相,油溶性高分子溶解在中间相,待溶剂挥发后可获得纳米胶囊,同时还可在中间相中加入油溶性药物。复乳液的尺寸一般大于单乳液,均匀性不如单乳液,所得纳米胶囊的尺寸通常达数百纳米。除了二次乳化,相分离也可用来制备复乳液。例如,O'/O/W 型复乳液是通过在 O/W 型乳液液滴中再加入一种与高分子不互溶的难挥发性油(O')(如食用油),随着低沸点有机溶剂的挥发,难挥发性油(O')缓慢从油相析出并与高分子发生相分离,难挥发性油由于疏水性更强而形成内相,最终得到油溶性药物纳米胶囊。W/O/W 型复乳液则是通过在 O/W 型乳液液滴中添加吸水性物质,使水分子扩散进入液滴并形成内相,最终可得水溶性药物纳米胶囊。由于相分离法所得复乳液由单乳液演变而来,因此在尺寸和均匀性方面均大有改善(见扩展阅读 2)。

(二) 自乳化/溶剂扩散法

自乳化/溶剂扩散法是将聚合物和药物溶解于易溶于水的有机溶剂(如丙酮、甲醇等)和难溶于水的有机溶剂(如二氯甲烷、氯仿等)形成的混合溶剂中作为油相,分散于大量水中后由于易溶于水的有机溶剂自发地从油相扩散进入水相,在两相界面产生湍流,从而产生液滴并最终形成纳米粒子的方法。例如,有研究人员采用该方法制备了负载难溶性药物冬凌草甲素(ORI)的 PLA 纳米球药物载体,其平均尺寸为 137.3 nm,包封率为 91.88%±1.83%,载药量为 2.32%±0.05%。该方法的优点是不需要表面活性剂,但该法制备的纳米药物载体的均匀性不如乳液-溶剂挥发法。

(三) 乳液交联法

乳液交联法是指在形成稳定纳米乳液后对高分子进行交联反应,使高分子在液滴中形成三维网状结构,从而将纳米乳液液滴转变成纳米凝胶的方法。根据高分子的溶解性,可分别通过乳液交联法制备油性纳米凝胶或反相乳液交联法制备水性纳米凝胶。交联剂可预先加入液滴中,待纳米乳液形成后,通过外部刺激(如温度、pH、光等)引发交联反应。对于非刺激响应型交联剂,则需在乳液形成后加入连续相,并通过扩散进入液滴中交联聚合物。与交联沉淀法一样,交联方式也有物理交联和化学交联之分。

五、喷雾干燥法

喷雾干燥法是指先将高分子与药物分子溶解到溶剂中,之后利用喷雾干燥设备使溶液雾化成微型液滴并经干燥形成纳米粒子的方法(图6-5)。该方法既适用于水溶性药物及高分子,也适用于油溶性药物及高分子,且无须使用表面活性剂。但制备纳米级的药物载体对设备要求高,价格昂贵。与乳液-溶剂挥发法一样,喷雾干燥法所得纳米粒子的尺寸也取决于液滴尺寸和高分子的浓度;而与自组织纳米沉淀法相比,这种基于液滴挥发的方法所得纳米药物载体的包封率更高。但是,这种方法一般要求雾滴中的溶剂在高温条件下瞬间蒸发,因此并不适用于不耐受高温的高分子及药物。

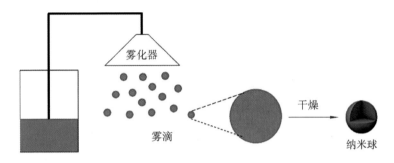

图 6-5　喷雾干燥法制备高分子纳米药物载体的示意图

Figure 6-5　Scheme of spray drying method for the preparation of polymer nano-drug carriers

六、层层自组装制备技术

高分子层层自组装技术是指将两种或多种高分子交替沉积到基底上,在纳米水平对纳米药物载体进行结构和功能控制的技术,是极有发展前景的新型纳米技术。以纳米粒子为基底核,利用层层自组装技术可制备纳米药物载体(图6-6)。该方法制备条件温和,较易制备多功能载体,并精确控制药物载体的结构,在缓释、控释尤其是程序化释放方面具有独特的优势,在癌症治疗方面具有巨大的前景。层层自组装沉积时的吸附力主要有静电作用、氢键、共价键、疏水作用等。通过静电作用进行聚电解质的层层自组装得到了最为广泛的研究,天然生物大分子(如多肽、蛋白质、核酸以及大多数多糖分子)在溶液中带有大量的电荷,因此很容易通过静电作用吸附。带电荷的水溶性药物分子可通过吸附的方式包覆到载体中,载药量高。疏水性药物分子则可预先包覆到基底核中,如表面带电荷的高分子纳米球/胶囊、胶束、介孔二氧化硅等。该技术所得的纳米药物载体可在不同的微区中负载不同的药物。例如,Ramasamy 等以脂质体胶束为基底核,通过聚乙二醇和聚赖氨酸层层自组装制备了纳米药物载体,其核中负载阿霉素,多层膜负载米托蒽醌。

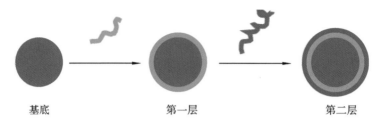

图 6-6　层层自组装制备高分子纳米药物载体的示意图

Figure 6-6　Scheme of layer-by-layer self-assembly technology for the preparation of polymer nano-drug carriers

第四节　高分子纳米药物载体的性能指标

高分子纳米药物载体的物理、化学、生物学性质对其药物递送及疾病诊断、治疗等功能的发挥有重要的影响。因此,如何有效、充分地评估高分子纳米药物载体的性能对载体的设计、筛选、优化具有关键的指导作用。高分子纳米药物载体的性能指标包括体外性能指标和体内性能指标。体外性能指标一般包括粒径及其分布、ζ 电位、形态结构、载药量、包封率、释放速率及响应性等;体内性能指标包括高分子纳米药物载体的体内分布、靶向性及生物安全性等。相对于体内性能指标,体外性能指标的测量更加便捷、迅速,且造成测量误差的因素较少。科研人员通过大量的研究已经初步总结了一些高分子纳米药物载体的体外性能指标与其体内性能指标的关系。这些经验和规律可以帮助我们利用体外的测量手段快速地筛选出符合体内应用需求的高分子纳米药物载体材料。本节将对测量高分子纳米药物载体体外和体内主要性能指标所使用的仪器和技术进行介绍。

一、粒径及其分布

高分子纳米药物载体的粒径及其分布对纳米药物的药代动力学、体内分布、透皮效率、滞留时间等有重要的影响。纳米材料的粒径及其分布的主要测量手段包括动态光散射(DLS)与扫描或透射电子显微镜。

动态光散射是通过测量因粒子布朗运动导致的散射光强度的波动,并通过斯托克斯-爱因斯坦方程计算出粒子平均粒径的技术。这项技术的优势包括可以得到溶液中纳米颗粒整体的粒径和分布情况、测量速率快、重复性强等,并且该技术测量的是纳米材料的水合粒径,可对高分子纳米药物载体包含其表面的亲水高分子层或吸附蛋白后的粒径进行测量,这些信息不容易从扫描或透射电子显微镜照片中获取。但 DLS 在应用过程中也存在一些问题,例如,由于散射光强正比于颗粒粒径的六次方,纳米颗粒溶液中存在的灰尘等大尺寸杂质会对溶液颗粒整体粒径测量造成重要影响,如果纳米材料的吸收光和入射激光重合将无法测量出粒径,对于非球形的纳米颗粒只能给出与其等同的球形纳米颗粒的粒径信息。此外,纳米颗粒在溶液中的稳定性、分散状态及测试的温度等因素也会影响最终的结果,因而需在特定的条件下进行测量。

除 DLS 外,我们也可以利用扫描或透射电子显微镜拍摄高分子纳米颗粒的照片,并在照片中测量纳米颗粒的粒径。这种测量方式一般需要在不同区域拍摄含有大量纳米颗粒的照片,并测量几百个纳米颗粒的粒径从而计算出纳米材料的平均粒径及其分布数据。这种测量技术的优势在于可以测出高分子纳米药物载体实心部分(比如胶束的内核部分)、非球形结构及颗粒细微结构部分(比如囊泡的空心部分)的尺寸并避免灰尘等大尺寸杂质造成的干扰。但该方法的问题在于测量用时较长且无法给出溶液中纳米颗粒整体的粒径信息;制备样品过程中纳米颗粒可能会由于浓度升高、干燥等因素发生形貌和尺寸的改变。此外,由于高分子纳米颗粒表面亲水部分在透射电子显微镜下衬度低,一般很难观测到,因而通过电子显微镜图片给出的粒径一般小于 DLS 给出的水合粒径。因此,将 DLS 技术和电子显微镜测量技术的测量结果相结合,可以得到更全面的高分子纳米药物载体的粒径和分布信息。

二、Zeta(ζ)电位

高分子纳米药物载体的电荷性质与材料的稳定性及细胞吞噬、体内分布、蛋白吸附等纳米颗粒与生物界面相互作用的机制相关,因此测量高分子纳米药物载体的电荷性质具有重要的意义。高分子纳米药物载体的 ζ 电位可以通过 ζ 电位仪进行测量。纳米颗粒的 ζ 电位是依据 Stern 双电层理论建立的模型中滑动面基于溶液中远离界面处的电位大小(图 6-7)。Stern 双电层理论指溶液中带电荷的纳米颗粒表面分为 Stern 层和扩散层:Stern 层是指紧密吸附在纳米颗粒表面的具有相反电荷的离子层;扩散层分为两层,一层为内侧靠近 Stern 层的可以稳定地与 Stern 层一起运动的含有离子的流体层,另一层为外侧的分散介质层。二者发生相对移动时的界面为滑动面,该处对远离界面的流体中某点的电位称为 ζ 电位。目前,最常用的 ζ 电位仪是基于电泳光散射技术的电位仪。其测量机制是溶液中不同电荷性质的纳米颗粒在电场作用下移动速率不同,导致其颗粒散射光频率产生多普勒频移,通过多散射光频率的分析可以计算溶液中纳米颗粒的 ζ 电位和电泳迁移率。纳米颗粒的 ζ 电位会随溶液 pH、离子强度等环境因素发生改变,因此测量时需明确所需的测量条件。

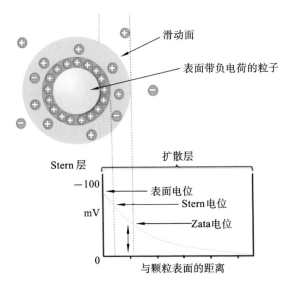

图 6-7 溶液相纳米颗粒表面双电层的示意图及相应层面的电位

Figure 6-7 Schematic showing the electric double layer of the NPs in aqueous solution

三、形态结构

高分子纳米药物载体形态结构的常用测量手段包括透射电子显微镜(TEM)、扫描电子显微镜(SEM)及原子力显微镜(AFM)等。

TEM具有非常高的分辨率,可对亚纳米到微米级别尺寸的物体进行成像,并可通过冷冻模式、扫描透射模式等不同的成像模式提供许多纳米结构和元素的信息,因此是最常用的测量高分子纳米药物载体形态结构的工具。TEM是通过照射在纳米颗粒上的聚集电子束透过样品后在物镜上聚焦而成像的。由于纳米颗粒中元素种类、样品密度、厚度等不同,照射在样品上的电子束会发生不同程度、不同角度的立体角散射,因而纳米颗粒的结构和材料的区别可以通过图片上形貌和衬度的不同体现出来。

为了增强高分子纳米颗粒在TEM下的衬度,常采用染色的制样方法。染色法总体可划分为正染和负染两种。正染是利用TEM下高衬度的材料对所需观察的纳米颗粒进行标记,从而使纳米颗粒在TEM图像中颜色变得更深的方法。例如,利用醋酸双氧铀和氨基的作用可以对蛋白质等含有氨基的高分子纳米颗粒进行标记。与正染相反,负染是通过提升样品外背景区域的衬度来提升材料样品在成像中对比度的方法。经过负染的样品在TEM下背景呈深色,而样品处由于染色剂较少呈现亮色。染色法可以提升某些高分子纳米颗粒甚至颗粒微观结构的衬度,从而更加清晰地利用TEM对其形态结构进行测量。

冷冻透射电子显微镜(Cryo-TEM)技术是观察溶液相中高分子纳米颗粒最直观的方法,因为其通过电子束对冷冻在液体中的纳米颗粒进行成像(图6-8(a))。2017年诺贝尔化学奖颁发给了发展测量生物大分子高分辨结构的Cryo-TEM技术的三位科学家,这也再次体现了Cryo-TEM在结构测量中的重要作用(见扩展阅读3)。

除了以上几种测量技术外,TEM还有许多不同模式可用于测量纳米颗粒的形态结构。例如利用高分辨TEM(HRTEM)可对纳米材料原子间的晶格进行成像,在含有无机纳米材料的无机/高分子复合纳米粒子的测量中发挥重要作用。同时,将电子断层扫描成像技术与图像分析的数学模型相结合可以重建纳米颗粒的三维立体结构图像,使我们对具有三维结构的纳米颗粒的形态有更加直观和准确的认识。此外,利用TEM的能量色散X射线谱(EDXS)及电子能量损失光谱(EELS)等技术可对纳米颗粒中的元素分布情况进行测量。

总之,TEM具有的高分辨、多功能测量能力已使其成为高分子纳米药物载体形态结构测量中不可或缺的技术手段。

SEM技术是一种利用电子束扫描纳米颗粒表面并对其表面形态结构进行成像的技术。通常来说,SEM的分辨率不如TEM,且某些导电性不好的材料需要在样品表面喷涂一层很薄的导电层来增加样品的导电性才能得到清晰的SEM图片。SEM相较TEM的优势在于可一次性装载更多的样品,考虑到在SEM和TEM测量过程中更换样品都需要真空环境,在一定时间内SEM可测量的样品数量更多。此外,SEM可以提供样品表面形态结构的更多信息。因此,在高分子纳米药物载体的测量过程中,SEM更适合对尺寸较大的导电聚合物材料或者无机/高分子复合纳米材料外部形态结构进行测量。

AFM是一种可对纳米颗粒表面结构进行高分辨三维成像的测量手段。其主要通过微悬臂(cantilever)和与悬臂相连的精细探针(fine probe)与颗粒表面作用收集相应的成像信息。除了可以测量纳米颗粒的形态,AFM还可以在测量过程中提供颗粒高度、软硬程度等信息。

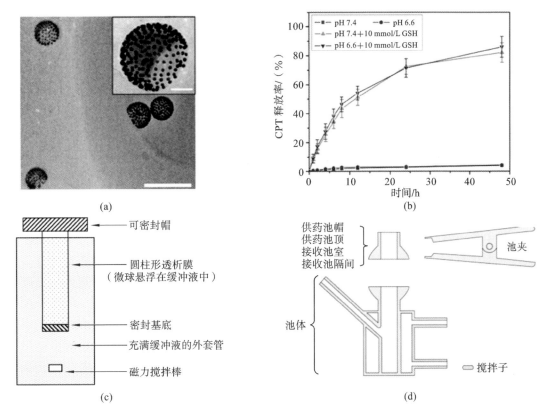

图 6-8　纳米颗粒的透射电镜图及药物释放的测量

（a）Cryo-TEM 测量纳米颗粒；（b）药物释放曲线示例；（c）透析法测量药物释放速率；（d）Franz 扩散池示意图

Figure 6-8　The TEM image and drug release measurement of nanoparticles

（a）Cryo-TEM image of nanoparticles；（b）Examples of drug release profile；（c）Drug release rate measured by dialysis；（d）Schematic showing the Franz diffusion cell

这些信息对分析环形、片形、碟形等二维高分子纳米材料的性能具有重要意义。此外，用于 AFM 的样品不需要表面修饰或者喷涂其他材料，且可以对 TEM 图片中衬度较低的纳米颗粒的形态进行准确的测量。基于这些优势，AFM 技术也是高分子纳米颗粒形态测量中常用的技术手段。

四、载药量与包封率

高分子纳米药物载体的载药量和包封率是决定载体性能的重要参数。载药量指药物占高分子纳米载药体系的质量分数，可通过式（6-1）计算：

$$C = \frac{M_{\mathrm{drug}}}{M_{\mathrm{drug}} + M_{\mathrm{carrier}}} \times 100\% \tag{6-1}$$

其中，C 代表载药量，M_{drug} 和 M_{carrier} 分别代表药物和高分子纳米药物载体的质量。

包封率是指负载在高分子纳米药物载体内的药物的质量占制备药物制剂时加入药物的总质量的比例，可通过式（6-2）计算：

$$\mathrm{EE} = \frac{M_{\mathrm{drug}}}{M_{\mathrm{total\ drug}}} \times 100\% \tag{6-2}$$

其中,EE 代表包封率,M_{drug} 和 $M_{total\ drug}$ 分别代表高分子纳米药物载体内负载的药物的质量和加入药物的总质量。

由上述公式可知,为了测量载药量和包封率,需要知道高分子纳米药物载体的质量、载体负载的药物质量及所用药物的总质量。若高分子纳米药物载体的合成效率是 100%,则高分子纳米药物载体的质量可用投入高分子材料的总质量进行计算。若合成效率低于 100%,则需要通过其他方法确定高分子材料的质量,例如冷冻干燥后利用天平、热重分析技术等称量,利用高分子材料质量与吸光强度的关系来确定样品中实际高分子质量等。为了测定溶液或药物制剂中药物的质量,通常需要建立药物浓度与吸光度、荧光强度等光学性质的标准曲线。常用的仪器包括紫外分光光度计、荧光分光光度计或高效液相色谱仪等。

高分子纳米药物载体中药物质量可用差量法、完全释放法及直接测量法测量。利用差量法测量时,高分子纳米药物载体中的药物质量等于所用药物总质量减去未负载到高分子纳米药物载体中的药物质量。某些药物在被负载到高分子纳米药物载体后荧光或吸收光谱的峰值和强度会发生改变,利用这些性质可以测量被负载到高分子纳米药物载体中的药物质量。但更多情况下,可利用高速离心或超滤离心等方法将负载药物的高分子纳米药物载体和游离的药物分离,并通过测定上清液或滤出液中药物的质量得到未被负载的药物质量。但遗留在上清液中的高分子纳米药物载体、滤膜对药物的吸附及药物自身在负载过程中的团聚、沉淀等因素会造成一定误差。对于一些制备过程中有损失的高分子纳米药物载体,可通过调节 pH、有机溶剂溶解等方法完全破坏载体,从而促使药物释放并对释放药物进行定量。若药物自身有特征吸收峰,也可直接通过吸收峰来测定高分子纳米药物载体中的药物含量。

五、药物体外释放

高分子纳米药物载体的药物释放效率与速率对药物代谢、穿越生理屏障、疾病部位滞留时间、靶向性能等有重要的影响。提升药物疗效的一个关键技术是实现药物的可控释放。高分子纳米药物载体的体外药物释放性能可在一定程度上反映其体内的释放效果,因而是设计和优化高分子纳米载药体系的重要参数。药物的释放效率和速率可从药物释放曲线中得出。药物释放曲线指释放的药物占药物总量的比例随时间变化的曲线。典型的药物释放曲线包括快速释放阶段、缓释阶段和平台阶段(图 6-8(b))。一些特别的响应性纳米药物载体,比如光响应性纳米药物载体会在施加响应性刺激时加快药物释放速率。为了测量药物释放曲线,需在测定前尽可能地除去溶液中未被负载到高分子纳米药物载体中的药物分子,并在释放过程中将所释放的药物同高分子纳米药物载体材料及其中未释放的药物分离。为了模拟体内环境,药物体外释放实验通常在 37 ℃的磷酸盐缓冲液(PBS)中进行,并定期更换溶解所释放药物的 PBS 以模拟体内药物从病灶处流失的情况。为了模拟肿瘤或皮肤微环境,或验证高分子纳米药物载体的响应能力,也可用具有酸性、氧化性(如过氧化氢)、还原性(如谷胱甘肽)等特定性质的溶液作为药物释放溶液。高分子纳米药物载体体外药物释放的测量方法包括透析法、Franz 扩散池法及高速或超滤离心法等。透析法和 Franz 扩散池法都是利用由药物在半透膜两侧存在浓度差导致的扩散作用将所释放的药物和高分子纳米药物载体材料及其负载的药物分离。在透析法中,高分子纳米载药体系被装载到透析袋中,并对大量溶液进行透析(图 6-8(c))。通过测量不同时间点透析袋外部溶液中增加的药物量或透析袋内减少的药物量,得出高分子纳米药物载体的药物释放曲线。Franz 扩散池可用于测量透皮给药的体外释放,一般由供药池、接收池和中间的半透膜组成(图 6-8(d))。半透膜可以用动物皮肤来替代。释放的药物可以从接收池中取样测定。除了以上两种方法外,超滤离心法和高速离心法也是常用的药物体外释放研究方法。在此方法中,高分子纳米药物载体和释放溶液混合,通过振荡或搅拌等方法来模拟体内释放环境并在特定时间点通过离心将高分子纳米药物载体和释放的药物分离。超滤离心管由内部的浓缩管和套在外部的收集管构成,其中浓缩管底部有超滤膜。在特定时间点,量取含有高分子纳米药物载体和释放药物的混合溶液放入上层浓缩液中,离心后高分子纳米药物载体和未释放的药物保持在上层浓缩液中,而释放的小分子药物透过超滤膜进入下层收集管中,从而与载体分离。通过测量收集管中的药物质量可确定药物释放量。而高速离心则把高分子纳米药物载体和释放药物的混合溶液直接通过离心分离,高分子纳米药物载体在离心后沉淀在离心管底部,通过测量上清液中药物的含量表征高分子纳米药物载体的体外药物释放曲线。高分子纳米药物载体的药物体外释放测量也存在一些误差,例如药品在透析袋、离心管壁上吸附等。此外,体外实验很难完全模拟体内的药物释放环境,因而体内实际的药物释放量仍需进一步的研究来确认。

六、刺激响应性

肿瘤微环境和皮肤微环境都呈弱酸性。肿瘤微环境的 pH 在 6.5 左右,皮肤的 pH 在 4 和 7.4 之间。因而 pH 响应的高分子纳米药物载体可用于促进药物在靶区域的释放或透皮给药的效率。为了模拟高分子纳米药物载体在肿瘤或皮肤微环境中的行为,需要制备适用于生物样品的不同 pH 的缓冲液。除 pH 以外,缓冲液还需具有一定的离子强度、不影响材料的其他性质、良好的溶解性等性质。常用的酸性缓冲液包括磷酸盐缓冲液、柠檬酸盐缓冲液、醋酸盐缓冲液等。通过与形态结构、尺寸、药物释放等体外测量技术相结合,可得到高分子纳米载药体系在弱酸性条件下的响应性能。

七、体内分布

高分子纳米载药体系会随着血液循环进入肿瘤和各正常器官中,其体内分布对治疗效果和毒副作用都有重要影响。高分子纳米载药体系的体内分布需关注如下重要因素:高分子纳米载药体系在肝、脾等正常器官中的分布情况,在肿瘤或血液中达到的峰浓度、达到峰浓度的时间以及高分子纳米载药体系的循环时间等。其测量方法主要分为动物标本分析和活体成像分析两大类。若使用动物标本分析测量高分子纳米载药体系的血液循环参数,可在给药后的特定时间点收集动物的血液标本并进行样品处理,利用高分子纳米药物载体或其负载药物的理化性质鉴定高分子纳米载药体系在血液中的浓度。但一般小鼠血液总共仅 2 mL 左右,因此取血次数和每次取血量都有限制。若使用动物标本分析法测量高分子纳米载药体系在各器官或肿瘤中的分布,则需要在特定时间点处死小鼠,取出相关器官或肿瘤组织进行分析。因而每只小鼠只能提供被处死时间点的药物分布信息。相对于动物标本分析法,活体成像分析法是一种非侵入式的测量手段,可以实时检测小动物体内高分子纳米载药体系的成像情况,但增加成像功能模块也为高分子纳米载药体系的制备提出了更高要求。常用的成像技术包括荧光成像、光声成像、磁共振成像(MRI)、正电子发射断层扫描(PET)、单光子发射计算机断层扫描(SPECT)等,其中荧光成像、光声成像、MRI 可以从图像中的信号强度半定量地测量高分子纳米载药体系的肿瘤富集和器官分布情况。其中,荧光成像、光声成像穿透深度较浅,但成像速度快,MRI 具有很高的穿透深度但成像速度慢。相对而言,PET 和 SPECT 具有很高的成像穿透深度且可以准确地定量高分子纳米载药体系在肿瘤和器官中的分布,但这两种技术需要使用具有放射性的同位素标记高分子纳米载药体系,且测试成本较高。由于各种活体成像技术都有各自的优缺点,在实验中应根据具体需求选用合适的技术。大部分活体成像手段需要在高分子纳米药物载体中引入具有相应功能的官能团,因而若官能团在体内酶、离子等的作用下脱落会造成纳米药物载体分布数据的误差。此外,若药物在进入疾病区域前释放也可能导致数据误差。因此,在测量高分子纳米载药体系的体内分布时应考虑这些因素的影响。

八、生物安全性

由于高分子纳米药物载体会在正常组织、器官中有一定程度的分布,因此其生物安全性是评价其性能的一个重要指标。前期研究中的生物安全性评价主要包括细胞实验和动物实验两个方面。为了研究高分子纳米药物载体材料在细胞层面的安全性,可将高分子纳米药物载体与正常细胞共孵育,通过 MTT、MTS、CCK-8 等方法检测载体材料对正常细胞增殖的影响。通常细胞实验确认了高分子纳米药物载体具有良好的生物相容性后,再通过动物实验来研究载体材料对心、肝、肾等重要脏器的影响。在动物实验中需要设置材料组和对照组。分别提取材料组和对照组中小动物的重要器官制备石蜡切片,进行苏木精-伊红染色后,通过光学显微镜观察来确定高分子纳米药物载体是否会造成材料组动物脏器发生病理变化。此外,通过血常规、生化等指标可以检测心、肝、肾等器官的功能情况,以进一步确定高分子纳米药物载体的生物安全性。只有在细胞和小动物层面体现出相当好的生物安全性的高分子纳米药物载体材料才有可能进入临床试验中。

第五节　高分子纳米药物载体在黑素瘤、银屑病等治疗中的应用

一、黑素瘤治疗药物简介

手术切除对黑素瘤早期患者有很好的治疗效果,其中Ⅰ期患者的 5 年总生存率高达95%。此外,放疗、化疗及最近发展迅速的肿瘤免疫疗法都被用于黑素瘤的临床治疗。然而,当患者体内的黑素瘤发生转移后,治愈率显著下降,3 年总生存率不到 15%,因而发展新型黑素瘤治疗方法具有重要意义。化疗是传统的癌症治疗手段。化疗药物中,达卡巴嗪(dacarbazine)是被美国食品药品监督管理局(FDA)批准的治疗转移性黑素瘤的标准药物,但没有数据确认该药物可延长患者的生存期。此外,其他一些化疗药物,如阿霉素(doxorubicin,DOX)、顺铂(cisplatin)、紫杉醇(paclitaxel,PTX)及紫杉烷类药物(taxanes)等,也已进行了临床试验或动物实验。近年来,黑素瘤的肿瘤免疫治疗也取得了巨大进展。早期用于治疗黑素瘤的免疫制剂包括干扰素-α(IFN-α)和白细胞介素-2(IL-2)等,但其在提升患者总生存率和总响应率等方面的效果并不理想。随后发展的伊匹单抗(ipilimumab)与纳武单抗(nivolumab)等单抗类药物使部分具有药物响应性的患者总生存率大大增高,但也存在毒副作用大、患者响应率低等问题,具体介绍可参见黑素瘤免疫治疗相关章节。

二、高分子纳米药物载体向黑素瘤递送药物的途径

高分子纳米药物载体的给药途径主要为注射给药和经皮给药。我们将在银屑病的治疗部分详细介绍高分子纳米药物载体的经皮给药途径,本部分将重点介绍高分子纳米药物载体注射给药的相关内容。注射给药是指直接将药物注射到血管、器官或组织中的给药方式,具有高药物利用率,可分为静脉注射、腹腔注射、肌内注射与皮下注射等。黑素瘤的药物递送研究主要采用静脉注射给药方式,其注射方式包括静脉推注与滴注两种。不同的注射方式将会影响高分子纳米药物载体的药物动力学参数甚至体内分布情况。由于药物直接进入血液循环系统,药物的生物利用度较高。然而,高分子纳米药物载体会吸附血液中的蛋白质,导致其表面物理、化学性质发生改变,促使其被体内单核-巨噬细胞系统清除后富集在肝脏、脾脏等器官中,最终导致肿瘤内的载体富集程度低并造成一定程度的毒副作用。这也是在高分子纳米药物载体领域亟须解决的关键问题之一。

三、提升高分子纳米药物载体在肿瘤富集的设计规律

高分子纳米药物载体可延长某些水溶性小分子药物的血液循环时间,解决疏水抗癌药物水溶性不好的问题,并提升药物的稳定性。传统理论认为,高分子纳米药物载体在肿瘤的富集基于肿瘤部位血管壁间隙及引流淋巴管的缺陷导致的载体材料在肿瘤处的高渗透长滞留(EPR)效应(图 6-9)。但正如上文所说,高分子纳米药物载体在作用于肿瘤细胞之前需要克服一系列生理屏障。这些屏障包括血清蛋白的吸附、肝脏与脾脏等对纳米药物的清除、纳米药物穿透肿瘤血管壁及最终进入肿瘤细胞等。为了克服这些生理屏障,高分子纳米药物载体必须具有特定的物理化学性质,从而使其适应人体各部位作用的机制。但由于体内环境和生理屏障的复杂性,目前大多数高分子纳米药物载体的设计仍无法完全满足克服这些生理屏障的需求。此外,不同生理屏障对高分子纳米药物载体理化性质的要求存在矛盾。例如,为了避免高分子纳米药物载体在血液中被起保护作用的单核-巨噬细胞系统当作异物清除,一般要求高分子纳米药物载体尺寸较小,但要想取得更长的肿瘤停留时间和药物作用时间,一般要求高分子纳米药物载体尺寸较大。这些相互矛盾的需求大大增加了高分子纳米药物载体的设计难度。虽然提升纳米药物在肿瘤富集的设计仍有待优化,但基于大量的研究结果,可以总结出一些载体设计的基本规律,主要包括高分子纳米药物载体的尺寸、表面化学性质等。

高分子纳米药物载体的尺寸是影响其药代动力学和体内分布的重要因素。总体而言,尺寸大于 100 nm 的纳米材料比尺寸较小的纳米材料更容易被单核-巨噬细胞从血液中清除,不利于纳米材料的肿瘤富集。而尺寸小于 5 nm 的纳米材料会被肾脏快速排出,缩短其血液循环时间。当纳米粒子尺寸为 5~100 nm 时,尺寸更小的纳米粒子通常表现出更好的肿瘤内扩散能力。但良好的肿瘤内扩散能力并不一定能带来更好的肿瘤富集效果,因为肿瘤内部和边缘之间存在的组织间质压力(interstitial fluid pressure)可以将纳米药物载体从肿瘤组织重新推回血管;因此,小尺寸的纳米材料在肿瘤中的停留时间较短。研究结果表明,某些黑素瘤内组织间质压力可高达 50 mmHg。鉴于肿瘤复杂的微环境,肿瘤富集效果最好的高分子纳米药物载体尺寸需要通过实验来确定。例如,Kataoka 等利用聚乙二醇聚谷氨酸嵌段共聚物(PEG-b-P(Glu))制备了平均粒径为 30 nm 的载药聚合物胶束。同时,他们还利用 PEG-b-P(Glu)与 P(Glu)均聚物共混的方法制备了平均粒径为 70 nm 的载药聚合物胶束。通过比较平

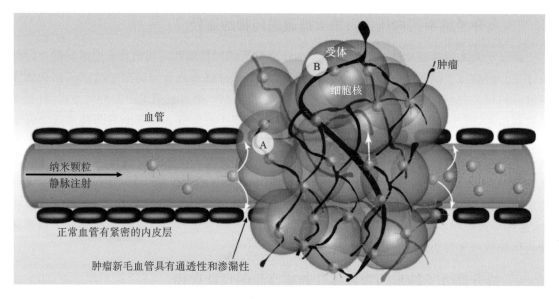

图 6-9　肿瘤 EPR 效应示意图

Figure 6-9　Schematic diagram of tumor EPR effect

均粒径为 30 nm、70 nm 的聚合物胶束以及被美国 FDA 批准用于临床的平均粒径为 80 nm 左右的载药脂质体(doxil)在黑素瘤淋巴转移模型中的富集情况,他们发现平均粒径为 30 nm 的聚合物胶束具有最深的肿瘤穿透深度、最好的肿瘤富集效果以及最好的化疗效果。这个例子说明粒径的调控对高分子纳米载药体系在黑素瘤中的治疗效果具有重要影响。但不同高分子材料的体内作用机制不能一概而论,需要针对不同的材料与肿瘤模型进行研究和探讨。

　　高分子纳米药物载体的表面化学性质也是影响其肿瘤富集效果的重要因素。相对于表面带正电荷或负电荷的纳米材料,表面电中性的纳米材料可以有效地减少血清蛋白的吸附,有利于延长其血液循环时间与提升其肿瘤富集效果。因此,高分子纳米药物载体表面常用 PEG 进行保护。研究显示,高分子纳米药物载体表面 PEG 的密度可以影响其血液循环时间和肿瘤富集情况。Wang 等利用聚乙二醇聚己酸内酯嵌段共聚物(PEG-b-PCL)与 PCL 均聚物共组装,通过调节嵌段共聚物中 PCL 的链长和 PCL 均聚物的比例,制备了一系列尺寸、表面 PEG 密度可调的聚合物胶束。随后,选择其中平均粒径在 100 nm 左右、具有不同 PEG 密度(0.19～0.86 PEG/nm^2)的聚合物胶束用于研究表面 PEG 密度对高分子纳米药物载体的体内分布和肿瘤富集情况的影响。结果表明,具有较高 PEG 密度的聚合物胶束血清蛋白吸附最少,循环时间最长。负载多西他赛(docetaxel)后,表面 PEG 密度最高的聚合物胶束对黑素瘤表现出了最好的治疗效果,小鼠存活期最长。除 PEG 外,两性离子配体和两性离子聚合物也是常用的表面修饰配体。两性离子配体指含有等量正负电荷的配体,整体显电中性。此外,聚多巴胺也常用于高分子纳米药物载体的表面修饰(见扩展阅读 4)。

　　虽然 PEG 和两性离子配体可以降低血清蛋白的吸附,但其与肿瘤细胞间的作用也会相应减弱。为了选择性地提升高分子纳米药物载体与肿瘤细胞间的作用,我们可以通过增加肿瘤靶向基团或引入刺激响应基团在肿瘤处特异性地改变载体表面理化性质等方法来实现。靶向基团通过增强高分子纳米药物载体与肿瘤细胞、组织上受体的相互作用提升材料在肿瘤的富集。常用的靶向基团包括小分子、糖、多肽、蛋白质等几种类别。黑素瘤细胞表面高表达的受体包括转铁蛋白受体(TfR)、叶酸受体(FR)、成纤维细胞生长因子受体(FGFR)、层粘连蛋白受体(LR)、生长抑素受体(SSTR)、sigma 受体、MC1R、CD44 等。Tu 等利用乙二胺修饰的透明质酸制备了负载顺铂的纳米载药体系。该纳米载药体系利用透明质酸与黑素瘤细胞表达的 CD44 之间的作用,增强了载体靶向能力,并可以在酸性或还原性环境中实现药物的释放。此外,黑素瘤新生血管内皮细胞上高表达的整合素也可以作为高分子纳米药物载体的靶向目标。常见的靶向基团包括 Arg-Gly-Asp(RGD),环形 Arg-Gly-Asp-D-Tyr-Lys(cRGDyK)等。Tu 等将维生素 E 琥珀酸酯与 PEG 的偶联物(D-α-tocopherol polyethylene glycol succinate, TPGS)与聚乳酸(PLA)通过二硫键连接,制备了可被肿瘤中还原性谷胱甘肽(GSH)断开的聚合物(TPGS-b-PLA)。他们将 TPGS-b-PLA 与可连接 RGD 的 PEG-b-PLA 共混,制备了负载抗癌药物 PTX、表面带有 RGD 的聚合物胶束。当胶束中的二硫键被肿瘤细胞中的 GSH 切断时,可释放出 PTX。实验结果表明,表面键合 RGD 的聚合物胶束比不含 RGD 的胶束及商用的 PTX 纳米制剂具有更好的肿瘤抑制效果,证实了 RGD 可提升高分子纳米药物载体对黑素瘤的靶向效果。在肿瘤处特异性地改变载体表面理化性质是指利用高分子纳米药物载体上的刺激响应基团在肿瘤微环境中发生的理化反应,使高分子纳米药物载体表面理化性质发生转变,从而使其在进入肿瘤前不被血清蛋白吸附,而在进入肿瘤后迅速与肿瘤细胞和组织作用,促进肿瘤内高分子纳米药物载体的富集。Cai 等制备了在肿瘤微酸性环境中响应脱掉表面 PEG 的高分子纳米药物载体,成功地向黑素瘤递送核酸类药物和光敏剂。脱掉 PEG 后,该高分子纳米药物载体的 ζ 电位提升到 20 mV,增强了高分子纳米药物载体与带负电荷的细胞膜的作用。目前,高分子纳米药物载体的黑素瘤靶向研究还存在一些问题,例如配体靶向性不足、靶向基团易被血清蛋白覆盖从而失去靶向能力等,因此仍需进一步的研究。

四、高分子纳米药物载体在黑素瘤化疗中的应用

高分子纳米药物载体的功能包括增加疏水药物的水溶性、降低药物的毒副作用、提升药物在肿瘤中的富集等。为了提高治疗效果,除提升高分子纳米药物载体的肿瘤富集效果以外,还应在载体到达肿瘤前维持载体的稳定性,减少或防止药物的提前释放,并使药物在肿瘤区域快速释放。维持高分子纳米药物载体血液稳定性的方法主要有高分子前药法、载体交联法、降低聚合物临界胶束浓度等。高分子链的运动性、吸附血清蛋白和血液剪切力的作用等因素可降低高分子纳米药物载体的稳定性,造成载体中药物的提前释放。此外,药物自身也可能由于扩散作用而提前与载体分离。这些都会降低药物的利用率(见扩展阅读 5)。

高分子前药法指将化疗药物通过响应性共价键键合到高分子上,制备高分子前药,再利用高分子前药来制备纳米药物载体的方法。由于药物直接键合在高分子链上,其扩散速率会降低,因而会大大减少由于扩散导致的药物提前释放。响应性基团的共价键具有在肿瘤微环境中断裂的能力。常被利用的肿瘤微环境包括微酸性、高活性氧含量、特定的酶、高谷胱甘肽浓度等。例如,Luan 等分别将 PEG 和 DOX 与 PTX 通过含有二硫键的分子键合,制备了两种两亲性高分子前药。将它们共组装可以形成负载有可精确调控 PTX 与 DOX 比例的聚合物胶束。该胶束在肿瘤微环境中的药物释放速率比正常条件下更快。

载体交联法指通过交联载体中的高分子链以增强载体的稳定性、减少药物提前释放的方法。其中,交联所需的共价键通常是可在肿瘤微环境中响应断裂的基团。Hennink 等将 DOX 通过腙键与甲基丙烯酰胺分子键合,构建了可在酸性条件下断裂的前药。通过 DOX 小分子

前药与含有甲基丙烯酸侧链的高分子共聚合得到了交联的载药高分子体系。该体系在正常血液(pH=7.4)中只释放 5% 的药物,而在酸性环境中可在相同时间内释放 100% 的药物。动物实验结果显示,该药物递送体系具有良好的黑素瘤抑制效果。

高分子纳米药物载体进入血液后会逐渐被清除,其血液浓度会在一定时间内持续降低。当浓度低至聚合物的临界胶束浓度以下时,高分子纳米药物载体的稳定性下降,容易导致载体结构的破坏和药物的提前释放。因此,降低聚合物的临界胶束浓度可提升高分子纳米药物载体的稳定性。Cao 等将超亲水的两电性聚合物和超疏水的磷脂分子结合,制备了两亲性聚合物分子,并利用其制备了亲疏水部分具有强对比极性的纳米胶束,用于递送化疗药物(图 6-10(a))。结果表明,该胶束的临界胶束浓度可低至 2.7×10^{-6} mmol/L,这一数值是常用的小分子表面活性剂十二烷基磺酸钠的 $1/10^6$,是大分子表面活性剂聚山梨酸酯 80 的 $1/10^4$。动物实验结果表明,利用这种具有强对比极性的聚合物胶束递送多西他赛对黑素瘤的治疗效果显著优于由聚山梨酸酯 80 制备的药物载体和商用多西他赛纳米制剂。

高分子纳米药物载体在肿瘤部位的药物释放速率也是取得良好治疗效果的关键因素。药物释放速率低将降低有效药物的浓度;药物释放速率太快,则可能导致药物从肿瘤部位流失而无法发挥作用。因此,选择最适合的药物释放速率对黑素瘤的治疗有重要意义。药物的释放机制包括药物从载体中扩散释放、载体在酸性环境或酶等的作用下发生结构破坏导致药物释放、药物与载体之间的共价作用力或非共价作用力被破坏导致药物释放等。如何实现可控的药物释放是高分子纳米载药体系治疗肿瘤的关键问题之一。

五、高分子纳米药物载体在黑素瘤光热、光动力疗法中的应用

光疗法是高效、精准的癌症治疗方法。光疗法主要包括光热疗法和光动力疗法。光热疗法是利用高分子纳米药物载体或药物的光热效应,将吸收的光能转化为热能,从而提升肿瘤组织局部温度来消灭肿瘤的方法。为了同时满足激光的高穿透性及对正常组织低伤害的要求,通常选用组织吸收较少的近红外 I 区(750~1000 nm)或 II 区(1000~1350 nm)激光作为光源。为了实现肿瘤光热治疗,在构建高分子纳米药物载体时需键合或负载具有光热转换效应的小分子、无机纳米材料或使用半导体聚合物作为载体材料。例如,Wang 等利用双乳液法制备了 PEG-b-PLGA 纳米泡(图 6-10(b)),并在纳米球的内核和膜中分别包覆了全氟戊烷和 IR780。其中,IR780 是疏水的小分子光热转换试剂,全氟戊烷是一种低沸点(29 ℃)的液体。在进行光热治疗时,全氟戊烷受热迅速汽化,从而使纳米泡转变为微米泡。尺寸变大的纳米泡不仅可以增强黑素瘤超声成像的信号强度,而且可以提升血管的通透性,使更多的纳米泡进入肿瘤,从而增强肿瘤光热治疗效果。除了提升高分子纳米药物载体的肿瘤富集效果外,提升纳米材料的光热转换效率、设计并利用穿透深度更深的激光光热体系、控制光热治疗对正常组织的伤害等都是高分子纳米药物载体肿瘤光热治疗需要探索的方向。光热治疗最大的问题是激光的穿透深度有限(一般为几毫米),仅可对皮肤浅表的黑素瘤进行治疗,难以实现对深层组织肿瘤的治疗。发展光热疗法和化疗、免疫治疗、手术、放疗等联合治疗的手段是解决光热治疗瓶颈问题的潜在方法之一。

肿瘤光动力疗法指利用在肿瘤处富集的高分子纳米药物载体在激光照射下产生活性氧并杀死肿瘤细胞的癌症治疗方法。活性氧的产生可以促使细胞产生氧化应激环境,并对 DNA、蛋白质等生物大分子造成损伤,最终导致肿瘤细胞死亡。为了实现肿瘤光动力学治疗,需要在

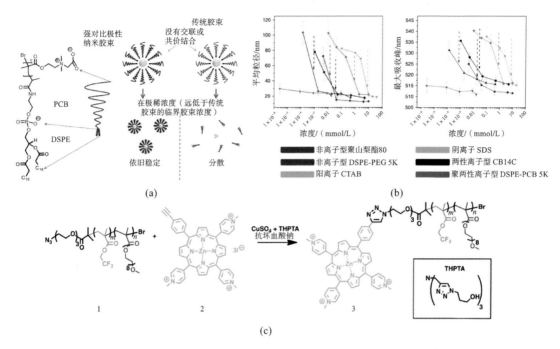

图 6-10 高分子纳米药物载体在化疗(a)、光热治疗(b)及光动力疗法(c)中的应用

Figure 6-10 **The application of polymer nano-drug carriers in chemotherapy (a),**
photothermal therapy (b) and photodynamic therapy (c)

高分子纳米药物载体上键合或负载光敏剂。光敏剂在激光照射下被激发后可通过能量转移(Ⅱ型)途径产生单线态氧或通过电子转移(Ⅰ型)途径产生自由基,其中经过Ⅱ型途径需要消耗氧气。一方面,鉴于肿瘤内的缺氧微环境,如何提供更多的氧气来源是Ⅱ型光动力疗法需要解决的关键问题之一。Pokorski 等利用末端带阳离子锌乙基苯基卟啉的聚甲基丙烯酸三氟乙酯聚乙二醇甲醚甲基丙烯酸酯的共聚物(poly(TFEMA-*co*-OEGMEMA))制备了聚合物胶束。其中,阳离子锌乙基苯基卟啉是光敏剂;含氟聚合物具有吸氧功能,可以在缺氧环境下提升Ⅱ型光动力疗法产生单线态氧的能力。另一方面,发展含有Ⅰ型光敏剂的高分子纳米药物载体也是解决光动力疗法的氧气依赖问题的方案之一。类似于光热疗法,光动力疗法的治疗效果受制于激光有限的穿透深度。除了发展联合疗法外,开发由其他穿透性更深的光源诱导的光动力疗法也是研究的重要方向。这些光源包括 X 射线、切连科夫辐射等。这些由新型光源诱导的光动力疗法将为深层转移黑素瘤的治疗提供新方案。

六、高分子纳米药物载体在黑素瘤放疗中的应用

放疗是临床上非常有效的癌症治疗手段。虽然有报道显示某些黑素瘤可以耐受辐射,但也有报道显示放疗对黑素瘤产生了良好的治疗效果。放疗利用放射线破坏细胞中的 DNA,使其无法增殖。如何减少放疗的副作用、增强治疗效果是放疗中需解决的关键问题。放疗分为通过外部照射放射线对肿瘤进行治疗和向体内注射带有放射性元素的药物制剂两种形式。对于利用外部放射线照射肿瘤的治疗方案,具有高原子序数的元素(如金、铋、铪等)可通过增强放射线在肿瘤区域的散射提高其对细胞的破坏效果。而对于向体内注射带有放射性元素的药物制剂的治疗方案,如何提升药物在肿瘤中的富集效果是提升治疗效果的关键。Deng 等将聚

乙二醇聚甲状腺素嵌段共聚物(PEG-*b*-poly(L-thyroxine),PEG-*b*-PThy)和碘-131(^{131}I)通过甲状腺素连接,制备了含有^{131}I的两亲性聚合物分子,并组装成高分子纳米材料。这种具有放射性的高分子纳米药物载体对黑素瘤具有良好的肿瘤抑制效果。

综上,高分子纳米药物载体可增强化疗、光热/光动力治疗、放疗等对黑素瘤的治疗效果。EPR效应是大多数抗肿瘤纳米药物载体的设计基础。但近期的一些结果表明,不同肿瘤的EPR效应会有差异,且患者的个体差异和肿瘤的不同阶段都可能对肿瘤的EPR效应产生影响。目前,通过纳米药物进行肿瘤治疗的瓶颈在于有限的肿瘤富集和治疗效果。此外,最新研究结果表明,某些纳米材料可能主要通过肿瘤血管壁中内皮细胞的转胞吞作用进入肿瘤组织,而不是通过传统EPR理论中血管壁上间隙进入肿瘤组织。这些新的结果还有待进一步研究确认,但EPR理论的发展也说明目前高分子纳米药物载体的设计策略有待进一步提高和完善。此外,高分子纳米药物载体的毒副作用仍需进一步研究。发展具有良好生物相容性和生物降解性的高分子纳米药物载体也是我们需要持续探索的方向。

七、银屑病治疗药物简介

银屑病的主要治疗手段包括使用外用药物、系统给药、光疗等。其中外用药物主要有糖皮质激素、维生素 D_3 衍生物、维甲酸类、钙调磷酸酶抑制剂等。系统药物主要有甲氨蝶呤、环孢素、维甲酸类等小分子药物及英夫利昔单抗等生物制剂。甲氨蝶呤等系统药物用于局部外部用药的研究也有相关报道。此外,虽然光疗以紫外线照射为主,但光敏剂与光动力联合疗法也在银屑病的治疗中有所应用。

八、银屑病的治疗方法及给药方式简介

对于轻至中度的寻常型银屑病,临床上主要采用外用药物治疗的方法或外用药物与系统给药或光疗相联合的方法进行治疗;对于一些伴有严重并发症的银屑病患者,则主要采用系统疗法;而对于上述疗法无效的情况,可考虑成本更高的生物制剂。其中,外用药物治疗主要以局部治疗的方式进行,而系统疗法通常以口服、皮下注射或静脉滴注等方式进行,其中局部治疗占80%以上。因此,我们将重点介绍高分子纳米药物载体在外用药物治疗中的应用。

九、高分子纳米药物载体提升药物皮肤穿透能力的设计规律

局部给药最大的问题是由于皮肤角质层对药物的穿透和吸收产生障碍,药物利用率低。特别是在银屑病中,皮肤角化过度和表皮增生导致的皮肤结构变化会进一步降低药物的穿透能力。高分子纳米药物载体可负载大量疏水药物,从而提升疏水药物的作用浓度,同时可利用自身的性质提升药物的皮肤穿透能力及皮肤停留时间,实现药物的可控、靶向释放,因而有助于银屑病的局部药物治疗。

纳米材料可以在皮肤内毛囊、汗腺等附属结构中释放药物从而提升药物的穿透深度,还可通过跨细胞途径和跨细胞间质途径进入皮肤。此外,近期发现的亲水性透皮通路也在纳米粒子进入皮肤的过程中起到了重要作用。由于纳米材料通过扩散作用进入皮肤,因而提升皮肤表面高分子纳米药物载体的浓度有利于增加皮肤中高分子纳米药物载体的扩散深度和药物浓度。皮肤中允许纳米材料通过的通道有一定尺寸限制,比如毛囊、汗腺等皮肤附属结构的尺寸为几微米到几十微米,纳米尺度的材料相对容易进入;而细胞间隙的尺寸仅为几纳米到几十纳

米。因此,构建小尺寸的高分子纳米药物载体可提升高分子纳米药物载体在皮肤中扩散的深度。除了尺寸以外,高分子纳米药物载体的透皮能力还与其变形能力和表面电荷性质相关。具有较强变形能力的高分子纳米药物载体可以通过改变自身形状进入细胞间隙,从而提升材料的扩散效率。而皮肤的酸性环境使表面带负电荷的材料容易在皮肤中聚集,导致尺寸增大,削弱其扩散能力。因此,表面电中性或带正电荷的高分子纳米药物载体具有更强的皮肤穿透能力。

十、高分子纳米药物载体在银屑病治疗中的应用

高分子纳米材料可负载药物并利用靶向功能延长药物在病灶中的停留时间,并作为化学增强剂提升药物的扩散效率。研究显示,在银屑病的皮肤炎症环境中,CD44蛋白在角质细胞上大量表达,而与之对应的透明质酸(HA)的表达降低。因此,CD44可以作为高分子纳米药物载体的靶点。Feng等制备了HA和磷脂分子的偶联物,并构建了负载姜黄素(curcumin)的高分子纳米药物载体(图6-11(a))。姜黄素可以抑制皮肤角质形成细胞的增殖。HA具有靶向CD44的作用,因此表面键合HA的高分子纳米药物载体较不含HA的载体具有更高的靶向能力,提高了姜黄素在皮肤中的富集,提升了其对银屑病的治疗效果。HA除具有靶向CD44的功能以外,还有很好的吸水保湿性能。Vicent等将连有银屑病治疗药物氟轻松

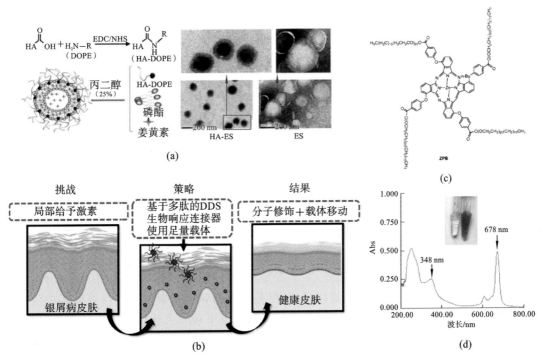

图 6-11 高分子纳米药物载体在银屑病治疗中的应用

(a)HA和磷脂分子偶联物制备的高分子纳米药物载体;(b)HA-PGA纳米材料提升药物皮肤穿透深度;(c)(d)光动力疗法在银屑病中的治疗;(c)酞菁锌-Brij 58偶联物的结构与(d)吸收峰

Figure 6-11 The application of polymer nanocarriers in psoriasis treatment

(a) Nanocarriers prepared by HA and phospholipid molecular conjugate; (b) The skin penetration depth of drugs enhanced by HA-PGA nanomaterials; (c)(d) Photodynamic therapy in the treatment of psoriasis, Structure (d) and absorption peak (d) of zinc phthalocyanine -Brij 58 conjugate

(fluocinolone acetonide)的聚-L-谷氨酸(PGA)与 HA-PGA 共组装,制备了高分子纳米载药体系(图 6-11(b))。该药物载体与单纯的 PGA-药物偶联物相比,可介导更大的皮肤穿透深度。其机制可能与 HA 的吸水作用提升了皮肤角质层及表皮层的水含量有关。在溶酶体酸性环境和组织蛋白酶 B 的共同作用下,药物可从载体中释放,实现对银屑病的治疗。

十一、高分子纳米药物载体增强光疗法在银屑病中的应用

除紫外线照射以外,近红外光的光动力疗法也在银屑病的治疗中有一定应用。Li 等利用两亲性酞菁锌-Brij 58 偶联物制备了平均粒径为 30 nm 左右的单分子胶束药物载体(图 6-11(c))。其中酞菁锌可吸收波长为 600~800 nm 的近红外光(图 6-11(d)),并可在近红外光照下产生单线态氧,实现对银屑病的治疗。

虽然高分子纳米药物载体可以在一定程度上提升药物的皮肤穿透能力,但是绝大部分高分子纳米药物载体仍停留在表皮上层,其皮肤穿透深度和药物递送效率仍然有限。为了进一步提升银屑病的治疗效果,可将高分子纳米载药体系和离子电渗疗法、微针等物理增强手段结合,提升药物的利用率和治疗效果。相关内容见本教材的银屑病章节。

第六节　挑战与展望

实现纳米药物的临床应用是纳米药物研究的目标,也是纳米药物研究的难点。目前,大部分被美国 FDA 批准用于临床的纳米药物的载体材料为脂质体。已有 19 种脂质体配方被批准用于各种疾病的治疗,其中包括 8 种用于癌症治疗的药物。许多基于高分子的载药体系具有很好的临床转化前景。如负载 PTX 的 PEG-b-PLA 胶束(Genexol-PM)已被批准用于乳腺癌的治疗,白蛋白-PTX 连接的纳米球(abraxane)被批准用于胰腺癌与卵巢癌的治疗。目前,仍没有基于高分子材料的纳米药物载体被批准用于黑素瘤或银屑病的治疗,但已有针对黑素瘤的高分子纳米载药系统进入临床试验阶段,如白蛋白-PTX 连接的纳米药物递送体系。

高分子纳米药物载体的临床转化是一个复杂的问题,涉及载体材料对药代动力学的改变,对药物肿瘤富集与治疗效果的提升,载体材料的降解、代谢,潜在的毒副作用,还有其标准化生产能力等诸多方面的问题。为了提升高分子纳米药物载体的临床转化潜力,在载体设计时应尽可能使用可降解、代谢的材料。此外,除了需要考虑纳米材料自身的成像、治疗功能外,还要重点研究其与生物系统相互作用的规律,例如提升材料的肿瘤富集效果或在银屑病中实现靶向、可控的药物释放等。同时,现有的动物模型并不能完全模拟人体黑素瘤或银屑病的特征,如何构建更加符合实际的动物模型来验证纳米药物的治疗效果也是需要重点研究的问题。纳米药物的开发是一个多学科交叉的研究方向,需要各学科、领域专家的共同努力来推进其临床转化进程。

相比于皮肤疾病治疗,应用于皮肤美容的高分子纳米药物载体的发展速度则快得多(见第九章),越来越多的含有高分子纳米药物载体的皮肤美容产品不断被开发出来并走向市场。

思　考　题

1. 比较高分子纳米药物载体与无机纳米药物载体的优缺点。

2. 哪些参数会影响高分子的临界胶束浓度?

3. 通过 DLS 测量的高分子纳米药物载体的粒径与通过 TEM 或 SEM 观察到的粒径有何区别?

4. 高分子纳米药物载体在黑素瘤的治疗中有何优势?

5. 高分子纳米药物载体在银屑病等皮肤疾病治疗中有何优势?

扩 展 阅 读

[1] Deng R, Derry M J, Mable C, et al. Using dynamic covalent chemistry to drive morphological transitions: controlled release of encapsulated nanoparticles from block copolymer vesicles[J]. J Am Chem Soc, 2017, 139(22): 7616-7623.

[2] Yu X, Zhao Z, Nie W, et al. Biodegradable polymer microcapsules fabrication through a template-free approach[J]. Langmuir, 2011, 27(16): 10265-10273.

[3] Helvig S, Azmi I D M, Moghimi S M, et al. Recent advances in cryo-TEM imaging of soft lipid nanoparticles[J]. AIMS Biophysics, 2015, 2(2): 116-130.

[4] Park J, Brust T F, Lee H J, et al. Polydopamine-based simple and versatile surface modification of polymeric nano drug carriers[J]. ACS Nano, 2014, 8(4): 3347-3356.

[5] Ali I, Rahis-Uddin, Salim K, et al. Advances in nano drugs for cancer chemotherapy[J]. Curr Cancer Drug Targets, 2011, 11(2): 135-146.

参 考 文 献

[1] Min Y, Caster J M, Eblan M J, et al. Clinical translation of nanomedicine[J]. Chem Rev, 2015, 115(19): 11147-11190.

[2] Gelderblom H, Verweij J, Nooter K, et al. Cremophor EL: the drawbacks and advantages of vehicle selection for drug formulation[J]. Eur J Cancer, 2001, 37(13): 1590-1598.

[3] Xing J, Zhang D, Tan T. Studies on the oridonin-loaded poly (D, L-lactic acid) nanoparticles *in vitro* and *in vivo*[J]. Int J Biol Macromol, 2007, 40(2): 153-158.

[4] Yoo H S, Oh J E, Lee K H, et al. Biodegradable nanoparticles containing doxorubicin-PLGA conjugate for sustained release[J]. Pharm Res, 1999, 16(7): 1114-1118.

[5] Bhadra D, Bhadra S, Jain S, et al. A PEGylated dendritic nanoparticulate carrier of fluorouracil[J]. Int J Pharm, 2003, 257(1-2): 111-124.

[6] Kono K, Kojima C, Hayashi N, et al. Preparation and cytotoxic activity of poly(ethylene glycol)-modified poly(amidoamine) dendrimers bearing adriamycin[J]. Biomaterials, 2008, 29(11): 1664-1675.

[7] Moura L A, Ribeiro F V, Aiello T B, et al. Characterization of the release profile of doxycycline by PLGA microspheres adjunct to non-surgical periodontal therapy[J]. J Biomat Sci Polym Ed, 2015, 26(10): 573-584.

[8] Nam Y S, Kim J W, Park J, et al. Tocopheryl acetate nanoemulsions stabilized with lipid-polymer hybrid emulsifiers for effective skin delivery [J]. Colloids Surf B

Biointerfaces,2012,94:51-57.

[9] Liang R,Dong L,Deng R,et al. Surfactant-free biodegradable polymeric nanoparticles generated from self-organized precipitation route: cellular uptake and cytotoxicity[J]. Eur Polym J,2014,57:187-201.

[10] Sadighian S, Hosseini-Monfared H, Rostamizadeh K, et al. pH-triggered magnetic-chitosan nanogels (MCNs) for doxorubicin delivery: physically vs. chemically cross linking approach[J]. Adv Pharm Bull,2015,5(1):115-120.

[11] Liang R,Wang J,Wu X,et al. Multifunctional biodegradable polymer nanoparticles with uniform sizes: generation and *in vitro* anti-melanoma activity [J]. Nanotechnology,2013,24(45):455302.

[12] Ventura C A,Tommasini S,Crupi E,et al. Chitosan microspheres for intrapulmonary administration of moxifloxacin: interaction with biomembrane models and *in vitro* permeation studies[J]. Eur J Pharm Biopharm,2008,68(2):235-244.

[13] Gormley A J,Chandrawati R,Christofferson A J,et al. Layer-by-layer self-assembly of polymer films and capsules through coiled-coil peptides[J]. Chem Mater, 2015, 27 (16):5820-5824.

[14] Liu Y, Li Y, He J, et al. Entropy-driven pattern formation of hybrid vesicular assemblies made from molecular and nanoparticle amphiphiles[J]. J Am Chem Soc, 2014,136(6):2602-2610.

[15] Wang S, Yu G, Wang Z, et al. Hierarchical tumor microenvironment-responsive nanomedicine for programmed delivery of chemotherapeutics[J]. Adv Mater,2018,30 (40):e1803926.

[16] D'Souza S S,DeLuca P P. Methods to assess *in vitro* drug release from injectable polymeric particulate systems[J]. Pharm Res,2006,23(3):460-474.

[17] Beriro D J,Cave M R,Wragg J,et al. A review of the current state of the art of physiologically-based tests for measuring human dermal *in vitro* bioavailability of polycyclic aromatic hydrocarbons (PAH) in soil[J]. J Hazard Mater, 2016, 305: 240-259.

[18] Qiu H,Gao Y,Boott C E,et al. Uniform patchy and hollow rectangular platelet micelles from crystallizable polymer blends[J]. Science,2016,352(6286):697-701.

[19] Bruschi M L. Strategies to modify the drug release from pharmaceutical systems[M]. London:Woodhead Publishing,2015.

[20] Proksch E. pH in nature,humans and skin[J]. J Dermatol,2018,45(9):1044-1052.

[21] Grumezescu A. Nanoscale fabrication, optimization, scale-up and biological aspects of pharmaceutical nanotechnology[M]. Amsterdam:Elsevier Academic Press,2018.

[22] Garbe C,Eigentler T K,Keilholz U,et al. Systematic review of medical treatment in melanoma:current status and future prospects[J]. Oncologist,2011,16(1):5-24.

[23] Avril M F, Aamdal S, Grob J T, et al. Fotemustine compared with dacarbazine in patients with disseminated malignant melanoma:a phase Ⅲ study[J]. J Clin Oncol,

2004,22(6):1118-1125.

[24] Liu Q,Das M,Liu Y,et al. Targeted drug delivery to melanoma[J]. Adv Drug Deliver Rev,2018,127:208-221.

[25] Golombek S K,May J N,Theek B,et al. Tumor targeting via EPR:strategies to enhance patient responses[J]. Adv Drug Deliver Rev,2018,130:17-38.

[26] Blanco E,Shen H,Ferrari M. Principles of nanoparticle design for overcoming biological barriers to drug delivery[J]. Nat Biotechnol,2015,33(9):941-951.

[27] Zhang Y R,Lin R,Li H J,et al. Strategies to improve tumor penetration of nanomedicines through nanoparticle design [J]. Wiley Interdiscip Rev Nanomed Nanobiotechnol,2019,11(1):e1519.

[28] Cabral H,Makino J,Matsumoto Y,et al. Systemic targeting of lymph node metastasis through the blood vascular system by using size-controlled nano carriers[J]. ACS Nano,2015,9(5):4957-4967.

[29] Du X J,Wang J L,Liu W W,et al. Regulating the surface poly(ethylene glycol) density of polymeric nanoparticles and evaluating its role in drug delivery *in vivo*[J]. Biomaterials,2015,69:1-11.

[30] Lu Y,Yue Z,Xie J,et al. Micelles with ultralow critical micelle concentration as carriers for drug delivery[J]. Nat Biomed Eng,2018,2(5):318-325.

[31] Ling X,Shen Y,Sun R,et al. Tumor-targeting delivery of hyaluronic acid-platinum (Ⅳ) nanoconjugate to reduce toxicity and improve survival[J]. Polym Chem,2015,6 (9):1541-1552.

[32] Guo Y,Niu B,Song Q,et al. RGD-decorated redox-responsive D-α-tocopherol polyethylene glycol succinate-poly(lactide) nanoparticles for targeted drug delivery [J]. J Mater Chem B,2016,4(13):2338-2350.

[33] Dai L,Li K,Li M,et al. Size/charge changeable acidity-responsive micelleplex for photodynamic-improved PD-L1 immunotherapy with enhanced tumor penetration[J]. Adv Funct Mater,2018,28(18):1707249.

[34] Talelli M,Iman M,Varkouhi A K,et al. Core-crosslinked polymeric micelles with controlled release of covalently entrapped doxorubicin[J]. Biomaterials,2010,31(30): 7797-7804.

[35] Zhao D,Wu J,Li C,et al. Precise ratiometric loading of PTX and DOX based on redox-sensitive mixed micelles for cancer therapy[J]. Colloid Surface B Biointerfaces,2017, 155:51-60.

[36] Liu M,Zhang P,Deng L,et al. IR780-based light-responsive nanocomplexes combining phase transition for enhancing multimodal imaging-guided photothermal therapy[J]. Biomater Sci,2019,7(3):1132-1146.

[37] Wallat J D,Wek K S,Chariou P L,et al. Fluorinated polymer-photosensitizer conjugates enable improved generation of ROS for anticancer photodynamic therapy [J]. Polym Chem,2017,8(20):3195-3202.

［38］ Liu Y,Bhattarai P,Dai Z,et al. Photothermal therapy and photoacoustic imaging via nanotheranostics in fighting cancer［J］. Chem Soc Rev,2019,48(7):2053-2108.

［39］ Ding H,Yu H,Dong Y,et al. Photoactivation switch from type Ⅱ to type Ⅰ reactions by electron-rich micelles for improved photodynamic therapy of cancer cells under hypoxia［J］. J Control Release,2011,156(3):276-280.

［40］ Rogers S J,Puric E,Eberle B,et al. Radiotherapy for melanoma:more than DNA damage［J］. Dermatology Research and Practice,2019,2019:9435389.

［41］ Gu X,Zhu Z,Fan Q,et al. Nanoagents based on poly(ethylene glycol)-*b*-poly (lthyroxine) block copolypeptide for enhanced dual-modality imaging and targeted tumor radiotherapy［J］. Small,2019,15(45):e1902577.

［42］ Sindhwani S,Syed A M,Ngai J,et al. The entry of nanoparticles into solid tumours ［J］. Nat Mater,2020,19(5):566-575.

［43］ Pradhan M,Alexander A,Singh M R,et al. Understanding the prospective of nano-formulations towards the treatment of psoriasis［J］. Biomed Pharmacother,2018,107:447-463.

［44］ Du H,Liu P,Zhu J,et al. Hyaluronic acid-based dissolving microneedle patch loaded with methotrexate for improved treatment of psoriasis［J］. ACS Appl Mater Interfaces,2019,11(46):43588-43598.

［45］ Jin Y,Zhang X,Zhang B,et al. Nanostructures of an amphiphilic zinc phthalocyanine polymer conjugate for photodynamic therapy of psoriasis［J］. Colloid Surface B Biointerfaces,2015,128:405-409.

［46］ Cevc G,Vierl U. Nanotechnology and the transdermal route a state of the art review and critical appraisal［J］. J Control Release,2010,141(3):277-299.

［47］ Zhang Y,Xia Q,Li Y,et al. CD44 assists the topical anti-psoriatic efficacy of curcumin-loaded hyaluronan-modified ethosomes:a new strategy for clustering drug in inflammatory skin［J］. Theranostics,2019,9(1):48-64.

［48］ Dolz-Pérez I,Sallam M,Masiá E,et al. Polypeptide-corticosteroid conjugates as a topical treatment approach to psoriasis［J］. J Control Release,2020,318:210-222.

［49］ Shetty P K,Venuvanka V,Jagani H V,et al. Development and evaluation of sunscreen creams containing morin-encapsulated nanoparticles for enhanced UV radiation protection and antioxidant activity［J］. Int J Nanomed,2015,10:6477-6491.

［50］ Ali I,Alsehli M,Scotti L,et al. Progress in polymeric nano-medicines for theranostic cancer treatment［J］. Polymers(Basel),2020,12(3):598.

(邓仁华　刘奕静　李钰策)

Chapter 6
Polymer Nano-Drug Carriers and Their Applications in Skin Disease Treatments

6.1 Overview of Nano-Drug Carriers

6.1.1 Introduction of nano-drug carriers

Nanoparticles (NPs) have been widely used as carriers for nano-drug delivery system. Drug molecules could be loaded inside or on the surface of carriers by physical adsorption, encapsulation or chemical bonding. Nano-drug delivery system is applicable to various administration routes including vein, muscles, skin, mucous membrane, oral, etc. It allows effective control of drug release rate, improving the biological membrane permeability, altering the body distribution, and elevating bioavailability, etc. Since the 1990s, with the rise and development of nanotechnology, nano-drug loading technology developed rapidly. The birth of nano-drug carrier is possibly because of the insolubility of about half of the drugs. This problem can be overcome by using nanocarriers, because most NPs can well disperse in water. Furthermore, the stability of the active drugs could be improved when the drugs are loaded inside the carriers. Moreover, it enables slow-release of drugs, which can prolong the duration of action and reduce dosing frequency of drugs. In addition, the drug-loaded NPs can enter target cells through endocytosis, thus improving the utilization of drugs.

Since the first nano-drug delivery system was reported in 1995, more than 50 systems are currently under clinical investigation, and the number is increasing. Improving the efficacy and reducing side effects of drugs are particularly required in clinical applications. Therefore, developing nano-drug carriers for targeted delivery and controlled release of drugs is one of the hot spots in biomedicine fields. Targeted delivery could be achieved by modifying carriers with specific substances or functional groups, and the release rate is controllable by employing physical, chemical and biological interactions. Such nano-drug carriers are helpful for improving pharmacokinetic parameters of drugs. In addition, diagnosis reagents, detection reagents and treatment drugs could be loaded in the same carrier, which could be used as a promising therapeutic agent.

6. 1. 2　Polymer nano-drug carriers

Natural and synthetic polymers are common materials for nano-drug carriers. The first polymer drug-loading system, penicillin-poly(vinyl amine) complex, was reported in 1962. In 1975, Ringsdorf proposed polymer drug carriers, in which small molecule drugs were combined with polymer carriers through covalent bonds. Compared with inorganic materials, polymers are able to undergo pH, temperature, light and other stimulus-responses, and polymers can be easily shaped into nanoparticles with different shape and size. In addition, there are a variety of polymers that are biocompatible and biodegradable, and low- or non-toxic.

6. 1. 3　Demand for polymer nano-drug carriers in skin disease treatment and cosmetic dermatology

Drug delivery is involved in the field of skin disease, cosmetic skin care, etc. For example, melanoma is a disease with an extremely high mortality rate. There is great significance to develop nano-drug delivery system with better curative effect and less toxic side effects for the treatment of melanoma. In addition, nano-drug delivery systems have also been used for the treatment of psoriasis and some other skin diseases or cosmetic skin care. Compared with traditional drugs in ointment or cream forms, nano-drug carriers have following advantages: effectively improve the dispersibility of undissolved active functional components in water, enhance the stability of the active components, promote penetration of functional components across cuticle barrier, realize the targeting transport and sustained release of functional components, and significantly increase the residence time of functional components in the skin, avoid inflammation and allergic reaction. Moreover, it enables synergies of different functional components. In recent years, more and more polymer nano-drug delivery systems have been developed for applications in the treatment of skin diseases and cosmetic skin care.

6. 2　Classification of Polymer Nano-Drug Carriers

6. 2. 1　Classified by chemical composition

Both natural and synthetic biocompatible, biodegradable polymers have been applied for nano-drug carriers. Among them, polysaccharides, poly(amino acids), and polyesters are the commonly used polymers.

6.2.1.1 Polysaccharides

Polysaccharides have been widely used as nano-drug carrier materials because they contain lots of highly active hydrophilic groups (such as hydroxyl, carboxyl, and amino) that could be easily modified, and some of them have the function of immunoregulation, antitumor and antiviral. Currently, polysaccharides including glucan, hyaluronic acid, heparin, alginate, chitosan, and mushroom polysaccharides, etc. have been used as nano-drug carriers. Hyaluronic acid is one of the widely used carrier materials due to its tumor targeting effect. However, the strong hydrophilicity, poor stability, and short biological half-life of hyaluronic acid limit its application in nano-drug carriers. For example, the drug loading is very low and drug is leaked too fast when using hyaluronic acid to load the water-soluble drugs. Chitosan is another commonly used carrier material, because it has good biological adhesive, exhibits different inhibition to bacteria, fungi and other microorganisms, has hemostatic function, can improve human immunity, and has antitumor effect. Furthermore, it can be broken down by lysozyme in the body. Due to their strong hydrophilicity, hyaluronic acid and chitosan were usually processed into nanogels, which can serve as drug carriers. In addition, nano-gels could be modified with functional inorganic nanoparticles such as gold, quantum dots and magnetic NPs to improve their functionality. Besides, they are often used as the outer layer of the hydrophobic polymers or inorganic nano-drug carriers to improve their hydrophilicity, stability, and targeting.

6.2.1.2 Poly(amino acids)

Poly(amino acids) contain multiple reactive sites, therefore, it is easy to manipulate their hydrophilicity, charge and targeted features through further modification. Poly (glutamic acid), polylysine, poly (styrene alanine) and poly (aspartic acid), etc. are commonly used for nano-drug carriers. Hydrophobic poly(amino acids) usually link with hydrophilic polymer block (such as poly (ethylene glycol)) forming amphiphilic block copolymer to prepare micelles, which can be used as nano-drug carriers. With the active groups such as carboxyl and amino groups, poly(amino acids) are capable of combining with drug molecules through either chemical bonding, physical embedding, or electrostatic adsorption. Therefore, the drugs can be loaded in different positions of the micelles. Amino acid copolymers can be synthesized by copolymerization of two or more amino acids. Due to their rich variety, amino acids with the desired structure and properties can be selected to prepare copolymers according to the requirements of different drugs.

6.2.1.3 Polyesters

Most aliphatic polyesters have low biological toxicity and good compatibility. Hydrophobic polyesters can be used as carriers in the forms of NPs or microcapsules. The aliphatic polyesters that have been approved for drug carriers by the Food and Drug

Administration (FDA) of the United States include poly(lactic acid) (PLA), poly(lactic-*co*-glycolic acid) (PLGA), polycaprolactone (PCL), etc. In the 1970s, Pitt and Schindler put forward that PCL can be used as drug delivery carries. At present, it has been widely used in biomedical fields.

PLA has the features of non-toxic, nonirritant, and no immunogenicity, and therefore is used as nano-drug carriers. However, the hydrophilicity of PLA is poor and its degradation speed is very slow. Oppositely, poly(glycolic acid) (PGA) has high polarity and faster degradation speed, but its crystallinity is high. Both PLA and PGA are limited in clinical application due to their features. PLGA is the copolymer of lactic acid and glycolic acid. The solubility, mechanical properties and degradation speed of PLGA can be manipulated by adjusting the ratio of these two monomers to obtain suitable carrier materials. Yoo et al. prepared PLGA NPs containing an anticancer drug doxorubicin. The drug encapsulation efficiency is as high as 96.6% and the drug loading is 3.45%. Moreover, doxorubicin can be slowly released in 25 days.

Besides, the hydrophobic polyesters are often linked with hydrophilic polymers to form amphiphilic block copolymer to prepare the micellar-typed nano-drug carriers. Poly(ethylene glycol) (PEG) is often used as the hydrophilic block, which can increase the solubility and stability of nano-drug carriers. In general, the phagocytosis speed increases with the hydrophobicity. Therefore, enhancing the surface hydrophilicity of the nano-drug carriers could be able to prolong the circulation time of drugs in the body.

6.2.2 Classified by morphology of carriers

According morphology, polymer nano-drug carriers can be classified into 3D macromolecules, polymer nano-spheres/capsules, polymer micelles/vesicles, polymer nano-gels and nano-emulsions, etc. (Figure 6-1).

6.2.2.1 3D macromolecules

Dendritic polymer is a kind of 3D macromolecule with multilevel branching structure, which is obtained by constantly repeating branched growing from the central molecule. Its size is typically between 5 and 50 nm with good uniformity and can be adjusted precisely. Both interior and surface of dendritic polymer can be designed by various functional groups, which are able to combine with drug molecules through physical or chemical interaction. The drugs combined via physical interaction could be released too fast and are easy to leak, while the drugs combined by chemical interaction are hard to be released. Grafting hydrophilic chains (e.g., PEG) on the surface of hydrophobic dendritic polymer can improve drug loading and the stability of the physical interaction-combined drugs. Polyamide-amine (PAMAM) is a kind of dendritic polymer nano-drug carrier material that has received a lot of studies. Bhadra et al. found that after grafting PEG on the PAMAM surface, the drug loading of an anticancer drug 5-fluorouracil (5-FU) was increased 12 times, the drug release rate was reduced to 1/6, the circulation time in blood was increased 3 times, and the efficacy is 10 times as much as 5-FU naked medicine. By regulating the surface degree of polymerization and grafting rate of PEG, the drug loading and the release rate of PAMAM could be controlled accurately. In addition, the release of chemical interaction-combined drugs can be improved by chemical bonds that are easy to fracture in the body. For example, drugs connected through ester bond are more likely to be released than via amide bond. More importantly, under the weak acid environment of the tumor, drug molecules can combine with dendritic polymer by the acid sensitive chemical interaction (e. g., hydrazone bond), which can realize stimulus responsive drug release, improve the cytotoxicity of drugs, and avoid the killing to normal cells. Kono et al. reported that the cytotoxicity of doxorubicin (DOX) bonded on the surface of PAMAM via hydrazone bond is 10 times better than that of drugs through amide bond connection. Similarly, proteins are also 3D macromolecules, and have been widely used as nano-drug carriers.

6.2.2.2　Polymer nano-spheres/capsules

Polymer nano-spheres (or nano-capsules) usually refer to solid or hollow zero-dimension NPs in range of tens to hundreds of nanometers formed by aggregating of hydrophobic polymers. PLA and PLGA are often used to prepare nano-spheres (or nano-capsules) to load drugs. Hydrophobic drugs can be loaded into the polymer matrix of polymer nano-spheres via hydrophobic interaction. *In vivo*, the drugs release slowly with gradual degradation of the polymers. Nano-capsules can be employed to encapsulate aqueous or oily solution of hydrophilic or hydrophobic drugs.

6.2.2.3　Polymer micelles/vesicles

Polymer micelles are spherical aggregates formed via self-assembly of amphiphilic block copolymers with hydrophobic chain as core and hydrophilic chain as corona. The hydrophobic chains commonly used include PLA, PLGA, PCL and poly(amino acids), etc., and PEG is used as the hydrophilic block. The size of polymer micelles is generally between 10-100 nm and it is usually monodispersed. Drugs are supposed to be loaded in the hydrophobic core of micelles via physical interaction while hydrophilic shell can maintain the stability of the micelles and prolong the circulation time *in vivo* as well. In addition, drug molecules also can be bonded onto hydrophobic chains of block copolymer through chemical interaction, followed by self-assembling into micelles. The size of the hydrophobic core and its interaction with drugs have important effects on drug loading. Currently, most polymer nano-drug carriers in clinical researches are polymer micelles.

Polymer vesicles are aggregates with capsule shape and bilayer structure formed via the self-assembly of amphiphilic block copolymers. Unlike the spherical micelles, vesicles are filled with water. The block ratio of hydrophobic chains to hydrophilic chains of block copolymer used for the preparation of micelles is smaller than that for vesicles. The size of vesicles is usually larger than that of micelles but the uniformity of the former is no better than that of the latter. Similar with polymer nano-capsules, vesicles are also a kind of nanoscale liquid capsule, which not only are able to load traditional small-molecule drugs but also can be used to deliver NPs and biological macromolecules such as protein and nucleic acid. Unlike nano-capsules, both the internal and external walls of vesicles are hydrophilic polymer chains. Vesicles are suitable for loading hydrophilic drugs. But owing to the restriction of the preparation methods, the encapsulation efficiecy of drugs is very low. Unlike the spherical micelles/NPs, the drugs loaded in the cavity of vesicles/nano-capsules not only can release slowly via penetrating their wall, but also are able to release instantaneously with the breaking up of the wall to achieve local high concentration of drugs. It allows to regulate and control the speed of drug release according to different requirements.

6.2.2.4　Polymer nano-gels

Polymer nano-gels are a kind of nanoscale dispersion system containing large amounts of liquid, in which polymer chains forming continuous network structure via physical or chemical cross-linking. Most of the common polymer nano-gels are hydrogels, and the water content is as high as about 90% in three-dimensional network structure of hydrophilic or amphiphilic polymers. To improve the performance of the nano-gels, functional inorganic NPs, including gold NPs, magnetic NPs, and quantum dots, etc. can be doped into nano-gels. The nonspherical gold NPs in nano-gels can be used as a thermal sensor applying to photodynamic therapy and photothermal therapy. Nano-gels containing magnetic NPs can be used to achieve drug targeting delivery under external magnetic field. In addition, quantum dots can be used for imaging, and therefore can be used to build integration of diagnosis and treatment platform.

6.2.2.5　Nano-emulsions

Nano-emulsions are stable dispersion systems, in which the oil phase in the form of nano-droplets disperse in water stabled by surfactants. Like nano-capsules, drugs are dissolved in oil droplets and the drug loading depends on the solubility of drugs in the oil phase. Diameter of oil droplets is between 1-100 nm and the uniformity is different owing to the preparation methods, but most of them are not good as spherical micelles. Cooking oil can be chosen as oil droplets and surfactant is supposed to be biodegradable amphiphilic polymer with good biocompatibility. Hydrophobic chains of surfactant in nano-emulsions face oil droplets while hydrophilic chains spread in the water phase, but the accumulate intensity of polymer chains is smaller than polymer nano-spheres/capsules and polymer micelles/vesicles. Therefore, the release speed of drugs from nano-emulsion could be very fast.

6.3　Preparation Technologies for Polymer Nano-Drug Carriers

Until now, few technologies have been developed in the preparation of polymer nano-drug carriers. Drugs can be loaded on/inside polymer carriers via bonded/adsorbed with polymers, embedded into the matrix of polymer NPs, or encapsulated inside polymer nano-capsules/vesicles/nano-emulsions. Among them, three-dimensional macromolecules, such as dendritic polymer and albumin, can combine with drug molecules via physical or chemical interactions to obtain nano-drug delivery system. Physical interaction mainly includes van der Waals force, hydrogen bonding, electrostatic interaction and hydrophobic interaction. Chemical interaction includes ester bond, amido bond, hydrazone bond, etc. Other types of polymer nano-drug carriers, such as spherical micelles, vesicles, and nano-spheres/capsules, can be classified as polymer aggregates. According to the morphologies of aggregates, their preparation methods are shown as follows.

6.3.1 Monomer polymerization

Polymer NPs can be directly obtained by polymerization of monomers, at the meantime, drugs are loaded. Emulsion polymerization is a commonly used method for the preparation of NPs. Specifically, drug molecules are dissolved in a monomer as the oil phase, then emulsified by an aqueous phase containing surfactants, followed by polymerization reaction to produce nano-drug delivery system. This method is suitable for hydrophobic polymers and drugs, and typically used for spherical nano-drug carriers. It should be pointed out that in some polymerization reactions, high temperature may affect the activity of the drugs. Besides, residual monomer, catalyst, surfactant, and initiator, etc. that could bring side effects are hard to be removed completely.

6.3.2 Solution self-assembly

In selective solvents, when the concentration of an amphiphilic block copolymer is above its critical micelle concentration (CMC), the block copolymer spontaneously aggregate into assemblies with hydrophobic chains as the core whereas hydrophilic chains as the corona. This process is known as solution self-assembly (Figure 6-2). According to the block ratio of hydrophilic block to hydrophobic block, assemblies of various morphologies, including spherical micelles, vesicles, or other shaped micelles can be obtained. During the self-assembly process, hydrophobic drugs can be loaded in the core of the spherical micelles or the wall of vesicles, whereas hydrophilic drugs can be encapsulated inside vesicles or linked on the surface of carriers. Solution self-assembly is a robust and simple method, and the surface of carriers are hydrophilic polymer chains, which are conducive to the stability, targeting, circulation *in vivo* of nano-drug delivery system. Due to these advantages, solution self-assembly has become the mostly used method for the preparation of nano-drug delivery systems in the clinical research at present. One of the disadvantages of this method is that the encapsulation efficiency of drugs is relatively low. Besides, CMC are very low for most copolymers; therefore, it costs lots of solvents in fabrication. In recent years, a method combining polymerization and self-assembly, i. e., polymerization induced self-assembly (PISA) is attracting increasing attention because of high concentration and tunable morphologies of assemblies (see extended reading 1).

6.3.3 Nano-precipitation

There are mainly two types of nano-precipitation methods: self-organizing nano-precipitation for the preparation of nano-spheres and cross-linking induced nano-precipitation for nano-gels.

6.3.3.1 Self-organizing nano-precipitation

Self-organizing nano-precipitation is a technique that takes advantage of the solubility difference of polymers and drug molecules in good and poor solvents to precipitate the polymers and drugs into NPs (Figure 6-3). Firstly, the polymers and drugs are dissolved in a water-miscible organic solvent (the good solvent), then water (the poor solvent) is slowly added to induce the precipitation of both of them to form a nano-drug delivery system. In contrast to solution self-assembly, this method is applied for hydrophobic polymers (e. g., PLA, PLGA, and PCL), and the obtained NPs are usually nano-spheres. The preparation conditions are mild (room temperature and atmospheric pressure) and the products are easy to be purified and no added additives. The size of NPs is closely related to the polymer and drug concentration. Particle size increases with the increase of polymer and drug concentration, and the NPs becomes less homogeneous. The encapsulation efficiency of drugs by using this method is also relatively low. Specific interactions between drug molecules and polymers can greatly improve the encapsulation efficiency.

6.3.3.2 Cross-linking induced nano-precipitation

Cross-linking can induce nano-precipitation of polymers into nano-gels in solution. This method is mainly aimed at the multifunctional hydrophilic polymers, such as polysaccharides and poly(amino acids), particularly, chitosan. According to the different mechanisms of cross-linking, it can be further divided into physical- and chemical-cross-linking induced nano-precipitation.

Ionic cross-linking is a commonly used physical-cross-linking method. Specifically, when chitosan is dissolved in an acid solution, the amine ($-NH_2$) is protonated to cationic $-NH_3^+$. In this case, the chitosan molecules would be cross-linked and gather into nano-gels via electrostatic interaction caused by the introduction of negatively charged anion cross-linking agent. The commonly used anionic cross-linking agents include sodium tripolyphosphate, sodium phosphate, sodium dodecyl sulfate. Among them, sodium tripolyphosphate is mostly used because of fast cross-linking speed and mild reaction conditions. Moreover, the obtained nano-gels are uniform in size, safe and non-toxic, and their surface charge are adjustable.

Chemical-cross-linking such as covalent cross-linking is one of the earlier methods used in the preparation of chitosan nano-gels. Chitosan molecules are cross-linked into nano-gels by forming covalent bonds between cross-linker and the functional groups on chitosan such as hydroxy and amino groups. Sadighian et al. prepared pH-responsive and magnetic chitosan nano-gels by using glutaraldehyde as cross-linking agent and discussed the effects of physical- and chemical-cross-linking on the performance of magnetic chitosan nano-gels as adriamycin targeting drug carriers. The chemical-cross-linked nano-gels have better stability, more controllable release property, but the residual cross-linking agents could be toxic and it means more workload for post-processing purification.

6.3.4 Emulsion based methods

Emulsion droplets can be applied as templates for the preparation of nano-drug carriers. Emulsion based methods include emulsion-solvent evaporation method, self-emulsion/solvent diffusion method and emulsion cross-linking method. The first two methods are mainly used for the preparation of nano-spheres/capsules, while the latter one is used for the preparation of nano-gels.

6.3.4.1 Emulsion-solvent evaporation method

Typically, the hydrophobic polymers and drugs are firstly dissolved in a water-immiscible and low boiling point organic solvent as the oil phase, then emulsified by an aqueous phase containing surfactants to form an oil-in-water (O/W) emulsion, followed by evaporation of the organic solvent to form a nano-drug delivery system (Figure 6-4). Organic solvents of the oil phase should be more volatile than water, such as dichloromethane, chloroform, toluene and ethyl acetate. Among them, the toxicity of ethyl acetate is very low. The distribution of drug molecules in the carriers depends on the hydrophobicity and the strength of interaction between them. If the interaction between drugs and carriers is very weak, the drugs with weak hydrophobicity tend to be distributed near the surface of the carriers. On the contrary, the drugs with strong hydrophobicity are distributed inside the carriers. Reversed-phase (W/O) emulsions can be applied to load hydrophilic drugs in hydrophilic polymer carriers, in which both the polymers and the drugs are firstly dissolved in water and the surfactant is dissolved in the oil phase. Reversed-phase emulsions require that the organic solvent is harder to evaporate than water.

The advantages of emulsion-solvent evaporation method are high encapsulation efficiency, precise control of drug loading, and this method is capable to load multiple drugs or testing reagents simultaneously. Hydrophobic biodegradable polymers such as PLA and PLGA can be used to prepare nano-drug carriers by this method. The size of the nano-drug carriers can be easily controlled by varying the size of the emulsion droplets and the concentration of the polymers. The size uniformity depends on the emulsification method, which is generally inferior to the spherical micelles, but better than NPs obtained by the self-organized nano-precipitation method. Majority surfactants in the products can be removed by centrifugation or dialysis, but few residuals are inevitable. To reduce the toxic and side effects of surfactants, nonionic surfactants such as poly(vinyl alcohol) (PVA) can be used.

Based on emulsion-solvent evaporation method, researchers also developed the double emulsion-solvent evaporation method, which can be used to prepare nano-capsules. Double emulsions are complex emulsions formed through further secondary emulsification of ordinary emulsion, which are also known as multilayer emulsions. If water-in-oil (W/O) single emulsion is secondary emulsified in water phase, W/O/W multiple emulsion will be achieved. On the contrary, O/W/O multiple emulsion is able to be obtained via secondary emulsification of O/W single emulsion in oil phase. The double emulsions contain internal phase, intermediate phase and external phase. W/O/W multiple emulsion has been applied for nano-drug carriers. Water-soluble drugs are dissolved in internal phase and oil-soluble polymers are dissolved in the intermediate phase. Nano-capsules can be obtained after complete evaporation of the organic solvent. At the same time, oil-soluble drugs can also be added in the intermediate phase. The size of the double emulsions is generally greater than single emulsions, while the uniformity is inferior to single emulsions. The size of capsules is usually hundreds of nanometers in size. Apart from secondary emulsification, phase separation also can be introduced to generate double emulsions. For example, a non-volatile poor solvent (O') can be added in the oil phase of the emulsion. With the evaporation of the organic solvent of the oil phase, phase separation between O' and polymer occurs, resulting in O'/O/W multiple emulsion. For instant, cooking oil can be served as the non-volatile poor solvent. However, by adding absorbent materials (such as sodium dioctyl sulfosuccinate) in the oil phase of O/W emulsion droplets, W/O/W multiple emulsion can be achieved. Specifically, the water molecules diffuse into the droplets and form the internal phase, which can be used to load water-soluble drugs. Both size and uniformity of the droplets could be improved by employing the phase strategy (see extended reading 2).

6.3.4.2 Self-emulsion/solvent diffusion method

A mixed solvent composed of a water-insoluble organic solvent and a water-soluble organic solvent (e. g., acetone, methanol) is used for the oil phase. After mixing with water, the water-soluble organic solvent spreads spontaneously from oil phase into aqueous phase, hence the turbulence occurs at the two-phase interface, resulting in the generation of droplets and eventually forming NPs of polymers and drugs after solvent evaporation. The advantage of this method is that no surfactant is required, but the uniformity of nano-drug carriers are not as good as that of emulsion-solvent evaporation method. PLA nano-spherical drug carriers loading insoluble drug oridonin (ORI) were prepared by this method, whose average size is 137.3 nm, the encapsulation efficiency is $91.88\% \pm 1.83\%$, and drug loading is $2.32\% \pm 0.05\%$.

6.3.4.3 Emulsion cross-linking method

It refers to the method that the polymer is cross-linked after the formation of stable nano-emulsion, so that the polymer forms a three-dimensional network structure in the droplet and the droplets of nano-emulsion are transformed into nano-gel consequently. According to the solubility of the polymer, oily nano-gels can be prepared by emulsion cross-linking method and aqueous nano-gels are able to be prepared by reverse emulsion cross-linking method. The cross-linking agents can be added to the droplets in advance. After the formation of the nano-emulsion, the cross-linking reaction can be initiated by external stimuli (e. g. , temperature, pH, light). For non-stimulus responsive cross-linking agents, they can be added into the continuous phase after the emulsion is formed and the polymer is cross-linked via the diffusion of cross-linking agents into the droplet. Like cross-linking nano-precipitation method, there are physical-cross-linking method and chemical-cross-linking method.

6.3.5 Spray drying method

Polymers and drug molecules are firstly dissolved in a volatile solvent, then the solution is sprayed into tiny droplets, followed by drying into a powder of NPs (Figure 6-5). This method is suitable for both hydrophobic and hydrophilic nano-drug delivery systems, and no surfactant is needed. However, the preparation of nanoscale drug systems requires high quality and expensive equipment. Similar with the emulsion-solvent evaporation method, the size of the NPs obtained by spray drying method depends on the size of the droplets and their concentration. Compared with self-organizing nano-precipitation method, this method has a higher encapsulation efficiency. But this method generally requires the solvent in fogdrop to evaporate instantaneously under high temperature condition, which is not suitable for high temperature intolerant polymers and drugs.

6.3.6 Layer-by-layer self-assembly technology

Polymer layer-by-layer self-assembly technology refers to the technology of alternating deposition of two or more kinds of polymers and drugs onto the substrate and controlling the structure and function of nano-drug carriers at the nanometer level. It is a new nanotechnology with great development prospects. The nano-drug carriers can be prepared by layer-by-layer self-assembly technology with NPs as substrate cores. The preparation condition of this method is mild. It is easy to prepare multifunctional carriers and the structure of the nano-drug carriers is precisely controlled. This method has unique advantages in the aspects of sustained release, controlled release, especially programmed release, which makes it have great prospects in the field of cancer treatment. The adsorption forces during layer-by-layer self-assembly deposition are mainly electrostatic interaction, hydrogen bond, covalent bond, hydrophobic interaction, etc. Layer-by-layer self-assembly of polyelectrolytes via electrostatic interaction has been most widely studied. Natural biological macromolecules, such as polypeptides, proteins, nucleic acids and most polysaccharide molecules, carry a large amount of electric charge in the solution. As a result, they are easily adsorbed by electrostatic interaction. Water-soluble drug molecules with charges can be loaded into the carriers by means of adsorption with high drug loading. Hydrophobic drug molecules are prior to be loaded into the substrate cores, such as charged surface of polymer NPs/capsules, micelles, and mesoporous silica. The nano-drug carriers obtained by this technology can load different drugs in different microdomain. For example, Ramasamy et al. prepared a nano-drug carrier through layer-by-layer self-assembly of poly (ethylene glycol) and polylysine with liposome micelles as the substrate cores. Moreover, the doxorubicin was loaded in core and mitoxantrone was loaded within multilayer films.

6.4 Characterization of Polymer Nano-Drug Carriers

The physical, chemical, and biological properties of the polymer nano-drug carriers affect their ability in drug delivery, disease diagnosis and treatment. Therefore, how to effectively evaluate the performance of polymer nano-drug carriers is essential in the design, screening, and optimization of carriers. Characterizations of polymer nano-drug carriers can be performed *in vitro* and *in vivo*. The *in vitro* characterizations include the particle size and its distribution, zeta (ζ) potential, morphology, drug loading content, encapsulation efficiency, release profile, and responsiveness, etc. The *in vivo* characterizations include the distribution, targeting, and biocompatibility. Compared with the *in vivo* characterizations, the *in vitro* characterizations are more convenient and rapid, and have fewer variabilities. Researchers have established the relationship between the *in vitro* and *in vivo* characterizations for some polymer nano-drug carriers. These experiences and principles help us to find the desired polymer nano-drug carrier materials quickly by *in vitro* experiments, thereby avoiding the use of animals. In this section, we will introduce the instruments and techniques for the evaluation of *in vitro*/*in vivo* characterizations.

6.4.1 Particle size and its distribution

The particle size and its distribution of polymer nano-drug carriers influence their pharmacokinetics,*in vivo* distribution, transdermal efficiency, and residence time. The main methods to evaluate the particle size and its distribution of nanomaterials are dynamic light scattering (DLS) and scanning or transmission electron microscopy.

DLS is a technology that measures the fluctuations in the intensity of scattered light caused by the Brownian motion of particles. The average particle size can be calculated by the Stokes-Einstein equation. This technology provides repeatable overall sizes and distributions of NPs in a short time. Besides, this method measures the hydrodynamic diameters of NPs, which is not easy to be provided by scanning or transmission electron micrographs. However, there are also some limitations for the DLS technique. For example, since the intensities of scattered light is proportional to the sixth power of particle sizes, the presence of large-sized impurities such as dust in the NP solution will significantly affects the overall particle size. If the absorption of the nanomaterial coincides with the incident laser, the particle size cannot be measured. Meanwhile, for non-spherical NPs, DLS can only provide the equivalent spherical sizes. Besides, the stability of NPs, temperature, and other factors can also affect the final result.

The size information of the NPs can be obtained from scanning or transmission electron microscopy as well. Generally, we need to calculate the average particle size and partide size distribution from a photograph of at least several hundreds of NPs. The advantage of these technologies is that they can provide the size for the solid part of nano-drug carrier (such as the core of a micelle), as well as the morphology of non-spherical or other structures (such as the hollow part of the vesicle), and avoid the influences of large sizes impurities. However, there are also some disadvantages. For example, these methods are time-consuming, and they cannot provide the overall particle size information. Moreover, the morphology and size of NPs may change with the increase of concentration or during sampling. Besides, since the hydrophilic parts are generally invisible under the transmission electron microscope due to their low contrast, the particle size given by the transmission electron microscope is usually smaller than the hydrodynamic diameter given by DLS. Therefore, combining the results of DLS and electron microscopy can provide a more comprehensive characterization of the particle size and distribution information of nano-drug carriers.

6.4.2　Zeta (ζ) potential

The charge properties of nano-drug carriers are related to the stability of materials and the interactions between the NPs and biological interfaces such as cell phagocytosis, distribution *in vivo*, and adsorption of protein. Therefore, it is meaningful to measure the charge properties of polymer nano-drug carriers. The charge properties of nano-drug carriers can be measured by zeta (ζ) potential. The ζ potential of a nano-drug carrier can be described by the Stern electric double layer theory (Figure 6-7). The Stern electric double layer theory indicated that the surface of charged NPs in solution could be divided into a Stern layer and a diffuse layer. The Stern layer refers to a layer of ions with opposite charges tightly adsorbed on the surface of NPs. The diffuse layer consists of two layers—a fluid layer containing ions that are close to the Stern layer and can stably move with the Stern layer, and a dispersion layer on the outer side. The interface between the two layers is the slipping plane, where the potential is called ζ potential. Most of ζ potential meters are based on electrophoretic light scattering technology. NPs with different charge properties in the solution move at different rates under the electric field, resulting in a Doppler shift in the frequency of the scattered light, and then the ζ potential can be calculated. The ζ potential of NPs varies with the surroundings of the solution, such as pH and ionic strength. Therefore these conditions should be constant during measurement.

6.4.3　Morphology

Microscopes, including transmission electron microscope (TEM), scanning electron microscope (SEM), and atomic force microscope (AFM), are used to measure the morphology of polymer nano-drug carriers.

TEM is the most commonly used tool to measure the morphological structure of polymer nano-drug carriers. It can image objects of several nanometers to micrometers with high resolution. It also provides nanostructure and elemental information through different imaging modes (e. g. , freezing mode and scanning transmission mode). During testing of TEM, the electron beams pass through the sample and focus on the object lens. The intensity and angle of electron beams vary with the differences in element, density, and thickness of NPs. As a result, different morphology and contrast in the image reflect the different structures and materials of the NPs.

Staining is usually used to improve the contrast of polymer NPs under TEM. There are two staining methods—positive staining and negative staining. In positive staining, the NPs are stained by high contrast materials, so that the NPs show darker appearances in the TEM image. For example, uranyl acetate can be used to stain proteins and other polymer NPs containing amino groups. Negative staining improves the contrast of the sample in the imaging by increasing the contrast of the background. The negatively stained sample displays a dark background in the TEM image, while the sample is bright due to the less stain. The staining method can improve the contrast of some polymer NPs as well as provide the microstructures of the particles.

Cryo-TEM is the direct method to observe polymer NPs in the solution phase. It uses electron beams to image the NPs frozen in the liquid(Figure 6-8(a)). Three scientists who developed Cryo-TEM technology to measure the high-resolution structure of biological macromolecules were awarded the 2017 Nobel Prize in Chemistry, demonstrating the critical role of Cryo-TEM in structural measurement (see extended reading 3).

Besides, there are other modes for TEM measurement. For example, high-resolution TEM (HRTEM) can image the lattice between atoms in nanomaterials, which enables us to characterize inorganic/polymer composite NPs. In addition, the combination of computerized tomography imaging technology and the mathematical model of image analysis can reconstruct the three-dimensional structure image of the NPs, so that we will have a more intuitive and accurate understanding of the morphology of the NPs with the three-dimensional structure. Furthermore, the TEM energy-dispersive X-ray spectroscopy (EDXS), electron energy loss spectroscopy (EELS) and other technologies enable us to measure the distribution of elements in NPs.

In short, the high-resolution and multifunctional measurement capabilities of TEM have made it an indispensable technique in the measurement of nano-drug carriers.

SEM is a technology that visualizes the surface topography of NPs using electron beams. Generally, the resolution of SEM is less than TEM. Moreover, materials with poor conductivity need to be covered with a thin gold layer on the surface of the sample to increase the conductivity. The advantage of SEM compared with TEM is that it can load more samples at one time. Considering that samples need to be vacuumed during the test process of SEM and TEM, SEM can check more samples than TEM in a certain period. In addition, SEM provides more information about the surface structure of NPs. Therefore, SEM is more suitable for the measurement of the external morphology of large-sized conductive materials or inorganic/polymer composite nanomaterials.

AFM can perform high-resolution three-dimensional imaging of the surface structure of NPs. It interacts with the particle surface through a cantilever and a fine probe connected to the cantilever to collect corresponding imaging information. Except for the morphology of NPs, AFM provides additional information such as particle height, softness, and hardness, which are of great significance for the analysis of two-dimensional polymer nanomaterials such as ring, sheet, and dish. Moreover, surface modification or spraying is not required during the sampling of AFM. For NPs with low contrast in TEM images, it also provides accurate morphology. Due to these advantages, AFM technique becomes an important technique for the measurement of the morphology of polymer NPs.

6.4.4 Drug loading content and encapsulation efficiency

The drug loading content and encapsulation efficiency are two important parameters to determine the drug delivery performance of polymer nano-drug carriers. Drug loading content refers to the mass fraction of drug in the polymer nano-drug, which can be calculated by equation 6-1:

$$C = \frac{M_{drug}}{M_{drug} + M_{carrier}} \times 100\% \qquad \text{(Equation 6-1)}$$

where C represents the drug loading content, M_{drug} and $M_{carrier}$ represent the mass of the drug and polymer nano-drug carrier, respectively.

Encapsulation efficiency refers to the ratio of drug loaded in the polymer nano-drug carrier to the total amount of the drug added during the preparation of the drug formulation, which can be calculated by equation 6-2:

$$EE = \frac{M_{drug}}{M_{total\ drug}} \times 100\% \qquad \text{(Equation 6-2)}$$

where EE is the encapsulation efficiency, M_{drug} and $M_{total\ drug}$ represent the mass of the drug in the polymer nano-drug carrier and the total mass of the added drug, respectively.

To measure the drug loading and encapsulation efficiency, we need to determine the mass of the polymer nano-drug carrier, loaded drug, and the total drug. Mass of polymer nano-drug should be determined since the yield of drug loading is usually less than 100%. The mass of nano-drug can be determined by a balance or thermogravimetric analysis after freeze-drying. To determine the concentration of drugs in solution, we can employ a standard curve method based on UV absorbance, fluorescence intensity, or high-performance liquid chromatography.

The amount of drugs in polymer nano-drug carriers can be determined by differential method, the complete release method, and the direct measurement method. The differential method calculates the loaded drug by the differences between the feeding and the remained drugs. For some drugs, we can utilize the fluorescence or absorption spectrum changes after being loaded in the polymer nano-drug carrier to check the loading efficiency. In more cases, methods such as high-speed or ultrafiltration centrifugation are used to separate nano-drug from free drugs and determine the unloaded drugs. However, the residual polymer nano-drug carrier in the supernatant, the absorption of the drug by the filter membrane, and the agglomeration and precipitation of the drug itself during the loading process will cause certain errors. We can also quantify the amount of drugs after completely destroying the carrier by adjusting the pH or dissolving in an organic solvent to promote drug release. The drug content can also be determined by the absorption peak directly if the drug has a characteristic absorption peak in the polymer nano-drug carrier.

6.4.5 *In vitro* drug release

The efficiency and rate of drugs release affect the metabolism, ability to pass through the physiological barrier, residence time at the disease site, and targeting performance of drugs. A key issue in improving the therapeutic effect of drugs is to achieve the controlled release of drugs. The *in vitro* drug release performance of polymer nano-drug carriers reflects the *in vivo* release to a certain extent. Therefore, it is an essential parameter for designing and optimizing carrier systems. The drug release curve refers to the relationship of the ratio of released drugs to the total amount of drugs over time. A typical drug release curve consists of a rapid release phase, a sustained release phase, and a plateau phase (Figure 6-8(b)). Some special responsive nano-drug carriers, such as light-responsive nano-drug carriers, could accelerate the drug release in response to the specific stimuli. To measure the drug release curve, we need to remove the free drug in the solution, and separate the released drug from the polymer nano-drug carrier material and the unreleased drug in the release process. *In vitro* drug release is usually performed in phosphate buffer solution (PBS) at 37 ℃ to simulate the internal environment. The PBS that dissolves the released drug is regularly replaced to simulate the loss of the drug from the disease site. Specific solutions such as acidic, oxidizing (e. g. , hydrogen peroxide), and reducing (e. g. , glutathione) solutions are also used to simulate the characteristics of tumor or skin microenvironment or to verify the responsibility of polymer nano-drug carriers. The *in vitro* drug release methods include dialysis method, Franz diffusion method, and high-speed or ultrafiltration centrifugation. Both the dialysis method and the Franz diffusion method separate the released drug from the nano-drug by the concentration difference of the drug on both sides of the semi-permeable membrane. In the dialysis method, nano-drug is put in a dialysis bag and dialysis towards large amounts of solution (Figure 6-8(c)). The drug release curve of the polymer nano-drug carrier is obtained by recording the amount of drug increased in the solution outside the dialysis bag. The Franz diffusion method, which composed of a drug supply pool, a receiving pool, and a semi-permeable membrane (Figure 6-8(d)), is employed to measure the transdermal drug release. The semi-permeable membrane is used for the simulation of skin, and the released drug is collected from the receiving pool. Except for the above two methods, ultrafiltration centrifugation and high-speed centrifugation are also used for *in vitro* drug release. In this method, nano-drug is mixed with the release solution with shaking and stirring to simulate the *in vivo* environment. Nano-drug and the released drug are separated by centrifugation at specific time points. The ultrafiltration centrifuge tube consists of an inner concentrating tube with an ultrafiltration membrane at the bottom and a collection tube. After centrifugation, the nano-drug and unreleased drug remain in the concentrating tube, and the released small molecule drugs pass through the ultrafiltration membrane and are collected in the collection tube. The amount of drug released can be determined by measuring the amount of the drug in the collection tube. High-speed centrifugation separates the mixed solution of nano-drug and released drug by direct centrifugation. After centrifugation, the nano-drug is precipitated on the bottom of the centrifuge tube. The *in vitro* drug release curve can be calculated by measuring the drug content in the supernatant. The adsorption of drugs on the wall of dialysis bags and centrifuge tubes may result in errors in the *in vitro* drug release. Besides, it is difficult to completely simulate the drug release environment *in vivo* by the above *in vitro* experiments. As a result, the actual *in vivo* drug release are still required.

6.4.6　Stimulus responsiveness

Both the tumor and the skin microenvironment are weakly acidic. The pH value of the tumor microenvironment is around 6.5, and that of the skin microenvironment is between 4 and 7.4. Therefore, pH-responsive polymer nano-drug carriers can be used to promote the release of drugs in targeted areas or transdermal delivery efficiency. Buffer solutions with different pH values are required to simulate the behavior of nano-drug carriers in tumor or skin microenvironment. Besides, the buffer solutions also need to have certain ionic strength and good solubility. Phosphate buffer solution, citrate buffer solution, and acetate buffer solution are the commonly used acidic buffer solutions. The pH responsibility of nano-drug carriers under weakly acidic conditions can be obtained by combining of morphology, size, and drug release.

6.4.7　Biodistribution

The nano-drug will enter the tumor and various healthy organs with the blood circulation. Therefore its biodistribution will influence the therapeutic effect and toxic side effects. By testing the *in vivo* biodistribution of nano-drug, we will obtain the distribution in healthy organs such as liver and spleen, the peak concentration in tumors or blood, the time to reach peak concentration, and the circulation time of nano-drug, etc. Its measuring method contains two aspects: animal sampling analysis and *in vivo* imaging analysis. The animal sampling analysis measures the blood parameters of the nano-drug. The concentrations of the nano-drug in the blood are determined by the physical and chemical properties of nano-drug carriers or the loaded drugs after collected blood samples of animals at specific time points. Unfortunately, the number of blood collections and the amount of blood taken each time are limited since one mice has only about 2 mL of blood. For the measurement of the distribution of the nano-drug in various organs or tumors, it is necessary to sacrifice mice at specific time points and take samples of organs and tumor tissues for analysis. Therefore, each mouse can only provide drug distribution information for one time point. In comparison, the *in vivo* imaging method is a non-invasive method, which enables us to detect the real-time distribution of nano-drug at different time points. The imaging techniques include fluorescence imaging, photoacoustic imaging, magnetic resonance imaging (MRI), positron emission tomography (PET), single photon emission computed tomography (SPECT), etc. Among them, fluorescence imaging, photoacoustic imaging, and MRI can semi-quantitatively measure the tumor enrichment and organ distribution of nano-drug by the signal intensity. Fluorescence imaging and photoacoustic imaging provides fast imaging but low penetration depth, while MRI can penetrate deeply, but take more time for imaging. In comparison, PET and SPECT have a high imaging penetration depth and a quantified distribution of nano-drug in tumors and organs accurately. However, these two technologies require to use radioactive isotope-labeled nano-drug and cost a lot. Appropriate technologies should be selected according to the specific requirements of each experiment since every imaging technology has its advantages and disadvantages. Most *in vivo* imaging methods need to introduce functional groups with corresponding functions into the polymer nano-drug carriers. Therefore, if the functional groups are cleaved by the enzymes or ions *in vivo*, it may cause errors in results. Besides, if the drug is released before entering the diseased area, it may also cause errors. Thus, these factors should be considered during the measurement *in vivo*.

6.4.8 Biocompatibility

Since polymer nano-drug carriers are distributed in both healthy tissues and organs, their biocompatibility is important to achieve a good therapeutic effect. Biocompatibility in pre-clinical trials mainly includes two aspects: *in vitro* and *in vivo*. For *in vitro* biocompatibility, the polymer nano-drug carriers can be incubated with normal cells, and the effect of carrier system on the proliferation of normal cells can be evaluated by the thiazole blue (MTT) method. After confirming that the polymer nano-drug carrier has a good *in vitro* biocompatibility, we will evaluate the *in vivo* biocompatibility by detecting its effect on the heart, liver, kidney, and other important organs. These organs were then extracted to prepare paraffin sections, stained with hematoxylin and eosin and observed on an optical microscope to check whether the polymer nano-drug carriers would cause pathological changes in the organs. In addition, the biomarkers of the heart, liver, kidney, and other organs were detected to further determine the biocompatibility of nano-drug. Only the polymer nano-drug carriers that exhibit considerable biocompatibility both *in vitro* and *in vivo* may be further evaluated in clinical trials.

6.5 Applications of Polymer Nano-Drug Carriers in Melanoma and Psoriasis Treatment

6.5.1 Introduction to the drugs for melanoma treatment

Surgery is a very effective treatment for early-stage melanoma patients, which results in the above 95% of 5-year overall survival rate of stage Ⅰ patients. Except for surgery, radiotherapy, chemotherapy, and rapidly evolving immunotherapy are also used in melanoma treatment. However, the 3-year survival rate of patients with metastatic melanoma are below 15%. Thus, developing a new melanoma treatment plan is of great significance. Chemotherapy is a traditional cancer treatment strategy. Dacarbazine (DTIC) is a standard chemotherapeutic drug that has been approved by the US FDA for metastatic melanoma treatment. Yet, there is no data to confirm that DTIC improves the survival of patients. In addition, there are some other chemotherapeutic drugs that have been tested in clinical or pre-clinical studies, such as doxorubicin (DOX), cisplatin, paclitaxel (PTX), and taxanes. Recently, great progress has been achieved in melanoma immunotherapy. Earlier immunotherapeutic agents, such as interferon-alpha (IFN-α) and interleukin-2 (IL-2), are not ideal for improving the overall survival or responsive rates of patients. The subsequent development of monoclonal antibody drugs, such as ipilimumab and nivolumab, significantly improves the overall survival rates of drug-responsive patients, yet problems such as high toxicity and low responsive rates still exist. The related content is discussed in melanoma immunotherapy related chapter.

6.5.2 Drug delivery routes of polymer nano-drug carriers for melanoma treatment

The main routes of drug delivery for polymer nano-drug carriers are injection and transdermal drug delivery. Since we are going to introduce the transdermal drug delivery of polymer nano-drug carriers in psoriasis treatment section, we will focus on relevant contents of the injection route for drug administration. Injection, characterized by high drug availability, refers to directly inject drugs to veins, organs, or tissues, which includes intravenous injection, intraperitoneal injection, intramuscular injection, subcutaneous injection, and others. In the study of drug delivery for melanoma, intravenous injection is mainly used, which includes intravenous injection and infusion. Different injection routes will influence the pharmacokinetic parameters and even the *in vivo* distribution of the polymer nano-drug carriers. Because the nano-drugs enter the circulatory system directly, their bioavailability is high. Yet, the adsorption of protein corona on the surfaces of nanomaterials will change their surface chemical and physical properties, resulting their blood clearance by the mononuclear phagocytic system in the body and their enrichment in liver, spleen and other organs, eventually leading to low tumor accumulation and toxic and side effects to some extent. This is also one of the key problems that researchers need to solve in the field of polymer nano-drug carriers.

6.5.3 The principle of designing polymer nano-drug carriers with improved tumor accumulation

Polymer nano-drug carriers can prolong the time of some water-soluble small molecule drugs in blood circulation, solve the problem of poor water-solubility of hydrophobic anticancer drugs, and improve the stability of drugs. According to the traditional theory, the enrichment of polymer nano-drug carriers in the tumor is based on the enhanced permeability and retention (EPR) effect, which refers to the presence of the wide fenestrations on tumor vessel walls and the defective lymphatic drainage (Figure 6-9). But the polymer nano-drug carriers need to overcome a number of physiological barriers before they can act on cancer cells. These barriers include the adsorption of serum proteins, the removal of nano-drugs by liver and spleen, and the passage of nano-drugs through tumor vessel walls and their internalization into tumor cells. To overcome these physiological barriers, polymer nano-drug carriers must have specific physical and chemical properties, so that they can adapt to the mechanism of action with various parts of bodies. However, because of the complexity of the *in vivo* environment and physiological barriers, the design of most current polymer nano-drug carriers is still unable to fully meet the needs of overcoming these physiological barriers. In addition, different physiological barriers have contradictory requirements for the physicochemical properties of nano-drug. For example, in order to avoid the removal of the polymer nano-drug carrier in the blood by the protective mononuclear phagocytic system as a foreign body, the size of the polymer nano-drug carrier is generally required to be small, but in order to achieve a longer tumor residence time and drug action time, the size of the polymer nano-drug carrier is generally required to be large. These conflicting demands greatly increase the difficulty of designing polymer nano-drug carriers. Although the design to promote tumor enrichment of nanomaterials remains to be optimized, based on a large number of research results, we can summarize some basic laws of carrier design, including the size and surface chemical properties of nanomaterials.

The size of polymer nano-drug carrier is an important factor affecting its pharmacokinetic dynamics and *in vivo* distribution. In general, nanomaterials larger than 100 nm are easier to be removed from the blood by macrophages and other mononuclear phagocytes than nanomaterials of smaller size, which negatively impacts their tumor accumulation. When the size of NPs is less than 5 nm, NPs will rapidly eliminate from bodies via the kidney, reducing their blood circulation time. When the size of NPs is between 5 nm and 100 nm, smaller NPs generally exhibit better intratumor diffusion. However, NPs with good diffusion ability do not necessarily bring higher tumor enrichment, because the interstitial fluid pressure existing between the tumor periphery and core can push the nano-drug carriers back to the blood vessels from the tumor tissues. Therefore, nanomaterials of small size have shorter tumor retention time. Studies have shown that the interstitial fluid pressure in some melanoma tissues can be as high as 50 mmHg. Because of the complex microenvironment of the tumor, the best sizes of the polymer nano-drug carriers for tumor accumulation should be determined by experiments. For example, Kataoka et al. prepared drug-carrying polymer micelles with an average particle size of 30 nm using PEG-*b*-P(Glu) block copolymer. At the same time, they also prepared drug-carrying polymer micelles with an average particle size of 70 nm by co-assembly of PEG-*b*-P (Glu) and P (Glu) homopolymer. By comparing the tumor accumulation of 30 nm, 70 nm of polymer micelles with the 80 nm the US FDA-approved liposome formulation (doxil) in melanoma lymphatic metastatic tumor model, they found that polymer micelles with an average particle size of 30 nm had the deepest tumor penetration depth, the highest tumor accumulation, and the best chemotherapeutic effect. This example shows that the regulation of particle size is of great significance for the treatment of melanoma with polymer nano-drug delivery system. However, the mechanism of different polymer materials interact with *in vivo* system may differ, so it is necessary to study and discuss different materials in distinct tumor models.

The surface chemical property of the polymer nano-drug carriers is also an important factor affecting its tumor accumulation. Compared with nanomaterials with positive or negative surface charges, nanomaterials with neutral surface can effectively reduce the adsorption of serum proteins, which can improve their blood circulation time and tumor accumulation effect. Therefore, PEG is commonly used to protect the surface of polymer nano-drug carriers. It has been shown that the density of PEG on the surface of polymer nano-drug carriers can influence their blood circulation time and tumor accumulation. Wang et al. used PEG-*b*-PCL block copolymers to co-assemble with PCL homopolymers to prepare a series of polymer micelles with tunable sizes and surface PEG densities by adjusting the PCL chain length and the ratios of PCL homopolymer in the assemblies. Subsequently, polymer micelles with an average size of about 100 nm and different PEG densities (0.19 - 0.86 PEG chains/nm^2) were selected to study the influence of surface PEG densities on the *in vivo* distribution and tumor accumulation of the polymer nano-drug carriers. The results showed that the polymer micelles with high PEG density had the least adsorption and the longest blood retention time. After loading docetaxel, the polymer micelles with the highest PEG density showed the best therapeutic effect on melanoma and the longest survival in mice. In addition to PEG, the zwitterionic small molecule and polymer ligands are also frequently used to modify the surface of polymer nano-drug carriers. The so-called zwitterionic ligands refer to ligands with equal positive and negative charges, resulting in a neutral charge (see extended reading 4).

Although PEG and zwitterionic ligands can reduce the adsorption of serum proteins, they also reduce the interaction between nanomaterials and tumor cells. To selectively enhance the interaction between the nano-drug carriers and tumor cells, we can add tumor targeting groups or introduce stimulus response groups to nano-drug carriers that specifically change the surface physicochemical properties at the tumor site. The target groups promote the accumulation of nanomaterials in tumors by enhancing the interaction between polymer nano-drug carriers and receptors on tumor cells and tissues. Commonly used target groups include small molecules, saccharides, peptides, proteins and other categories. The receptors highly expressed on the surface of melanoma cells include transferrin receptor (TfR), folic acid receptor (FR), fibroblast growth factor receptor (FGFR), laminin receptor (LR), somatostatin receptor (SSTR), sigma receptor, MC1R, CD44, etc. Tu et al. prepared a nano-drug delivery system loaded with cisplatin by using ethylenediamine modified hyaluronic acid. The nano-drug delivery system enhances the targeting ability by using the interaction between hyaluronic acid and CD44 expressed on melanoma cells, and can achieve responsive drug release in acidic or reductive environments. In addition, integrins, which are highly expressed on melanoma neovascular endothelial cells can also be used as targets for polymer nano-drug carriers. Common targeting groups include Arg-gly-Asp (RGD), circular Arg-Gly-Asp-D-Tyr-Lys (cRGDyK), etc. Tu et al. prepared block copolymers by conjugation D-α-tocopherol polyethylene glycol succinate with PLA through disulfide bonds, which were cleavable by GSH in tumor cells(TPGS-b-PLA). The co-assembly of TPGS-b-PLA and PEG-b-PLA can produce PTX-loaded polymer nano-micelles with or without RGD on the surfaces. The cleavage of disulfide bonds in polymer micelles by GSH in tumor cells triggered the release of PTX. The experiment results showed that polymer nano-micelles with RGD targeting groups have better tumor inhibition effect than those without RGD and commercial PTX nanoformulations, which confirmed that RGD can improve the melanoma targeting ability of polymer nano-drug carriers. Changing the physical and chemical properties of polymer nano-drug carriers specifically in tumor is the use of the stimuli-responsive groups on nano-drug carriers that can have physical or chemical reactions in the tumor microenvironment to change their surface physical and chemical properties, which prevents polymer nano-drug carriers from serum protein absorption before entering tumors, and promotes the interaction between polymer nano-drug carriers and tumor tissues or tumor cells after they enter tumors, leading to their enhanced tumor accumulation. Cai et al. successfully delivered nucleic acid drugs and photosensitizer to melanoma by using the pH-responsive polymer nano-drug carriers that can detach PEG on the surface in tumor acidic microenvironment. After the removal of PEG, the zeta potential of the polymer nano-drug carrier was increased to 20 mV, enhancing the interaction between polymer nano-drug carrier and the negatively charged cell membrane. At present, there are still some problems in the research of melanoma targeting polymer nano-drug carriers, such as insufficient targeting ability of ligands, and the shelter of targeting groups by serum proteins causing the loss of the targeting ability. Therefore, further research is still needed for the targeting ability of polymer nano-drug carriers.

6.5.4 The application of polymer nano-drug carriers in the chemotherapy of melanoma

The functions of polymer nano-drug carriers mainly include improving the water-solubility of hydrophobic drugs, reducing the toxic and side effects of drugs, and enhancing the enrichment of drugs in tumors. Besides, enhancing the tumor accumulation of the polymer nano-drug carriers, maintaining the stability of the polymer nano-drug carriers before it reaches the tumor, reducing or preventing the early release of the drugs, and fast releasing drug in the tumor area can all improve the therapeutic effect. The methods to maintain the blood stability of polymer nano-drug carriers include using polymer prodrugs instead of small molecular drugs, designing cross-linked nano-drug carriers and reducing critical micelle concentration of polymers. The factor of the motility of the polymer chains, the effect of serum protein adsorption and blood shear force, can destabilize the polymer nano-drug carriers, resulting in the early release of drugs from carriers. In addition, the drug itself may be separated from the carriers in advance by diffusion. All of these factors can reduce the bioavailability of drugs (see extended reading 5).

Polymer prodrug method is to conjugate chemotherapeutic drugs to the polymers through the responsive covalent bond, which were used to make nano-drug carriers. Because the drugs conjugated on polymer chains have slower diffusion rates, which reduce the diffusion-driven premature drug release. The covalent bonds of responsive groups can break in the tumor microenvironment. The commonly used tumor microenvironment includes acidic pH, high reactive oxygen species concentration, certain enzymes, and high glutathione concentration. For example, Luan et al. prepared two amphiphilic polymer prodrugs by linking PEG and DOX or PTX via disulfide bonds, respectively. Their co-assembly can form polymer micelles with precisely regulated PTX/DOX loading ratios. The drug release rate from the micelles in the reductive tumor microenvironment was faster than that under normal conditions.

Cross-linking the polymer nano-drug carriers is a method to enhance the stability of the carriers and reduce the premature release of drugs from the carriers. Among them, the covalent bonds required for cross-linking can usually break by responding to certain characters in the tumor microenvironment. Hennink et al. constructed a small molecule prodrug that could break under acidic pH condition by bonding DOX to methylacrylamide via a hydrazone bond. The copolymerization of DOX prodrug and the polymer containing the side chains of methacrylic acid generated the cross-linked polymer nano-drug delivery system. The system released only 5% of the drug in the normal blood pH (pH=7.4), while it could release 100% of the drug in the acidic environment in the same time period. The results of animal experiments showed that the drug delivery system has a good inhibitory effect on melanoma.

After entering the blood, the polymer nano-drug carriers will be gradually cleared *in vivo*, and its blood concentration will decrease continuously in a certain period of time. When the concentration is lower than the critical micelle concentration of the polymers, the stability of the polymer nano-drug carrier decreases, which easily leads to the destruction of the structure of the carrier and the premature release of the drug. Therefore, reducing the critical micelle concentration of the polymers can improve the stability of the nano-drug carriers. Cao et al. synthesized amphiphilic polymer molecules by combining the super-hydrophilic zwitterionic polymers with the super-hydrophobic lipid molecules. The amphiphilic polymers could be used to prepare micelles with strong contrast polarity between their hydrophobic and hydrophilic components, which were used to deliver chemotherapy drugs (Figure 6-10(a)). The results showed that the critical micelle concentration of the micelle could be as low as 2.7×10^{-6} mmol/L, which is $1/10^6$ of sodium dodecyl sulfonate, a commonly used small molecule surfactant, and $1/10^4$ of polysorbate 80, a large molecule surfactant. The results of animal experiments showed that docetaxel delivered by the polymer micelles with strong contrast polarity showed significant better treatment effect than drugs delivered by nano-drug carriers prepared from polysorbate 80 and commercial docetaxel nano-formulation.

The drug release rate of the polymer nano-drug carriers in tumors is also a key factor to obtain a good therapeutic effect. If the drug release rate is low, the effective drug concentration will be reduced. If the drug is released too fast, it may quickly leave tumors and become ineffective. Therefore, a suitable drug release rate has an important impact on the treatment of melanoma. The mechanism of drug release includes drug diffusion from the carriers, drug release due to the destructions of nano-drug carriers by responding to acidic pH or certain enzymes, and drug release due to interruption of covalent or non-covalent interactions between the drug and the carrier. How to achieve controlled drug release is one of the key problems of the polymer nano-drug delivery system in the field of tumor treatment.

6.5.5 The application of polymer nano-drug carriers in photothermal and photodynamic therapy of melanoma

Phototherapy is a highly effective and accurate cancer therapy. Phototherapy mainly includes photothermal therapy and photodynamic therapy. Photothermal therapy is to use the photothermal effect of polymer nano-drug carriers or the encapsulated drugs to transform the absorbed light energy into heat energy, so as to improve the local temperature of tumor tissues to eliminate tumors. To meet the requirements of deeper penetration and low damage to normal tissue, the NIR I (750-1000 nm) or II (1000-1350 nm) lasers with less tissue absorption are usually selected as the light source. To realize the photothermal tumor treatment, the construction of polymer nano-drug carriers requires conjugation or loading small molecules, inorganic nanomaterials with photothermal conversion effect, or using semiconductor polymers as the carrier materials. For example, Wang et al. prepared nanobubbles with PEG-*b*-PLGA by double emulsion method (Figure 6-10 (b)), which contained perfluoropentane and IR780 in the core and membrane of the nano-spheres, respectively. Among them, IR780 is a hydrophobic small molecule photothermal conversion agent, and perfluoropentane is a low boiling point (29 ℃) liquid. During photothermal treatment, perfluoropentane is heated and vaporized rapidly, thus transforming the nanobubbles into microbubbles. The enlarged nanobubbles can not only enhance the signal intensity of melanoma ultrasound imaging, but also improve the vascular permeability, so that more nanobubbles can enter the tumor and enhance the photothermal treatment effect. In addition to improving the tumor enrichment effect of polymer nano-drug carriers, improving the photothermal conversion efficiency of polymer nano-drug carriers, designing and utilizing laser with deeper penetration depth, and controlling the damage of photothermal therapy to normal tissues are all the directions that need to be explored in the photothermal tumor therapy of polymer nano-drug carriers. The biggest problem of photothermal therapy is the limited penetration depth of laser, which is only a few millimeters. It can only be used to treat melanoma in the superficial skin, and it is difficult to achieve the treatment of tumors in deep tissues. The development of combination therapy of photothermal therapy with chemotherapy, immunotherapy, surgery, and radiotherapy is one of the potential methods to solve the bottleneck problem of photothermal therapy.

Tumor photodynamic therapy refers to a cancer treatment method that uses polymer nano-drug carriers enriched at the tumors to generate reactive oxygen species under laser irradiation and kill tumor cells. The production of reactive oxygen species inside cells can promote cells to produce oxidative stress environment and damage biological macromolecules such as DNA and protein, eventually leading to the death of tumor cells. To realize tumor photodynamic therapy, it is necessary to conjugate or load photosensitizers in polymer nano-drug carriers. When the photosensitizers are excited by a laser, it can generate singlet oxygen through the energy transfer (type Ⅱ) pathway or free radicals through the electron transfer (type Ⅰ) pathway. The type Ⅱ pathway requires oxygen consumption. On the one hand, in view of the hypoxic microenvironment within the tumor, how to provide more oxygen sources is one of the key issues that need to be addressed for type Ⅱ photodynamic therapy. Pokorski et al. prepared polymer micelles using fluoropolymers of poly(TFEMA-*co*-OEGMEMA) with terminal cationic zinc-ethyl phenyl porphyrin, in which cationic zinc-ethyl phenyl porphyrin is the photosensitizer; fluoropolymers have the ability to absorb oxygen and enhance the ability of type Ⅱ photodynamic pathway to produce singlet oxygen under hypoxic environment. On the other hand, the development of polymer nano-drug carriers containing type Ⅰ photosensitizers is another solution to the problem of oxygen dependence in photodynamic therapy. Similar to photothermal therapy, the effectiveness of photodynamic therapy is limited by the laser's limited penetration depth. In addition to the development of combination therapy, the development of photodynamic therapy induced by other light sources with deeper penetration is also an important research direction. These sources include X-ray, Cerenkov radiation, and etc. These new light-source-induced photodynamic therapies will provide new strategies to treat deep metastatic melanoma.

6.5.6 The application of polymer nano-drug carriers in the radiotherapy of melanoma

Radiotherapy is a very effective treatment for cancer in clinic. Although it has been reported that some melanoma can tolerate radiation, it has also been reported that radiotherapy has a good therapeutic effect on melanoma. Radiotherapy uses radiation to destroy DNA in cells, making them unable to proliferate. However, how to reduce the side effects of radiotherapy and enhance the therapeutic effect are the key problems to be solved in radiotherapy. Radiotherapy can be divided into two categories: treating tumors by external radiation and injecting radioactive drugs into the body. For the external radiation therapy, elements with high atomic number (e. g., gold, bismuth, and hafnium) can enhance the destruction effect of radiation by enhancing the scattering of radiation in the tumor area. For the injection of radioactive drugs, how to improve the tumor accumulation of drugs is the key to improve the therapeutic effect. Deng et al. synthesized the amphiphilic polymer by coupling PEG-b-poly(L-thyroxine) and radioactive iodine-131 (^{131}I) and assembled them into polymer nanomaterials. This kind of polymer nano-drug carrier containing radioactivity has a good tumor inhibition effect on melanoma.

In conclusion, polymer nano-drug carriers can enhance the therapeutic effect of chemotherapy, photothermal/photodynamic therapies, radiotherapy and other therapies of melanoma. The EPR effect is the basis for the design of most antitumor nano-drugs. Recently, there are some results suggesting that EPR effects may vary from tumors to tumors, patients to patients, and different tumor stages. At present, the bottleneck problems of tumor therapy of nano-drug lie in the limited tumor accumulation and therapeutic effect. In addition, the latest research results indicated that some nanomaterials may enter tumor tissues mainly through the trans-endocytosis process through the endothelial cells in tumor vascular walls, rather than through the leakiness in the vascular walls in the traditional EPR theory. These new results need to be further studied and confirmed, but the development of EPR theory also indicates that the current design strategies of polymer nano-drug delivery system need to be further improved. In addition, the toxic and side effects of polymer nano-drug carriers require further study. The development of polymer nano-drug carriers with good biocompatibility and biodegradability is also the direction that demands continuous investigation.

6.5.7 Introduction to the drugs for psoriasis treatment

The main treatment methods for psoriasis include using local topical drugs or systemic administrated drugs, phototherapy, and others. Topical drugs include glucocorticoids, vitamin D_3 derivatives, retinoid acids, calcineurin inhibitors, and so on. Systemic drugs mainly include small molecule drugs such as methotrexate, cyclosporin, retinoic acid and biological drugs such as infliximab. Systemic drugs (e. g. , methotrexate) used as local topical drugs have also been reported. In addition, clinical phototherapy mainly uses UV light, photodynamic therapy with photosensitizers have also been applied in the treatment of psoriasis.

6.5.8 The brief introduction of therapeutic strategies and drug administration routes of psoriasis

For mild to moderate psoriasis vulgaris, topical drug therapy or topical drugs combined with systematic drugs or phototherapy are the main therapeutic strategies. Systematic drug therapy is mainly used for psoriasis patients with severe complication. In cases that these therapies do not work, higher-cost biological therapies may be considered. Among them, topical drug therapy is mainly carried out in the form of local therapy, while systemic drug therapy is usually carried out in the form of oral administration, intramuscular injection or intravenous injection. Local treatment accounts for more than 80% of them. Therefore, we will focus on introducing the applications of polymer nano-drug carriers in topical drug therapy.

6.5.9 The design principles of polymer nano-drug carriers for improving the skin penetration ability of drugs

The biggest problem of local topical drug administration is that the stratum corneum of the skin prevents penetration and absorption of the drugs, resulting in low drug availability. Especially in psoriasis, the skin structure changes caused by skin keratinization and epidermal hyperplasia further reduce the drug penetration ability. Polymer nano-drug carriers can be loaded with a large number of hydrophobic drugs, so as to improve the action concentration of hydrophobic drugs. At the same time, they can use their own properties to improve the skin penetration ability and skin residence time of drugs, and achieve controlled and targeted release of drugs, thus contributing to local drug therapy for psoriasis.

Nanomaterials can increase the penetration of drugs by releasing drugs inside the skin's affiliated structures such as wrinkles and hair follicles. They can also enter the skin through intracellular and intercellular pathways. In addition, the recently finding showed that hydrophilic transdermal pathway also plays an important role in the process of NPs entering the skin. Since nanomaterials can enter the skin through diffusion, increasing the concentration of nanomaterials on the skin surface is beneficial to increase their diffusion depth and drug concentration in the skin. There are certain size restrictions on the passage of nanomaterials in the skin. For example, the sizes of hair follicles, sweat glands and other skin accessory structures are several to dozens of microns, which easily allow nanomaterials to enter. However, the sizes of the intercellular space are only a few to dozens of nanometers. Therefore, the construction of small-sized polymer nano-drug carriers can improve the diffusion depth of nanomaterials in the skin. In addition to the size, the transdermal capability of the polymer nano-drug carriers is also related to its deformation capability and surface charge properties. The easily deformable polymer nano-drug carriers can enter the intercellular space by changing its own shape, thus improving the diffusion efficiency of the nanomaterials. The acidic environment of the skin makes the negatively charged nanomaterials to aggregate in the skin, resulting in increased size, thus reducing its ability to diffuse. Therefore, the polymer nano-drug carriers with neutral or positively charged surfaces have stronger skin penetration capability.

6.5.10 Application of nano-polymer drug carriers in the treatment of psoriasis

polymer nanomaterials can load drugs and use their targeting ability to improve the residence time of drugs in lesions, and as chemical enhancers to improve the diffusion efficiency of drugs. Studies have shown that in the inflammatory skin environment of psoriasis, CD44 protein is highly expressed, while the expression of its corresponding hyaluronic acid (HA) is decreased. Therefore, CD44 can be used as a target of polymer nano-drug carriers. Feng et al. prepared a conjugate of HA and phospholipid molecules and constructed a curcumin-loaded polymer nano-drug carriers (Figure 6-11(a)). Curcumin can inhibit the proliferation of skin keratinocytes. HA can target CD44, thus, polymer nano-drug carriers with conjugated HA on surfaces have a higher targeting ability than HA free polymer nano-drug carriers, which improves the enrichment of curcumin in the skin and the therapeutic effect of curcumin on psoriasis. In addition to CD44 targeting, HA has excellent water-absorbing and moisturizing properties. Vicent et al. prepared the polymer nano-drug delivery system (Figure 6-11(b)) by co-assembly of poly-L-glutamate (PGA) with conjugated psoriatic drug, fluocinolone acetonide, and HA-PGA. The drug delivery system have greater skin penetration depth than a PGA-drug conjugate. The mechanism may be related to the increase of water content in stratum corneum and epidermis due to the water absorption of HA. Under the combined action of acid and enzyme, the drug can be released from the carriers to achieve the treatment of psoriasis.

6.5.11 The applications of polymer nano-drug carriers in enhancing the phototherapy of psoriasis

Besides using ultraviolet light, photodynamic therapy using near-infrared light has also been used in the treatment of psoriasis. Li et al. prepared a single molecule micelle drug carrier (Figure 6-11(c)) with a size of about 30 nm by using the amphiphilic zinc phthalocyanine -Brij 58 conjugate. Zinc phthalocyanine can absorb near-infrared light of 600-800 nm (Figure 6-11(d)), and can produce singlet oxygen under near-infrared light to realize the treatment of psoriasis.

Although polymer nano-drug carriers can improve the skin penetration ability of drugs to a certain extent, most polymer nano-drug carriers still remain in the upper epidermis, and their skin penetration depth and drug delivery efficiency are still limited. To further improve the therapeutic effect of psoriasis, combining polymer nano-drug delivery system with ionosmosis therapy, microneedles and other physical enhancement method can improve the utilization rate and therapeutic effect of drugs. The relevant content is discussed in other chapters about psoriasis in this textbook.

6.6   Challenges and Perspectives

The clinical translation of nano-drug is the final goal of the research on nano-drug, which is also a major difficulty in the research on nano-drug. Currently, most of the FDA-approved nano-drug carriers for clinical application are liposome formulation. Currently, there are 19 liposome formulations that have been approved for the treatment of various diseases, including eight drugs for cancer treatment. Many polymer-based drug delivery systems are promising for clinical transformation. For example, PTX-loaded PEG-*b*-PLA micelles (Genexol-PM) have been approved for the treatment of breast cancer, and nano-spheres of albumin-PTX-conjugates (abraxane) have been approved for the treatment of pancreatic and ovarian cancer. Currently, no polymer-based nano-drug carriers have been approved for the treatment of melanoma or psoriasis, but some polymer-based nano-drug delivery systems for melanoma have entered the clinical trial stage, such as the albumin-PTX-conjugated nano-drug delivery system.

The clinical translation of polymer nano-drug carriers is a complex question, which involves the change of pharmacokinetic of drug loaded in nano-drug carriers, the enhanced tumor accumulation of drug and therapeutic effect, the degradation and metabolism, potential toxic and side effects of the carrier materials, and its standardized production capacity. To improve the clinical translation potential of polymer nano-drug carriers, degradable and metabolic materials should be used as much as possible in the design of the carriers. In addition, besides introducing imaging and therapeutic functions to the nanomaterials, we should focus on investing the principles of interaction between nanomaterials and biological systems. At the same time, the currently used animal models cannot completely simulate the characteristics of human melanoma or psoriasis, and how to build a more realistic animal model to verify the therapeutic effect of nano-drug is also a problem that needs to be solved. The development of nano-drug is an interdisciplinary research direction, which requires the joint efforts of experts from all disciplines and fields to promote its clinical translation process.

Compared with the skin disease treatment, polymer nano-drug carriers for cosmetic dermatology were developed much faster (see chapter 9). More and more cosmetic dermatology products containing polymer nano-drug carriers have been developed and entered the market.

Questions

1. Please compare the advantages and disadvantages of polymer nano-drug carriers with inorganic ones.

2. Which parameters affect CMC of block copolymers?

3. Please compare the size of polymer nano-drug carriers measured by DLS with that observed under TEM or SEM.

4. Please describe the advantages of polymer nano-drug carriers in the treatment of melanoma.

5. Please describe the advantages of polymer nano-drug carriers in the treatment of psoriasis.

Extended reading

[1] Deng R, Derry M J, Mable C, et al. Using dynamic covalent chemistry to drive morphological transitions: controlled release of encapsulated nanoparticles from block copolymer vesicles[J]. J Am Chem Soc, 2017, 139(22): 7616-7623.

[2] Yu X, Zhao Z, Nie W, et al. Biodegradable polymer microcapsules fabrication through a template-free approach[J]. Langmuir, 2011, 27(16): 10265-10273.

[3] Helvig S, Azmi I D M, Moghimi S M, et al. Recent advances in cryo-TEM imaging of soft lipid nanoparticles[J]. AIMS Biophysics, 2015, 2(2): 116-130.

[4] Park J, Brust T F, Lee H J, et al. Polydopamine-based simple and versatile surface modification of polymeric nano drug carriers[J]. ACS Nano, 2014, 8(4): 3347-3356.

[5] Ali I, Rahis-Uddin, Salim K, et al. Advances in nano drugs for cancer chemotherapy[J]. Curr Cancer Drug Targets, 2011, 11(2): 135-146.

(Deng Renhua   Liu Yijing   Li Yuce)

第七章
生物医用高分子在黑素瘤免疫治疗中的应用

第一节　黑素瘤免疫治疗概述

肿瘤免疫治疗是运用免疫学原理,采取主动或被动的方式来增强机体的抗肿瘤免疫应答,以达到抑制肿瘤生长、清除肿瘤细胞目的的方法。2011年之后,肿瘤免疫治疗已逐渐成为医学领域的研究热点(图7-1)。肿瘤免疫治疗主要由三大部分组成:①非特异性免疫治疗,主要是指使用重组白细胞介素-2(interleukin-2,IL-2)及干扰素等细胞因子,激活或促进患者免疫细胞杀伤功能的治疗;②主动特异性免疫治疗,主要是指使用自身肿瘤细胞、肿瘤蛋白、多肽片段或肿瘤载体制成肿瘤疫苗来免疫患者,激活自体免疫,从而增强抗肿瘤效应的治疗;③被动免疫治疗,包括过继性细胞免疫治疗以及单克隆抗体治疗(见扩展阅读1)。

抗肿瘤免疫反应是一系列逐步发生的事件(图7-2)。简言之,肿瘤细胞的坏死或凋亡诱导肿瘤抗原的释放,所释放的抗原通常被抗原呈递细胞(antigen-presenting cells,APCs)捕获。随后,APCs在主要组织相容性复合体Ⅰ(major histocompatibility complex Ⅰ,MHC-Ⅰ)类分子和主要组织相容性复合体Ⅱ(MHC-Ⅱ)类分子上呈现抗原肽,以激活淋巴结中的未成熟T细胞。活化的T细胞通过T细胞受体(T cell receptor,TCR)和MHC抗原肽复合物之间的相互作用进入肿瘤微环境(tumor microenvironment,TME),并靶向肿瘤细胞。肿瘤特异性T细胞一经识别,可通过诱导细胞凋亡来清除肿瘤细胞。肿瘤细胞的死亡导致额外的肿瘤抗原的释放,从而进一步加强肿瘤免疫周期的后续循环。以上过程称为肿瘤免疫循环。在肿瘤免疫周期中,存在众多发挥作用的因素,这为肿瘤的治疗提供了广泛的潜在治疗靶点(见扩展阅读2)。

目前,美国食品药品监督管理局(Food and Drug Administration,FDA)批准用于黑素瘤免疫治疗的药物如下:细胞因子IL-2;免疫检查点抑制剂,如伊匹单抗 ipilimumab(Yervoy),其作用靶点为细胞毒性T细胞相关蛋白4(cytotoxic T lymphocyte-associated protein 4,CTLA-4),帕博利珠单抗 pembrolizumab(Keytruda),其作用靶点为程序性细胞死亡蛋白1(programmed cell death protein 1,PD-1),及纳武单抗 nivolumab(Opdivo),其作用靶点为PD-1。相关内容在前文中已详细介绍,请参照第2章第2节。

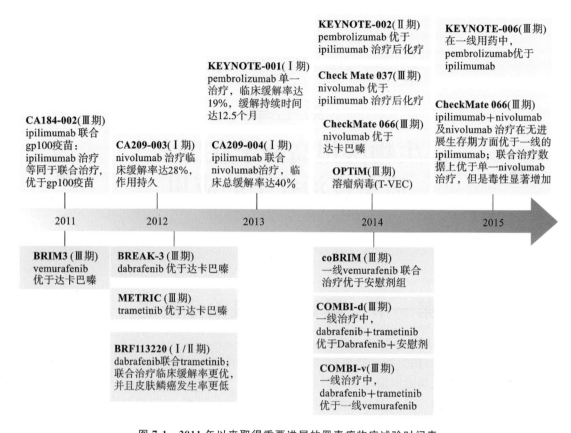

图 7-1　2011 年以来取得重要进展的黑素瘤临床试验时间表

Figure 7-1　The seminal timeline chart for practice-changing clinical trials in advanced-stage melanoma since 2011

除了已获得美国 FDA 批准的免疫治疗药物外,还有一些新的黑素瘤免疫治疗药物正处于研究阶段,如单克隆抗体 varlilumab、单克隆抗体 MGA271、细胞因子和肿瘤疫苗等(见扩展阅读 3)。例如,通过靶向 CD27 来加强 T 细胞、自然杀伤细胞(natural killer cell,NK 细胞)的免疫效应的单克隆抗体 varlilumab 正处于治疗转移性黑素瘤的临床试验 I 期。CD27 是 T 细胞的共刺激受体,属于肿瘤坏死因子 α(tumor necrosis factor α,TNF-α)受体超家族成员,在 T 细胞的生存、活化及 NK 细胞的增殖、细胞毒活性中发挥重要作用。抗 B7-H3 的单克隆抗体 MGA271 目前正处于黑素瘤治疗的临床试验 I 期。B7-H3 是 B7 受体家族成员,表达于 APCs 和其他非淋巴组织细胞。B7-H3 对 T 细胞的调节功能目前还存在一定的争议:一些研究表明 B7-H3 是共刺激受体,而另一些研究显示,B7-H3 对受体有抑制效应。此外,一些细胞因子,如粒细胞-巨噬细胞集落刺激因子(granulocyte-macrophage colony-stimulating factor,GM-CSF)、IL-2、白细胞介素-15(interleukin-15,IL-15)、白细胞介素-18(interleukin 18,IL-18)、白细胞介素-21(interleukin-21,IL-21)等,均具有抗肿瘤效应,目前在黑素瘤的治疗中正处于临床试验阶段。

肿瘤疫苗是黑素瘤免疫治疗的另一重要内容,目前已经取得了一些研究进展。肿瘤细胞表面的抗原通常通过多种机制来进行修饰,抑制机体内的免疫细胞对其进行识别,阻碍了机体对肿瘤细胞的清除。黑素瘤疫苗是利用黑素瘤相关抗原(如肿瘤细胞、肿瘤相关蛋白或多肽、表达肿瘤抗原的基因)制备而成的。这些黑素瘤疫苗注射到肿瘤或患者体内后,由 APCs 摄取

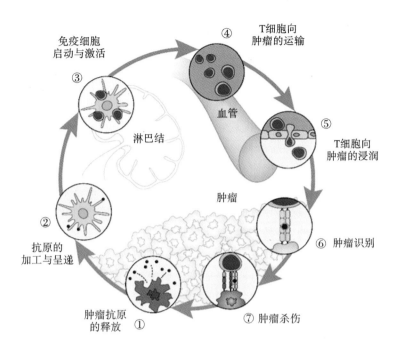

图 7-2 肿瘤免疫循环示意图

抗肿瘤免疫反应的产生是一系列的阶段性事件,包括肿瘤抗原的释放,抗原的加工与呈递,APCs 和 T 细胞的启动与激活,抗原特异性细胞毒性 T 细胞(cytotoxic T lymphocytes,CTLs)向肿瘤部位的运输和浸润,以及对肿瘤细胞识别和清除。

Figure 7-2 Illustration of the tumor immune cycle

The production of anti-tumor immune response is a series of stepwise events, including antigen release by tumor cells, antigen processing and presentation by APCs, priming and stimulation of APCs and T cells, transportation and infiltration of CTLs to the tumor site, and the recognition and eliminating of tumor cells.

并呈递给免疫细胞,使机体 T 细胞致敏、活化,从而克服肿瘤引起的免疫抑制状态,增强免疫原性,产生抗原特异性细胞免疫反应来杀伤黑素瘤细胞,进而抑制黑素瘤的生长、转移及复发。MAGE、gp100、Melan A、NY-ESO 等是常用于制备黑素瘤疫苗的肿瘤抗原,它们能够激活黑素瘤抗原特异性免疫反应来诱导机体抗黑素瘤效应,有望成为黑素瘤免疫治疗的有效靶点。

APCs 是指能够摄取、加工处理抗原,并将处理过的抗原呈递给 T 细胞的一类免疫细胞。树突状细胞(dendritic cells,DCs)是一类功能最强的抗原呈递细胞,是肿瘤免疫治疗的启动子和重要靶点,在固有和适应性免疫激活中发挥着重要作用。DCs 主要通过两种途径介导抗原呈递:①通过胞吞作用摄取外源性抗原蛋白,蛋白分子在溶酶体中降解为多肽片段,并由 MHC-Ⅱ类分子呈递给辅助性 T(T-helper,Th)细胞,如 $CD4^+$ T 细胞;②通过降解 DCs 胞质中的内源性抗原蛋白,降解所产生的多肽片段与 MHC-Ⅰ类分子结合,呈递给 $CD8^+$ T 细胞,从而激活 CTLs,进一步浸润肿瘤组织,识别肿瘤细胞表面表达的 MHC-Ⅰ抗原复合物,启动对肿瘤细胞的杀伤。诱导肿瘤特异性 CTLs 的产生并对肿瘤细胞特异性杀伤是实现肿瘤有效免疫治疗的重要途径。同时,活化的 $CD8^+$ T 细胞不仅能够直接杀死肿瘤细胞,还可获得持久的记忆表型,对预防肿瘤的复发具有重要意义。此外,$CD4^+$ T 细胞通过增强肿瘤部位 CTLs 的克隆性扩增和促进记忆表型的产生和维持,促进有效的抗肿瘤反应的获得。DCs 通过 MHC-Ⅰ/Ⅱ类分子的抗原呈递诱导 Th 细胞和 CTLs 的产生和活化,这已成为肿瘤疫苗临床试验的理论基础。

根据黑素瘤抗原的不同,黑素瘤疫苗可分为肿瘤抗原肽疫苗、肿瘤相关抗原疫苗和肿瘤DNA疫苗。以多肽为抗原而形成的疫苗称为肿瘤抗原肽疫苗,其可通过活化DCs来激活患者自身的免疫系统,从而产生针对黑素瘤细胞的主动免疫反应。黑素瘤抗原肽疫苗在杀伤肿瘤细胞的过程中具有特异性高、毒副作用很小等优势。肿瘤相关抗原(tumor-associated antigen,TAA)是由肿瘤细胞产生的抗原,可在宿主内触发免疫反应。全肿瘤细胞裂解物(tumor cell lysate,TCL)作为肿瘤抗原已被应用于肿瘤疫苗的研制。与特定的蛋白或者多肽肿瘤抗原相比,全肿瘤细胞来源的抗原在肿瘤疫苗中具有诸多优势:可通过诱导CTLs反应和CD4⁺ T细胞的活化来提供潜在肿瘤抗原的全面来源,其所包含的多种肿瘤抗原可同时靶向肿瘤细胞,从而避免肿瘤抗原缺失导致的免疫豁免。然而,含有抗原和细胞因子的可溶性肿瘤细胞裂解物本质上是不稳定的,容易产生DCs摄取不良、抗原交叉呈递效率低和CTLs反应诱导受限等问题。

基因相关的肿瘤免疫治疗已成为许多癌症治疗研究的热点方向,具有从源头上有效地治疗疾病、消除或预防遗传性疾病的能力,在黑素瘤治疗中表现出了巨大的潜力。DNA疫苗涉及使用抗原编码的DNA诱导免疫反应,在癌症和传染病领域已得到了广泛的应用。DCs是人体内最有效的抗原呈递细胞,在DNA疫苗中发挥着重要作用。抗原编码的DNA需要被体内的APCs(如DCs、巨噬细胞和B细胞)识别,随后利用其蛋白酶体复合物来转染APCs,并将表达的抗原蛋白切割成小肽片段,最后将所得的小抗原片段与MHC-Ⅰ类和MHC-Ⅱ类分子结合,并呈递给T细胞。同时,DCs表面相关的甘露糖受体(mannose receptors,MRs)可识别细胞表面或病原体细胞壁上的多种糖分子,通过参与受体介导的吞噬作用来维持内环境的稳定,并将固有免疫与适应性免疫结合,构成机体的免疫防御系统。此外,从分子水平上干预肿瘤信号转导通路可为抗肿瘤治疗提供一种新思路。PUMA(p53上调的凋亡调控因子)是Bcl-2蛋白家族中的一员,是p53的下游基因,具有促凋亡作用。PUMA可诱导多种肿瘤细胞凋亡,从而抑制肿瘤细胞增殖。

近年来,发展预防或治疗性疫苗的策略主要包括改善体内特定DCs的抗原呈递效率和延长疫苗活性两个方面。随着人们对肿瘤免疫反应认识的深入和肿瘤免疫治疗的迅速发展,免疫佐剂作为一种免疫增强剂在肿瘤疫苗设计中得到了广泛的应用。免疫佐剂可非特异性地通过上调免疫细胞表面分子的表达、促进固有免疫应答等方式增强机体特异性免疫。有效的肿瘤疫苗需要合适的佐剂来增强抗原呈递效率、抗原免疫原性和抗原诱导的免疫效应。抗原和免疫佐剂的共呈递有望增强肿瘤特异性T细胞的免疫应答,可降低肿瘤免疫逃逸的可能性,并减少对单一抗原的免疫耐受性。Montanide ISA 51和720是被临床认可的免疫佐剂,通过刺激体液免疫反应和细胞免疫反应增强肿瘤细胞的免疫原性。另外,单磷酰脂质A(monophosphoryl lipid A,MPLA)是一种Toll样受体4(Toll-like receptors 4,TLR4)激动剂,通常被用于增强抗病毒和抗肿瘤的免疫反应。APCs中TLR的刺激可激活细胞内信号通路,最终诱导炎症细胞因子、趋化因子、干扰素和协同共刺激分子的上调,为T细胞刺激提供适当的环境。然而,MPLA具有较长的疏水性烷基链,这导致其水溶性较差,且限制了其在肿瘤疫苗中的广泛应用。因此,开发更高效的载体用于肿瘤抗原和免疫佐剂的共呈递具有重要的意义。

与传统疗法相比,用于黑素瘤治疗的免疫疗法在客观缓解率、疾病进展时间和患者总生存率等方面有了相当大的改善。然而,不同的免疫疗法也各有其局限性。例如,在免疫检查点阻断方面,免疫疗法取得了前所未有的成功;但不幸的是,只有小部分患者对免疫疗法有反应。临床结果表明,只有 15% 的患者可响应伊匹单抗,不超过 40% 的患者响应抗-PD-1(anti-programmed cell death protein 1,aPD-1)/程序性死亡因子配体 1(programmed death-ligand 1,PD-L1)抗体。肿瘤相关抗原疫苗存在稳定性差、半衰期短和在血浆中容易降解、基因片段摄取率低、易被核酸酶降解等问题。此外,由于不可控的组织累积和不确定的免疫治疗药物的组成及生物活性,大多数免疫治疗策略面临免疫相关不良事件的风险,如低钾血症、垂体炎、心肌炎、糖尿病和甲状腺功能障碍等。当发生免疫相关不良事件时,许多患者不得不停止治疗,这进一步限制了免疫治疗的效果。因此,提高免疫治疗反应率、减少毒副作用对免疫治疗具有重要的意义。

生物医用高分子材料的发展及其在黑素瘤免疫治疗中的应用为清除黑素瘤免疫治疗的各种障碍带来了希望。例如,高分子材料可防止抗原肽被蛋白酶降解;可在抗原和免疫佐剂的共呈递中控制抗原的释放并延长抗原的呈递时间;可作为基因载体,增强结构可塑性、精确性;可抵抗核酸酶降解,增强基因的稳定性和降低毒性等。除了通过包封肿瘤抗原和基因来辅助黑素瘤的免疫治疗外,对于其他黑素瘤成分,辅助使用生物医用高分子材料也可强化机体特异性免疫应答从而起到有效的抗肿瘤作用。将黑素瘤免疫治疗与生物医用高分子材料结合,可将现有利用黑素瘤抗原、基因片段和其他黑素瘤成分进行免疫治疗的方式进行优化,有望解决黑素瘤免疫治疗的现存问题。

第二节 用于黑素瘤免疫治疗的生物医用高分子载药体系

生物医用高分子材料可在克服与免疫疗法相关的关键挑战中发挥重要作用。该类材料可通过改善药物的循环次数、组织归巢、组织穿透等来改善其在体内的生物分布,并通过抗原的缓慢释放和产生免疫记忆提高肿瘤免疫治疗的可持续性,从而促进免疫佐剂材料或其他肿瘤治疗方式协同治疗,产生更有效的黑素瘤免疫治疗(见扩展阅读 4)。根据其大小,用于黑素瘤免疫治疗的高分子载体材料可分为聚合物纳米材料、聚合物微米材料和聚合物宏观尺寸材料。

一、聚合物纳米材料

随着纳米技术的飞速发展,聚合物纳米材料作为治疗药物的载体在肿瘤诊断和治疗中得到了广泛的应用。聚合物纳米材料可保护药物分子不被降解,可改变细胞摄取、体内分布、代谢和清除的途径等,可增强药物的有效性和减少药物的副作用。聚合物纳米材料是肿瘤免疫治疗中最常用的载体材料。除了上述所提到的优势外,聚合物纳米材料还可以通过增加 APCs 对抗原的摄取、增强 APCs 对抗原的呈递、诱导 CTLs 应答、传递细胞因子和抗体来调节免疫抑制 TME。根据聚合物纳米材料的形态,聚合物纳米材料可分为聚合物纳米颗粒、纳米凝胶、纳米囊泡和纳米胶束等。

(一) 聚合物纳米颗粒

聚合物纳米颗粒在黑素瘤免疫治疗中已被广泛地研究。其中,聚乳酸-羟基乙酸(poly(lactic-co-glycolic acid),PLGA)纳米颗粒具有良好的安全性、易合成性和适应性等优势,已成为药物传递和免疫治疗的重要材料。而且,PLGA 纳米颗粒易于结合或修饰药物、细胞因子、抗体和其他免疫调节剂等,因此产生了一系列基于 PLGA 纳米颗粒的肿瘤免疫治疗策略。

PLGA 纳米颗粒通过包覆抗原来形成肿瘤疫苗,可提高抗原的呈递效率,保护药物分子不被降解。例如,Sasada 等采用 PLGA 纳米颗粒经皮共递送黑素瘤特异性抗原肽(TRP2 和 GP100)和弗氏完全佐剂(Freund's complete adjuvant,FCA),可在黑素瘤荷瘤小鼠体内诱导强效的 CTLs 反应。包覆模式抗原卵清蛋白(ovalbumin,OVA)、免疫佐剂聚肌胞苷酸(polyinosinic:polycytidylic acid,poly(I:C))和瑞喹莫德(TLR7/8 激动剂,R848)的 PEG 修饰的 PLGA 纳米颗粒,可触发核内体的 TLRs,并诱导表达 OVA 的黑素瘤小鼠产生有效的抗肿瘤免疫反应。PLGA 纳米颗粒可包覆小分子抑制剂来实现对黑素瘤的免疫治疗。例如,Lavasanifar 等在 2010 年采用 PLGA 纳米颗粒将 STAT3 的小分子抑制剂 JSI-124 递送到肿瘤和免疫抑制的 DCs,在体外通过 JSI-124 在肿瘤细胞和免疫抑制的 DCs 中调节抗黑素瘤免疫响应。PLGA 纳米颗粒共同递送抗癌药物紫杉醇(paclitaxel,PTX)和免疫刺激剂脂多糖的无毒衍生物(SP-LPS),实现化疗和免疫治疗的联用,从而增强其体外对黑素瘤细胞的杀伤效应。此外,包覆 TLR7/8 激动剂的 PLGA 纳米颗粒使 DCs 通过 MHC-Ⅰ过程来增强共刺激分子的表达和抗原的呈递,在黑素瘤模型中具有显著的黑素瘤预防和治疗效果。PLGA 纳米颗粒还可用于递送免疫检查点抑制剂。例如,Wang 等采用 PLGA 纳米颗粒共同递送 aPD-1 和抗 OX40(一种刺激性抗体来激活成本化受体),其在两种黑素瘤模型中均有明显的黑素瘤治疗效果。2017 年,Goldberg 等开发了 aPD-1 修饰的 PLGA 纳米颗粒来靶向 T 细胞,并同时释放 R848 和 SD-208(转化生长因子-β(TGF-β)受体抑制剂),以打破 TGF-β 的免疫抑制作用,从而增强其抗肿瘤反应。此外,PLGA 纳米颗粒还可用于调控肿瘤相关巨噬细胞(tumor-associated macrophages,TAMs),从而激活机体抗肿瘤免疫。例如,2018 年,Chen 等利用 PLGA 纳米颗粒来递送活性氧(reactive oxygen species,ROS)生成物,使 TAMs 向 M1 表型极化,随后招募协调 CTLs,从而有效地抑制肿瘤的发展,并在一定程度上预防肿瘤的复发。

另外,利用 PLGA 纳米颗粒可实现肿瘤免疫治疗,与化疗、光热治疗、光动力治疗、放射治疗等肿瘤治疗策略联合,从而实现对黑素瘤的有效治疗。一些研究小组将光热转换材料加入 PLGA 纳米颗粒中,以实现光热治疗(photothermal therapy,PTT)和免疫治疗的联合应用,并进一步联合免疫检查点抑制剂建立黑素瘤的光热免疫协同治疗。2018 年,You 等报道了一种结合 PD-1 阻断剂和光热消融治疗黑素瘤的策略,构建了 aPD-1 和中空金纳米壳共包覆的 PLGA 纳米颗粒。研究结果表明,该复合纳米颗粒具有较强的抗肿瘤效应,可消除大部分原发肿瘤,并能显著抑制远端未治疗的原发肿瘤的生长。Yang 等在 2019 年构建了具有核壳结构的 PLGA 纳米颗粒,以 aPD-1 和全氟戊烷(perfluorinated pentane,PFP)液体作为核,以 PLGA 作为壳层,其中 PLGA 纳米颗粒的表面用聚乙二醇(poly(ethylene glycol),PEG)和 gly-argy-asp-ser(GRGDS)肽进行修饰,并在 PLGA 纳米颗粒的壳中包覆氧化铁纳米颗粒。该杂化纳米颗粒表现出了优异的黑素瘤光热免疫协同治疗效果。2018 年,Kim 等设计了一种层层杂化的 PLGA 纳米颗粒,该纳米颗粒通过封装红外染料 IR-780 碘化物和化疗药物伊马替尼,实现黑素瘤的协同 PTT 和光动力治疗(photodynamic therapy,PDT)。该纳米颗粒产生的热效应和 ROS,能有效地杀伤黑素瘤细胞并下调肿瘤内调节性 T 细胞(regulatory cell,Treg)的功能。2017 年,Wang 等报道了一种肿瘤放疗与免疫治疗协同应用的策略:首先对肿瘤进行放疗,随后用 PLGA 纳米颗粒选择性地捕获肿瘤抗原,以供 DCs 呈递,从而激活机体抗原特异性抗肿瘤反应(图 7-3)。放疗与免疫检查点抑制剂抗程序性细胞死亡蛋白 1(anti-programmed cell death protein 1,aPD-1)的协同应用,可实现显著的远端肿瘤的消融。

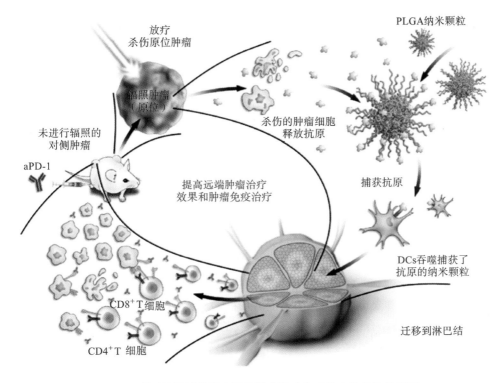

图 7-3　利用抗原捕获纳米颗粒提高肿瘤免疫治疗效果的示意图

Figure 7-3　Schematic depiction of utilizing of antigen-capture nanoparticles (AC-NPs) to improve cancer immunotherapy

　　然而,PLGA 的降解产物是酸性的,这可能会降低所封装药物的稳定性并在与其邻近的组织产生轻微炎症。除了 PLGA 纳米颗粒外,还有许多其他的聚合物纳米颗粒已被用于免疫治疗,如聚丙烯硫化物(polypropylene sulfide,PPS)纳米颗粒、聚丙烯聚乙二醇(polypropylene poly(ethylene glycol),PPG)纳米颗粒、聚己内酯(polycaprolactone,PCL)纳米颗粒等。PPS 是一种机械强度良好的有机热塑性材料,易被活性氧(reactive oxygen species,ROS)降解,可用于药物递送领域。Hubbell 等制备的粒径为 30 nm 的 PPS 纳米颗粒可有效地靶向淋巴结中的 DCs(CD11c$^+$),从而在肿瘤引流淋巴结内累积。同时,共包覆黑素瘤抗原和免疫佐剂 CpG 寡脱氧核苷酸(CpG oligonucleotide,CpG ODN)或紫杉醇的 PPS 纳米颗粒,可增加肿瘤内抗原特异性 CD8$^+$ T 细胞,从而刺激有效的抗肿瘤免疫响应,抑制黑素瘤的生长。Florindo 等构建了甘露糖功能化脂肪族聚醚基纳米颗粒,实现了黑素瘤相关抗原、TLR 配体 poly(I:C) 和 CpG ODN 的共载;该纳米颗粒可用于靶向抗原呈递细胞,可有效增强 Th1 免疫反应,在治疗和预防模型中可有效地抑制黑素瘤的生长。

(二)纳米凝胶

　　纳米凝胶是黑素瘤免疫治疗的主要载体材料。纳米凝胶由天然聚合物(如多糖、多肽和核酸)、合成聚合物(如聚乙二醇(PEG)和聚 N-异丙基丙烯酰胺(PNIPAM))或其组合制成,是目前在黑素瘤免疫治疗中研究得较多的纳米材料。与上述讨论的聚合物纳米颗粒相比,纳米凝胶具有柔性,可改善纳米颗粒的体内循环、体内生物分布,并具有免疫佐剂效应。例如,Ma 等合成了一种具有两亲性且 pH 敏感的半乳糖右旋视黄醛纳米凝胶,通过负载模式抗原 OVA 构建了一种自佐剂肿瘤疫苗。该疫苗可促进 DCs 的成熟、抗原的摄取和胞质抗原的释放,从而进一步增强 MHC-I 抗原呈递,引发较强的抗黑素瘤免疫反应。Nostrum 等用阳离子葡聚糖纳米凝胶作为载体,通过二硫键结合模型抗原 OVA,从而构建肿瘤疫苗。该疫苗联合免疫佐剂 poly(I:C),在肿瘤预防模型和治疗模型中产生了强烈的抗肿瘤免疫反应,有效地抑制了肿瘤的发生和发展。Wang 等通过沉淀聚合的方法合成了一种以多肽为化学交联剂,以 N-异丙基丙烯酰胺(NIPAAM)为支架的酶响应多肽-交联纳米凝胶。该纳米凝胶可高效地包封肿瘤转移抑制肽 P-5m,对转移性黑素瘤具有显著的抑制作用。

(三)纳米囊泡

纳米囊泡具有核壳结构,其壳层通常由两亲性材料(如脂类、聚合物或蛋白质)自组装而成,其内核是亲水储层。用于黑素瘤免疫治疗的纳米囊泡主要有三种:聚合物纳米囊泡、聚电解质多层纳米囊泡、DNA 纳米囊泡。聚合物纳米囊泡由两亲性嵌段共聚物的双层膜组成,可将药物包封在囊泡膜内或水相内核。例如,Moon 等采用单层膜阳离子脂质体和透明质酸构建交联的多层脂质体聚合物纳米囊泡,通过协同递送模式抗原 OVA、免疫佐剂 CpG ODN 和化疗药物米托蒽醌,从而实现增强的抗肿瘤免疫反应。Qiu 等将 PEG 与弱阳离子聚合物复合制备了聚合物纳米囊泡,该囊泡可递送编码 IL-12 的质粒,从而有效地抑制肿瘤生长。Stephan 等还开发了一种聚合物囊泡,该囊泡的核由 DNA 混合的聚氨基酯水凝胶形成,壳层由可与 T 细胞靶向配体结合的聚谷氨酸组成,合成的 DNA 纳米载体可对特异性 T 细胞进行原位编程。最近,Wilson 等构建了内溶聚合体来增加刺激性激动剂环鸟苷-磷酸腺苷-磷酸(cyclic guanosine monophosphateadenosine monophosphate,cGAMP)的活性,从而抑制肿瘤生长、延长机体生存时间,并增加免疫记忆。聚电解质多层(polyelectrolyte multilayer,PEM)纳米囊泡与聚合物纳米囊泡类似,其壳层由静电吸附的聚阳离子和聚阴离子组成。Jewell 等使用阳离子的聚(β-氨基酯)和 TLRs 激动剂 CpG ODN 通过静电相互作用制备了聚电解质多层纳米囊泡,以激发机体较强的抗黑素瘤免疫反应。DNA 纳米囊泡主要由 DNA 组成,在酶的作用下通过滚环扩增形成笼状纳米结构,可对不同药物分子进行包覆。2016 年,Gu 等以包含了间隔 CpG 序列和酶切位点的单链 DNA 长链为原料,制备了 DNA 纳米茧并包覆 aPD-1。在蛋白水解酶的作用下,该 DNA 纳米茧释放 CpG ODN 和 aPD-1,可用于肿瘤切除术后预防性复发治疗,在转移性黑素瘤模型中显著抑制了转移性结节的形成(图 7-4)。

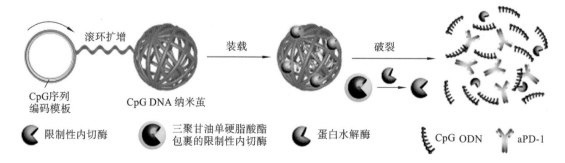

图 7-4 炎症条件下 DNA 纳米茧传递 CpG ODN 和 aPD-1 的示意图

Figure 7-4 Schematic illustration of delivery of CpG ODN and anti-PD-1 antibody (aPD-1) by DNA nanococoons under an inflammation condition

（四）纳米胶束

纳米胶束是两亲性聚合物分子在水中自组装形成的结构。由于聚合物的组成、长度和与载体介质的相互作用不同，胶束具有丰富的形貌。胶束可共包覆不同的亲、疏水性药物，可直接调节免疫系统或作为肿瘤疫苗纳米载体。Li 等将 PEG 与 IDO（indoleamine 2，3-dioxygenase）抑制剂 NLG919 偶联所形成的前药自组装形成胶束，并包覆化疗药物紫杉醇；该复合胶束可以有效地逆转肿瘤免疫抑制，显著地提高对黑素瘤的治疗效果。Li 等报道了一种共负载光敏剂和可降低 PD-1 与 PD-L1 相互作用的小干扰 RNA（small interfering RNA，siRNA）的具有 pH 响应的阳离子胶束，用于实现黑素瘤的光动力协同免疫治疗。与单纯的光动力治疗相比，该多功能杂化胶束可显著抑制黑素瘤的生长和转移（图 7-5）。Gao 等合成的聚合物复合胶束不仅能增强抗原呈递和交叉呈递，而且可通过刺激干扰素基因的刺激因子途径来提高其抗肿瘤免疫效应，与免疫检查点抑制剂协同作用，从而实现对黑素瘤的治疗。

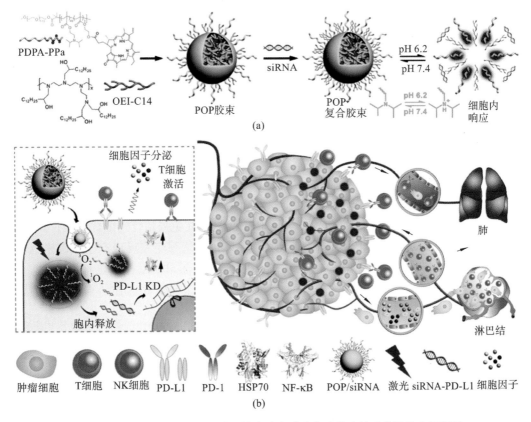

图 7-5 联合 PD-L1 阻断剂用于增强的光动力肿瘤免疫治疗的酸激活胶束示意图

Figure 7-5 Schematic illustration of the acid-activatable micelleplexes for PD-L1 blocker-enhanced photodynamic cancer immunotherapy

通过调控多肽的组成，可调控基于两亲性多肽的胶束的长度和聚合物序列等，从而有效地调控其在淋巴结中的累积、细胞摄取及免疫原性。此外，基于多肽的胶束可以很容易地沿着其冠状突起显示抗原，与抗原在胶束的不同位置结合，从而增加其抗原呈递能力，提高其疫苗效应。例如，Ma 等报道了基于聚乙二醇-b-聚（L-赖氨酸）-b-聚（L-亮氨酸）（PEG-PLL-PLLeu）杂化多肽的自组装阳离子胶束。该多肽胶束可同时封装 OVA 和 TLR3 激动多聚肌苷酸

(polyinosinic acid,PIC),作为一种简单有效的疫苗递送系统,以协同增强肿瘤特异性 CTLs 反应。

二、聚合物微米材料

聚合物微米材料在肿瘤免疫治疗中发挥着重要作用。聚合物微米材料的尺寸一般大于 1 μm,可与单个细胞相互作用;可激活、扩大免疫细胞群;与聚合物纳米材料相比,可提高药物(如抗体、细胞因子等)的递送效率;微尺度材料易变形,可调节其吞噬及在体内的分布。聚合物微米材料在肿瘤免疫治疗中的应用主要体现在两个方面:作为人工抗原呈递细胞(aAPCs),用于引发和扩增 T 细胞群;作为免疫治疗的药物(如抗体、细胞因子)载体,以增强对黑素瘤的免疫治疗效果。聚合物微米材料有望克服聚合物纳米材料在肿瘤免疫治疗中面临的问题(如组织归巢、体内循环等)。用于黑素瘤免疫治疗的聚合物微米材料主要有 PLGA、PLGA 杂化物、PLA 和聚苯乙烯等。从形貌上来区分,主要有聚合物微球和聚合物微胶囊。

(一)聚合物微球

在黑素瘤免疫治疗研究中,最常用的不可降解的聚合物微球材料是聚苯乙烯。Xie 等在聚苯乙烯微球表面修饰了 HLA-A2/肽四聚体和抗小鼠 CD28 单克隆抗体;该材料在 HLA-A2/Kb 转基因小鼠中能有效地进行抗原特异性 CTLs 增殖,识别人靶细胞表面内源性表达的肿瘤抗原,并以抗原特异性的方式杀伤肿瘤细胞。Liang 等在聚苯乙烯微球表面共包覆 H-2Kb-Ig/pTRP2 二聚体复合物、抗 CD28 抗体、4-1BBL 分子和 CD83 分子。该聚苯乙烯微球可从 C57BL/6 小鼠脾细胞中扩增出 pTRP2 特异性 CTLs,从而靶向黑素瘤细胞。

在黑素瘤免疫治疗研究中,最常用的可降解的聚合物微球材料是 PLGA。在 21 世纪初,研究人员发现 PLGA 微球可以稳定地包裹免疫调节物质(如人类乳头瘤病毒 16 E7、质粒 DNA),并安全、有效地递送给人体,这奠定了 PLGA 微球在免疫治疗中的优先地位。此后,人们对使用 PLGA 微球传递抗原、细胞因子和抗体来增加或增强免疫反应产生了越来越浓厚的兴趣。例如,2017 年,Schneck 等构建了基于 PLGA 并结合 aPD-1 检查点抑制剂的 aAPCs。该 aAPCs 可激活 CD8$^+$ T 细胞,并诱导 CD8$^+$ T 细胞最大限度地分泌 IFN-γ,从而延缓了黑素瘤的发生与发展。

(二)聚合物微胶囊

聚合物微胶囊具有核壳结构,因此有多相储存空间,从而可储存并递送高负载的亲水和疏水药物。亲水性区域可用来储存抗体、细胞因子和其他处于活性状态的蛋白质,可克服药物在包覆过程中暴露在有机溶剂中所造成的不稳定或失活。此外,由聚电解质层制成的微胶囊与类似材料制备的均质微球相比,微胶囊可改善抗原呈递,增强机体免疫应答。Andry 等报道了可降解的羟乙基淀粉(hydroxyethyl starch,HES)微胶囊,其粒径为 4~15 μm;负载牛血清白蛋白后可用于黑素瘤免疫治疗,增强抗原的呈递效应。此外,Ma 等利用一种通用的疫苗接种策略,在角鲨烯乳液的油水界面周围的球形纳米粒子上组装构建了一种粒径约为 10 μm 的 Pickering 乳液。Pickering 乳液保留了力依赖的变形能力和所呈递抗原的横向流动性,使其具有可调节的细胞吞噬及体内分布、较高的生物安全性和抗原负载能力。Pickering 乳液的核、壳和表面为抗原、佐剂和其他免疫调节剂等提供了有效的负载位点,随后呈递给 APCs 来增强黑素瘤疫苗的持久性和有效性。

三、聚合物宏观尺度材料

与浸润组织和细胞的微纳材料不同的是,宏观尺度材料具有较大的尺寸,可通过植入或局部注射作用于机体,从而招募并重新编程细胞来实现原位扩张 T 细胞,持续递送治疗药物;该材料也可用作合成的功能性免疫组织类似物(如人工淋巴结),因此受到了越来越多的关注。与系统给药相比,植入或局部注射的毒性低,可激活局部的免疫反应(见扩展阅读 5)。目前的研究中,用于黑素瘤免疫治疗的宏观尺度材料主要有高分子支架、水凝胶和聚合物微针等。

(一)高分子支架

生物高分子支架是一种特殊的免疫治疗材料,可以提供与周围微环境持续相互作用的结构和体积,克服免疫原性较差的问题,从而进一步提高免疫治疗效率,降低成本及毒副作用。较常用的高分子支架材料有 PLGA、聚乙烯-醋酸乙烯(poly(ethylene-vinyl acetate),PEVA)、胶原蛋白等。例如,Mooney 等开发了负载细胞因子 GM-CSF、危险信号和肿瘤抗原的微孔 PLGA 基质,来构建肿瘤疫苗,从而模拟对细菌感染的免疫反应。PLGA 支架释放 GM-CSF,作为被招募的 DCs 的居所,与抗原肿瘤裂解液和佐剂 CpG ODN 共同刺激、激活 DCs 并显著增强其对淋巴结的定位,产生特异性的抗黑素瘤免疫反应。

(二)水凝胶

与可植入高分子支架相比,水凝胶材料通常更柔软,更易于注射或喷射给药,使用方便且适用范围广。由于其可设计的机械和物理化学性质,水凝胶可控制各种治疗药物(如小分子药物、大分子药物)在不同时间和空间上的释放,从而保护药物免受机体降解,提高药物利用效率。其在空间和时间可调的交联、可降解性及药物的可控释放等特性,为其在细胞和各种免疫调节剂的输送中的应用提供了良好的基础。常用的水凝胶材料有合成聚合物水凝胶(如PEG)、海藻酸水凝胶、多肽水凝胶、天然提取物水凝胶(如透明质酸、壳聚糖、胶原蛋白等)。

一方面,水凝胶可用于递送免疫细胞因子,如 GM-CSF、TLR3 激动剂 poly(I:C)、肿瘤抗原及免疫检查点抑制剂等。例如,2014 年 Wang 等构建了一种可注射型温敏 PEG-PLGA 水凝胶。该水凝胶通过控制释放趋化剂 GM-CSF 来募集 DCs 和巨噬细胞,从而有效地提高机体的抗黑素瘤免疫效应。2015 年,Mooney 等发表了一项关于海绵状大孔海藻酸水凝胶的研究。该水凝胶以肿瘤细胞作为抗原,以 GM-CSF 作为 DCs 增强因子,以 CpG ODN 作为 DCs 激活因子,可诱发传统 DCs 和浆细胞样 DCs 组成的局部浸润,随后在黑素瘤模型中诱导有效、持久和高特异性的抗肿瘤 T 细胞反应。

另一方面,水凝胶可用于共递送免疫细胞因子、肿瘤全抗原或免疫检查点抑制剂。例如,Wang 等制备了一种可注射和自组装的聚(L-缬氨酸)凝胶,并用该水凝胶负载肿瘤细胞裂解物和免疫增强剂 TLR3 激动剂 poly(I:C),可引起 CTLs 免疫应答,从而获得良好的黑素瘤免疫治疗效果。Wang 等用多肽在水溶液中自组装形成了一种可注射的 PEG-b-聚(L-丙氨酸)水凝胶。将肿瘤细胞裂解液、GM-CSF、免疫检查点抑制剂(抗-CTLA-4/PD-1 抗体)共包覆于该水凝胶后,对黑素瘤有较好的免疫治疗效果。这种水凝胶联合免疫治疗不仅能显著增加小鼠脾脏和肿瘤内活化的效应因子 $CD8^+$ T 细胞,而且能降低 Treg 的比例。

通过响应 TME 中的酸性、升高的 ROS、温度等来构建响应性水凝胶,可有效地控制释放黑素瘤免疫治疗因子,从而实现增强的黑素瘤免疫治疗。2019 年,Gu 等构建了一个原位形成的双响应凝胶,用于局部协同递送脱甲基剂 zebularine(Zeb)和 aPD-1。先将 aPD-1 负载于

pH 敏感的 $CaCO_3$ 纳米颗粒中,再将上述 $CaCO_3$ 纳米颗粒和 Zeb 封装在 ROS 响应的水凝胶中,从而构建 ROS/pH 双响应凝胶。该水凝胶可响应肿瘤内的酸性和 ROS,控制药物释放,延长药物在肿瘤内的保留时间,从而有效地增强抗黑素瘤免疫反应。此外,2018 年,Gu 等构建了一种具有 ROS 响应的可注射聚多肽水凝胶;该水凝胶可有效负载并持续释放 aPD-L1 和 IDO 免疫抑制酶 D-1MT,能有效地降低局部 ROS 水平和促进免疫治疗因子的释放,从而增强体内抗黑素瘤免疫治疗效应。此外,Gu 等开发了喷雾型生物响应性纤维蛋白水凝胶,其中包含了预先负载 aCD47 抗体的 $CaCO_3$ 纳米颗粒;该纤维蛋白水凝胶可清除手术伤口中的 H^+,使肿瘤相关的巨噬细胞极化到 M1 表型(图 7-6);该免疫治疗纤维蛋白凝胶可"唤醒"宿主的固有和适应性免疫,从而抑制手术后肿瘤的局部复发和潜在的转移扩散。Lee 等设计了负载免疫调节因子 OVA 表达质粒 pOVA 的纳米级复合物和 GM-CSF 免疫增强因子的可智能注射左旋多巴和聚己内酯-丙交酯功能化的透明质酸的水凝胶;该水凝胶通过高效招募免疫细胞来有效地消除黑素瘤。

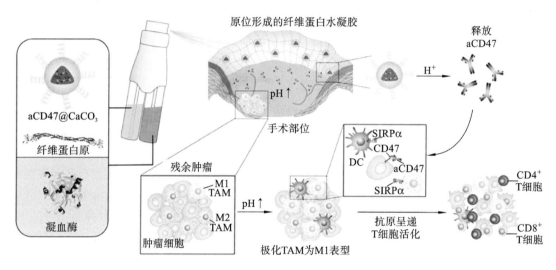

图 7-6　含有 aCD47@CaCO₃ 纳米颗粒的原位喷涂生物响应性纤维蛋白水凝胶在肿瘤切除后使用的示意图

Figure 7-6　Schematic showing the *in situ* sprayed bioresponsive fibrin hydrogel containing aCD47@CaCO₃ nanoparticles within the post-surgery tumor bed

此外,水凝胶还可联合免疫治疗与其他治疗方式,从而实现黑素瘤的免疫协同治疗。2018 年,Gu 等通过将 ROS 响应的连接剂与聚乙烯醇(poly(vinyl alcohol),PVA)交联得到 ROS 可降解水凝胶,并用其共包覆吉西他滨(gemcitabine,GEM)和 aPD-L1。基于肿瘤 TME 中丰富的 ROS,该水凝胶通过 ROS 响应控制释放化疗药物和 aPD-L1,实现了黑素瘤化疗与免疫治疗联合应用策略,从而增强了机体抗肿瘤免疫反应,有效地抑制了肿瘤的复发。同年,Yang 等构建了以合成的两亲性多肽 RADA₃₂(序列为 RADARADARADARADA)通过自组装形成的纳米纤维水凝胶,并用该纳米纤维水凝胶成功包覆化疗药物阿霉素(doxorubicin,DOX)和具有抗肿瘤作用的蜂毒肽。通过响应 TME,该水凝胶可有效控制释放其负载的药物,调节固有免疫细胞,消耗 M2 肿瘤相关巨噬细胞,从而实现黑素瘤的化疗与免疫治疗联合应用。2019 年,Lv 等设计了负载自交联 CpG ODN 纳米颗粒和光敏剂 IR820 的聚乙二醇水凝胶,实现光热免疫协同治疗;该水凝胶通过光热杀伤黑素瘤细胞,并诱导被杀伤的黑素瘤细胞释放黑素瘤相关抗原,从而有效地激发特异性抗肿瘤免疫反应。与单独的光热治疗相比,该水凝胶不仅能发挥有效的光热治疗作用清除原发肿瘤,同时也能激活机体全身抗肿瘤免疫响应,可实现更有效的全身协同的黑素瘤治疗。

（三）聚合物微针

微针技术是一种增强的经皮药物递送方式。在近 25 年中,微针阵列被广泛关注。微针是微米大小的针头,一般其长度为 $100 \sim 1000 \ \mu m$。微针经皮穿过角质层时,产生水孔,从而显著提高药物的渗透率。微针的类型主要包括固体微针、涂层微针、空心微针和可溶性微针。

固体微针可用于预处理皮肤以形成导管从而提高药物的渗透性;涂层微针将涂在微针表面的药物输送到皮肤;空心微针可通过微针空心将药物注入皮肤;可溶性微针通常是指可溶性聚合物微针,其可将封装在微针中的药物递送并完全溶解到皮肤内部。近年来,微针在透皮免疫调节中具有显著优势:①体积小;②无痛和微创;③可降低注射后微生物入侵的感染风险;④多功能和精确交付表皮;⑤方便,不需要专业培训进行管理,可提高患者的依从性和可负担性。固体微针、涂层微针、空心微针在疟疾、麻疹、流感、艾滋病等疾病的免疫治疗领域均有研究。可溶性微针(尤其是可溶性聚合物微针)在目前黑素瘤免疫治疗中得到了广泛的研究。

2013 年,Kissenpfennig 等采用可溶性甲基乙烯基醚-马来酸酐共聚物为微针基质,并在微针中负载包覆了抗原的 PLGA 纳米颗粒。一方面,该可溶性微针可靶向皮肤连续的 DCs 网状结构;皮肤 DCs 原位摄取抗原后,将负载抗原的 PLGA 纳米颗粒递送至皮肤引流淋巴结,从而显著促进 T 细胞的活化及增殖。该可溶性微针在小鼠体内可产生有效的抗原特异性细胞免疫响应,产生抗原特异性毒性 CD8$^+$ T 细胞,从而有效地抑制黑素瘤的生长。另一方面,该可溶性微针可使 PLGA 纳米颗粒包覆的抗原保留在皮肤层,从而提高抗原的稳定性。

从 2016 年开始,Gu 课题组构建了基于透明质酸(hyaluronic acid,HA)的不同微针,并研究了其对黑素瘤的免疫治疗效果。研究发现,可控释放机制能有效提高其对黑素瘤的免疫治疗效果并有效减少其毒副作用。首先,Gu 课题组构建了负载具有 pH 敏感性能的葡聚糖纳米颗粒的 HA 微针,其中葡聚糖纳米颗粒中共包覆葡萄糖氧化酶(glucose oxidase,GOx)、过氧化氢酶(catalase,CAT)和 aPD-1(图 7-7)。GOx 将葡萄糖和氧气转化为葡萄糖酸和过氧化氢。上述反应产生的过氧化氢在 CAT 的作用下被分解,从而进一步促进葡萄糖的降解,从而实现 aPD-1 在葡聚糖纳米颗粒中的可控持续释放。与瘤内分别注射同剂量的 aPD-1、不可控降解的微针相比,该 HA 微针可有效地激活机体抗黑素瘤免疫反应。同年,Gu 课题组构建了基于 HA 微针的黑素瘤协同免疫治疗策略。免疫抑制酶 IDO 的抑制剂 1-MT 通过共价键与 HA 连接后形成两亲性结构,通过自组装形成纳米颗粒并包覆 aPD-1。随后,他们制备了负载纳米颗粒的 HA 微针,该微针穿过角质层后,可局部共递送 aPD-1 和 1-MT,使其累积到局部黑素瘤周围的皮肤 DCs 网络中,从而延长药物在肿瘤部位的保留时间,并缓解系统给药可能引起的毒副作用。在 TME 中透明质酸酶的作用下,HA 发生降解,从而释放 aPD-1 和 1-MT。aPD-1 和 1-MT 的协同作用,可诱导强而持久的抗黑素瘤免疫响应。2017 年,Gu 等将黑色素和黑素瘤全抗原疫苗加入 HA 微针中。在近红外光照射下,微针在局部产生热量,可进一步增强 DCs 对抗原的吞噬、增加极化的 T 细胞的浸润、局部细胞因子的分泌,从而激活更强的抗肿瘤疫苗效应。2019 年,Hahn 等利用 HA 微针负载接枝了细胞毒性 T 细胞表位肽的 HA,可有效增强特异性 CTLs 的反应,从而抑制黑素瘤的生长。

2017 年,Jewell 等采用层层自组装的方法,在 PLA 微针阵列上交替吸附带正电荷的黑素瘤抗原和带负电荷的免疫佐剂 CpG ODN,其中聚电解质多层膜可达 128 层,厚度约 200 nm。

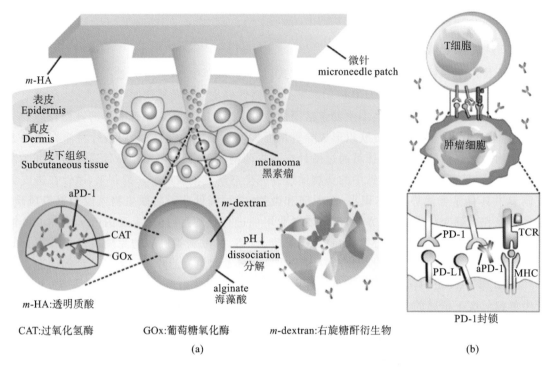

CAT:过氧化氢酶　　　　　GOx:葡萄糖氧化酶　　　　　m-dextran:右旋糖酐衍生物

(a)　　　　　　　　　　　　　　　　　　　　　(b)

图 7-7　负载抗程序性细胞死亡蛋白-1(aPD-1)的具有 pH 敏感性能的葡聚糖纳米颗粒的 HA 微针

Figure 7-7　Schematic of the MN patch-assisted delivery of aPD-1 for the skin cancer treatment

该 PLA 微针在体内可促进肿瘤特异性 CD8$^+$ T 细胞的有效增殖。2018 年,Lee 等采用 pH 响应的低聚磺胺甲嘧啶(oligo sulfamethazine)共轭的聚 β-氨基酸酯聚氨酯(poly(β-amino ester urethane))和一种合成的双链 RNA 免疫刺激佐剂 poly(I:C),通过层层自组装的方法构建负载纳米 DNA 疫苗的聚碳酸酯微针阵列,实现了免疫佐剂 poly(I:C)和卵清蛋白表达质粒(plasmid expressing ovalbumin,pOVA)的共递送,有效地抑制黑素瘤的生长和体内肺转移。2020 年,Lee 等构建聚多肽纳米复合物鸡尾酒微针,以阳离子聚多肽和 PEG 作为基质,采用高转染阳离子两亲性结合物共递送免疫佐剂 poly(I:C)和 pOVA,从而实现黑素瘤的免疫治疗。Wu 等构建了一种核壳结构的微针,共递送 aPD-L1 和 1-MT,用于黑素瘤的免疫治疗。其中,aPD-L1 通过较强的静电相互作用吸附到带电的壳层,并使其浓缩在微针尖端;PVA 是微针的主体,作为微针核壳结构中的核,具有丰富的氢键。PVA 与 1-MT 形成的较强的氢键相互作用,可抑制 1-MT 的结晶化。因此,1-MT 以过饱和的状态形成了均相药物-聚合物溶液,从而使 1-MT 以较高的载药量包覆于均一的微针中。与肿瘤内注射相同剂量的药物相比,包覆药物的具有核壳结构的微针具有较好的黑素瘤抑制效率。

第三节　挑战与展望

生物医用高分子材料可以保护负载的药物分子、黑素瘤抗原及免疫刺激因子免受周围生物环境的影响(如被各种酶降解等),同时延长其生物半衰期,并降低其系统毒性。高分子纳米药物载体也可以将负载的黑素瘤抗原靶向递送给专职 APCs,以提高抗原的呈递效率,从而提高黑素瘤抗原特异性 T 细胞的活化效率。高分子载体能够实现黑素瘤抗原和免疫佐剂的共递送,能够进一步提高抗原特异性 T 细胞的免疫效应,并能与其他免疫治疗方法协同作用,提高对黑素瘤的治疗效果。因此,高分子载体在黑素瘤免疫治疗中有很好的应用前景。虽然生物医用高分子在黑素瘤免疫治疗领域的研究已经取得了一定的进展,但是距离实现大规模的临床应用还有一段距离。一些基本的科学问题(如在不同器官中的分布及其代谢途径,急性毒性、亚慢性毒性、慢性毒性、遗传毒性和生殖毒性等)尚需要进一步解决。随着对各种高分子材料特性理解的深入,根据临床不同需求,制备不同纳米、微米材料或宏观尺度材料将进一步提高黑素瘤免疫治疗效果。

思 考 题

1. 如何实现亲、疏水性不同的抗原肽和(或)药物的共递送,从而提高黑素瘤抗原肽疫苗的免疫效应?

2. 如何实现纳米药物载体的 DCs 靶向?

3. 如何利用高分子材料激活机体免疫系统,实现原位黑素瘤和远端转移瘤的预防及治疗?

4. 如何利用高分子材料实现多种治疗方法的联合,提高黑素瘤的预防和治疗效果?

5. 在黑素瘤免疫治疗中,生物医用高分子材料的哪些性质是需要改进的? 可举例说明。

扩 展 阅 读

[1] 张叔人. 肿瘤免疫治疗进展[M]. 北京:中国协和医科大学出版社,2017.

[2] Gong N, Zhang Y, Zhang Z, et al. Functional nanomaterials optimized to circumvent tumor immunological tolerance[J]. Adv Funct Mater,2019,29(3):1806087.

[3] 刘宝瑞. 肿瘤个体化与靶向免疫治疗学[M]. 北京:科学出版社,2017.

[4] Sun Q, Barz M, De Geest B G, et al. Nanomedicine and macroscale materials in immuno-oncology[J]. Chem Soc Rev,2019,48(1):351-381.

[5] Shields C W 4th, Wang L L, Evans M A, et al. Materials for immunotherapy[J]. Adv Mater,2020,32(13):e1901633.

参 考 文 献

[1] Luke J J, Flaherty K T, Ribas A, et al. Targeted agents and immunotherapies: optimizing outcomes in melanoma[J]. Nat Rev Clin Oncol,2017,14(8):463-482.

[2] Zhang Z, Tongchusak S, Mizukami Y, et al. Induction of anti-tumor cytotoxic T cell responses through PLGA-nanoparticle mediated antigen delivery[J]. Biomaterials, 2011,32(14):3666-3678.

[3] Rosalia R A, Cruz L J, van Duikeren S, et al. CD40-targeted dendritic cell delivery of PLGA-nanoparticle vaccines induce potent anti-tumor responses[J]. Biomaterials,2015, 40:88-97.

[4] Solbrig C M, Saucier-Sawyer J K, Cody V, et al. Polymer nanoparticles for immunotherapy from encapsulated tumor-associated antigens and whole tumor cells

[J]. Mol Pharm,2007,4(1):47-57.

[5]   Min Y,Roche K C,Tian S,et al. Antigen-capturing nanoparticles improve the abscopal effect and cancer immunotherapy[J]. Nat Nanotechnol,2017,12(9):877-882.

[6]   Molavi O,Mahmud A,Hamdy S,et al. Development of a poly(D,L-lactic-*co*-glycolic acid) nanoparticle formulation of STAT3 inhibitor JSI-124: implication for cancer immunotherapy[J]. Mol Pharm,2010,7(2):364-374.

[7]   Roy A,Singh M S,Upadhyay P,et al. Combined chemo-immunotherapy as a prospective strategy to combat cancer:a nanoparticle based approach[J]. Mol Pharm,2010,7(5):1778-1788.

[8]   Kim H,Niu L,Larson P,et al. Polymeric nanoparticles encapsulating novel TLR7/8 agonists as immunostimulatory adjuvants for enhanced cancer immunotherapy[J]. Biomaterials,2018,164:38-53.

[9]   Mi Y,Smith C C,Yang F,et al. A dual immunotherapy nanoparticle improves T-cell activation and cancer immunotherapy[J]. Adv Mater,2018,30(25):e1706098.

[10]   Schmid D,Park C G,Hartl C A,et al. T cell-targeting nanoparticles focus delivery of immunotherapy to improve antitumor immunity[J]. Nat Commun,2017,8(1):1747.

[11]   Shi C,Liu T,Guo Z,et al. Reprogramming tumor-associated macrophages by nanoparticle-based reactive oxygen species photogeneration[J]. Nano Lett,2018,18(11):7330-7342.

[12]   Luo L,Yang J,Zhu C,et al. Sustained release of anti-PD-1 peptide for perdurable immunotherapy together with photothermal ablation against primary and distant tumors[J]. J Control Release,2018,278:87-99.

[13]   Ou W,Jiang L,Thapa R K,et al. Combination of NIR therapy and regulatory T cell modulation using layer-by-layer hybrid nanoparticles for effective cancer photoimmunotherapy[J]. Theranostics,2018,8(17):4574-4590.

[14]   Napoli A,Valentini M,Tirelli N,et al. Oxidation-responsive polymeric vesicles[J]. Nat Mater,2004,3(3):183-189.

[15]   Thomas S N,Vokali E,Lund A W,et al. Targeting the tumor-draining lymph node with adjuvanted nanoparticles reshapes the anti-tumor immune response [J]. Biomaterials,2014,35(2):814-824.

[16]   Silva J M,Zupancic E,Vandermeulen G,et al. *In vivo* delivery of peptides and toll-like receptor ligands by mannose-functionalized polymeric nanoparticles induces prophylactic and therapeutic anti-tumor immune responses in a melanoma model[J]. J Control Release,2015,198:91-103.

[17]   Rodell C B,Arlauckas S P,Cuccarese M F,et al. TLR7/8-agonist-loaded nanoparticles promote the polarization of tumour-associated macrophages to enhance cancer immunotherapy[J]. Nat Biomed Eng,2018,2(8):578-588.

[18]   Umeki Y,Mohri K,Kawasaki Y,et al. Induction of potent antitumor immunity by sustained release of cationic antigen from a DNA-based hydrogel with adjuvant activity

[J]. Adv Funct Mater,2015,25(36):5758-5767.

[19] Wang C,Li P,Liu L,et al. Self-adjuvanted nanovaccine for cancer immunotherapy:role of lysosomal rupture-induced ROS in MHC class Ⅰ antigen presentation [J]. Biomaterials,2016,79:88-100.

[20] Fan Y,Kuai R,Xu Y,et al. Immunogenic cell death amplified by co-localized adjuvant delivery for cancer immunotherapy[J]. Nano Lett,2017,17(12):7387-7393.

[21] Gao M, Zhu X, Wu L, et al. Cationic polyphosphazene vesicles for cancer immunotherapy by efficient *in vivo* cytokine IL-12 plasmid delivery [J]. Biomacromolecules,2016,17(6):2199-2209.

[22] Smith T T,Stephan S B,Moffett H F,et al. *In situ* programming of leukaemia-specific T cells using synthetic DNA nanocarriers[J]. Nat Nanotechnol,2017,12(8):813-820.

[23] Shae D,Becker K W,Christov P,et al. Endosomolytic polymersomes increase the activity of cyclic dinucleotide STING agonists to enhance cancer immunotherapy[J]. Nat Nanotechnol,2019,14(3):269-278.

[24] Tsai S J , Andorko J I , Zeng X , et al. Polyplex interaction strength as a driver of potency during cancer immunotherapy[J]. Nano Res,2018,11(10):5642-5656.

[25] Wang C,Sun W,Wright G,et al. Inflammation-triggered cancer immunotherapy by programmed delivery of CpG and anti-PD1 antibody[J]. Adv Mater,2016,28(40):8912-8920.

[26] Kuai R,Ochyl L J,Bahjat K S,et al. Designer vaccine nanodiscs for personalized cancer immunotherapy[J]. Nat Mater,2017,16(4):489-496.

[27] Chen Y,Xia R,Huang Y,et al. An immunostimulatory dual-functional nanocarrier that improves cancer immunochemotherapy[J]. Nat Commun,2016,7:13443.

[28] Wang D,Wang T,Liu J,et al. Acid-activatable versatile micelleplexes for PD-L1 blockade-enhanced cancer photodynamic immunotherapy[J]. Nano Lett,2016,16(9):5503-5513.

[29] Luo M,Wang H,Wang Z,et al. A STING-activating nanovaccine for cancer immunotherapy[J]. Nat Nanotechnol,2017,12(7):648-654.

[30] Luo Z,Li P,Deng J,et al. Cationic polypeptide micelle-based antigen delivery system:a simple and robust adjuvant to improve vaccine efficacy[J]. J Control Release,2013,170(2):259-267.

[31] De Temmerman M L, Rejman J, Vandenbroucke R E, et al. Polyelectrolyte LBL microcapsules versus PLGA microparticles for immunization with a protein antigen [J]. J Control Release,2012,158(2):233-239.

[32] Devy J,Balasse E,Kaplan H,et al. Hydroxyethylstarch microcapsules:a preliminary study for tumor immunotherapy application[J]. Int J Pharm,2006,307(2):194-200.

[33] Xia Y,Wu J,Wei W,et al. Exploiting the pliability and lateral mobility of pickering emulsion for enhanced vaccination[J]. Nat Mater,2018,17(2):187-194.

[34] Kosmides A K,Meyer R A,Hickey J W,et al. Biomimetic biodegradable artificial

antigen presenting cells synergize with PD-1 blockade to treat melanoma [J]. Biomaterials,2017,118:16-26.

[35] Bencherif S A,Warren Sands R,Ali O A,et al. Injectable cryogel-based whole-cell cancer vaccines[J]. Nat Commun,2015,6:7556.

[36] Liu Y,Xiao L,Joo K I,et al. *In situ* modulation of dendritic cells by injectable thermosensitive hydrogels for cancer vaccines in mice[J]. Biomacromolecules,2014,15 (10):3836-3845.

[37] Song H,Huang P,Niu J,et al. Injectable polypeptide hydrogel for dual-delivery of antigen and TLR3 agonist to modulate dendritic cells *in vivo* and enhance potent cytotoxic T-lymphocyte response against melanoma [J]. Biomaterials, 2018, 159: 119-129.

[38] Ruan H,Hu Q,Wen D,et al. A dual-bioresponsive drug-delivery depot for combination of epigenetic modulation and immune checkpoint blockade [J]. Adv Mater,2019,31(17):e1806957.

[39] Yu S,Wang C,Yu J,et al. Injectable bioresponsive gel depot for enhanced immune checkpoint blockade[J]. Adv Mater,2018,30(28):e1801527.

[40] Chen Q,Wang C,Zhang X,et al. *In situ* sprayed bioresponsive immunotherapeutic gel for post-surgical cancer treatment[J]. Nat Nanotechnol,2019,14(1):89-97.

[41] Duong H T T,Thambi T,Yin Y,et al. Degradation-regulated architecture of injectable smart hydrogels enhances humoral immune response and potentiates antitumor activity in human lung carcinoma[J]. Biomaterials,2020,230:119599.

[42] Jin H,Wan C,Zou Z,et al. Tumor ablation and therapeutic immunity induction by an injectable peptide hydrogel[J]. ACS Nano,2018,12(4):3295-3310.

[43] Dong X,Liang J,Yang A,et al. Fluorescence imaging guided CpG nanoparticles-loaded IR820-hydrogel for synergistic photothermal immunotherapy[J]. Biomaterials,2019, 209:111-125.

[44] Wang C,Ye Y,Hochu G M,et al. Enhanced cancer immunotherapy by microneedle patch-assisted delivery of anti-PD1 antibody[J]. Nano Lett,2016,16(4):2334-2340.

[45] Zaric M,Lyubomska O,Touzelet O,et al. Skin dendritic cell targeting via microneedle arrays laden with antigen-encapsulated poly-D, L-lactide-*co*-glycolide nanoparticles induces efficient antitumor and antiviral immune responses[J]. ACS Nano,2013,7(3): 2042-2055.

[46] Ye Y,Wang J,Hu Q,et al. Synergistic transcutaneous immunotherapy enhances antitumor immune responses through delivery of checkpoint inhibitors[J]. ACS Nano, 2016,10(9):8956-8963.

[47] Ye Y,Wang C,Zhang X,et al. A melanin-mediated cancer immunotherapy patch[J]. Sci Immunol,2017,2(17):eaan5692.

[48] Kim H,Seong K Y,Lee J H,et al. Biodegradable microneedle patch delivering antigenic peptide-hyaluronate conjugate for cancer immunotherapy[J]. ACS Biomater

Sci Eng,2019,5(10):5150-5158.

[49] Zeng Q,Gammon J M,Tostanoski L H,et al. *In vivo* expansion of melanoma-specific T cells using microneedle arrays coated with immune-polyelectrolyte multilayers[J]. ACS Biomater Sci Eng,2017,3(2):195-205.

[50] Duong H T T,Yin Y,Thambi T,et al. Smart vaccine delivery based on microneedle arrays decorated with ultra-pH-responsive copolymers for cancer immunotherapy[J]. Biomaterials,2018,185:13-24.

[51] Duong H T T,Yin Y,Thambi T,et al. Highly potent intradermal vaccination by an array of dissolving microneedle polypeptide cocktails for cancer immunotherapy[J]. J Mater Chem B,2020,8(6):1171-1181.

[52] Yang P,Lu C,Qin W,et al. Construction of a core-shell microneedle system to achieve targeted co-delivery of checkpoint inhibitors for melanoma immunotherapy[J]. Acta Biomater,2020,104:147-157.

（刘倩倩　谢君　刘奕静）

Chapter 7
Applications of Biomedical Polymers in Immunotherapy of Melanoma

7.1   Overview of Immunotherapy for Melanoma

Tumor immunotherapy is a method to achieve the purpose of inhibiting tumor growth and removing tumor cells in an active or passive way to enhance the body's anti-tumor immune response by applying immunological principles. It has gradually become a research hotspot in the medical field since 2011 (Figure 7-1). Tumor immunotherapy mainly consists of three parts: ① Non-specific immunotherapy, mainly refers to the use of recombinant interleukin-2 (IL-2), interferon and other cytokines, to activate or promote the killing function of the patient's immune cells. ② Active specific immunotherapy, mainly refers to the use of tumor cells, tumor proteins, peptides or tumor carriers to make tumor vaccines to immunize patients, to activate autoimmunity and enhance anti-tumor effect. ③ Passive immunotherapy, including adoptive cell immunotherapy and monoclonal antibody therapy (see extended reading 1).

The generation of anti-tumor immune response, which is known as the tumor immune cycle, is a series of progressive events from the release of tumor antigens to tumor-specific immune generation (Figure 7-2). In brief, necrosis or apoptosis of tumor cells induces the release of tumor antigens, which are usually captured by antigen-presenting cells (APCs). Then, APCs present antigenic peptides in major histocompatibility complex I (MHC-I) and major histocompatibility complex II (MHC-II) to activate immature T cells in lymph nodes. Activated T cells enter the tumor microenvironment (TME) and target tumor cells through the interaction between T cell receptors (TCRs) and MHC antigen-peptide complexes. Once being recognized, tumor-specific T cells can eliminate tumor cells by inducing apoptosis. The death of tumor cells leads to the release of additional tumor antigens, which further enhance the subsequent revolutions of this tumor immune cycle. Many factors that come into play in the tumor immune cycle provide a wide range of potential therapeutic targets for the treatment of tumors (see extended reading 2).

The drugs approved by the Food and Drug Administration (FDA) of the United States for melanoma immunotherapy are IL-2 and immune checkpoint inhibitors, such as ipilimumab (trade name: Yervoy; target: cytotoxic T lymphocyte-associated protein 4, CTLA-4), pembrolizumab (trade name: Keytruda; target: programmed cell death protein 1, PD-1) and nivolumab (trade name: Opdivo; target: PD-1). Please refer to chapter 2, section 2 for details in the previous article.

In addition to the US FDA-approved immunotherapies, several new melanoma immunotherapies are in research phase, such as the monoclonal antibody varlilumab, the monoclonal antibody MGA271, cytokines and tumor vaccine (see extended reading 3). For example, the monoclonal antibody varlilumab, which targets CD27 to enhance the immune response of T cells and natural killer (NK) cells, is used in the treatment of tumors such as melanoma. CD27 is a costimulatory receptor of T cells and a member of tumor necrosis factor α (TNF-α) receptors superfamily. It plays an important role in the survival and activation of T cells and in the proliferation and cytotoxic activity of NK cells. Varlilumab is currently in phase I of clinical trials for the treatment of metastatic melanoma. MGA271 is a monoclonal antibody against B7-H3, which is currently in phase I of clinical trials for the treatment of melanoma. B7-H3, a member of B7 receptors family, expresses in APCs and other non-lymphoid tissue cells. The regulatory function of B7-H3 on T cells is still controversial. Some studies have shown that B7-H3 is a costimulatory receptor, while others have shown that B7-H3 has inhibitory effect on the receptor. In addition, some cytokines, such as granulocyte-macrophage colony-stimulating factor (GM-CSF), IL-2, interleukin-15, (IL-15), interleukin-18 (IL-18), interleukin-21 (IL-21), have anti-tumor effect and are currently in clinical trials for the treatment of melanoma.

The tumor vaccine is another important part of the melanoma immunotherapy, and some research has been done. Antigens on the surface of tumor cells are usually modified through a variety of mechanisms to inhibit the recognition by immune cells in the body, which hinders the clearance of tumor cells by the body. The melanoma vaccine is made of melanoma antigen such as tumor cells, tumor-associated proteins or peptides, genes that express tumor antigens. These vaccines are collected by APCs and presented to immune cells, further sensitize and activate T lymphocytes to overcome the immunosuppressive state caused by tumors, enhance immunogenicity and produce antigen-specific cellular immune response to kill melanoma cells, thereby inhibiting the growth, metastasis and recurrence of melanoma. MAGE, gp100, Melan A and NY-ESO are commonly used tumor antigens for the preparation of melanoma vaccine. They can activate the tumor-associated antigen (TAA) specific immune response to induce the anti-melanoma effect in the body, and they are expected to be effective targets for melanoma immunotherapy.

DCs are the most powerful antigenic antigens, which are thought to be the promoter of tumor immunotherapy as well as an important target for tumor immunotherapy, and they play a key role in the innate and adaptive immune activation. DCs are mainly used in two ways to mediate antigens presentation. In one way, DCs obtain exogenous antigen proteins through the cytoplasm. Then, the proteins molecules were decomposed into polypeptide fragments in the lysosomes and were proposed to the $CD4^+$ auxiliary T(T-helper, Th) cells, such as $CD4^+$ T lymphocytes by MHC-Ⅱ. In the other way, the endogenous antigen proteins in the DCs are degraded by protease. The peptide fragments of the degradation were combined with MHC-Ⅰ molecules and were proposed by the $CD8^+$ T lymphocytes to activate the antigen-specific cell toxicity T lymphocytes (CTLs). CTLs can infiltrate tumor tissue and identify the MHC-Ⅰ antigen complexes expressed on the surface of the tumor cells, thus kill tumor cells. It is an important way to achieve effective immune treatment against tumors that tumor-specific CTLs are induced and play specific killing effect on tumor cells. Moreover, the activation of $CD8^+$ T lymphocytes not only directly kill tumor cells, but also obtain a persistent memory phenotype, which is of great significance to prevent the recurrence of tumors. In addition, $CD4^+$ T lymphocytes are also essential to the effective anti-tumor response for its effect of enhancing the cloning of CTLs and promoting the production and maintenance of memory phenotypes. DCs induce the production and activation of Th cells and CTLs by the antigen presentation of MHC-Ⅰ/Ⅱ, which has become the theoretical basis for the clinical trials of antigen based vaccines.

According to the antigen of melanoma, the melanoma vaccines can be divided into the antigen peptide vaccine, the tumor-associated antigen vaccine and the DNA vaccine. The vaccine, formed by polypeptide as an antigen, is called the melanoma antigen peptide vaccine, which can activate the patient's immune system by activating DCs, thus produce active immunity against melanoma cells. The melanoma antigen peptide vaccine has the advantages of high specificity and low toxicity in the process of killing tumor cells. TAA is an antigen protein produced by tumor cells that can trigger an immune response in the host. The tumor cell lysate (TCL) is used as a tumor antigen for the development of tumor vaccines. Compared with specific proteins or polypeptide tumor antigens, the antigen of the whole tumor cell source has many advantages as a vaccine. It can induce the activation of CTLs and $CD4^+$ T lymphocytes to provide a comprehensive source of potential tumor antigen, which can target tumor cells simultaneously, thereby avoiding the immune privilege caused by the absence of tumor antigens. However, the soluble tumor cell lysate that contains antigen and cell factor is essentially unstable. The TCL is easy to produce problems such as poor DCs intake, low antigen cross delivery efficiency and limitation of the induction of CTLs.

Gene related tumor immunotherapy has become the focus of many cancer treatments. It can effectively treat disease from the source and eliminate or prevent hereditary diseases. Recent studies have shown that it has great potential in the treatment of melanoma. DNA vaccines are involved in the use of immune responses induced by DNA encoded by antigen. DNA vaccines have been widely used in the field of cancer and infectious diseases. The DNA encoded by antigen needs to be identified by APCs, such as DCs, macrophages and B lymphocytes, and then transfect APCs with its protease complex. The antigen protein is cut into small peptide fragments, which are presented to T lymphocytes and combined with MHC- I and MHC- II . Moreover, the surface related mannose receptors (MRs) of DCs can recognize a variety of sugar molecules on the cell surface or the cell wall of pathogens, which maintain the stability of the internal environment by participating in receptor-mediated phagocytosis, and combine innate immunity with acquired immunity to form the immune defense system of the body. In addition, studies on tumor signaling pathways indicate that molecular intervention of these signaling pathways provides a new idea for anti-tumor therapy. PUMA (the regulatory factors of apoptosis upregulated by p53), a member of the Bcl-2 protein family, is a downstream gene of p53 and has a pro-apoptotic effect. PUMA can induce the apoptosis of various tumor cells and inhibit the proliferation of tumor cells.

The recent strategies of preventive vaccines or therapeutic vaccines focus on improving the delivery of antigens and the extension of vaccine activity by the specific DCs. With the rapid development of the tumor immune response and tumor immunotherapy, immunoadjuvant as an immune enhancer has been widely used in the tumor vaccine. Immunoadjuvant can nonspecifically enhance the body's specific immunity by up-regulating the surface molecules expression of the immune cells and promoting the innate immune response. Effective tumor vaccines usually require appropriate adjuvants to enhance antigen presentation efficiency, antigen immunogenicity and antigen-induced immune effects. The co-delivery of antigen and immunoadjuvant is expected to enhance the immune responses of the tumor-specific T lymphocytes, which can reduce the risk of immune escape and reduce the immune tolerance for single antigen peptides. Montanide ISA 51 and 720 are clinically approved as immunoadjuvants, which enhance the immunogenicity of tumor cells by stimulating humoral and cellular anti-tumor immune response. In addition, monophosphate A (MPLA), activator of Toll-like receptors 4 (TLR4), is commonly used to enhance the immune response against viral infections and tumors. The stimulation of TLR could activate the internal signaling pathway in APCs and ultimately induce inflammatory cytokines, chemokines, interferons and synergistic costimulatory molecules, which provide the appropriate environment for the T lymphocytes stimulation. But the poor water solubility of MPLA resulted of the long hydrophobic alkyl chain has limited its extensive application in tumor vaccines. Therefore, it is of great significance to develop higher effect carriers for the co-delivery of tumor antigen and immunoadjuvant.

Compared with traditional therapies, immunotherapy has shown considerable improvement in objective response rates, time of disease progression and overall survival rate of patients. However, different immunotherapies also have their limitations. For example, immune checkpoint blocking has had unprecedented success, but unfortunately, only a small percentage of patients respond to immunotherapy. Clinical results indicate that only 15% of the patients respond to ipilimumab (a monoclonal antibody against human CTLA-4) and no more than 40% of the patients respond to anti-PD-1/PD-L1 antibodies. Tumor-associated antigen vaccine faces with instability, short half-life and easy to degrade in plasma, low uptake rate of gene fragments, easy to be degraded by nucleases, etc.

Furthermore, owing to the uncontrolled tissue accumulation and constitutive bioactivity of immunotherapeutic agents, most immunotherapy strategies share the risk of immune-related adverse events (IRAEs), including hypokalemia, hypophysitis, myocarditis, diabetes mellitus and thyroid dysfunction. As a result, many patients have to discontinue treatment when IRAEs occur, which further limits the outcome of immunotherapy. Therefore, it is very necessary to improve the response rate of immunotherapy while reducing the side effects.

It is hopeful to remove various obstacles in the melanoma immunotherapy with the development of biomedical polymer materials. For example, biomedical polymer materials can prevent proteases from degrading antigenic peptides, and can control release antigen and prolong antigen presentation in the co-delivery of antigen and immunoadjuvant for tumor vaccine. As a gene carrier, the delivery system loaded gene fragments has the advantages of high plasticity, accurate structure, resistance to nuclease degradation, stability and low toxicity. In addition to the adjuvant immunotherapy of melanoma by encapsulating tumor antigens and genes, the adjuvant use of biomedical polymer materials for other melanoma components can also enhance the body's specific immune response and thus play an effective anti-tumor effect. Combining melanoma immunotherapy with biomedical polymer materials can optimize the existing methods of using melanoma antigens, gene fragments and other melanoma components for immunotherapy, promising to solve the existing problems of melanoma immunotherapy.

7.2 Biomedical Polymer Drug Delivery System for Immunotherapy of Melanoma

Biomedical polymer materials can play an important role in overcoming key challenges associated with immunotherapies, which can change biological distribution of drugs in the body by improving the cycles, organization homing and tissue penetration of the drugs. The synergistic effect of immunoadjuvants and immunotherapy can be enhanced through the slow release of antigen and improving the immune memory, which results in the sustainability of tumor immunotherapy (see extended reading 4). According to their size, polymer materials used in melanoma immunotherapy can be divided into polymer nanomaterials, polymer micromaterials and macroscale polymer materials.

7.2.1 Polymer nanomaterials

With the rapid development of nanotechnology, polymer nanomaterials have been widely used in tumor diagnosis and treatment as the carrier of therapeutic drugs. Polymer nanomaterials can protect drug molecules from degradation and alter pathways of cell uptake, *in vivo* distribution, metabolism and clearance to enhance the effectiveness and reduce the side effects of the drug. Polymer nanomaterials are the most commonly used carrier materials in tumor immunotherapy. In addition to the advantages mentioned above, polymer nanomaterials can also increase the uptake and the presentation of antigens by APCs, induce CTLs responses and deliver cytokines and antibodies to regulate immunosuppressive TME. According to the morphology of polymer nanomaterials, they can be divided into solid nanoparticles (NPs), nanogels, nanovesicles, nano-micelles, etc.

7.2.1.1 Solid NPs

Solid NPs have been extensively researched in melanoma immunotherapy to enhance the anti-melanoma immune response. Among them, solid poly(lactic-*co*-glycolic acid) (PLGA) NPs have become an important material for drug delivery and immunotherapy due to their good biosafety, synthetic ability and adaptability. A series of tumor immunotherapy strategies have been developed based on PLGA NPs for its easiness to bind and modify drugs, cytokines, antibodies and other immunomodulators.

On the one hand, PLGA NPs can encapsulate antigens to form anti-tumor vaccines, thereby improving the efficiency of antigen presentation and the stability in physiological environment. Sasada et al. used PLGA NPs to co-deliver melanoma-specific antigen peptides (TRP2 and GP100) and Freund's complete adjuvant (FCA) to induce a strong CTLs response in melanoma-bearing mice. PEG modified PLGA NPs loaded with mode antigen ovalbumin (OVA), immunoadjuvant muscle cytidine acid(polyinosinic: polycytidylic acid, poly(I: C)) and Resiquimod (TLR7/8 agonist, R848), can trigger endosomal TLRs to induce an effective anti-tumor immune response in mice bearing OVA-expressing melanoma tumors. On the other hand, PLGA NPs can load with small molecule inhibitors to realize the immunotherapy of melanoma. In 2010, Lavasanifar et al. used PLGA NPs to deliver JSI-124, a small molecule inhibitor of STAT 3, to tumor cells and immunosuppressed dendritic cells, thereby modulating the anti-melanoma immune response in tumor cells and immunosuppressed dendritic cells *in vitro* through JSI-124. Moreover, PLGA NPs can deliver anticancer drug paclitaxel (PTX) and non-toxic derivative of lipopolysaccharide (SP-LPS) for the combination with chemotherapy and immunotherapy to enhance its killing effect on melanoma cells *in vitro*. Furthermore, PLGA NPs loaded with TLR7/8 agonists can enable DCs to enhance the expression of co-stimulatory molecules and antigen presentation through the MHC-I process, thereby achieving significant effects on the prevention and treatment melanoma models. Besides, PLGA NPs can deliver immune checkpoint inhibitors. Wang et al. demonstrated that PLGA NPs co-delivered aPD-1 and anti-OX40, a stimulant antibody that activates the costalized receptor, has therapeutic results in two melanoma models. In 2017, Goldberg et al. developed aPD-1-decorated PLGA NPs that target T cells and simultaneously release R848 and SD-208 (transforming growth factor-β (TGF-β) receptor inhibitors) to break the immunosuppressive effects of TGF-β and potentiate its anti-tumor response. In addition, PLGA NPs can also be used to regulate tumor-associated macrophages (TAMs) to activate anti-tumor immunity. In 2018, Chen et al. employed PLGA NPs to deliver reactive oxygen species (ROS) generating products to polarize TAMs toward the M1 phenotype and subsequently recruit coordinated CTLs to effectively prevent tumor progression and recurrence.

What's more, PLGA NPs incorporated therapeutic agents to realize the combination of tumor immunotherapy with chemotherapy, photothermal therapy, photodynamic therapy, radiation therapy and other tumor treatment strategies, so as to achieve effective treatment of melanoma. Several research groups have added photothermal conversion materials to PLGA NPs to achieve the combination of photothermal therapy (PTT) and immune therapy, which can be further combined with immune checkpoint inhibitors for the treatment of melanoma. In 2018, You et al. reported a therapeutic strategy combining PD-1 blocker and photothermal ablation for melanoma, where aPD-1 peptide and hollow gold nanoshells were co-encapsulated into PLGA NPs, which showed a strong anti-tumor effect, eliminated most of the primary tumors and also significantly inhibited the growth of distally untreated primary tumors. In 2019, Yang et al. constructed multifunctional PLGA NPs with core-shell structure encapsulated with aPD-1 and perfluorinated pentane (PFP) liquid in the core. The modification of PLGA NPs with polyethylene glycol (PEG) and gly-argy-asp-ser (GRGDS) peptides act as encapsulating shell, while iron oxide NPs were loaded in the shell. The hybrid nanoparticles showed an excellent synergistic effect in the treatment of melanoma. In 2018, Kim et al. designed a layer-by-layer hybrid PLGA NP encapsulated the infrared dye IR-780 iodide and the chemotherapy drug imatinib to achieve the anti-tumor effect of PTT and PDT as well as the down-regulation of Treg in tumors. In 2017, Wang et al. reported a synergistic strategy of tumor radiation therapy and immunotherapy. The tumor was first treated with radiation, then the released tumor antigens were selectively captured with PLGA NPs for DCs presentation, resulted in activating the body's antigen-specific anti-tumor response (Figure 7-3). Combined with the immune checkpoint inhibitor anti-programmed cell death protein 1 (aPD-1), significant distal tumor ablation can be achieved.

However, the degradation products of PLGA are acidic, which may reduce the stability of the encapsulated drugs and cause mild inflammation in adjacent tissues. In addition to PLGA NPs, there are many other solid NPs that have been applied in immunotherapy, such as polypropylene sulfide (PPS) NPs, polypropylene poly(ethylene glycol) (PPG) NPs, polycaprolactone (PCL) NPs, and PEG NPs. PPS is a kind of mechanically robust and organic thermoplastic material and has been a promising oxidation-responsive material for drug delivery applications due to the degradation by ROS. Hubbell et al. reported that PPS

NPs with a particle size of 30 nm could effectively target DCs (CD11c⁺) in lymph nodes, thus accumulating in tumor draining lymph nodes. PPS NPs co-coated with melanoma antigen and immunoadjuvants CpG or paclitaxel can increase tumor antigen specific CD8⁺ T cells, thus stimulating an effective anti-tumor immune response and inhibiting melanoma growth. Florindo et al. constructed mannosel-functionalized aliphatic polyester-based NPs that co-loaded melanoma-associated antigens and TLR ligands poly (I: C) and CpG oligonucleotide for targeting to antigen-presenting cells, which effectively enhanced the Th1 immune response and effectively inhibited the growth of melanoma in the treatment and prevention model.

7.2.1.2　Nanogels

Nanogels are the main carrier materials for melanoma immunotherapy. Nanogels are made from natural polymers (e. g., polysaccharides, peptides and nucleic acids), synthetic polymers (e. g., poly(ethylene glycol) and PNIPAM) and their combinations. Compared with solid NPs, nanogels possess characteristically soft, which can improve the circulation and biological distribution of NPs *in vivo* and have the effect of immunoadjuvant. Ma et al. synthesized an amphiphilic pH-sensitive galactosyl dextran-retinal nanogel loaded OVA antigen to construct a self-adjuvant tumor vaccine to promote DCs maturation, antigen uptake and cytoplasmic antigen release, which further augmenting MHC-I antigen presentation and eliciting potent anti-melanoma immune response. Nostrum et al. constructed a tumor vaccine by using cationic dextran nanogel as carrier conjugated model antigen OVA via disulfide bonds. The vaccine combined with immunoadjuvant poly (I:C) can produce a strong anti-tumor immune response in tumor prevention model and treatment model, which can effectively inhibit tumor genesis and development. Wang et al. demonstrated an enzyme-responsive polypeptide-crosslinked nanogel by using polypeptides as chemical crosslinking agents and N-isopropyl acrylamide (NIPAAM) as scaffold by precipitation polymerization. The nanogel can encapsulate the tumor metastasis inhibitor peptide P-5m with high loading capacity, thereby showing significant inhibitory effect on metastatic melanoma.

7.2.1.3　Nanovesicles

Nanovesicles are particles with core-shell structures, whose shells are typically self-assembled from amphiphilic materials such as lipids, polymers, and proteins and the cores are a reservoir of water-rich hydrophilic components. There are three main types of nanovesicles used in melanoma immunotherapy: polymer nanovesicles, polyelectrolyte multilayer nanovesicles, and DNA nanovesicles. Polymer nanovesicles are composed of bilayer membranes of amphiphilic block copolymers, which can encapsulate drugs in the vesicle membrane or aqueous phase core. For example, Moon et al. used monolayer cationic liposomes and hyaluronic acid to construct cross-linked multilayer liposome polymer nanovesicles, which achieved enhanced anti-tumor immune response by synergistic delivery of mode antigen OVA, immunoadjuvant CpG oligonucleotide (CpG ODN) and chemotherapy drug mitoxantrone. Qiu et al. fused PEG with weak cationic polymer to form polymer nanovesicles, which delivered plasmids encoding for IL-12, resulted in improved tumor growth inhibition. Stephan et al. also developed a polymer nanovesicle for *in-situ* programming of specific T cells by using synthetic DNA nanocarriers. The nanocarriers consist of a DNA-mixed poly(β-amino ester) hydrogel in its core and a PGS shell conjugated to a T cell-targeting ligand. Recently, Wilson et al. constructed an insoluble polymer to increase the activity of the stimulant agonist cyclic guanosine monophosphateadenosine monophosphate (cGAMP), which can inhibit tumor growth, prolong the survival time of the body and increase immune memory. Polyelectrolyte multilayer (PEM) nanovesicles are similar to polymer nanovesicles in that their shells are composed of electrostatic adsorption of polycation and polyanion. Jewell et al. used cationic poly (β-amino ester) and TLRs agonist CpG ODN to prepare the polyelectrolyte multilayer nanovesicles through electrostatic interaction in order to stimulate the body's strong anti-melanoma immune response. DNA nanovesicles are mainly composed of DNA, which can be rolled into a cage-like nanostructure through enzyme action and be used to encapsulate various drug molecules. In 2016, Gu et al. prepared DNA nanococoons from long strand of DNA containing the spacer CpG sequence and the restriction site to encapsulate aPD-1 for prophylactic relapse treatment after tumor resection (Figure 7-4), which significantly inhibited the formation of metastatic nodules in the model of metastatic melanoma.

7.2.1.4　Nano-micelles

Nano-micelles are self-assembled structures of amphiphilic polymer molecules in water. The micelles have a variety of morphologies due to the various polymer compositions, lengths and interactions with the carrier mediums. Micelles can encapsulate both hydrophilic and hydrophobic drugs in a single system, which can directly regulate the immune system as a part of a combinatorial approach to reduce tumor burden and/or be used as tumor vaccine nanocarriers against cancer. Li et al. reported a self-assembled micelles based on the prodrug formed by the coupling of PEG and IDO-inhibitor NLG919 and combined with chemotherapeutic drug paclitaxel, which can effectively reverse tumor immunosuppression and significantly improve the therapeutic effect on melanoma. An pH-activated cationic micelle was reported for photodynamic therapy mediated cancer immunotherapy, which was integrated photosensitizer and small interfering RNA (siRNA) to reduced the PD-1 and PD-L1 interaction. Compared with photodynamic therapy alone, this multifunctional hybrid micelle remarkably augmented efficacy for melanoma inhibition and distant metastasis (Figure 7-5). Gao et al. used synthetic micelles not only to enhance antigen delivery and cross-presentation, but also to enhance the anti-tumor immune effect of the interferon gene by stimulating its stimulator pathway and synergistic immune checkpoint inhibition, which can enable the treatment of melanoma.

It is possible to prepare very homogeneous polypeptide-based micelles that can effectively regulate their accumulation, cell uptake and immunogenicity in lymph nodes due to the well controlling of the lengths and polymer sequences of peptides. Moreover, poly peptide-based micelles can easily display antigens along their corona, increasing their abilities of antigen presentation and permit the incorporation of antigens at various locations throughout the micelles, which have been shown to dictate vaccine potency. Ma et al. reported a self-assembled cationic micelle based on poly(ethylene glycol)-*b*-poly(L-lysine)-*b*-poly(L-leucine) (PEG-PLL-PLLeu) hybrid polypeptide, which could be used as a simple and effective vaccine delivery system. Furthermore, the polypeptide-based micelle encapsulate both OVA and TLR3-activated polyinosinic acid (PIC) to synergically enhance tumor-specific CTLs responses.

7.2.2 Polymer micromaterials

Polymer micromaterials (generally larger than 1 μm in size) can interact with a single cell, which play an important role in tumor immunotherapy. Moreover, polymer micromaterials with selectivity and tunability can activate and expand the immune cell population, improve drug (e.g., antibodies, cytokines) delivery compared with polymer nanomaterials, and adjust their phagocytosis and distribution *in vivo* for its easy to deformation. The applications of polymer micromaterials in tumor immunotherapy are mainly reflected in two aspects. One is that as artificial antigen presenting cells (aAPCs), they are used to induce and amplify T cell populations. The other is that they enhance the immunotherapy of melanoma as immunotherapeutic drug carriers, such as antibodies, cytokines and antigens. Polymer micromaterials are expected to overcome the challenges of polymer nanomaterials in tumor immunotherapy, such as tissue homing and circulation *in vivo*. Polymer micromaterials used in melanoma immunotherapy mainly include PLGA, PLGA hybrid materials, PLA and polystyrene. There are mainly polymer microspheres and polymer microcapsules in morphology.

7.2.2.1 Polymer microspheres

Polystyrene is the most commonly used non-degradable polymer microspheres material in immunotherapy research for melanoma. Xie et al. used polystyrene microspheres and modified HLA-A2/peptide tetramer and anti-mouse CD28 monoclonal antibody on its surface. In HLA-A2/Kb transgenic mice, they could effectively proliferate antigen-specific CTLs, recognize endogenous tumor antigens expressed on the surface of human target cells and kill tumor cells in an antigen-specific way. Liang et al. amplified pTRP2-specific CTLs from C57BL/6 mouse spleen cells by co-coating H-2Kb-Ig/pTRP2 dimer complex, anti-CD28 antibody, 4-1BBL and CD83 on the surface of polystyrene microspheres to target melanoma cells.

PLGA is the most commonly used degradable polymer microspheres material in research for melanoma immunotherapy. In the early 2000s, researchers demonstrated that PLGA microspheres can stably encapsulate immunomodulatory substances (e.g., human papillomavirus 16 E7 and plasmid DNA) and deliver them safely and effectively to humans, which established the priority of PLGA microspheres in immunotherapy for melanoma. Since then, there have been growing interest in using PLGA microspheres to deliver antigens, cytokines and antibodies to increase or enhance the immune response. In 2017, Schneck et al. constructed PLGA-based artificial antigen presenting cells that are combined with anti-PD1 checkpoint inhibitors, which activated CD8$^+$ T lymphocytes and induced CD8$^+$ T lymphocytes to secrete IFN-γ to the maximum extent, thereby delaying the occurrence of melanoma.

7.2.2.2 Polymer microcapsules

Polymer microcapsules have a core-shell structure, which provides a multiphase storage space for the storage and delivery of highly loaded hydrophilic and hydrophobic drugs. The hydrophilic domain can be used to store antibodies, cytokines and other proteins in the active state, overcoming the instability or inactivation caused by unavoidable exposure to organic solvents during drug coating. Moreover, the microcapsules made of polyelectrolyte layer can improve the antigen delivery and enhance the immune response compared with the homogeneous microspheres prepared by similar materials. For example, Andry et al. reported that degradable hydroxyethyl starch (HES) microcapsules with sizes of 4-15 μm, which loaded with bovine serum albumin for the melanoma immunotherapy to enhance the antigen presentation effect. Otherwise, Ma et al. constructed a Pickering emulsion with a particle size of about 10 μm by assembling spherical nanoparticles around the oil-water interface of the squalene emulsion as a common vaccination strategy. The Pickering emulsion retains the force-dependent deformability and lateral mobility of the presented antigen, resulted in adjustable phagocytosis and *in vivo* distribution as well as high biosecurity and antigen-loading capacity. The core, shell, and surface of the Pickering emulsion provide various effective loading sites for antigens, adjuvants and other immunomodulators, which are then presented to APCs to enhance the durability and effectiveness of the melanoma vaccine.

7.2.3 Macroscale polymer materials

Unlike micromaterials or nanomaterials that can infiltrate tissue and cells, macroscale polymer materials with large size, can be implanted or local injected into the body to recruit and reprogram cells for *in-situ* expansion of T cells and continuously deliver therapeutic drugs. Furthermore, macroscale polymer materials can be used as the synthetic functional immunohistochemical analogues (e. g. , artificial lymph nodes), therefore, the materials draw more and more attentions. Compared with systemic administration, implantation or local injection is less toxic and can activate a more local immune response (see extended reading 5). At present, macroscale materials used in melanoma immunotherapy mainly include polymer scaffolds, hydrogels and polymer microneedles, etc.

7.2.3.1 Polymer scaffolds

As special materials for immunotherapy, polymer scaffolds can provide the structure and volume of continuous interaction with the surrounding microenvironment, which can overcome the problem of poor immunogenicity and further improve the efficiency of immunotherapy, while reducing the cost and toxic side effects. Commonly used polymer materials include PLGA, poly(ethylene-vinyl acetate) (PEVA), collagen, etc. Mooney et al. developed a microporous PLGA matrix loaded with granulocyte-macrophage colony-stimulating factor (GM-CSF), danger signals and tumor antigens to construct tumor vaccines, which mimicked an immune response to bacterial infection. The PLGA scaffold releases GM-CSF, acts as a home for the recruited DCs, and together with antigenic tumor lysate and adjuvant CpG ODN to stimulate the activation of DCs, which significantly enhances its localization to lymph nodes resulted in a specific anti-melanoma immune response.

7.2.3.2　Hydrogels

Compared with implantable polymer scaffolds, hydrogels are generally softer, can be injected or sprayed conveniently, which have been widely applied in melanoma immunotherapy. Due to their adjustable mechanical and physicochemical properties, hydrogels can control the release of various therapeutic drugs (e.g., small molecule drugs, large molecule drugs) at different time and space, therefore protect the drugs from degradation by the body. Their cross-linking structures, degradability and controllable drug release property in time and space provide a good foundation for application in delivery of cell and various immunomodulators. Hydrogel materials include synthetic polymer hydrogels (e.g., PEG), alginate hydrogels, polypeptide hydrogels, natural extract hydrogels (e.g., hyaluronic acid, chitosan, and collagen).

On the one hand, hydrogels can be used to deliver immune cytokines such as GM-CSF, TLR3 agonist poly (I:C), tumor antigens, and immune checkpoint inhibitors. For example, Wang et al. constructed an injectable temperature-sensitive PEG-PLGA hydrogel in 2014, which can recruit DCs and macrophages through controlled release of GM-CSF, resulted in improving the immune effect against melanoma. In 2015, Mooney et al. reported a study on a spongy macroporous alginate hydrogel. The hydrogel used tumor cells as antigen, GM-CSF as DCs enhancer and CpG ODN as DCs activator. Local infiltration consisting of conventional DCs and plasmacytoid DCs can be induced followed by effective, persistent and highly specific anti-tumor T cell responses in melanoma models.

On the other hand, hydrogels can be used for the co-delivery of immune cytokines, tumor total antigens or immune checkpoint inhibitors. Wang et al. prepared an injectable and self-assembled polypeptide poly(L-valine) gel loaded with tumor cell lysates as antigens and TLR3 agonist poly(I:C) as immune enhancer, which can induce immune response in CTLs achieving good anti-melanoma effect. Wang et al. self-assembled an injectable PEG-*b*-poly (L-alanine) hydrogel in aqueous solution using polypeptides. Tumor cell lysate, GM-CSF and immune checkpoint inhibitor (anti-CTLA-4/PD-1 antibody) were co-coated in the hydrogel, which showed a good immunotherapeutic effect on melanoma. This hydrogel combined with immunotherapy could not only significantly increase the activated effector CD8$^+$ T cells in the spleen and tumor of immunized mice, but also reduce the proportion of Treg.

Hydrogels can be constructed to respond to TME acidity, increased ROS and temperature, etc. , which can control the release of melanoma immunotherapy factors and realize enhanced melanoma immunotherapy. In 2019, Gu et al. constructed an *in-situ* formed dual response hydrogel for local collaborative delivery of demethylating agent zebularine (Zeb) and aPD-1. aPD-1 was first loaded in pH-sensitive CaCO$_3$ NPs and then encapsulated with Zeb in a ROS-responsive hydrogel to construct the ROS/pH dual response hydrogel. By taking advantage of the acidic and ROS-rich tumor microenvironment within the tumor, the drug release was controlled and the retention time of the drug was prolonged, thus effectively enhancing the anti-melanoma immune response. In addition, in 2018, Gu et al. demonstrated a ROS-responsive injectable polypeptide hydrogel to release aPD-L1 and IDO immunosuppressive enzyme D-1MT, which could effectively reduce the local ROS level and promote the release of immunotherapeutic factors, thereby enhancing the anti-melanoma effect *in vivo*. Moreover, Gu et al. developed a spray-type bioresponsive fibrin hydrogel containing aCD47 antibody loaded CaCO$_3$ NPs, which can remove H$^+$ from surgical wounds and polarize tumor associated macrophages to M1 phenotype (Figure 7-6). The results showed that the immunotherapeutic fibrin hydrogel could "awaken" the innate and adaptive immunity of the host to inhibit the local recurrence and potential metastatic spread of the tumor after surgery. In addition, Lee et al. designed hydrogels that can intelligent inject levodopa- and poly(ε-caprolactone-*co*-lactide) ester-functionalized hyaluronic acid, which loaded with immunoregulatory factor OVA expressing plasmid (pOVA) and GM-CSF immunoenhancing factors. The hydrogels can effectively eliminated melanoma in mice though recruiting immune cells.

Otherwise, hydrogels can be used to treat melanoma in combination with immunotherapy and other therapies. In 2018, Gu et al. obtained a ROS-degradable hydrogel by cross-linking the unstable ROS-responsive linker with poly(vinyl alcohol) (PVA), while loading with gemcitabine (GEM) and anti-PD-L1 blocking antibody (aPD-L1). Due to the abundant ROS in the TME, this hydrogel realized the combined chemotherapy and immunity therapy strategy by controlling the release of chemotherapeutic drugs and ICB inhibitors, which enhanced the postoperative ICB and inhibited tumor recurrence. In the same year, Yang et al. used a synthetic amphiphilic polypeptide RADA$_{32}$ (with the sequence of RADARADARADARADA) to self-assemble into a nanofiber hydrogel encapsulated with doxorubicin (DOX) and melittin for a potent chemoimmunotherapy against melanoma through the active regulation of TME. Due to its controlling drug release property and its abilities to regulate innate immune cells, deplete M2-like TAMs, and direct resist cancer and stimulate immune, the hydrogel exhibited potent anti-cancer efficacy for subcutaneous and metastasis tumors. In 2019, Lv et al. designed a poly(ethylene glycol) hydrogel loaded with self cross-linking CpG ODN NPs and photosensitizer IR820 for the combination of photothermal therapy and immunotherapy. The hydrogel can induce melanoma-related antigen release from the killed tumor cells through photothermal killing of melanoma cells, which can effectively stimulate specific anti-tumor immunity, activate the body's systemic anti-tumor immune responses while effectively removing the primary tumor by hyperthermia and achieving a more effective systemic therapeutic effect than single phototherapy.

7.2.3.3　Polymer microneedles

Microneedle technology is a method of enhancing transdermal drug delivery and has received a lot of attentions for nearly 25 years. Microneedles are micron-sized needles with a general length of 100-1000 μm, which can penetrate vertically into the epidermal layer of the skin. When the microneedles pass through the cuticle layer, aqueous holes can be created, which can significantly increase drug permeability. The types of microneedles are mainly divided into solid microneedles, coated microneedles, hollow microneedles and soluble microneedles.

Solid microneedles can be used to pretreat the skin to form a catheter, thus improving drug permeability, while coated microneedles deliver the drug on the surface of the microneedles to the skin. Hollow microneedles can be used to infuse drugs into the skin through a microneedle hollow. Soluble microneedles are generally soluble polymer microneedles that encapsulate the drug and completely dissolve in the skin. In recent years, microneedles have demonstrated significant advantages in transdermal immune regulations: ①small size; ②painless and minimally invasive; ③lower risk of infection from microbial invasion; ④versatile and precise delivery to epidermis; ⑤convenient, do not need professional training for management, improve patient compliance and affordability. Solid microneedles, coated microneedles and hollow microneedles have been studied in the field of immunotherapy for malaria, measles, influenza, AIDS and other diseases. Soluble microneedles, especially soluble polymer microneedles are currently widely investigated in melanoma immunotherapy.

In 2013, Kissenpfennig et al. used soluble methyl vinyl ether-maleic anhydride copolymer as microneedle matrixes to deliver antigen-loaded PLGA NPs to the continuous DCs network of the skin. After *in-situ* antigen uptake, cutaneous DCs delivers antigen-loaded PLGA NPs to cutaneous drainage lymph nodes, which significantly improves T cells activation and proliferation. Moreover, effective antigen-specific cellular immune response can be produced in mice producing antigen-specific toxic CD8$^+$ T lymphocytes, which can effectively inhibit the growth of melanoma. Furthermore, the antigens loaded in PLGA NPs can be retained in the skin layer to improve the stability of antigens.

Since 2016, Gu's research group has constructed different microneedles based on hyaluronic acid (HA) for melanoma immunotherapy. They found that the controllable release mechanism plays an important role in improving the efficacy of immunotherapy for melanoma with significant reduction of toxic and side effects. Firstly, Gu et al. developed a kind of HA microneedles loaded with pH-sensitive dextran NPs encapsulating with glucose oxidase (GOx), catalase (CAT) and aPD-1 (Figure 7-7). GOx converted blood glucose and oxygen into gluconic acid and hydrogen peroxide. The hydrogen peroxide produced by the above reaction was decomposed under the action of CAT, which further promoted the degradation of glucose and realized the controlled and continuous release of aPD-1 from dextran NPs. Compared with intratumoral injection of the same dose of aPD-1 and non-degradation microneedles, these HA microneedles can effectively activate the anti-melanoma immunity. In the same year, Gu et al. constructed a synergistic immunotherapy strategy based on HA microneedles. Inhibitor 1-MT of immunosuppressant enzyme IDO was linked to HA through covalent bond to form an amphiphilic structure, which formed NPs through self-assembling and loaded aPD-1. Subsequently, HA microneedles loaded with NPs were prepared, and accumulated into the cutaneous DCs network around local melanoma through the corneum, thus improving the retention time of the drug in the tumor site and alleviating the toxic side effects caused by systemic administration. Due to the function of hyaluronidase in TME, HA was degraded to release aPD-1 and 1-MT. The synergistic effect of aPD-1 and 1-MT can induce a strong and persistent anti-melanoma immune response. In 2017, Gu et al. added melanin and melanoma total antigen vaccines to HA microneedles. Under the irradiation of near-infrared light, the heat was generated locally, which could further improve the phagocytosis of antigens by DCs, increase the infiltration of polarized T cells and local cytokines secretion, therefore activating stronger anti-tumor vaccine effect. In 2019, Hahn et al. used HA microneedles to load HA grafted with cytotoxic T cell epitope peptides, which could effectively improve the responses of specific CTLs and inhibit the growth of melanoma.

In 2017, Jewell et al. demonstrated PLA microneedle array coated with alternate adsorption with positively charged melanoma antigen and negatively charged immunoadjuvant CpG through layer-by-layer self-assembling. The polyelectrolyte multilayers could be up to 128 layers with a thickness of about 200 nm and effectively promote the proliferation of tumor-specific $CD8^+$ T lymphocytes *in vivo*. In 2018, Lee et al. demonstrated DNA nanovaccine based on polycarbonate microneedle array, which was obtained by the layer-by-layer self-assembly of ultra-pH-responsive OSM-(PEG-PAEU) and poly(I: C). The co-delivery of immune adjuvant poly(I: C) and plasmid expressing ovalbumin (pOVA) can effectively inhibit the growth of melanoma cells and lung metastasis *in vivo*. In 2020, Lee et al. constructed a cocktail of polypeptides nanocomplex microneedle, the microneedle used cationic polypeptides and PEG as the matrixes and highly transfected cationic amphiphilic binder to co-deliver immunoadjuvant poly (I: C) and pOVA, which realized the immunotherapy of melanoma. Wu et al. constructed a core-shell microneedle to deliver aPD-L1 and 1-MT for immunotherapy of melanoma. Through strong electrostatic interaction, the aPD-L1 was adsorbed on the shell and concentrated in the tip of the microneedle. The crystallization of 1-MT was inhibited by the hydrogen bond interaction between PVA and 1-

MT, so that 1-MT was supersaturated to form homogeneous drug-polymer solution and loaded in homogeneous microneedles with high drug load. PVA, as the core of the microneedles with abundant hydrogen bonds, inhibits its crystallization through hydrogen bond interaction with 1-MT, so that 1-MT is supersaturated to form homogeneous drug-polymer solution and loaded in homogeneous microneedles with high drug loading efficiency. Compared with intratumoral injection with the same dose, microneedles with core-shell structure show better melanoma inhibition efficiency.

7.3   Challenges and Perspectives

Biomedical polymers can protect the loaded drugs, melanoma antigens and immune stimulators from the surrounding biological environment (e. g. , being reduced by various enzyme degradation), while extending their biological half-life and reducing the systemic toxicity. The polymer nano-drug carriers can also deliver the loaded melanoma antigens to the specialized APCs to improve the delivery efficiency of the antigens, thereby improving the activation efficiency of the melanoma antigen specific T cells. Otherwise, the polymer carriers can achieve the co-delivery of melanoma antigens and immunoadjuvants, further improve the immune effect of the antigen specific T cells and have synergistic effect with other immune therapies. Therefore, carriers based on biomedical polymers have a great application prospect in the immune treatment of melanoma. Although biomedical polymers have made some progress in the field of immunotherapy of melanoma, there are still some basic scientific problems (e. g. , the biodistribution in various organs and their metabolic pathways; the acute toxicity, subchronic toxicity, chronic toxicity, genotoxicity, and reproductive toxicity) need to be solved before clinical application. With the further understanding of the properties of various polymer materials, the design of various nanomaterials, micromaterials or macroscale polymer materials based on different clinical needs will further improve the efficacy of melanoma immunotherapy.

Questions

1. How to co-deliver antigenic peptides and/or drugs with different hydrophilic and hydrophobic properties to improve the immune effect of the melanoma antigenic peptide vaccines?

2. How to achieve DCs targeting of nano-drug carriers?

3. How to use polymer materials to activate the immune system, so as to realize the prevention and treatment of melanoma *in-situ* and distal metastases?

4. How to use polymer materials to realize the combination of multiple therapeutic methods, so as to improve the prevention and treatment effect of melanoma?

5. What properties of biomedical polymer materials need to be improved in the

immunotherapy of melanoma? Illustrate by example.

Extended Reading

［1］ 张叔人.肿瘤免疫治疗进展[M].北京:中国协和医科大学出版社,2017.

［2］ Gong N,Zhang Y,Zhang Z,et al. Functional nanomaterials optimized to circumvent tumor immunological tolerance[J]. Adv Funct Mater,2019,29(3):1806087.

［3］ 刘宝瑞.肿瘤个体化与靶向免疫治疗学[M].北京:科学出版社,2017.

［4］ Sun Q,Barz M,De Geest B G,et al. Nanomedicine and macroscale materials in immuno-oncology[J]. Chem Soc Rev,2019,48(1):351-381.

［5］ Shields C W 4th,Wang L L,Evans M A,et al. Materials for immunotherapy[J]. Adv Mater,2020,32(13):e1901633.

(Liu Qianqian　Xie Jun　Liu Yijing)

第八章
透皮给药技术

第一节 透皮给药概述

透皮给药(transdermal drug delivery，TDD)是指使药物透过皮肤被递送至局部靶组织或进一步经淋巴管、毛细血管进入相应淋巴结或体循环，从而发挥局部或全身治疗作用的一种给药途径。与口服、皮下注射、皮内注射、静脉注射等传统给药方式相比，透皮给药可避免口服给药所引起的胃肠道不良反应并可避过肝脏的首过效应，且多为无创或微创，疼痛感轻微、不遗留针头、操作简便并可自行使用，可有效提高患者的用药依从性。此外，透皮给药可控性强，可灵活调整给药剂量及给药时间，使得用药安全性有所保障。目前，已有超过20种药物获得美国食品药品监督管理局批准用于透皮给药，全球透皮给药市场每年高达320亿美元。

第二节 透皮给药的生理与组织学基础

一、皮肤屏障与药物透皮途径

皮肤屏障是阻碍透皮给药的重要生理结构。角质层是皮肤屏障的主要组成部分，厚度为 $10 \sim 20~\mu m$，由死细胞构成，结构致密，主要成分为角蛋白和脂质。在其下的颗粒层，细胞通过紧密连接，进一步阻碍药物的渗透(详见第一章中皮肤的屏障功能、皮肤屏障及本章扩展阅读1)。

在皮肤屏障完整的情况下，药物穿透皮肤屏障经皮吸收主要有3条途径(图8-1)。

（一）跨细胞途径

药物穿过角质形成细胞到达活性表皮，然后被真皮层中的毛细血管吸收进入体循环，此途径需经多次水/脂分配，只占药物经皮吸收的极小一部分。

（二）跨细胞间质途径

药物穿过角质形成细胞之间的脂质双分子层，为药物经皮吸收的主要途径。绝大多数小分子药物通过此途径被吸收，脂溶性药物更易通过此途径被透皮吸收。

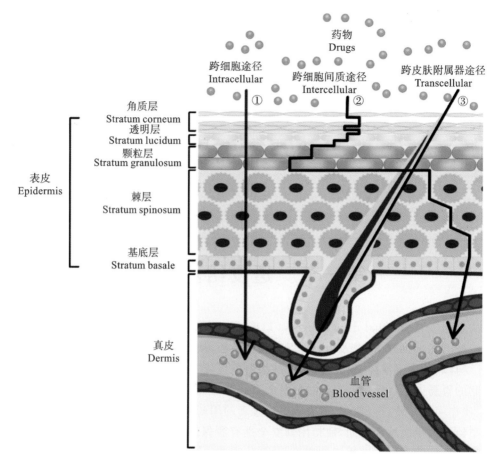

图 8-1 药物透皮途径示意图

注：①跨细胞途径：药物穿过角质细胞。②跨细胞间质途径：药物穿过角质形成细胞之间的脂质双分子层。③跨皮肤附属器途径：药物经皮肤附属器被吸收。

Figure 8-1 Illustration of drug transdermal pathways

①Intracellular pathway：drugs pass through keratinocytes. ②Intercellular pathway：drugs pass through the lipid bilayer between keratinocytes. ③Transcellular pathway：drugs are absorbed through the skin appendages.

(三)跨皮肤附属器途径

药物也可通过皮肤附属器(如毛囊、皮脂腺和汗腺)途径被吸收,该途径是离子型和极性大分子药物及纳米药物经皮吸收的主要途径。

二、皮肤的淋巴引流与血液循环

皮肤中血管和淋巴管的存在是透皮给药引起系统性效应的组织学基础。皮肤血管分布于真皮及皮下组织,在皮肤附属器部位毛细血管尤为丰富,这为大分子药物和纳米药物通过跨皮肤附属器途径进入血液循环提供了有利条件。皮肤毛细淋巴管起始于真皮乳头层,其通透性较强;药物在透皮后可随皮肤组织液通过毛细淋巴管引流至淋巴结中。另外,药物也可以作用于皮肤中的细胞,通过细胞的迁移来间接产生系统性效应。例如,疫苗可作用于皮肤中的抗原呈递细胞(如表皮中的朗格汉斯细胞和真皮中的树突状细胞),这些免疫细胞可以进一步迁移至淋巴结,从而产生系统性的免疫效应。

第三节 影响透皮给药的因素

一、皮肤因素

（一）厚度

不同年龄、性别、部位、种族和个体的皮肤厚度可有一定差异。例如，眼睑处的皮肤厚度约为 0.5 mm，而掌跖部位的皮肤厚度可达 3~4 mm。一般情况下，皮肤较厚处角质层也较厚，此时药物渗透就较难。

（二）皮肤的结构

皮肤屏障的完整性、皮肤是否角化过度以及皮肤结构分子的排列和流动性等均会影响药物透皮的难易程度。例如，在特应性皮炎等皮肤屏障被破坏的疾病中，药物透皮效率增强。而在鸡眼、胼胝和足癣等角化过度的疾病中，角质层增厚，药物透皮效率减弱。角质层中脂质的排列也会影响药物渗透。各种内外因素导致角质层中蛋白质和脂质分子的排列结构、流动性发生变化时，皮肤的通透性也会发生相应的改变。

（三）水合度

当角质水合度高时，多种药物的渗透性将增强。基于此原理，对特定药物进行包封或湿敷来增强药物的渗透性已成为目前临床的常规操作。

（四）血供

通常，皮肤的血供不直接影响药物透皮能力。然而，血供越丰富的区域，药物在透皮后转运至循环系统的效率越高。当皮肤充血时，血流速度增快，经表皮到达真皮的药物将更快被运走，浅层和深层的浓度差增大，药物则更容易向深处渗透。

二、药物因素

（一）药物的脂水分配系数

一般认为 $\log P$（P 为脂水分配系数）为 0~5 的药物的透皮能力较强。$\log P$ 为 2 左右的药物的透皮能力最强。这样的药物既可以透过脂质双分子层亲水的头层，又可穿过疏水的尾层。

（二）分子量和分子结构

生理条件下，分子量较小（$M_w < 500$）的药物更易穿透皮肤。但并非分子量越小透皮效率更高，透皮效率还与分子的结构和形状等相关。例如，最近的一项研究探讨了棒状、球状和三角状的银纳米颗粒的透皮效率，其研究结果表明，这三类纳米颗粒的透皮效率顺序是棒状>球状>三角状。

（三）浓度

一般情况下，药物浓度越高，透皮效率就越高。然而，某些药物在高浓度时对皮肤刺激性明显或对角蛋白有凝固作用，反而影响了皮肤的通透性，导致吸收不良。浓度与药物的溶解度相关。因此，当药物在水和油中的溶解度都在 1 mg/mL 以上时，其透皮效率较佳。

（四）药物剂型

外用药物的剂型对透皮吸收有明显的影响。一般认为凝胶、乳剂、软膏、硬膏和霜剂中的药物渗透效率优于粉剂和水溶液。

此外,药物的解离度、熔点和 pH 等也会影响其透皮效率。

三、环境因素

（一）温度

环境温度升高时,物质扩散速度加快,皮肤血管扩张,皮肤的吸收能力也增强。研究表明,温度从 26 ℃增至 35 ℃时,表皮的水扩散速度可增加一倍。另一项研究发现,当温度从 32 ℃上升至 37 ℃时,芬太尼的体外透皮效率也翻倍。

（二）湿度

一方面,当环境湿度升高时,角质层与外界环境水分浓度差减小,皮肤对水分吸收减少,反之则对水分吸收增加;另一方面,环境湿度也可通过影响角质层的水合度来影响药物的透皮吸收。

第四节　透皮给药技术的发展历程

一、透皮给药技术的发展历程简介

透皮给药技术源远流长。早在春秋战国时期,《五十二病方》中便记载了脂膏、猪膏、豹膏、蛇膏等 30 余种膏方。相比之下,透皮给药技术在现代医学中的发展时间并不长。19 世纪 70 年代,山莨菪碱贴片才被作为首种透皮给药贴片被美国 FDA 批准用于晕车治疗。迄今为止,透皮给药技术历经了四代发展。

（一）第一代透皮给药技术:基于被动扩散的透皮给药

第一代透皮给药技术通过筛选合适的药物或对已有药物进行简单的化学修饰来达到透皮给药效果。第一代透皮药物限于具有高度亲脂性、$\log P$ 常大于 4、分子量不超过 400 的药物,以便通过皮肤屏障迅速扩散。因此,第一代透皮药物的种类十分有限。

（二）第二代透皮给药技术:基于无创促渗手段的透皮给药

第二代透皮给药技术的研究重点是通过使用促渗剂或纳米药物载体(如脂质体、微乳和凝胶等)来改善药物透皮能力,使其易于渗透皮肤或使用热穿孔(使用热能加快药物渗透并使皮肤更具通透性)、电穿孔(利用高压短电脉冲短暂增加皮肤渗透性)、离子促渗(使用低电压电流使药物通过皮肤)及非空化超声(利用超声的机械效应和热效应促进药物透皮)等外部驱动来可逆地提高皮肤对药物的通透性。第二代透皮给药技术的优势是暂时改变皮肤对药物的通透性,不破坏皮肤结构的完整性和皮肤屏障功能,安全、无创。尽管如此,第二代透皮给药技术仍有其局限性:一方面,无创促渗手段虽然能在一定程度上提高药物的给药效率,但药物总体生物利用度仍低下;另一方面,生物制剂的兴起给透皮给药带来了新的挑战(见扩展阅读 2)。2015—2018 年,美国 FDA 批准的所有药物中,近 30%是生物制剂。目前,绝大多数生物制剂为多肽骨架,其中多肽骨架的单克隆抗体已有超过 50 种获批,它们已成为重要的临床治疗手段。TNF-α、IL-17A、IL-23 和 IL-4/IL-13 的单克隆抗体已在银屑病、特应性皮炎等多种皮肤疾病中广泛应用。生物制剂分子量大(单克隆抗体约含 500 个氨基酸残基,分子量约为 150000)、稳定性差,因此第二代透皮给药技术还难以满足生物制剂的透皮需求。

(三) 第三代透皮给药技术:微创透皮给药

第三代透皮给药技术通过表皮在微创操作下形成的微通道来促进药物的递送。例如,通过射频消融、超声和激光等方式破坏角质层,形成微通道。由于形成的微通道尺寸远大于药物分子的尺寸,故各种亲水性、疏水性药物及蛋白质、DNA 等大分子生物制剂均可有效通过。但这些透皮给药方式往往依赖于笨重昂贵的设备和专业技术人员的操作,且具有一定的疼痛感。微针阵列是近些年来兴起的另一种微创透皮给药技术,它是由微米级别的小针形成的矩阵阵列,可分为固体微针、中空微针、涂层微针、可溶性微针、溶胀微针(又称水凝胶微针或相转化微针)等多种类型。由于微针的长度一般为 $50\sim1000~\mu m$,不触及真皮神经,故疼痛感往往较轻微。微针阵列作为一种新型的药物传递方法,具有无痛、定位准确、微创、安全高效、携带方便、患者可自行使用等优点,对于大分子、核酸类、多肽类、蛋白类、疫苗等生物制品的给药尤其具有优势,已成为第三代透皮给药技术中最具潜力的微创给药方式。第三代透皮给药技术虽然可短暂地损伤皮肤屏障,但这种损伤往往可由机体快速自行修复。

(四) 第四代透皮给药技术:基于反馈控释智能硬件的透皮给药

第四代透皮给药技术在个体化治疗和多学科交叉的背景下应运而生。该给药技术基于软性超薄可穿戴硬件、生物电子设备和药物所集成的贴片。该贴片可紧密地贴合皮肤,通过生物传感器监测生理信号(如血压和体温)、电生理信号(如心电图和脑电图)和生化信号(如汗液和体液的 pH、血糖和血氧水平),并将这些信号传递至制动器,从而依据需求控制释放相应药物,形成生物传感器-制动器反馈环路。目前,第四代透皮给药技术仍处于早期研发阶段(详见第十章可穿戴皮肤器件与电子皮肤相关内容)。

二、理想的透皮给药技术

透皮给药技术历经四代发展,已取得诸多瞩目成果,开发了诸多临床应用,但当前技术仍具有其局限性。理想的透皮给药技术应具有以下特点:

(1) 微创、无痛、安全、方便;

(2) 适用于疏水性、亲水性药物和大分子药物(如多肽、蛋白质、RNA、DNA 等);

(3) 保证药物性质稳定、剂量充足;

(4) 具有可控且理想的释放速度;

(5) 可自用,不遗留尖锐针头。

第五节 基于生物医用高分子的透皮给药技术

生物医用高分子在透皮给药领域已有数十年的应用,横跨第二代至第四代透皮给药技术。本节从基于生物医用高分子的促渗剂、纳米粒子、微针三个方面全面介绍生物医用高分子在透皮给药技术领域的应用。

一、基于生物医用高分子的促渗剂

促渗剂指能够可逆地降低皮肤对药物的阻力,加速药物穿透皮肤,去除后皮肤能恢复正常屏障功能的一类化学物质。传统的小分子化学促渗剂包括溶剂(乙醇、吡咯烷酮(吡咯烷酮羧酸钠)、亚砜(二甲基亚砜(DMSO)和癸甲基亚砜))、脂肪酸、表面活性剂、萜烯、月桂氮䓬酮等。促渗剂促渗机制多样,包括增加溶解度、增加对角质层的渗透性、使角质层晶体结构液态化、使角质层的脂质溶解等。二甲基亚砜(DMSO)、二甲基甲酰胺(DMF)和噁唑烷酮等具有皮肤刺激性的促渗剂目前已较少使用,而更温和的促渗剂脂肪酸、尿素和吡咯烷酮则仍有广泛应用。然而,传统的化学促渗剂仅适用于小分子药物,对生物制剂等大分子药物的促渗作用十分有限。相比而言,高分子促渗剂(如透明质酸、树枝状聚合物、环糊精、壳聚糖及其衍生物、皮肤促渗肽等)则在促进大分子药物和纳米粒子的透皮方面具有独特的优势。

(一)透明质酸

透明质酸(HA)是人体固有的一种线性多糖,大量存在于细胞外基质中。其具有极佳的生物相容性、可降解性、非免疫原性和低毒性。HA可作为促渗剂增强小分子药物(如双氯芬酸、布洛芬、克林霉素和环孢素)的渗透性,也可修饰在大分子和纳米颗粒表面,以增强其透皮能力。例如,HA和人类生长激素(hGH)的共轭物在小鼠皮肤上的渗透能力要比游离hGH更强。将HA与纳米氧化烯Ce6颗粒共轭亦可显著促进其透皮作用。透明质酸作为促渗剂的主要机制如下:①增加角质层的水合度,使脂质双分子层疏松,进而使亲水性药物具有更大的渗透性;②与HA接触可导致角质层中的角蛋白从 α-螺旋结构变为 β-折叠结构,脂质双分子层变得无序;③在活体皮肤细胞(例如角质形成细胞和成纤维细胞)上表达的HA受体可能参与HA和其所结合药物的主动转运。

(二)树枝状聚合物

树枝状聚合物是一类合成的超支化聚合物。它们的核心和高度功能化的分支可以通过宿主-客体相互作用和化学共轭来搭载亲水性和亲脂性药物,从而形成具有高载药量和高单分散性的通用平台。聚酰胺树枝状大分子(PAMAM)作为化学促渗剂,已被用于多种小分子药物在大鼠皮肤或猪皮中的透皮给药研究,包括盐酸坦舒洛辛(一种选择性的 α1A肾上腺素受体拮抗剂,用于尿潴留)、酮洛芬和二氟尼、8-甲氧基补骨脂素、核黄素(维生素 B_2)、5-氟尿嘧啶等。不同的树枝状聚合物促进药物透皮的机制取决于它们的大小(由分支代数决定)和电荷:①相对较小的树枝状聚合物可快速扩散、通过角质层,并通过改变脂质双分子层的溶解度、极性和结构完整性而充当药物渗透的流体;②阳离子树枝状聚合物可通过形成纳米孔来破坏脂质双分子层,从而促进药物的渗透;③某些树枝状化合物可参与跨细胞途径的药物渗透。

(三)环糊精

环糊精(CDs)是环状寡糖,其 α-D-吡喃葡萄糖的重复单元通过 α-1和 α-4位的碳原子相互连接。环糊精具有圆锥形的结构,在圆锥的外部具有亲水性羟基,在内腔表面分布有亲脂性骨架碳和醚性氧,故而在内腔搭载亲脂性药物。环糊精分子量大(分子量:1134.98)且 $\log P$ 低($-3\sim0$),故其自身透皮能力并不强。然而,环糊精可以与难溶性亲脂性药物形成复合物,从而增加其溶解性和稳定性,进而增高其皮肤渗透率。一般认为,环糊精不增加药物跨角质层的渗透性,因此环糊精-药物复合物的透皮运输仍较困难。提高其透皮效率的方案包括在表面进行亲脂性基团修饰或与小分子化学促渗剂合用等。

（四）壳聚糖及其衍生物

壳聚糖是一组由 β-(1-4)-连接的 D-葡萄糖胺和 N-乙酰基-D-葡萄糖胺沿着主链随机分布组成的阳离子多糖。只有低分子量的壳聚糖才能增加皮肤通透性。低分子量壳聚糖可促进抗肿瘤药物黄芩苷透过小鼠皮肤,核磁共振光谱显示壳聚糖与角质层中的角蛋白和糖蛋白均无静电相互作用。因此,角质层通透性增加可能由壳聚糖和脂质双分子间的偶极-偶极作用和范德华相互作用所引起。其他具有促渗作用的壳聚糖衍生物包括 N-三甲基壳聚糖和 N-精氨酸壳聚糖等。

（五）促渗肽

促渗肽是一类少于 30 个氨基酸残基的短肽。与上述化学促渗剂不同,促渗肽属于生物促渗剂,具有很好的生物相容性和低毒性,可用于促进多肽、蛋白质、核酸、纳米粒子以及其他生物活性分子的透皮给药。促渗肽可通过与药物物理混合、形成融合蛋白、共价连接和修饰载体等多种方式促进药物透皮吸收。目前,已有多种促渗肽制剂进入临床研究阶段。其中,RT-001 用于促渗肉毒菌素 A 治疗面部皱纹和 AZX-100 类似物用于促进 HSP20 的渗透和吸收预防皮肤瘢痕的临床研究已进入 Ⅱ 期临床研究阶段。

二、基于生物医用高分子的纳米粒子

利用聚合物纳米粒子搭载药物是第二代透皮给药技术中的重要策略。聚合物纳米粒子不仅可以减少药物的降解,增强药物跨皮渗透能力,还可以达到控制释放的效果。聚合物纳米粒子通常在毛囊中积累,通过跨皮肤附属器途径实现透皮。聚合物纳米粒子可分为天然聚合物纳米粒子(如壳聚糖、白蛋白纳米粒子)和合成聚合物纳米粒子(如聚乳酸-羟基乙酸(PLGA)、树枝状聚合物纳米粒子)。纳米粒子在透皮给药技术中的应用详见第六章高分子纳米药物载体及其在皮肤疾病治疗中的应用。

三、基于生物医用高分子的微针

（一）微针发展历程简介

微针(MNs)是一种新兴的微创透皮给药技术,可分为固体微针、中空微针、涂层微针、可溶性微针、溶胀微针(又称水凝胶微针或相转化微针)等多种类型(图 8-2)。微针可通过在皮肤上形成微米级的孔洞,将药物导入,从而提高药物的透皮效率。1998 年,美国佐治亚理工学院 Prausnitz 博士的研究团队利用反应离子刻蚀技术制造出以硅为基质材料的长约 150 μm,尖端曲率半径小于 1 μm 的固体微针阵列,并首次进行了皮肤渗透试验。研究结果表明,应用此种微针后可以使钙黄绿素(模型药物)的经皮药物渗透率提高 1000 倍。此后,固体微针发展迅猛,出现了以二氧化硅、玻璃、镍、钛等为基质材料的多种微针,尤其在美容领域,已形成多款商品化产品。固体滚轮微针作为光动力治疗中光敏剂的促渗手段已被写入美国皮肤外科学会 2016 版光动力指南中。然而,固体微针依赖"扎针-涂药"两步给药法,操作烦琐且剂量难以把控,针体反复使用有产生感染的风险。因此,后续在固体微针基础上发展出了涂层微针与中空微针等。涂层微针将药物涂抹在固体微针表层,扎入皮肤后药物可溶解扩散,从而实现一步给药并能显著提高药物的利用效率。2002 年,获得美国 FDA 批准的 Macroflux(Zosano Pharm

微针类型 Microneedle types	示意图 Schematic illustration
固体微针 Solid MNs	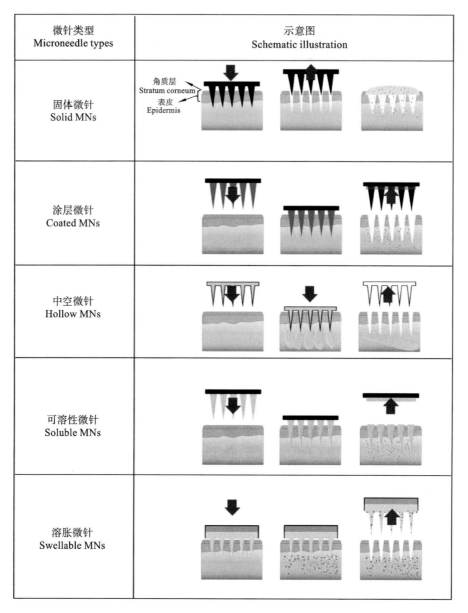
涂层微针 Coated MNs	
中空微针 Hollow MNs	
可溶性微针 Soluble MNs	
溶胀微针 Swellable MNs	

图 8-2　不同类型微针透皮给药示意图

Figure 8-2　Schematic illustration of transdermal administration of different types of microneedles

公司生产)是最早获批的微针器械,也是涂层微针的典型代表。然而,涂层微针也存在诸如载药量小等问题。中空微针是微米级别的矩阵注射器,典型代表为 2009 年获美国 FDA 批准的 Micronjet(NanoPass Technologies)。以上三种类型的微针大多基于金属、陶瓷、玻璃和硅等材质,生物相容性较差、遗留尖锐针头且需专业技术人员操作。近年来,基于生物医用高分子的可溶性微针和溶胀微针的问世克服了这些缺陷。可溶性微针在扎入皮肤后即可溶解,能在实现一步给药的同时,拥有相对较高的载药量和极佳的组织相容性,且经济有效,可自行使用且不遗留尖锐针头。溶胀微针在与皮肤中的组织液接触后发生溶胀而非溶解,从而释放药物。药物释放后可将微针拔出,从而避免聚合物沉积于皮层。由于溶胀微针吸收组织液,故也可用于皮肤组织液的提取。

聚合物微针的制备方法包括微成型(MM)、热压印(HE)、滴气吹塑(DAB)、电绘图(ED)、注射成型(IM)、激光微加工(LMM)、拉制光刻(DL)、光刻(PL)、包模造模法(IM)、连续液态界面制造成型(CLIP)、浸渍法、溶剂铸造、X射线法和3D打印等。应根据微针的类型、基质材料和药物性质选择恰当的制备方法。例如,溶胀微针的制备过程常需高温或紫外线处理,故应当考虑合成过程对药物的潜在影响。

因为生物医用高分子在固体微针和中空微针中仅有少量应用,且其优势相对其他材料不明显,所以本节主要集中讨论生物医用高分子作为涂层微针、可溶性微针和溶胀微针的基质在皮肤疾病中的应用。

(二)影响聚合物微针基质材料选择的因素

聚合物微针基质材料的选择除需考虑生物安全性和稳定性外,还应考虑以下因素。

1. 力学强度

微针的力学强度由微针壁厚、壁角、尖端半径、长度、针间距离和聚合物组成等决定。不同类型聚合物的力学强度不同,所负载的药物和纳米粒子也会影响微针的力学强度。例如,在我们的一项研究中,当透明质酸微针中负载368 μg光敏剂ALA时,其杨氏模量从58.9 MPa下降至40.0 MPa。而在我们的另一项研究中,当透明质酸微针中负载4 μg金纳米笼时,透明质酸微针的杨氏模量从68.9 MPa增高至224.9 MPa。

2. 基质溶解性/溶胀性

微针的溶解性或溶胀性是影响药物释放速率的重要因素。在设计微针时,需要根据药物的释放需求来选择基质材料。某些皮肤疾病的治疗中,需要药物迅速释放来快速达到有效局部浓度或血药浓度,例如化疗药物、光敏剂、光热剂、镇痛药物、止痒药物等。而另一些疾病则更适合长期缓慢释放药物,如银屑病、湿疹等炎症性疾病。此外,在皮肤疾病免疫治疗中,还需要考虑免疫事件发生的时序,根据药物具体作用机制来决定药物释放的时间和速度。值得注意的是,即使是治疗同一种疾病,由于药物性质的不同,其释放的需求也不同。例如,抗生素分为浓度依赖型和时间依赖型。在治疗皮肤感染时,前者需迅速释放药物以达到有效的药物浓度,而后者需相对缓慢释药,以保证有效抗菌药物浓度的作用时间。水溶性多糖和其类似物,如透明质酸(HA)、聚乙烯吡咯烷酮(PVP)、葡聚糖、羟丙基甲基纤维素(HPMC)、羟丙基纤维素(HPC)、羧甲基纤维素(CMC)和支链淀粉可迅速、完全溶解于水中,故常用于制备需要迅速释放药物的微针。而聚乳酸(PLA)、聚乳酸-羟基乙酸(PLGA)、聚碳酸酯(PC)、聚羧乙酸(PGA)、聚己内酯(PCL)、壳聚糖、蚕丝等不溶于水,但可在体内缓慢降解,常用于制备需缓慢释放药物的微针。聚合物的溶胀是聚合物基质持续给药的另一重要机制。基于可溶胀聚合物的溶胀微针可吸收大量水而不溶于水,其扩散由药物分子和聚合物的膨胀和交联结构所决定。常用的溶胀聚合物包括聚甲基丙烯酸羟乙酯(PHEMA)、聚苯乙烯-聚丙烯酸(PS-b-PAA)二嵌段、聚乙烯醇(PVA)、聚甲基乙烯醚-马来酸(PMVE/MA, Gantrez)、透明质酸丙烯酸酯等。

3. 靶向性

一些高分子材料本身具备靶向性质,如透明质酸(HA)可以选择性地结合癌细胞的CD44受体。而一些聚合物表现出氧化还原响应行为,可用于针对特定细胞或组织。

4. 响应性释放

聚合物微针可被设计成对特定环境或特定信号做出响应。常见的响应诱发信号包括特定的 pH、血糖浓度、低氧、温度、光、机械作用力及酶或受体。有研究表明,基于阴离子和阳离子聚合物的溶胀微针表现出对 pH 敏感的溶胀和响应性释放能力。例如,阳离子聚合物聚乙二醇-*b*-聚(β-氨基酯)在微酸性环境(pH 为 6.5～7.0)中比 pH＝7.4 时释放药物快 4 倍。McCoy 等通过交联聚甲基丙烯酸羟乙酯(PHEMA)和乙二醇二甲基丙烯酸酯制备了具有光响应性的水凝胶微针,获得了长时间的光响应药物释放(可达 160 h)。一些聚合物在低温下可高度溶胀,而当温度上升至一定值时则产生收缩。例如,聚甲氧基二甘醇甲基丙烯酸酯(PmDEGMA)和聚甲氧基三甘醇甲基丙烯酸酯(PmTEGMA)表现出热响应性药物释放。超过临界温度时,药物分子被挤压出收缩的凝胶从而引发药物释放。此外,聚合物微针可与具有控释、靶向功能的纳米粒子相结合,因此在透皮给药方面具有广阔的应用前景(见扩展阅读 3)。

(三) 微针在皮肤疾病透皮给药中的应用

基于生物医用高分子的微针目前在皮肤美容、皮肤炎症性疾病、皮肤肿瘤、皮肤感染中已有广泛的研究(见扩展阅读 4)。表 8-1 总结了近年来聚合物微针在上述疾病中的应用研究。在这些研究中,聚合物微针给药往往表现出比传统给药更佳的预防或治疗效果。

表 8-1　基于生物医用高分子的微针在皮肤疾病中的应用总结

药　　物	高分子基质/涂层	微针类型	疾病/应用模型	控制类型
ALA	HA	可溶性微针	小鼠皮下肿瘤光动力治疗	速溶
a-PD1	HA 与 MBA 交联物	可溶性微针	小鼠黑素瘤免疫治疗	pH 敏感性右旋糖酐纳米粒子控释
a-PD1＋1-MT	HA	可溶性微针	小鼠黑素瘤免疫治疗	缓释
肿瘤抗原＋CpG	immune polyelectrolyte multilayers (iPEMs)	涂层微针	黑素瘤肿瘤疫苗	—
DOX＋金纳米笼	HA	可溶性微针	小鼠黑素瘤化疗＋光热治疗	速溶
搭载 STAT3 siRNA 的 PEI	HA,右旋糖酐,PVP	可溶性微针	小鼠黑素瘤基因治疗	速溶
DOX＋ LaB6	PVA/PVP(底座＋针体),PCL(针尖)	可溶性微针	小鼠皮下肿瘤模型	NIR 敏感性控释
雷帕霉素	PVP	可溶性微针	体外血管异常模型	速溶
甲氨蝶呤	HA	可溶性微针	小鼠银屑病模型	速溶
博来霉素	HA	可溶性微针	体外增生性瘢痕模型	速溶
硫酸庆大霉素	PEG	可溶性微针	体外抗菌模型	缓释

续表

药　物	高分子基质/涂层	微针类型	疾病/应用模型	控　制　类　型
纳米银	CMC	可溶性微针	体外抗菌模型	—
绿茶提取物	HA	可溶性微针	大鼠伤口感染模型	—
伏立康唑	PGA	涂层微针	体外抗真菌模型	—
两性霉素 B	Gantrez AN-169	涂层微针	体外抗真菌模型	—
两性霉素 B	PGA	涂层微针	体外抗真菌模型	—
咪康唑	Gantrez AN-169	涂层微针	体外抗真菌模型	—
伊曲康唑	PGA	涂层微针	体外抗真菌模型	—
克林霉素	m-HA/DE(底座)RR-PVA(针体)	可溶性微针	小鼠痤疮丙酸杆菌感染模型	ROS 依赖性控释;缓释
阿昔洛韦	Gantrez S-97	可溶性微针	体内外扩散模型(潜在的抗病毒应用)	—
贻贝黏蛋白质外壳和丝纤蛋白内核		溶胀微针	大鼠伤口愈合模型	—

注:ALA,艾拉,一种光动力治疗药物;a-PD1,anti-PD-1 antibody,抗 PD-1 抗体,一种免疫治疗药物;HA,hyaluronic acid,透明质酸;MBA,N,N′-methylenebis(acrylamide);1-MT,1-methyl-DL-tryptophan,一种 IDO 抑制剂;CpG,一种 Toll 样受体激动剂,具有免疫佐剂效应;PEI,polyethylenimine,聚乙烯亚胺;PVA,poly(vinyl alcohol),聚乙烯醇;PVP,poly(vinyl pyrrolidone),聚乙烯吡咯烷酮;PEG,poly(ethylene glycol),聚乙二醇;PGA,poly(glycolic acid),聚乙醇酸;CMC,carboxymethyl cellulose,羧甲基纤维素;m-HA/DE,methacrylate hyaluronic acid/diatomaceous earth,甲基丙烯酸透明质酸/硅藻土;LaB6,lanthanum hexaboride 六硼化镧,一种光敏材料;RR-PVA,reactive oxygen species(ROS)-responsive poly(vinyl alcohol),活性氧敏感型聚乙烯醇;PCL,polycaprolactone,聚己酸内酯;Gantrez AN-169,一种甲基乙烯醚和马来酸酐的共聚物;Gantrez S-97,一种甲基乙烯醚和马来酸的共聚物。

第六节　挑战与展望

目前,第一代及第二代透皮给药技术已在临床实践中广泛应用,但促渗效率总体较为低下且难以满足生物制剂等大分子的透皮给药需求。第三代透皮给药技术通过表皮在微创操作下形成的微通道来促进药物的递送,适用于包括生物制剂在内的大多数药物。大多数第三代透皮给药技术依赖于笨重昂贵的设备和专业技术人员的操作,而微针凭借其简便的用药方式和广泛的适用性,已成为第三代透皮给药技术中最具潜力的微创给药方式。

尽管基于生物医用高分子的微针近年来发展迅速,但目前尚无获批的医用聚合物微针产品。聚合物微针在皮肤疾病中的应用研究仅有一项进入临床研究阶段(透明质酸可溶性微针用于斑块型银屑病的研究,NCT02955576)。相对来说,中空微针流感疫苗 Intanza® 早在 2009 年即获得美国 FDA 批准上市,多项基于中空微针的各类疫苗也已进入临床Ⅱ期或者Ⅲ期研究。

聚合物微针虽然具备诸多优势,但仍存在较多问题,如聚合物沉积于皮层、量产效率低、产品重现性低(残留不均,载药量不均一)、生产成本高等。此外,尽管有研究证明可以通过简单的方式将微针面积做得更大且不影响患者自用,低载药量仍是限制聚合物微针临床应用的一大因素。

另外,皮肤疾病有3000余种,但是由于动物模型的限制,许多研究停留在体外细胞水平甚至皮肤模拟物水平,诸多效应难以得到直观的动物水平的验证。近期研究表明,微针给药后,药物会分布至淋巴结、肝、肾、脾。因此,微针给药的药代动力学和安全性还有待进一步研究。聚合物微针在皮肤疾病中的应用研究仍任重道远。

基于反馈控释智能硬件的第四代透皮给药技术目前仍处于早期研发阶段,但我们有理由相信聚合物微针与智能硬件的结合将为透皮给药开启新的篇章。

思 考 题

1. 各类透皮给药技术可否用于组织液的提取和液体活检?它们分别具有哪些优势和局限性(见扩展阅读5)?

2. 生物大分子的透皮给药与小分子药物的透皮给药相比,有哪些注意事项?

3. 透皮给药技术可否用于细胞甚至组织的递送?有哪些应用前景?

4. 以微针在抗肿瘤中的应用为例,微针所载化疗药物和免疫检查点抑制剂的理想释放模式如何?应如何结合高分子材料进行设计?

5. 3D打印技术在透皮给药中有哪些应用前景?

扩 展 阅 读

[1] Yang R, Wei T, Goldberg H, et al. Getting drugs across biological barriers [J]. Adv Mater, 2017, 29(37): e1606596.

[2] Anselmo A C, Gokarn Y, Mitragotri S. Non-invasive delivery strategies for biologics [J]. Nat Rev Drug Discov, 2019, 18(1): 19-40.

[3] Singh P, Carrier A, Chen Y, et al. Polymeric microneedles for controlled transdermal drug delivery[J]. J Control Release, 2019, 315: 97-113.

[4] Sabri A H, Ogilvie J, Abdulhamid K, et al. Expanding the applications of microneedles in dermatology[J]. Eur J Pharm Biopharm, 2019, 140: 121-140.

[5] Mandal A, Boopathy A V, Lam L K W, et al. Cell and fluid sampling microneedle patches for monitoring skin-resident immunity[J]. Sci Transl Med, 2018, 10(467): eaar2227.

参 考 文 献

[1] Carter P, Narasimhan B, Wang Q. Biocompatible nanoparticles and vesicular systems in transdermal drug delivery for various skin diseases[J]. Int J Pharm, 2019, 555: 49-62.

[2] 赵辨. 中国临床皮肤病学[M]. 南京:江苏科学技术出版社, 2009.

[3] Kennedy J, Larrañeta E, McCrudden M T C, et al. *In vivo* studies investigating biodistribution of nanoparticle-encapsulated rhodamine B delivered via dissolving

microneedles[J]. J Control Release,2017,265:57-65.

[4] Ripolin A,Quinn J,Larrañeta E,et al. Successful application of large microneedle patches by human volunteers[J]. Int J Pharm,2017,521(1-2):92-101.

[5] Anselmo A C,Gokarn Y,Mitragotri S. Non-invasive delivery strategies for biologics [J]. Nat Rev Drug Discov,2019,18:19-40.

[6] Singh P,Carrier A,Chen Y,et al. Polymeric microneedles for controlled transdermal drug delivery[J]. J Control Release,2019,315:97-113.

[7] Sabri A H,Ogilvie J,Abdulhamid K,et al. Expanding the applications of microneedles in dermatology[J]. Eur J Pharm Biopharm,2019,140:121-140.

[8] Chang H,Zheng M,Chew S W T,et al. Advances in the formulations of microneedles for manifold biomedical applications[J]. Adv Mater Technol,2020,5(4):1900552.

[9] Lee K J,Jeong S S,Roh D H,et al. A practical guide to the development of microneedle systems—in clinical trials or on the market[J]. Int J Pharm,2020,573:118778.

[10] Lee H,Song C,Baik S,et al. Device-assisted transdermal drug delivery[J]. Adv Drug Deliv Rev,2018,127:35-45.

[11] Matriano J A,Cormier M,Johnson J,et al. Macroflux® microprojection array patch technology:a new and efficient approach for intracutaneous immunization[J]. Pharm Res,2002,19(1):63-70.

[12] Ye Y,Yu J,Wen D,et al. Polymeric microneedles for transdermal protein delivery[J]. Adv Drug Deliv Rev,2018,127:106-118.

[13] Zhu J,Dong L,Du H,et al. 5-aminolevulinic acid-loaded hyaluronic acid dissolving microneedles for effective photodynamic therapy of superficial tumors with enhanced long-term stability[J]. Adv Healthc Mater,2019,8(22):e1900896.

[14] Wang C,Ye Y,Hochu G M,et al. Enhanced cancer immunotherapy by microneedle patch-assisted delivery of anti-PD1 antibody[J]. Nano Lett,2016,16(4):2334-2340.

[15] Ye Y,Wang J,Hu Q,et al. Synergistic transcutaneous immunotherapy enhances antitumor immune responses through delivery of checkpoint inhibitors[J]. ACS Nano,2016,10(9):8956-8963.

[16] Zeng Q,Gammon J M,Tostanoski L H,et al. *In vivo* expansion of melanoma-specific T cells using microneedle arrays coated with immune-polyelectrolyte multilayers[J]. ACS Biomater Sci Eng,2017,3(2):195-205.

[17] Dong L,Li Y,Li Z,et al. Au nanocage-strengthened dissolving microneedles for chemo-photothermal combined therapy of superficial skin tumors[J]. ACS Appl Mater Interfaces,2018,10(11):9247-9256.

[18] Pan J,Ruan W,Qin M,et al. Intradermal delivery of STAT3 siRNA to treat melanoma via dissolving microneedles[J]. Sci Rep,2018,8(1):1-11.

[19] Mao J,Wang H,Xie Y,et al. Transdermal delivery of rapamycin with poor water-solubility by dissolving polymeric microneedles for anti-angiogenesis[J]. J Mater Chem B,2020,8(5):928-934.

[20] Du H,Liu P,Zhu J,et al. Hyaluronic acid-based dissolving microneedle patch loaded with methotrexate for improved treatment of psoriasis [J]. ACS Appl Mater Interfaces,2019,11(46):43588-43598.

[21] Xie Y,Wang H,Mao J,et al. Enhanced *in vitro* efficacy for inhibiting hypertrophic scar by bleomycin-loaded dissolving hyaluronic acid microneedles[J]. J Mater Chem B, 2019,7(42):6604-6611.

[22] Gittard S D,Ovsianikov A,Akar H,et al. Two photon polymerization-micromolding of polyethylene glycol-gentamicin sulfate microneedles[J]. Adv Eng Mater,2010,12(4): B77-B82.

[23] Park S Y,Lee H U,Lee Y C,et al. Wound healing potential of antibacterial microneedles loaded with green tea extracts[J]. Mater Sci Eng C Mater Biol Appl, 2014,42:757-762.

[24] Boehm R D,Daniels J,Stafslien S,et al. Polyglycolic acid microneedles modified with inkjet-deposited antifungal coatings[J]. Biointerphases,2015,10(1):011004.

[25] Boehm R D,Miller P R,Schell W A,et al. Inkjet printing of amphotericin B onto biodegradable microneedles using piezoelectric inkjet printing[J]. JOM,2013,65(4): 525-533.

[26] Sachan R,Jaipan P,Zhang J Y,et al. Printing amphotericin B on microneedles using matrix-assisted pulsed laser evaporation[J]. Int J Bioprint,2017,3(2):4.

[27] Boehm R D,Miller P R,Daniels J,et al. Inkjet printing for pharmaceutical applications [J]. Mater Today,2014,17(5):247-252.

[28] Boehm R D,Jaipan P,Skoog S A,et al. Inkjet deposition of itraconazole onto poly (glycolic acid) microneedle arrays[J]. Biointerphases,2016,11(1):011008.

[29] García L E G,MacGregor M N,Visalakshan R M,et al. Self-sterilizing antibacterial silver-loaded microneedles[J]. Chem Commun,2019,55(2):171-174.

[30] Zhang Y,Feng P,Yu J,et al. ROS-responsive microneedle patch for acne vulgaris treatment[J]. Adv Therap,2018,1(3):1800035.

[31] Chen M C,Lin Z W,Ling M H. Near-infrared light-activatable microneedle system for treating superficial tumors by combination of chemotherapy and photothermal therapy [J]. ACS Nano,2016,10(1):93-101.

[32] Pamornpathomkul B,Ngawhirunpat T,Tekko I A,et al. Dissolving polymeric microneedle arrays for enhanced site-specific acyclovir delivery[J]. Eur J Pharm Sci, 2018,121:200-209.

[33] Jeon E Y,Lee J,Kim B J,et al. Bio-inspired swellable hydrogel-forming double-layered adhesive microneedle protein patch for regenerative internal/external surgical closure [J]. Biomaterials,2019,222:119439.

[34] 郭彬彬,周文虎,丁劲松.生物促渗剂在经皮给药系统中的应用研究进展[J].中国新药杂志,2018,27(3):314-321.

[35] Marwah H,Garg T,Goyal A K,et al. Permeation enhancer strategies in transdermal

drug delivery[J]. Drug Deliv,2016,23(2):564-578.

[36] Watkinson A C,Kearney M C,Quinn H L,et al. Future of the transdermal drug delivery market-have we barely touched the surface[J]. Expert Opin Drug Deliv,2016, 13(4):523-532.

[37] Alkilani A Z,McCrudden M T,Donnelly R F. Transdermal drug delivery:innovative pharmaceutical developments based on disruption of the barrier properties of the stratum corneum[J]. Pharmaceutics,2015,7(4):438-470.

[38] Rzhevskiy A S,Singh T R R,Donnelly R F,et al. Microneedles as the technique of drug delivery enhancement in diverse organs and tissues[J]. J Control Release,2018, 270:184-202.

[39] Kováčik A,Kopečná M,Vávrová K. Permeation enhancers in transdermal drug delivery:benefits and limitations [J]. Expert Opin Drug Deliv,2020,17(2):145-155.

[40] Ali A,Ahmed S. A review on chitosan and its nanocomposites in drug delivery[J]. Int J Biol Macromol,2018,109:273-286.

[41] Ma G,Wu C. Microneedle,bio-microneedle and bio-inspired microneedle:a review[J]. J Control Release,2017,251:11-23.

[42] Rai V K,Mishra N,Yadav K S,et al. Nanoemulsion as pharmaceutical carrier for dermal and transdermal drug delivery:formulation development,stability issues,basic considerations and applications[J]. J Control Release,2018,270:203-225.

[43] Saghazadeh S,Rinoldi C,Schot M,et al. Drug delivery systems and materials for wound healing applications[J]. Adv Drug Deliv Rev,2018,127:138-166.

[44] Sanjay S T,Zhou W,Dou M,et al. Recent advances of controlled drug delivery using microfluidic platforms[J]. Adv Drug Deliv Rev,2018,128:3-28.

[45] Shende P,Sardesai M,Gaud R S. Micro to nanoneedles:a trend of modernized transepidermal drug delivery system[J]. Artif Cells Nanomed Biotechnol,2018,46(1): 19-25.

[46] Zhang Y,Feng P,Yu J,et al. ROS-responsive microneedle patch for acne vulgaris treatment[J]. Adv Therap,2018,1(3):1800035.

[47] Zhu J,Tang X,Jia Y,et al. Applications and delivery mechanisms of hyaluronic acid used for topical/transdermal delivery—a review[J]. Int J Pharm,2020,578:119127.

[48] Tak Y K,Pal S,Naoghare P K,et al. Shape-dependent skin penetration of silver nanoparticles:does it really matter? [J]. Sci Rep,2015,5:16908.

（朱今巾）

Chapter 8
Transdermal Drug Delivery

8.1　Introduction of Transdermal Drug Delivery

Transdermal drug delivery (TDD) refers to a skin-mediated approach to administration that allows drugs to be delivered to target tissues through the skin or further into the systemic circulation and corresponding lymph nodes through capillaries and lymphatic vessels, resultantly exerting a local or systematic therapeutic effect. Compared with traditional administration approaches (e. g. , oral administration, subcutaneous injection, intradermal injection, and intravenous injection), TDD has its distinctive advantages: ① TDD can avoid the gastrointestinal adverse reactions and the first-pass effect of liver caused by oral administration. ② In contrast with traditional injections, TDD is mostly non-invasive or minimally invasive, with little pain, no needles left, easy operation and self-operation, which may effectively improve patients' medication compliance. Finally, TDD is highly controllable because the dosage and time of administration can be flexibly adjusted to ensure the safety of medication. So far, the US Food and Drug Administration has approved more than 20 drugs for TDD, bringing a global TDD market worth up to ＄32 billion annually.

8.2　Physiological and Histological Background of TDD

8.2.1　Skin barrier and TDD pathways

The skin barrier is a critical physiological structure that hinders TDD. The stratum corneum, a dense structure consisting of dead cells (mainly containing keratin and lipids), is the main component of the skin barrier, with a thickness of 10-20 μm. In the stratum granulosum below, cells are tightly connected to further obstruct the drug penetration (see 1.2.1 Barrier function, 2.1.1 Skin barrier and extended reading 1 in this chapter for details).

There are three main pathways for transdermal absorption of drugs passing through the intact skin barrier (Figure 8-1).

8.2.1.1 Intracellular pathway

Drugs pass through keratinocytes to the active epidermis, and then is absorbed by capillaries in the dermis into the systemic circulation. It requires multiple water/lipid distributions and only accounts for a very small part of the drug's transdermal absorption.

8.2.1.2 Intercellular pathway

Drugs pass through the lipid bilayer between keratinocytes, and this is the major pathway for transdermal drug absorption. Most small-molecule drugs are absorbed through this pathway, especially accessible for fat-soluble small-molecule drugs.

8.2.1.3 Transcellular pathway

Drugs are absorbed through the skin appendages (e. g. , hair follicles, sebaceous glands, and sweat glands), and this is the main pathway of transdermal absorption of ionic and polar macromolecular drugs and nano-drugs.

8.2.2 Lymphatic drainage and blood circulation of the skin

Blood vessels and lymphatic vessels in the skin are the histological structure foundation for ensuring the systematic effect of transdermal administration. Blood vessels are distributed in the dermis and subcutaneous tissues, and the capillaries are particularly abundant around the skin appendages, which provide favorable conditions for macromolecular drugs and nano-drugs entering the systemic circulation through the transcellular pathway. The skin capillary lymphatic vessels originate from the dermal papilla layer with high permeability. After penetrating into the skin, drugs can be drained into the lymph nodes along with the skin tissue fluid through the skin capillary lymphatic vessels. Besides, drugs can also act on cells in the skin, and indirectly produce systemic effects through cell migration. For example, the vaccine can work on antigen-presenting cells in the skin, such as Langerhans cells in the epidermis and dendritic cells in the dermis, which can further migrate to the lymph nodes, thereby producing a systemic immune effect.

8.3 Factors Impacting TDD

8.3.1 Factors relevant to skin

8.3.1.1 Skin thickness

The skin thickness of individuals of different ages, genders, locations, and ethnicities may vary. For example, the thickness of the skin at the eyelid is about 0.5 mm, while that at the palm and plantar part can be up to 3-4 mm. In general, the stratum corneum is thicker where the skin is thicker, making it more difficult for drug penetration.

8.3.1.2　The structure of the skin

The efficiency of TDD depends on the integrity of the skin barrier, whether the skin is hyperkeratotic, or the arrangement and fluidity of the skin structure molecules. For example, in diseases where the skin barrier is damaged (e. g., atopic dermatitis), the transdermal efficiency of drugs is enhanced. However, it decreases in hyperkeratotic diseases (e. g., corns, calluses, and tinea pedis) due to the thickened stratum corneum. Besides, when various internal and external factors lead to changes in the arrangement structure and fluidity of proteins and lipid molecules in stratum corneum, the skin permeability will also change accordingly.

8.3.1.3　Degree of hydration

When the degree of keratin hydration is high, the penetration of many drugs will be strengthened. Based on this principle, it has become a routine clinical practice to enhance the penetration of drugs by encapsulating or compressing specific drugs.

8.3.1.4　Blood supply

The blood supply of the skin does not directly affect the transdermal capacity of drugs, but the more abundant the blood supply is, the more efficient the drugs are transported to the circulatory system after passing through the skin. When the skin is congested, the blood flow speed increases, giving rise to a faster transport of the drug through the epidermis to the dermis. At the same time, the concentration difference between the superficial layer and the deep layer increases, so the drug is more likely to penetrate downward.

8.3.2　Factors relevant to drug

8.3.2.1　Lipid-water partition coefficient of drugs

Drugs with $\log P$ (P refers to the lipid-water partition coefficient) between 0 and 5 are generally considered to have comparatively strong transdermal capacity. The transdermal ability of drugs with $\log P$ at about 2 is the strongest one. Such drugs can penetrate both the hydrophilic head layer of the lipid bilayer and the hydrophobic tail layer.

8.3.2.2　Molecular weight and molecular structure of drugs

In physiological conditions, drugs with a low molecular weight ($M_W < 500$) are more likely to penetrate the skin. But it is not true that drugs with smaller molecular weight will induce higher transdermal efficiency, because the transdermal efficiency is also related to the molecular structure and shape.

8.3.2.3　Drug concentration

In general, enhanced drug concentration will increase the transdermal efficiency. However, some drugs have obvious skin irritation effect or coagulation effect on keratin at high concentration, which reduces skin permeability and results in poor drug absorption. In addition, the concentrations are related to the solubility of drugs. To achieve an ideal transdermal efficiency, a drug is generally supposed to possess a solubility above 1 mg/mL both in water and oil.

8.3.2.4　The dosage form of drugs

The dosage form of topical medication has a significant effect on transdermal absorption. It is generally believed that the efficiency of drug penetration in gels, emulsions, ointments, plasters and creams is superior to that in powders and aqueous solutions.

In addition to the factors mentioned above, the dissociation degree, melting point and pH of drugs also affect its transdermal efficiency.

8.3.3　Environmentally relevant factors

8.3.3.1　Temperature

When the environment temperature rises, the skin's absorption capacity is increased because of the accelerated material diffusion speed and dilated skin blood vessels. A study found that when the temperature was increased from 26 ℃ to 35 ℃, the dispersion of epidermal water could double. Another study found that when the temperature rised from 32 ℃ to 37 ℃, the *in vitro* transdermal efficiency of fentanyl also doubled.

8.3.3.2　Humidity

On the one hand, increasing the environment humidity reduces the moisture concentration difference between the stratum corneum and the external environment, leading to decreased skin's absorption of moisture from the external environment. On the other hand, the environment humidity can affect the transdermal absorption of drugs by changing the hydration of the stratum corneum.

8.4　Development of TDD Technology

8.4.1　A brief introduction of the history of TDD technology

TDD technology has a long history. As early as the Spring and Autumn Period and Warring States Period, more than 30 kinds of prescriptions of plasters were recorded in the *Preions for Fifty-Two Diseases*. In contrast, the development history of TDD technology in modern medicine is not long. It was not until the 1870s that the anisodamine patch was approved by the US FDA for motion sickness as the first transdermal patch. So far, TDD technology has undergone four generations.

8.4.1.1　The first generation: passive diffusion-based TDD

The first generation of TDD technology selects suitable drugs or simply chemically modifies existing drugs to achieve transdermal effects. The first generation of TDD drugs are generally highly lipophilic, with $\log P > 4$, small molecular weight ($M_W < 400$) so that they spread quickly through the skin barrier. Therefore, the categories of the first generation of TDD drugs are extremely limited.

8.4.1.2 The second generation: non-invasive penetration promotion method-based TDD

The second generation of TDD technology focuses on two innovations. ① It improves the transdermal ability of drugs with application of penetration enhancers or nano-drug carriers (e.g., liposomes, microemulsions and gels). ② It uses thermal perforation (accelerating drug penetration and making the skin more permeable with the thermal energy), electroporation (using high voltage short electrical pulses to temporarily increase skin permeability), ionophoresis (using low voltage current to pass drugs through the skin), and non-cavitation ultrasound (relying on the mechanical and thermal effects of ultrasound to promote drug transdermal ability) and other external drives to reversibly improve the skin's permeability to drugs. The second generation of TDD technology only temporarily alters the skin's permeability to drugs without damaging the integrity of the skin structure and skin barrier function, which is safe and non-invasive. Nevertheless, the second generation of TDD technology still has its limitations. On the one hand, although the non-invasive penetration promotion method can improve the drug delivery efficiency to a certain extent, the overall bioavailability of drugs is still low. On the other hand, the rise of biologicals has brought new challenges to TDD(see extended reading 2). From 2015 to 2018, nearly 30% of all drugs approved by the US FDA were biologicals. At present, the vast majority of biologicals are peptide scaffolds, of which more than 50 monoclonal antibodies have been approved and become critical treatments in clinical practice. Monoclonal antibodies of TNF-α, IL-17A, IL-23 and IL-4/IL-13 have been widely used in various dermatological diseases such as psoriasis and atopic dermatitis. Biologicals have a large molecular weight (e.g., a monoclonal antibody has about 500 amino acid residues with a molecular weight of about 150000) and poor stability. Therefore, it is difficult to meet the transdermal requirements of biologicals through the second generation of TDD technology.

8.4.1.3 The third generation: minimally invasive TDD

The third generation of TDD technology promotes the delivery of drugs by microchannels on the epidermis formed by minimally invasive, such as the destruction of the stratum corneum by radio frequency ablation, ultrasound, and laser to form microchannels. Since the size of the formed microchannels is much larger than the size of the drug molecules, various hydrophilic and hydrophobic drugs, proteins, DNAs and other large molecular biologicals can effectively pass. However, these transdermal administration approaches often rely on bulky and expensive equipments and technical personnel to operate, as well as causing some pain to patients. Hopefully, in recent years, the rise of microneedles (MNs) has thrown new light on the TDD field. MNs are matrix arrays formed by micrometer-level small needles, which include solid MNs, hollow MNs, coated MNs, soluble MNs, swellable MNs (also known as hydrogel MNs or phase-transition MNs), etc. MNs are generally 50-1000 μm long, which is often hard to reach the dermal nerve, so the pain is often mild. As a novel drug delivery approach, microneedle array has advantages of painlessness, accurate positioning, minimally invasive, safe and efficient, easy to carry, and patients can use it by themselves. MNs are especially suitable for the administration of biologicals (e. g., macromolecules, nucleic acids, peptides, proteins, vaccines), and have become the most potential minimally invasive drug delivery method in the third generation of TDD technology. Although the third generation of TDD technology can transiently damage the skin barrier, the damage will be quickly repaired by self.

8.4.1.4　The fourth generation: controlled and feedback-guided intelligent device-based TDD

The fourth generation of TDD technology emerged in the context of individualized treatment and multidisciplinary intersection. It is based on a patch which is integrated with soft ultra-thin wearable intelligent device, bioelectronic devices and drugs. The patch can closely adhere to the skin to monitor the physiological signals (e. g., blood pressure and body temperature), electrophysiological signals (e. g., electrocardiogram and electroencephalogram) and biochemical signals (e. g., pH values of sweat and body fluid, levels of blood glucose and blood oxygen) through biosensors. These signals are transmitted to the actuator to control the release of the corresponding drugs according to demand, forming a biosensor-actuator feedback loop. Currently, the fourth generation of TDD technology is still in the early research stage (see chapter 10 Wearable Skin Devices and Electronic Skin for details).

8.4.2　Ideal TDD technology

With the development of four generations, TDD technology has achieved many remarkable results and clinical applications, but the current technology still has its limitations. The ideal TDD technology should have the following characteristics.

(1) Be minimally invasive, painless, safe and convenient.

(2) Be suitable for administration of hydrophobic, hydrophilic drugs and macromolecular drugs (e. g., peptides, proteins, RNAs, DNAs);

(3) Ensure the stability of the drug properties and adequate dosage.

(4) Ensure controllable and ideal release speed.

(5) Be accessible to self-administration without leaving sharp needles.

8.5　TDD Technology Based on Biomedical Polymers

Biomedical polymers have been applied to TDD for several decades, from the second to the fourth generation of TDD technology. This section will introduce the application of biomedical polymers in the field of TDD technology from three parts: penetration enhancers, nanoparticles (NPs) and microneedles (MNs) based on biomedical polymers.

8.5.1 Penetration enhancers based on biomedical polymers

Penetration enhancers are a kind of chemical substances that can reversibly reduce the resistance of the skin to drugs and accelerate the penetration of drugs through the skin. After removing them, the skin can restore the normal barrier function. Traditional small molecule chemical penetration enhancers include solvents (e. g., ethanol, pyrrolidone (sodium pyrrolidone carboxylate), sulfoxides (dimethyl sulfoxide (DMSO) and decyl methyl sulfoxide)), fatty acids, surfactants, terpenes, azone, etc. They work in a variety of ways, including increasing solubility of drugs and penetration of drugs to the stratum corneum, liquidizing the stratum corneum crystal structure, and dissolving the lipid of the stratum corneum. The skin irritant penetration enhancers such as dimethyl sulfoxide (DMSO), dimethylformamide (DMF) and oxazolidinones are currently rarely utilized, while the more moderate penetration enhancers such as fatty acids, urea and pyrrolidone are still widely used. However, traditional chemical penetration enhancers are only suitable for small molecular weight drugs, and they are very limited for the penetration of macromolecular drugs such as biologicals. Comparatively, the polymer penetration enhancers (e. g., hyaluronic acid, dendrimers, cyclodextrins, chitosan and its derivatives, and skin-penetrating peptides) have distinct advantages in promoting the penetration of macromolecular drugs and NPs.

8.5.1.1 Hyaluronic acid

Hyaluronic acid (HA) is a linear polysaccharide inherent in the human body, particularly abundant in the extracellular matrix. It has excellent biocompatibility, degradability, non-immunogenicity and low toxicity. HA can enhance the penetration of small molecule drugs (e. g., diclofenac, ibuprofen, clindamycin and cyclosporine), and be modified on the surfaces of macromolecules and NPs to enhance their transdermal ability as well. For example, the conjugate of HA and human growth hormone (hGH) penetrates the skin of mice more strongly than free hGH. Conjugation of HA and nano-alkylene oxide Ce6 particles can also significantly promote the transdermal effect. HA plays the role of penetration enhancer mainly through the following mechanisms: ① increasing the hydration of the stratum corneum, loosening the lipid bilayer, and making the hydrophilic drug more permeable; ② changing the keratin in the stratum corneum from α-helix to β-sheet, making the lipid bilayer disordered; ③ relying on HA receptors expressed on living skin cells (e. g., keratinocytes and fibroblasts) which are probably involved in the active transport of HA and the binding drugs.

8.5.1.2 Dendrimers

Dendrimers are a class of synthetic hyperbranched polymers. Their core and highly functional branches can carry hydrophilic and lipophilic drugs through host-guest interactions and chemical conjugation, consequently developing a universal platform with high drug loading and high monodispersity. Polyamide dendrimer (PAMAM), a chemical penetration enhancer, has been used for transdermal administration researches of various small molecular drugs (e. g. , tamsulosin hydrochloride (a selective alpha 1A adrenergic receptor antagonist for urinary retention), ketoprofen and diflunisal, 8-methoxypsoralen, riboflavin (vitamin B_2), 5-fluorouracil) in the skin of rat or pig. The mechanisms by which different dendrimers promote drug transdermal delivery depend on their sizes (determined by branch algebra) and charge. ① The relatively small dendrimers can quickly diffuse through the stratum corneum and change the solubility, polarity and structural integrity of the lipid bilayer to act as a fluid for drug penetration. ② The cationic dendrimers can form nanopores to destroy the lipid bilayer and promote drug penetration. ③ Certain dendrimers can participate in drug penetration through transcellular pathway.

8.5.1.3　Cyclodextrins

Cyclodextrins (CDs) are cyclic oligosaccharides whose repeating units of α-D-glucopyranose are connected to each other through carbon atoms in the α-1 and α-4 positions. The structures of CDs are shaped like a cone, with hydrophilic hydroxyl groups on the outside of the cone and lipophilic framework carbon and etheric oxygen distributed on the surface of inner cavity, in which lipophilic drugs can be carried in the inner cavity. CDs have a large molecular weight(M_W=1134.98) and a low log$P$ value (-3 to 0), so its transdermal ability is not strong. But they can bind to poorly soluble lipophilic drugs to increase their solubility and stability, thus increasing their skin permeability. However, in general, CDs do not increase the permeability of drugs across stratum corneum, which is still not easy for transdermal transport of cyclodextrin-drug complexes. Solutions to improve its transdermal efficiency include modification of lipophilic groups on the surface or combination with small molecule chemical penetration enhancers.

8.5.1.4　Chitosan and its derivatives

Chitosan are a group of cationic polysaccharides consisting of β-(1-4)-linked D-glucosamine and N-acetyl-D-glucosamine that are randomly distributed along the main chain. Among them, only relatively low molecular weight chitosan can increase the permeability of the skin, such as promoting the penetration of baicalin (an anti-tumor drug) into mouse skin. Nuclear magnetic resonance (NMR) spectroscopy shows that chitosan have no electrostatic interaction with keratin or glycoprotein in the stratum corneum, so the increased permeability of the stratum corneum may be ascribed to the dipole-dipole and van der Waals interaction between chitosan and lipid biomolecules. Other chitosan derivatives with penetration promoting effect include N-trimethyl chitosan, N-arginine chitosan and so on.

8.5.1.5　Skin-penetrating peptides

Skin-penetrating peptides are short peptides with less than 30 amino acid residues. Unlike the aforementioned chemical penetration enhancers, skin-penetrating peptides belong to biological penetration enhancers with good biocompatibility and low toxicity. They can be used to promote the transdermal administration of peptides, proteins, nucleic acids, nanoparticles, and other biologically active molecules by physical mixing, formation of fusion proteins, covalent connection, modification of carriers. Presently, a variety of skin-penetrating peptide preparations are undergoing the clinical trial, among which the clinical trial of RT-001 for the penetration of botulinum toxin A in treating facial wrinkles, and AZX-100 analogs for the penetration and absorption of HSP20 to prevent skin scars have entered phase Ⅱ clinical trail.

8.5.2　NPs based on biomedical polymers

The use of polymer NPs to carry drugs is an important strategy in the second generation of TDD technology. Polymer NPs can not only reduce the degradation of drugs and enhance the transdermal penetration ability of drugs, but also achieve controlled drug release. Polymer NPs usually accumulate in hair follicles and achieve transdermal delivery through the transcellular pathway. Polymer NPs encompass natural polymer NPs (e. g. , chitosan, albumin NPs) and synthetic polymer NPs (e. g. , PLGA, dendrimer NPs). The application of NPs in TDD technology is detailed in Chapter 6.

8.5.3　MNs based on biomedical polymers

8.5.3.1　Developmental history of MNs

MNs is an emerging minimally invasive TDD technology, which includes solid MNs, hollow MNs, coated MNs, soluble MNs, swellable MNs (also known as hydrogel MNs or phase-transition MNs), etc. MNs can deliver drugs through the formation of micron-level holes in the skin, improving the efficiency of drug penetration. In 1998, the research team of Dr. Prausnitz of the Georgia Institute of Technology in the United States applied reactive ion etching technology to fabricate a solid MNs array using silicon as the host material, with the length of about 150 μm and a tip curvature radius of less than 1 μm. Later, they used this MNs array to conduct a skin penetration test for the first time. The results showed that the application of MNs can increase the percutaneous drug penetration rate of calcein (model drug) by 1000 times. Since then, solid MNs have developed rapidly, and a variety of MNs using metal, silica, glass, nickel, and titanium as host materials have shown up. In particular, in the cosmetic field, all kinds of commercial MNs have been extensively used. The application of solid roller MNs has been included in the 2016 edition of the Photodynamic Guidelines of the American Academy of Dermatology as a means of promoting penetration of photosensitizers in photodynamic therapy. However, solid MNs rely on two steps of "needle sticking and drug application", which are troublesome to operate. Moreover, the drug dosage is difficult to control and the repeated use of the needle is prone to infection risks. Therefore, coated MNs and hollow MNs are evolved on the basis of solid MNs. The coated MNs smear drugs on the surface of the solid MNs, and drugs can be dissolved and diffused after MNs piercing into the skin, thereby achieving one-step administration and significantly improving the efficiency of drug utilization. Macroflux (produced by Zosano Pharm), which was approved by the US FDA in 2002, is the earliest approved MN device and a typical representative of coated MNs. Nonetheless, coated MNs also face challenges such as small drug loading. Hollow MNs are micron-level matrix syringes, the typical representative of which is Micronjet (produced by NanoPass Technologies) approved by the US FDA in 2009. Most of the above three categories of MNs are made of metal, ceramics, glass or silicon, so they generally are poorly biocompatible, easy to leave needle tips and call for professional involvement. In recent years, the advent of soluble MNs and swellable MNs based on biomedical polymers has overcome these deficiencies. Soluble MNs dissolve subsequent to penetrating into the skin, achieving the one-step administration. Furthermore, they have relatively high drug loading and excellent tissue compatibility. Additionally, they are quite cost-effective and can be operated by patients without leaving sharp needles. The swellable MNs swell and release drugs after contacting with the tissue fluid in the skin. After drugs are released, the MNs can be pulled out to prevent the polymer from depositing in the skin. Since the swellable MNs absorb tissue fluid, they can also be used for skin tissue fluid extraction.

Production strategies of polymer MNs include micro-molding (MM), hot embossing (HE), drip blow molding (DAB), electrographic drawing (ED), injection molding (IM), laser micromachining (LMM), drawing lithography (DL), lithography (PL), overmolding (IM), continuous liquid interface production (CLIP), dipping, solvent casting, X-ray and 3D printing. The appropriate production method should be selected according to the category of MNs, host materials and drug properties. For example, the process of swellable MNs synthesis often requires high temperature or UV, so the potential impact of the corresponding generation process on drugs should be considered.

This section focuses on the application of biomedical polymers as the host materials of coated MNs, soluble MNs and swellable MNs in skin diseases, because biomedical polymers have only a few applications in solid MNs and hollow MNs, and its advantages are less obvious compared to other materials.

8.5.3.2 Factors affecting the selection of host materials used in polymer MNs

The selection of host materials used in polymer MNs should consider the following factors in addition to biological safety and stability.

1. Mechanical strengths

The mechanical strengths of the MNs are determined by the wall thickness, wall corner, tip radius, length, distance between the needles and polymer composition of the MNs, so different categories of polymers differ in mechanical strengths. The carried drugs and NPs also pose effects to the mechanical strengths of the MNs. For example, in one of our research, when 368 μg photosensitizer ALA was loaded into the hyaluronic acid MNs, the Young's moduli of the MNs decreased from 58.9 MPa to 40.0 MPa. While in another research, 4 μg AuNC was loaded into hyaluronic acid MNs and the Young's moduli of the MNs increased from 68. 9 MPa to 224. 9 MPa.

2. Solubility/swelling ability of host materials

The solubility or swelling ability of the MNs is of importance to drug release rate. When designing a MN, the host material needs to be tailored to the drug release requirements. In the treatment of some skin diseases, the rapid release of drugs is required to quickly reach the effective local concentration or blood concentration, such as chemotherapy drugs, photosensitizers, photothermal agents, analgesic drugs, and anti-itch drugs. While in inflammatory diseases management,such as psoriasis and eczema, it is proper for long-term slow release of drugs. In addition, in the immunotherapy of skin diseases, it is necessary to consider the time course of the immune events and the specific mechanism of drugs to determine the time and speed of drug release. Of note, even for the treatment of the same disease, the requirement for drug release is also different due to the diverse nature of drugs. For example, antibiotics are classified into "concentration-dependent" and "time-dependent". When treating skin infections, the former needs to release drugs quickly to reach the effective drug concentration, while the latter needs to release drugs relatively slowly to ensure the action time with effective drug concentration. Water-soluble polysaccharides and their analogues, such as hyaluronic acid (HA), poly (vinyl pyrrolidone) (PVP), dextran, hydroxypropyl methyl cellulose (HPMC), hydroxypropyl cellulose (HPC), carboxymethyl cellulose (CMC) and amylopectin can be quickly and completely dissolved, so they are often used to prepare MNs that require rapid drug release. Conversely, poly(lactic acid) (PLA), poly(lactic-co-glycolic acid) (PLGA), polycarbonate (PC), poly (glycolic acid) (PGA), polycaprolactone (PCL), chitosan and silk are insoluble in water but can be slowly degraded in the body, which are often used to prepare MNs that need to be slowly released. The swelling property of the polymers is another important mechanism for the continuous administration. The swellable MNs made of swellable polymers can absorb a large amount of water without dissolving, and its diffusion is determined by the swelling ability and cross-linked structure of the drug molecules and polymers. Common swellable polymers include poly(hydroxyethyl methacrylate) (PHEMA), polystyrene-$block$-poly(acrylic acid) (PS-b-PAA), poly (vinyl alcohol) (PVA), poly (methyl vinyl ether-maleic acid) (PMVE/MA, Gantrez), hyaluronic acid acrylate, etc.

3. Targeting ability

Some polymer materials have natural targeting properties (e. g., HA can selectively bind to the CD44 receptor of cancer cells). Besides, other polymers can target specific cells and/or tissues through redox reactions.

4. Responsive release

Polymer MNs can be designed to respond to specific environments or specific signals. Common response-evoked signals include specific pH, blood glucose concentration, hypoxia, temperature, light, mechanical force, and enzymes or receptors. Swellable MNs based on anionic and cationic polymers exhibit pH-sensitive swelling property and responsive release capabilities. For example, the cationic polymer PEG-*b*-poly(β-amino ester) releases the drug 4 times faster in a slightly acidic environment (pH is 6.5-7.0) than that in the environment with pH $=$ 7.4. McCoy et al. prepared photoresponsive swellable MNs by cross-linking poly(2-hydroxyethyl methacrylate) (PHEMA) and ethylene glycol dimethacrylate, which obtained a long-term release (up to 160 h) of light-responsive drug. Some polymers swell highly at low temperature, but shrink when the temperature rises to a certain value. For example, poly (methoxydiethylene glycol methacrylate) (PmDEGMA) and poly (methoxytriethylene glycol methacrylate) (PmTEGMA) show heat-responsive drug release. When the temperature is above the critical temperature, the drug molecules are squeezed out of the contracted gel and released. Importantly, polymer MNs can be combined with NPs with controlled release and targeting functions, which is highly promising in TDD (see extended reading 3).

8.5.3.3 Applications of MNs in transdermal administration of skin diseases

MNs based on biomedical polymers have been extensively studied in cosmetic field, skin inflammatory diseases, skin tumors, and skin infections (see the corresponding section for details). Table 8-1 summarizes the application studies of polymer MNs in the above fields in recent years (see extended reading 4). In these studies, polymer MNs generally exhibited a better preventive or therapeutic effect than traditional administration of vaccines or drugs.

Table 8-1 Summary of application of MNs based on biomedical polymers in skin diseases

Drugs	Polymers	MNs types	Diseases or application models	Control categories
ALA	HA	Soluble	Photodynamic therapy of subcutaneous tumors in mice	Instant
a-PD1	Cross-linked product of HA and MBA	Soluble	Immunotherapy of mouse melanoma	pH-sensitive dextran NPs controlled release
a-PD1＋1-MT	HA	Soluble	Immunotherapy of mouse melanoma	Sustained release
Tumor antigen＋CpG	immune polyelectrolyte multilayers (iPEMs)	Coated	Melanoma vaccine	—

Continued

Drugs	Polymers	MNs types	Diseases or application models	Control categories
DOX+AuNC	HA	Soluble	Mouse melanoma chemotherapy + photothermal therapy	Instant
PEI with STAT3 siRNA	HA，dextran，PVP	Soluble	Gene therapy for melanoma in mice	Instant
DOX+LaB6	PVA/PVP (base + needle matrix) PCL (needle tip)	Soluble	Mouse subcutaneous tumor model	NIR sensitive controlled release
Rapamycin	PVP	Soluble	*In vitro* vascular abnormality model	Instant
Methotrexate	HA	Soluble	Mouse psoriasis model	Instant
Bleomycin	HA	Soluble	*In vitro* hypertrophic scar model	Instant
Gentamicin sulfate	PEG	Soluble	*In vitro* antibacterial model	Sustained release
Nano silver	CMC	Soluble	*In vitro* antibacterial model	—
Green tea extract	HA	Soluble	Rat wound infection model	—
Voriconazole	PGA	Coated	*In vitro* antifungal model	—
Amphotericin B	Gantrez AN-169	Coated	*In vitro* antifungal model	—
Amphotericin B	PGA	Coated	*In vitro* antifungal model	—
Miconazole	Gantrez AN-169	Coated	*In vitro* antifungal model	—
Itraconazole	PGA	Coated	*In vitro* antifungal model	—

Continued

Drugs	Polymers	MNs types	Diseases or application models	Control categories
Clindamycin	m-HA/DE(base) RR-PVA (needle matrix)	Soluble	Mouse *Propionibacterium acnes* infection model	ROS dependent controlled release; Sustained release
Acyclovir	Gantrez S-97	Soluble	*In vivo* and *in vitro* diffusion models (potential antiviral applications)	—
Mussel mucilage protein shell and silk fibroin core		Swellable	Rat wound healing model	—

Note: ALA, a drug used in photodynamic therapy; a-PD1(anti-PD-1 antibody), a drug used in immunotherapy; HA (hyaluronic acid); MBA, N, N'-methylenebis (acrylamide); 1-MT(1-methyl-dl-tryptophan), an IDO inhibitor; CpG, a Toll-like receptor agonist with immune adjuvant effect; PEI (polyethylenimine); PVA (poly (vinyl alcohol)); PVP (polyvinylpyrrolidone); PEG (polyethylene glycol); PGA (polyglycolic acid); CMC (carboxymethyl cellulose); m-HA/DE (methacrylate hyaluronic acid /diatomaceous earth); LaB6 (lanthanum hexaboride); RR-PVA (reactive oxygen species (ROS)-responsive poly(vinyl alcohol)); PCL (polycaprolactone); Gantrez AN-169: a copolymer of methyl vinyl ether and maleic anhydride; Gantrez S-97: a copolymer of methyl vinyl ether and maleic anhydride.

8.6 Challenges and Perspectives

At present, the first and second generations of transdermal drug delivery technology have been widely used in clinical practice, but the efficiency is generally low and it is difficult to meet the requirements of transdermal drug delivery of macromolecules such as biologicals. The third generation of transdermal drug delivery technology promotes drug delivery through minimally invasive microchannels formed on the epidermis, and is suitable for most drugs, including biologicals. However, most of the third generation of transdermal drug delivery technologies rely on cumbersome and expensive equipments and the operation of professional technicians, thus microneedles have become the most potential minimally invasive drug delivery methods in the third generation of transdermal drug delivery due to its simple medication method and wide applicability.

Although microneedles based on biomedical polymers have developed rapidly in recent years, there are currently no approved polymer microneedle products, with only one application study of polymer microneedles (hyaluronic acid soluble microneedles for the study of plaque psoriasis (NCT02955576)) in skin diseases entering the clinical trail stage. In contrast, the hollow microneedles influenza vaccine Intanza® was approved by the US FDA as early as 2009, and various types of vaccines based on hollow microneedles have entered phase Ⅱ or phase Ⅲ of clinical trial as well.

While polymer microneedles have numerous advantages, they are not without shortcomings, such as polymer deposition in the skin, low mass production efficiency, low product reproducibility (uneven residue, uneven drug loading), and high production costs. In addition, even if studies have shown that microneedles can be made larger in a simple way without troubling patients using by self, low drug loading is still a major challenge which hinders the clinical application of polymer microneedles.

In addition, many studies remain at the cell level *in vitro* and even at the level of skin simulant, and many mechanisms are difficult to verify intuitively at the animal level due to the limitations of animal models even if there are more than 3000 kinds of skin diseases to be deeply studied. Furthermore, recent studies have shown that drugs will reside in the lymph nodes, liver, kidneys, and spleen after microneedle administration, which need further research on the pharmacokinetics and safety of microneedle administration. In conclusion, the research on the application of polymer microneedles in skin diseases is still a daunting task and has a long way to go.

The fourth generation of transdermal drug delivery technology based on controlled and feedback-guided intelligent device is still in the early stage of development, but it is reasonable to expect that the combination of polymer microneedles and intelligent device will open a new chapter of transdermal drug delivery.

Questions

1. Can transdermal drug delivery technologies be used for the extraction of tissue fluid and liquid biopsy? What might be the advantages and limitations of each technology? (see extended reading 5)

2. What should be taken into particular consideration for the transdermal delivery of biomacromolecules compared to small molecule drugs?

3. Can transdermal drug delivery technologies be used for the delivery of cells or even tissues? What are the application prospects?

4. Taking the application of microneedles in tumor therapy as an example, what are the ideal release modes of chemotherapeutic drugs and immune checkpoint inhibitors respectively? How can we design polymer microneedles to meet these modes?

5. What are the prospects of 3D printing technology in transdermal drug delivery?

Extended Reading

[1]　Yang R, Wei T, Goldberg H, et al. Getting drugs across biological barriers [J]. Adv Mater, 2017, 29(37): e1606596.

[2]　Anselmo A C, Gokarn Y, Mitragotri S. Non-invasive delivery strategies for biologics

［J］. Nat Rev Drug Discov,2019,18(1):19-40.

［3］ Singh P,Carrier A,Chen Y,et al. Polymeric microneedles for controlled transdermal drug delivery［J］. J Control Release,2019,315:97-113.

［4］ Sabri A H,Ogilvie J,Abdulhamid K,et al. Expanding the applications of microneedles in dermatology［J］. Eur J Pharm Biopharm,2019,140:121-140.

［5］ Mandal A,Boopathy A V,Lam L K W,et al. Cell and fluid sampling microneedle patches for monitoring skin-resident immunity［J］. Sci Transl Med,2018,10(467): eaar2227.

（**Zhu Jinjin**）

第九章
生物医用高分子在皮肤美容中的应用

第一节 皮肤美容概述

皮肤美容学(cosmetic dermatology)是一门以医学美学为指导、皮肤科学理论为基础,运用医学与美学相结合的技术手段,研究人体皮肤的解剖结构与生理机能和实施维护、改善、修复与塑造人体皮肤健与美及规律性的科学,它是美容医学的一个临床应用主干学科。皮肤美容主要涉及皮肤美容基础理论、皮肤保健与美容、毛发保健与美容、激光与光子美容治疗技术、美容应用技术、皮肤外科学、美容中医学及常见损容性皮肤疾病治疗等。

皮肤美容的历史由来已久。在中国,有文献记载,皮肤美容从大禹时期(公元前 2277—公元前 2213 年)就开始了。相传大禹 50 岁后,眼角、额头相继出现皱纹,当时有人建议用蜡脂涂抹脸部以淡化皱纹;但是,蜡接触皮肤后会变硬。经过多次试验,最后有人建议以小麦磨粉和成团敷面,该方法获得成功,这便是上古文献中"禹选粉"的传说。到了唐代,医学家孙思邈在《千金要方》中提出了皮肤美容药方 80 余个,这是中国已知最早的美容处方的文献。明代李时珍在他的《本草纲目》中也记载了 700 多个美容药方。

在西方国家,史料记载,最早有意识地使用化妆品的是古埃及人。古埃及人酷爱芳香制品,他们不断从印度、阿拉伯等地搜集天然香料,用其制造香水和化妆品。古埃及人极其重视肌肤的健康与美丽,在沐浴后要涂抹大量的香油、香水或油膏来滋润皮肤;为了抵御炎热干燥的气候,将动物油脂涂抹在皮肤上来防止皮肤干燥。

现代皮肤美容的发展,主要分为五个阶段。第一阶段:普通油脂护肤时代,特点是只利用化妆品的纯物理性质达到保湿和防止皲裂的作用,这些化妆品主要取自天然未加工(最多加热)过的油脂,如动物油。第二阶段:油水混合物护肤时代,这一时代的产品是工业集成化生产的第一代化妆品,同样具有保湿和防止皲裂的作用,但比起第一代更加卫生、方便、纯净,代表产品有凡士林。第三阶段:天然植物化妆品时代,这一时代的产品是高科技植物提纯技术生产的第一代化妆品,其特点是卫生、方便、美观、纯度高,有一定功效,原料复杂繁多,代表产品有早先的黄瓜洗面奶等。第四阶段:生物激素生态化妆品时代,这一时代的产品是高科技生物工程技术生产的第一代化妆品,其特点是卫生、方便、美观、纯度高、功效强、原料复杂繁多、容易吸收、香味醇正。第五阶段：纳米技术天然精华化妆品时代，这一时代的产品是分子微化处理技术生产的第一代化妆品，也是现代化工科技在化妆品领域的应用。

第二节　生物医用高分子在皮肤屏障修复中的应用

人体皮肤屏障(图 9-1)分为解剖屏障和功能性屏障，皮肤最外层的结构是表皮的角质层，角质层形成角质层表皮通透性屏障，可防止水和电解质的损失。其他的保护或屏障作用包括免疫防御，紫外线防护和抗氧化损伤防护。许多炎症性皮肤疾病患者存在显著的皮肤屏障结构和功能障碍，患者皮损处角质层含水量下降，油脂含量减少，经皮水分丢失增加。反复慢性炎症导致患者皮肤屏障破坏，慢性光损伤是加重皮肤屏障破坏的重要诱发因素。皮肤屏障受损时，短时间紫外线照射后皮肤会出现红斑、水肿、水疱及色素沉着，长时间紫外线照射造成皮肤增厚、弹性纤维损伤、出现皱纹等损容性改变。可以通过现有的生物医用高分子材料进行皮肤屏障的修复。

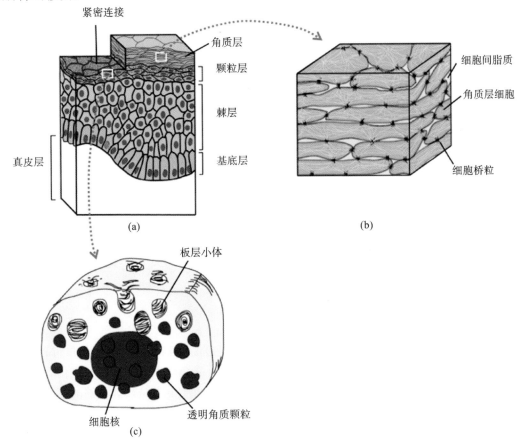

图 9-1　皮肤屏障

(a)表皮的结构，红线表示颗粒层紧密连接；(b)颗粒层细胞放大视图；(c)角质层的"砖和泥"结构

Figure 9-1　Skin barrier

(a)The structure of the epidermis (the red line represents tight junctions in the stratum granulosum)；(b)Magnified view of the cells in the stratum granulosum；(c)The "bricks and mortars" structure of the stratum corneum

（一）透明质酸（hyaluronic acid，HA）

HA 是一种直链非硫酸化的糖胺聚糖聚合物，是细胞外基质（ECM）的主要成分。ECM 是影响细胞新陈代谢最为关键的调节器。HA 的分子量大小对其各种功能至关重要。组织中高分子量的 HA 片段反映了完整的组织、抗血管生成和免疫抑制状态；而分子量较小的 HA 片段通常是炎症和血管生成的诱因，被认为是压力信号。由于其超强的保水能力，HA 负责维持皮肤的含水量。此外，HA 还参与伤口愈合和老化过程。

（二）抗氧化剂

临床上常用的抗氧化剂有果酸、水杨酸等。果酸于 1974 年被引入皮肤治疗领域，用于治疗鱼鳞病，它是指一类 α-羟基酸（alpha hydroxyacids，AHAs）；果酸是一个家族，包括羟基乙酸、酒石酸、柠檬酸、乳酸等。水杨酸最初提取自柳树。外用水杨酸或果酸治疗可以明显改善红斑、炎性丘疹以及色素沉着；其机制在于抗氧化剂外用于皮肤时，果酸激活细胞离子通道 TRPV3，钙离子过量进入细胞使之凋亡，从而软化角质层、加速角质层脱落，使得角质形成细胞中的黑素一同脱落，露出颜色更浅的肤色。长时间使用，可刺激真皮层胶原蛋白和黏多糖合成，皮肤皱纹变浅，对光老化皮肤造成的（因真皮胶原蛋白变性、减少）皱纹效果更佳。此外，抗氧化剂的使用可以软化角质，促进药物渗透，从而提高外用药疗效。

（三）肉毒毒素

肉毒毒素是革兰阳性厌氧芽孢肉毒梭菌产生的一种外毒素，通过抑制神经递质乙酰胆碱从外周轴突末端的释放而引起的化学反应来刺激神经。目前，有 A 型肉毒毒素（BoNTA）和 B 型肉毒毒素（BoNTB）在临床使用。Botox®（美国加利福尼亚州尔湾市的 Allergan 公司）是 A 型肉毒毒素，目前被美国食品药品监督管理局（FDA）批准用于多种适应证（包括眼睑痉挛和斜视）。肉毒毒素已被批准用于化妆品中，也被批准用于手足多汗症。肉毒毒素注射治疗可以用来改善玫瑰痤疮患者的顽固性面部潮红，以及因皮肤屏障破坏、慢性光损伤引起的额面部的皱纹。

第三节　生物医用高分子在皮肤缺损修复中的应用

一、皮肤替代材料

皮肤是人体的最大器官，比身体的任何其他部位更容易受到伤害。小的伤口可以在几天内自然愈合，严重Ⅲ度烧伤的大创面可能威胁患者生命。在急性大面积创伤和烧伤、老年和糖尿病患者中，仅靠正常的创面愈合反应和皮肤固有的组织再生能力是远远不够的，这对皮肤修复是一大挑战。生物医用高分子材料是医学与高分子科学有机结合而产生的具有特殊功能的天然及合成高分子生物材料，可以通过组成和结构控制使其具有不同的理化性质，以满足不同需求，而且具有易于加工成型、便于消毒灭菌、生物相容性好等优点。生物医用高分子材料的应用已遍及整个医学领域，现将与皮肤缺损修复的替代材料有关的生物医用高分子材料概括如下。

1. 天然生物医用高分子材料

组织工程支架的设计是为了模拟活体细胞外基质在组织中的功能。因此，研究人员已经探索出使用细胞外基质蛋白作为组织工程支架的材料,如胶原蛋白、明胶(胶原蛋白的水解形式)、弹性蛋白和透明质酸等。这些材料作为皮肤组织工程支架材料可以结合其他天然聚合物纤维蛋白(如血凝蛋白)和普鲁兰(真菌产生的天然生物聚合物)等,从而发挥协同作用。

2. 合成生物医用高分子材料

合成生物医用高分子材料是经过化学聚合反应生成的,如聚乳酸(PLA)、聚乳酸-羟基乙酸(PLGA)、聚氨酯(PU)等。尽管它们可能缺乏天然生物医用高分子材料中固有的细胞相互作用机制,但它们在成分与可重复性等方面的精确可控性,及其与天然生物医用高分子材料良好的结合能力,使它们非常适用于皮肤再生领域。

3. 天然和合成复合支架

许多研究者已经开始利用天然材料和合成材料的独特结合,探索制作复合组织工程支架。天然生物医用高分子材料具有机械性能差、降解速度快等缺点,这些缺点阻碍了其在临床中的应用。相比之下,大多数合成生物医用高分子材料具有良好的力学和物理性能(在生产过程中可以控制),与天然生物医用高分子材料相比,降解速度较慢。复合材料不仅具有天然材料固有的生物相容性,同时可弥补其缺乏足够的机械强度等不足。不同的合成和天然成分的结合,使得复合支架表现出更好的可控降解率和化学性能。同时还需要皮肤细胞生物学和原位制造技术(如 3D 打印等技术)的协同攻关。跨学科的交流与合作对组织再生至关重要,皮肤修复与再生也不例外。

二、皮肤移植材料

对于缺乏皮肤组织供区、皮肤损伤处无法修复或是不愿意接受供区损伤的患者,均需使用异体、异种组织或组织代用品来修复损伤。异体皮肤移植(allograft)和异种皮肤移植(xenografts)仍然是现今解决患者自体皮肤来源不足或者暂无接受自体皮肤移植条件等问题的主要方法。它们不仅可以防止电解质、蛋白质等体内成分的丢失,也可以减少创面病原微生物的污染,减轻创面疼痛,提高患者对其他治疗的顺应性,同时也可以提高自体皮肤移植的成功率。然而,异体、异种组织往往存在免疫排斥、吸收、变形或生物力学性能不够理想等问题。为此,按不同需要制作的生物医用高分子材料作为皮肤组织的移植材料,在临床应用中一直发挥着重要作用。

1. 暂时性皮肤移植材料

胶原类生物医用高分子材料是目前研究的热点。目前已经研发出透明聚合物膜、泡沫聚合物膜、水胶体、水凝胶贴片、无定形水凝胶、海绵泡沫类等材料。通过自聚和交联重建胶原可形成具有一定强度和稳定性的结构材料,具有高亲水性、无毒、体内生物相容性与降解性良好等生物特性。以胶原为主体材料,人们已发展出以组织工程学技术为特征的人工皮肤移植材料,如 Biobrane®、Dermagraft® 等。

2. 半永久皮肤移植材料

目前研究较为深入的生物医用材料还有 Integra® 等。它是牛胶原蛋白-鲨鱼硫酸软骨素组成的胶原支架,表面黏附一层硅胶薄膜。该材料可移植于血供丰富、无感染的创面,起到一种类似真皮替代物的作用。随着 10 天至 3 周的血液循环建立,去掉硅胶薄膜后可再移植一层 0.020 cm(即 0.008 英寸)的自体表皮。这种在人工合成材料上形成真皮,再行自体表皮移植的复合方法,有别于暂时性皮肤移植材料的使用方法。这是暂时性皮肤移植材料和永久性皮肤移植材料的一种结合,已真正形成了具有永久性的皮肤移植材料。在此,暂时性皮肤移植材料和永久性皮肤移植材料的研究融合在了一起。

3. 永久性皮肤移植材料

永久性皮肤移植材料为 Epicel®,它也被称为"试管皮肤"。1975 年 Rhinewald 和 Green 发明了在体外进行人工表皮细胞培养的表皮替代材料;该材料缺乏真皮成分,因此它移植后的创面有易感染、易破溃、易形成瘢痕等缺点。但 Epicel® 移植于已建立血液循环的 Integra®、Alloderm® 等人工真皮替代材料上,在长期临床观察中显示出了良好的效果。

随着生物学和生物工程技术的不断飞速发展,在皮肤替代品市场多元化的今天,临床医生应根据创面情况选择最适合的皮肤替代品进行治疗和应用。理想的皮肤替代品应包含的属性如下:促进组织再生;减少色素沉着;具有屏障保护和抗感染功能;可使附件结构(如毛囊和汗腺等)再生;易于处理和应用;保质期长。然而,现有的皮肤替代物与人们的期望还有一定距离,怎样才能发挥皮肤替代物的优点,并克服其不足之处,是未来研究的主要方向。

第四节　生物医用高分子在皮肤抗衰老中的应用

一、除皱

胶原纤维是真皮结缔组织中最丰富的成分,胶原纤维主要含胶原蛋白。真皮中的胶原蛋白主要为Ⅰ型胶原蛋白(85%～90%)、Ⅱ型胶原蛋白(8%～11%)和Ⅴ型胶原蛋白(2%～4%)。弹性纤维在维持皮肤弹性中起着重要作用,弹性纤维由弹性蛋白和丝状蛋白组成。弹性纤维和胶原纤维缠绕在一起以保持皮肤的完整性、强度与弹性。受到外界环境以及光老化损伤后,胶原蛋白与弹性蛋白结构遭到破坏,导致皮肤弹性下降,皱纹产生。

为了防止皱纹的产生与消除皱纹,在医学与化学及皮肤美容等领域产生了许多方法,如物理方法,包括激光、生物电等。在此,我们主要讨论化学相关的抗皱方法。

1. 肉毒毒素

肉毒毒素是肉毒梭菌产生的大分子蛋白聚合物,能够安全有效地治疗上、中、下面部的皱纹。使用肉毒毒素 3～7 天后,肌肉会发生麻痹,皱纹消失;3～6 个月后,突触再生逆转麻痹作用(图 9-2)。肉毒毒素是一种安全性很高的药物,其应用于美容领域是相对安全的。但是,其需要按照剂量范围使用,以优化患者的满意度并保持自然的效果。

2. 透明质酸

透明质酸(hyaluronic acid,HA)是一种直链非硫酸化的糖胺聚糖聚合物,是细胞外基质(extracellular matrix,ECM)的主要成分。皮肤中的透明质酸总量超过 50%;由于透明质酸具有强大的保水能力,其可以增加皮肤含水量,有助于在视觉上增加皮肤光泽。表皮中的透明质酸会随着年龄增加而减少。紫外线也会导致透明质酸与水分的流失,使皮肤产生皱纹。

外用透明质酸的抗皱效果是分子量依赖性的,这可能是由不同分子量的透明质酸通过角质层的经皮吸收不同所致。在一项临床试验中,76 名 30～60 岁有眼周皱纹的女性患者使用含不同分子量透明质酸(50、130、300、800、2000)的 0.1%乳膏配方,每日 2 次。60 天后观察到,使用含有低分子量透明质酸的乳霜配方的女性,皮肤水合度、皮肤弹性和眼部皱纹的减少

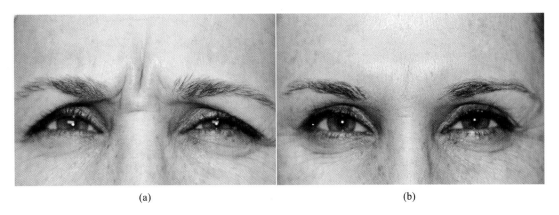

(a)   (b)

图 9-2　注射肉毒毒素(Botox)前后眉间纹和眉间复合肌变化

(a)注射前；(b)注射后 1 个月

Figure 9-2　Dynamic frown lines with glabellar complex muscle contraction

before and one month after onabotulinum toxin A(Botox) treatment

(a)Before；(b)After

有更大程度的改善。鉴于 HA 分子量依赖的经皮吸收特性，并且超小透明质酸分子能更好地经皮吸收，因此含有纳米透明质酸的外用配方的快速抗皱和皮肤修复效果更好。

透明质酸也可用于软组织填充。2007 年后，透明质酸软组织填充已经成为流行的非手术性美容手段之一，仅次于肉毒毒素皮肤填充治疗。真皮透明质酸填充很少引起过敏反应，副作用小，相对无痛，但不能长期维持效果，需要反复填充(图 9-3)。透明质酸软组织填充可能引起炎症、肿胀、淤青和不对称，这取决于注射技术；通常需要在面部的不同部位注射不同剂量的透明质酸，并加以按摩以防面部凹凸不平。使用透明质酸进行填充已成为祛除静态皱纹的主要手段，填充后可在几个月甚至更长时间内刺激体内胶原蛋白合成。透明质酸酶(hyaluronidase,HYase)可降解透明质酸，其在治疗透明质酸注射术后并发症(如血管栓塞)方

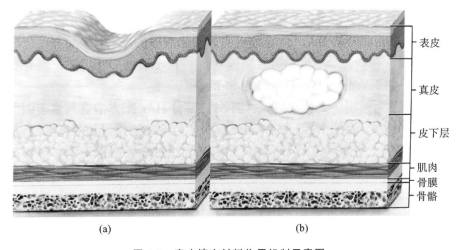

表皮

真皮

皮下层

肌肉
骨膜
骨骼

(a)   (b)

图 9-3　真皮填充材料作用机制示意图

(a)填充前；(b)填充后

Figure 9-3　Illustration showing mechanism of dermal filler materials

(a)Before；(b)After

面有显著效果。

3. 聚乳酸

聚乳酸是一种体积刺激剂,而不是直接作为填充物质使用。不同于透明质酸、胶原蛋白和羟基磷酸钙等,这种材料的优点之一是刺激胶原蛋白产生,以维持较长时间的抗皱效果。但是,聚乳酸的注射可能会引起皮下结节产生,需要少量多次注射。经常注射的区域是脸颊、下巴和太阳穴等部位,并在这些区域进行扇形注射。然而,由于其自身不作为填充物质,故无法预测可能产生的效果,在注射时需要控制使用量。

二、可穿戴聚合物

随着人们对运动手环等可穿戴器件需求的增长,越来越多的聚合物结合柔性电子技术应用于可穿戴的便携式设备,用于生命健康监测,如心率、脉搏、体温、血压及汗液中的生物指标的检测(图 9-4)。可穿戴聚合物的要求:①可以实现不同功能器件的集成的功能型材料;②可以同时满足柔性电子器件对机械稳定性的要求和与皮肤亲和性的需求。

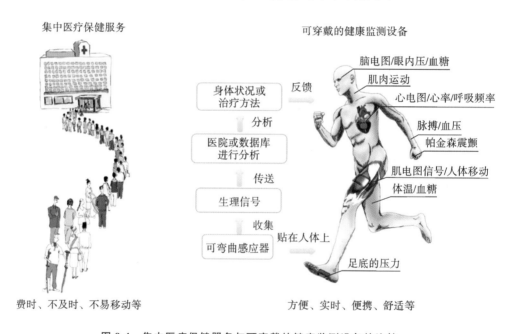

图 9-4 集中医疗保健服务与可穿戴的健康监测设备的比较

可穿戴的健康监测设备为便携式医疗保健提供了一种便捷的方式,促进了临床实践中传统诊断方法从集中医疗保健服务向分散医疗保健服务的转变。

Figure 9-4 Comparison of centralized healthcare service and wearable health monitor devices

Wearable health monitor devices provide a convenient way for portable healthcare and promote the movement of conventional diagnosis methods in clinical practice from centralized healthcare service towards decentralized healthcare delivery.

目前,柔性电子器件搭载在可穿戴聚合物(如聚二甲基硅氧烷(PDMS))等薄膜贴片上,可实现对日常生理指标的检测。例如,日常监测皮肤温度、皮肤的 pH 及钙离子水平。可通过蓝牙将该类柔性电子器件连接到无线设备上进行检测,具有较高灵敏度与可重复性。基于碳纳米管与金纳米线等制作的层状网络可以实现对体液中尿素水平产生很好的线性响应,可作为传感器应用于各种生物医学检测。聚对苯二甲酸乙二醇酯(PET)薄膜搭载了载有葡萄糖氧化酶的空心球状纳米粒子后,可实现对葡萄糖水平的检测。

还有其他可穿戴聚合物制作成的薄膜可以实现与皮肤的贴合,用于药物的递送及疾病治疗。聚酰亚胺(PI)薄膜与聚对二甲苯薄膜可联合应用,用于可搭载柔性电子器件(如 LED 灯及可皮下植入的微阵列注射器),实现血压监测与药物注射。负载有纳米粒子的琼脂糖水凝胶可与具备加热功能的柔性电子器件复合,搭建有效的温控给药平台。该平台可应用于皮肤慢性创伤及烧伤等的治疗,保持伤口水分,防止病原体损害,促进药物及生长因子的透皮给药。

第五节　生物医用高分子在毛发美容中的应用

一、护发产品

护发产品中的生物医用高分子材料多见于调理剂中,用于满足以下一种或多种功能:改善干、湿梳理性,使毛发光滑,保护并重新调整毛干受损区域;减少毛发孔隙,赋予头发光泽和丝滑感;针对热损伤和机械性损伤提供保护、滋润作用;增加蓬松感和浓密感,消除静电等。因此,一些常见的生物医用高分子材料(表 9-1)被添加到护发产品中,以满足上述要求。

表 9-1　护发产品中生物医用高分子材料的种类和作用

种　类	作　用
有机硅(二甲硅油,聚二甲基硅氧烷醇等)	赋予头发柔顺感与光泽感,改善干梳理性
阳离子聚合物(聚季铵盐-10,阳离子瓜尔胶衍生物等)	使头发更柔软、顺滑,更易梳理,同时减少静电,还可以作为头发清洁剂中的表面活性剂
羟乙基纤维素	改善物质的分散性和泡沫的稳定性,改善物质的黏度和流动性
PEG-2M	帮助各种阳离子、油脂等调理成分在头发及皮肤上吸附成膜,使头发光滑易梳理
壳聚糖	改善头发梳理性,使头发富有弹性和光泽
黄原胶	稳定乳液和泡沫,并帮助去除污垢

二、生发产品

传统生发产品配方中的常见聚合物有藻类多糖、黏多糖、右旋糖酐 40 等。它们通常充当头发的营养物质,并帮助头发生长。近年来,已有学者尝试将某些药物(如 5α 还原酶抑制剂,传统中药)负载到纳米胶囊中以靶向毛囊来进行生发治疗(如天然聚合物壳聚糖包衣的度他雄胺纳米胶囊)。

第六节 生物医用高分子在功能性护肤品中的应用

一、保湿产品

保湿产品中生物医用高分子材料的种类和作用见表 9-2。

表 9-2 保湿产品中生物医用高分子材料的种类和作用

种　类	作　用
神经酰胺脂质体	神经酰胺可防止皮肤中水分向环境的流失,减少经皮水分丢失(transepidermal water loss,TEWL),从而增加角质层含水量
透明质酸	透明质酸可以从基底层、大气和表皮下方中吸水,以增加皮肤水合作用
胶原蛋白	胶原蛋白分子中包含的天然保湿因子(如甘氨酸、羟脯氨酸和羟赖氨酸)可保持皮肤水分。胶原蛋白分子外部的亲水基团(如羟基和羧基)使其易于与水形成氢键,从而改善皮肤的储水能力
β-葡聚糖	β-葡聚糖可以在皮肤上形成一层薄膜,锁住水分并防止水分流失
聚谷氨酸	聚谷氨酸有强大的吸水性,可以抑制透明质酸酶的活性,具有极强的保湿能力
有机硅(二甲硅油,辛甲基聚硅氧烷等)	有机硅有助于形成保护性的湿润屏障,可以改善并保护皮肤干燥区域
甲壳素	甲壳素与蛋白质和脂质相互作用,形成附着在角蛋白和脂质上的保护膜,保持皮肤水分
其他(普鲁兰多糖,银耳多糖,酸豆多糖,菌核树胶等)	成膜保湿

二、美白产品

美白产品中生物医用高分子材料的种类和作用见表 9-3。

表 9-3 美白产品中生物医用高分子材料的种类和作用

种　类	作　用
胶原蛋白	胶原蛋白中的酪氨酸残基与皮肤中的酪氨酸竞争,与酪氨酸酶的活性中心结合,抑制酪氨酸酶催化皮肤中酪氨酸向多巴转化,从而防止皮肤中产生黑素,达到美白的效果

种　　类	作　　用
聚谷氨酸	聚谷氨酸可以显著抑制酪氨酸酶的活性,从而抑制皮肤黑素的产生
丝素蛋白	丝素蛋白可以阻止紫外线

三、防晒产品

紫外线吸收剂是防晒产品中的活性成分,可以防止有害的 UVB(290～320 nm)和 UVA(320～400 nm)到达皮肤表层以下的活性层。为了提高效率,紫外线吸收剂必须保留在皮肤最表层作为保护膜,并且在整个紫外线照射期间保持光稳定。同时,要避免皮肤渗透和紫外线吸收剂的光分解。通常,皮肤渗透会减少预期的紫外线保护,而光分解会导致颜色和外观的变化,增加防晒产品的光毒性,并且不能排除紫外线吸收剂分解产物的潜在过敏可能。

最常用的紫外线吸收剂是亲脂分子,其分子量相对较低。虽然采取了增加光稳定剂和使用高分子量紫外线滤光剂等措施来减少皮肤吸收,但它们仍然能够穿透皮肤并被系统吸收一部分,因此有必要开发新的不穿透皮肤的紫外线吸收剂配方。

在这种情况下,将紫外线吸收剂封装在不同结构中是一个有用的策略,以防止皮肤渗透和增强防晒活性的光保护潜力。封装材料包括许多超分子体系,如固体脂质纳米颗粒、纳米结构脂质载体、纳米乳液、聚合物纳米颗粒、二氧化硅纳米颗粒、树枝状聚合物等。下面将介绍防晒产品中的新型纳米载体。

1. 固体脂质纳米颗粒

固体脂质纳米颗粒(solid lipid nanoparticles,SLNs)是开发出来的第一代脂质纳米颗粒。将油/水纳米乳的液体脂质(油)替换为生理上耐受良好、可生物降解的熔融乳化脂质,这种脂质在室温和体温下均为固体。通常,该类纳米颗粒包含一个亲水的外壳和一个疏水的核,其中可封装疏水化合物。纳米颗粒的平均粒径在 40～1000 nm 之间。

SLNs 具有抗紫外线的特性,可以单独用作物理防晒剂。SLNs 可作为 3,4,5-三甲氧基苯甲酰甲壳素和维生素 E 防晒剂的载体,以增强紫外线防护效果。但是,它们也有一些不足:①由于脂质体物理状态的复杂性,在储存或使用过程中容易出现药物泄漏现象,稳定性较差;②药物在固体脂质基质中的溶解度有限,导致载药量有限;③SLN 虽然是生物基的,但很容易溶解,因此不适合油基配方。

2. 纳米结构脂质载体

纳米结构脂质载体(nanostructured lipid carriers,NLCs)被认为是第二代脂质纳米颗粒。NLCs 的开发是为了克服 SLNs 的缺点。NLCs 是在 SLNs 的基础上将固态油脂替换为固态油脂和液态油脂的混合物,其具有更加不规则的缺陷型结构,从而产生更大的空间来容纳更多的活性物质,有效地提高了其包覆率及在长期储存过程中活性物质的稳定性。NLCs 属于无定形的不完整结晶,相比于 SLNs 更便于活性成分的包覆。目前,NLCs 包覆活性成分的结构主要有 3 种,即无定型(amorphous type)、缺陷型(imperfect type)和复合型(multiple type)。

与 SLNs 相比,NLCs 的不规则结构有助于创造更大的空间,对生物活性化合物的载药能力更高。SLNs 的其他局限性,例如在储存过程中降低颗粒浓度和排出药物,也能通过 NLCs

的制备得到解决。NLCs 由具有生物降解性的生理性脂质配制而成,显示出非常低的毒性。NLCs 为双相药物释放模式,具有可调节的药物释放特性。在这种情况下,药物首先以突释方式释放,然后以恒定速率持续释放。此外,它们还有其他一些优点:由于闭塞性而增加了皮肤的水合作用,并且小巧的尺寸确保了与角质层的紧密接触,从而增加了药物在皮肤中的渗透量。在储存过程中稳定掺入药物,并增强了紫外线防护系统,减少了副作用。使用 NLCs 负载防晒剂,可大大提高体系防晒效果,降低防晒剂对皮肤的刺激性,减少化学防晒剂的使用剂量,同时提高防晒体系配伍性和稳定性。

3. 纳米乳液

纳米乳液是表面活性剂与油相及水相的复合物,有水包油、油包水和双连续纳米乳液等不同类型。其尺寸从 50 nm 到 200 nm 不等,具有非常低的油/水界面张力和被单分子层磷脂包围的亲脂性核心。这些特征使其更适合于亲脂性化合物的递送。通常,纳米乳液具有低黏度、高动力学稳定性、高界面面积和高增溶能力等特性。在化妆品配方中,纳米乳液能够让有效成分快速渗透和主动运输,并与皮肤水合。

4. 聚化物纳米颗粒

聚化物纳米颗粒(polymeric nanoparticles,PNs)是指直径达到亚微米级的聚合物胶体载体。根据它们的结构、组成和分布,可以将它们分为纳米胶囊(NCs)和纳米球(NSs)。在前者中,活性化合物被包裹在胶囊的内部空腔中;而在后者中,它们被吸附在表面。NC 的脂质壁层使亲脂性化合物持续释放并保护它们避免光降解。PNs 的性能取决于聚合物的组成、有机溶剂和表面活性剂的用量,这些因素会影响其粒径、表面性能和释放速率等参数。

PNs 的主要优点是能够控制/持续释放紫外线吸收剂,从而延长其在皮肤上的停留时间,提高防晒产品的光稳定性,防止皮肤吸收。

5. 二氧化硅纳米颗粒

二氧化硅纳米颗粒(silica nanoparticles,SNs)可以将紫外线吸收剂限制在中空的二氧化硅基质中,或者将紫外线吸收剂的前体限制在二氧化硅基质中,用于化学结合紫外线吸收剂。它们的粒径在 10 nm 和 10 μm 之间不等。最近报道的一种新型紫外线吸收剂是基于 BP-3 的前体在阳光照射下的光化学转化。紫外线吸收剂可根据需要由其前体产生,在需要的时间、地点和程度上提供保护,随着紫外线照射量的增加而增强其阻挡紫外线的能力。研究采用溶胶-凝胶技术,将 BP-3 的硅基前体和烷氧硅烷聚合,然后被 SN(平均粒径为 100~1000 nm)封装。与未封装的 BP-3 相比,封装将最终产品的吸光度提高了 3 倍,从而提高了 BP-3 前体的转化效率。从化学的角度来看,紫外线吸收剂被封装在刚性基质中,可通过限制反应初始阶段形成的自由基的迁移率来提高光转化效率。此外,紫外线吸收剂与防晒配方的其他成分之间的这种物理屏障可以防止化学配伍禁忌。从生物学的角度来看,限制在硅基质中可降低紫外线吸收剂潜在的毒性和致敏性。最后,由于二氧化硅是一种天然的化学惰性材料,相对于分子吸收剂,只要紫外线吸收剂不释放,这种超分子防晒剂对环境的影响也大大减小。

6. 树枝状聚合物

树枝状聚合物是一种高度分支的球状胶束状单分子纳米结构以及多价纳米颗粒,直径范围一般为 2~20 nm。连续系列的分支以树枝状方式嫁接到核上。该类聚合物通常采用三维球状结构,具有单分散性、多价和稳定性等特性,是具有一定精确度和选择性的理想载体。树枝状聚合物提供从内核的控制释放,药物一般被负载到聚合物的内部以及附着在其表面。

　　树枝状聚合物具有明确的三维结构和多种表面官能团,可以将药物包裹在树枝状聚合物结构内,也可以在药物与树枝状聚合物末端官能团之间形成静电/共价键。文献报道过两种药物传递机制。第一种机制是药物和树枝状聚合物之间的共价键在体内存在酶或键断裂所需的环境时发生断裂。药物释放的第二种方式不依赖于外部因素的物理条件、温度和 pH 的改变。

第七节　生物医用高分子在激光美容中的应用

　　经过多年的发展,激光美容已在临床上广泛应用。皮肤具有高散射的特性,这是由其本身的结构和不同成分的折射率不同所决定的。入射激光穿透皮肤时可发生反射、折射、散射和吸收。散射和吸收尤为重要:散射光与入射光相互重叠时,皮下组织光能叠加,光被靶组织吸收引起靶组织损伤。然而,皮肤的高散射特性降低了光在组织中的穿透深度,到达皮肤中靶组织的光较入射光减少,靶组织吸收能量减少。增加激光的能量密度可以增加目标发色团的能量吸收,但同时也会增加皮肤损伤(如水疱、色素沉着、瘢痕等)的风险。最近的一些研究表明,光透明剂可以减少组织中光的散射,增强激光的穿透深度,因此在皮肤激光美容方面有一定应用前景,可以增强皮肤深部皮损的治疗效果,减少清除靶组织所需的能量,从而减少激光所致的皮肤损伤(图 9-5);除此之外,激光手术常引起一些皮肤的损伤(如红斑、水肿等),这时可以使用医用敷料来促进皮肤愈合。在激光手术中,减少皮肤的散射和预防激光治疗后的皮肤损伤尤为重要,下面我们将主要介绍光透明剂和医用敷料在激光手术中的应用。

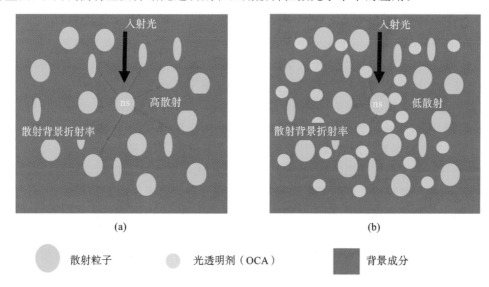

图 9-5　光透明剂引入后折射率匹配致散射降低示意图

Figure 9-5　Illustration showing the decrease of scattering caused by the refractive index matching after the OCA entering

一、光透明剂的应用

1. 光透明剂的种类和光透明作用机制

光透明剂是一种高折射率、高渗透性、生物相容性好的化学试剂,这种试剂对组织的作用是可逆的。目前,光透明作用的可能机制主要有三种:①折射率匹配:光透明剂渗透到组织中以提高组织间质液的折射率,使各组织成分的折射率相匹配,降低组织中光的散射,增强光的穿透深度。②脱水:高渗的光透明剂进入组织中导致水分丢失,从而降低组织折射率不匹配的程度。③胶原纤维解离:一些光透明剂进入组织后可以破坏胶原纤维,降低胶原组织的光散射(胶原纤维是真皮的主要散射源)。

光透明剂主要有以下几类:①醇类:如甘油、聚乙二醇、聚丙二醇甘露醇、山梨醇和木糖醇。②糖类:如葡萄糖、果糖、核糖和蔗糖。③有机酸类:如油酸和亚油酸。④其他有机溶剂:如二甲基亚砜和噻酮。⑤X线造影剂:如碘海醇。虽然这些光透明剂被认为是无毒的,但是长期使用可能导致组织水肿和刺激,局部血流阻滞,组织压缩甚至坏死(如皮肤注射光透明剂)。光透明剂的渗透取决于许多因素,包括光透明剂的类型、折射率、浓度以及生物组织暴露于该制剂的时间,还包括生物组织的原始浊度及其对特定光透明剂的渗透性。

2. 促进光透明剂渗透的方式

角质层的屏障功能阻止了光透明剂的渗透,故需要更久的皮肤光透明作用时间,但长时间的高渗光透明剂的应用可能导致皮肤损伤。可以加速光透明剂渗透的方法如下:①化学促渗剂:氮酮、油酸、二甲基亚砜、丙二醇和噻酮等可增强光透明剂的渗透性,目前这些促渗剂在体内应用较少,其安全性和促渗效果还有待进一步研究。②物理方法剥离角质层:如胶带剥脱、微晶磨皮。③其他因素:光热、激光、离子、超声等辅助应用。这些方法虽然能提高光透明作用的效果,缩短光透明剂的作用时间,但是可能产生其他副作用。例如,一些化学促渗剂对人体有毒性,物理方式也可导致皮肤受损。

3. 光透明剂在皮肤激光中的应用

目前,光透明剂尚未应用于临床中,但其对于改善激光治疗有着广阔的前景。针对皮肤组织的光透明研究主要是离体实验,少数为在体实验(动物实验)。光透明剂安全性和生物相容性问题以及离体组织和在体组织的药物代谢差距,限制了其在临床试验上的应用。离体实验的给药方式通常为离体组织浸泡,而在体实验的给药方式通常为表面涂抹和皮下注射。甘油、糖、聚乙二醇、丙二醇或乙酸的溶液对组织有可逆清除作用,可用于在体实验,但浓度不宜过高,避免组织损伤和坏死。甘油是在体实验常用的光透明剂,当其浓度大于30%时,可引起皮肤水肿等不良反应。在体应用噻酮、碘海醇效果较好,无明显不良反应。许多研究表明,光透明剂的应用可以提高体内外皮肤的光透明效应,增加分子光学成像的探测深度。关于光透明剂与激光联合应用的研究较少,但曾有报道表明,光透明剂(聚丙烯乙二醇和聚乙二醇的混合物)与激光联合治疗人体皮肤文身与对照组相比效果更佳,损伤较少;但该结果的样本量少,需要进一步研究。光透明剂在人体的应用还存在诸多挑战,寻找一种毒性小、生物相容性好、直接涂抹于皮肤、代谢迅速的光透明剂对激光美容有重要意义。

二、医用敷料在激光手术后修复中的应用

1. 医用敷料的定义和分类

医用敷料是一种可以贴合伤口、控制感染、促进皮肤损伤修复、避免瘢痕形成的医用材料。医用敷料分为被动、互动和生物活性创面敷料。根据原料、物理性质、结构不同,其对应的功能和适用的伤口类型也不同。①被动敷料:如纱布、薄纱,用于覆盖伤口,恢复结构功能。②互动敷料:如薄膜、泡沫、水凝胶和水胶体,防止伤口中细菌渗透。③生物活性创面敷料:如胶原蛋

白、透明质酸、壳聚糖、海藻酸盐和弹性蛋白,具有生物相容性、生物降解性、无毒性,可单独和联合试用。互动敷料和生物活性敷料属于新型敷料,可以防止伤口脱水,促进愈合。水凝胶敷料被视为伤口敷料的理想材料。纳米技术也被应用于医用敷料中,有机和非有机的纳米颗粒(如聚合物纳米颗粒(NPs)和银纳米颗粒(silver NPs))负载生长因子、抗菌剂和药物可促进伤口愈合。相关报道表明,已有多种医用敷料应用于皮肤烧伤中,如含银磺胺嘧啶的纳米片基超薄膜、一氧化氮(nitric oxide,NO)释放聚合膜、含酪氨酸(如环肽抗生素)的壳聚糖基成膜凝胶层等;这些敷料无明显毒性,可抑制炎症、减少瘢痕、促进上皮化和肉芽组织再生。

2. 激光手术后并发症与早期医用敷料的应用

在激光手术时,激光装置、治疗方式、术前评估、参数设置是否合理、操作是否恰当、患者病史(如异常瘢痕、过度日晒等)或用药史(如阿司匹林、非甾体抗炎药等)等均为影响激光手术后并发症的因素。这些并发症包括皮肤早期并发症(红斑、水肿、感染)、中期并发症(色素沉着、色减)、晚期并发症(瘢痕等)。激光手术后早期使用医用敷料可以改善早期并发症,减小中晚期并发症的风险,术后前两周是伤口护理的关键时期。用于激光手术后修复的医用敷料如下:①开放式敷料:可直接涂抹在皮肤表面的软膏,易于护理,可促进创面愈合,如优色林,但有增加痤疮、粟丘疹、感染的风险。②封闭式敷料:可以为伤口提供湿润的愈合环境,效果好;但费用较高,用时较长,不易贴合皮肤,无吸收层。激光手术后面部护理常用敷料为复合泡沫(Flexzan 和 Revitaderm)、水凝胶(2nd Skin)、聚合物膜(Silon TSR)和聚合物网(N-terface 和 Mepitel)。临床上,通常建议激光手术后至少使用 24 h 封闭式敷料,不超过 4 天,第 5 天改为开放式敷料,以帮助降低感染率。激光手术后前一周使用医学敷料的目的是防止皮肤感染,避免环境刺激,实现再上皮化。

综上,新型医用敷料在临床应用中前景广阔,然而,在敷料的药物渗透和活性、保水性和透气性,贴合皮肤等方面还需进一步提高。

第八节　挑战与展望

随着现代科学技术的发展,尤其是生物技术的重大突破,生物医用高分子材料在美容领域的应用将更加广泛,需求量也越来越大。新型生物医用高分子材料具有良好的生物相容性、一定的生物活性和无毒副作用等优点,新型材料不断出现,为皮肤美容带来了更多新的选择。国内外许多研究团队对生物高分子材料的研究为其在皮肤修复、功能性化妆品、皮肤填充物、辅助激光治疗等方面的应用提供了更多的参考数据。关于生物高分子材料在人体皮肤和组织中的安全性、组织相容性以及与皮肤组织间的作用机制等有待进一步研究,另外生物高分子材料商业化的应用仍需进一步探索。相信随着更多相关研究的开展,生物高分子材料在皮肤美容中的应用前景将更加广阔,生物高分子材料能得到更为迅速的发展,从而推动美容事业的发展。

思　考　题

1. 生物医用高分子替代材料应具有哪些特点?
2. 如何利用生物医用高分子材料对皮肤屏障进行修复?

3. 激光美容治疗中,生物医用高分子材料能起到哪些作用?

4. 生物医用高分子材料可以应用于哪些功效性护肤品中?

5. 防晒产品中的纳米脂质载体的作用有哪些?

扩 展 阅 读

[1] Draelos Z D. Cosmetic dermatology: products and procedures[M]. Hoboken N J: Blackwell Publishing Ltd. ,2010.

[2] Baran R,Maibach H I. Textbook of cosmetic dermatology[M]. 4th ed. London:Informa Healthcare,2010.

[3] Sarbana K. Lasers in dermatological practice [M]. New York:Mcgraw-hill Education,2014.

[4] 赵长生,孙树东. 生物医用高分子材料[M].2 版. 北京:化学工业出版社,2016.

[5] Carruthers J,Carruthers A. 软组织填充剂与医学美容——美容皮肤科实用技术[M]. 刘秉慈,译. 北京:人民军医出版社,2007.

参 考 文 献

[1] 向雪岑. 美容皮肤科学[M]. 北京:科学出版社,1998.

[2] 李树莱,白义杰. 美容皮肤科学[M]. 南昌:江西高校出版社,1999.

[3] 张其亮. 美容皮肤科学[M]. 北京:人民卫生出版社,2002.

[4] 张其亮,张静,陈红清. 概述美容皮肤科学定义、研究范围与体系结构[J]. 中国实用美容整形外科杂志,2004,15(6):332-333.

[5] Del Rosso J Q. Medical treatment of rosacea with emphasis on topical therapies[J]. Expert Opin Pharmacother,2004,5(1):5-13.

[6] Egawa G,Kabashima K. Barrier dysfunction in the skin allergy[J]. Allergol Int, 2018, 67(1):3-11.

[7] 吴艳,牛悦青,陈璨,等. 皮肤屏障与玫瑰痤疮相关性的研究进展[J]. 皮肤病与性病, 2011,33(2):77-78.

[8] Kullavanijaya P,Lim H W. Photoprotection[J]. J Am Acad Dermatol,2005,52(6):937-958.

[9] Cao X,Yang F,Zheng J,et al. Intracellular proton-mediated activation of TRPV3 channels accounts for the exfoliation effect of pseudo-hydroxyl acids on keratinocytes [J]. J Biol Chem,2012,287(31):25905-25916.

[10] Sun G,Zhang X,Shen Y,et al. Dextran hydrogel scaffolds enhance angiogenic responses and promote complete skin regeneration during burn wound healing[J]. Proc Natl Acad Sci,2011,108(52):20976-20981.

[11] Abdullahi A,Amini-Nik S,Jeschke M G. Animal models in burn research cell[J]. Cell Mol Life Sci,2014,71(17):3241-3255.

[12] Orgill D P. Excision and skin grafting of thermal burns[J]. N Engl J Med,2009,360 (9):893-901.

[13] Rheinwald J G，Green H. Serial cultivation of strains of human epidermal keratinocytes：the formation of keratinizing colonies from single cells[J]. Cell，1975，6 (3)：33-43.

[14] Sdobnov A Y，Darvin M E，Genina E A，et al. Recent progress in tissue optical clearing for spectroscopic application[J]. Spectrochim Acta A Mol Biomol Spectrosc，2018，197：216-229.

[15] Khan M H，Chess S，Choi B，et al. Can topically applied optical clearing agents increase the epidermal damage threshold and enhance therapeutic efficacy？[J]. Lasers Surg Med，2004，35(2)：93-95.

[16] 沈艳杰，曹建文. 我国医用敷料行业的发展及其临床护理应用[J]. 解放军护理杂志，2012，29(7)：27-30.

[17] Sdobnov A Y，Lademann J，Darvin M E，et al. Methods for optical skin clearing in molecular optical imaging in dermatology [J]. Biochemistry（Mosc），2019，84：S144-S158.

[18] Zhu D，Larin K V，Luo Q，et al. Recent progress in tissue optical clearing[J]. Laser Photon Rev，2013，7(5)：732-757.

[19] Costantini I，Cicchi R，Silvestri L，et al. In-vivo and ex-vivo optical clearing methods for biological tissues：review[J]. Biomed Opt Express，2019，10(10)：5251-5267.

[20] Tredget E E，Shupp J W，Schneider J C. Scar management following burn injury[J]. J Burn Care Res，2017，38(3)：146-147.

[21] Rahmani Del Bakhshayesh A，Annabi N，Khalilov R，et al. Recent advances on biomedical applications of scaffolds in wound healing and dermal tissue engineering [J]. Artif Cells Nanomed Biotechnol，2018，46(4)：691-705.

[22] Saghazadeh S，Rinoldi C，Schot M，et al. Drug delivery systems and materials for wound healing applications[J]. Adv Drug Deliv Rev，2018，1(127)：138-166.

[23] Mofazzal Jahromi M A，Sahandi Zangabad P，Moosavi Basri S M，et al. Nanomedicine and advanced technologies for burns：preventing infection and facilitating wound healing[J]. Adv Drug Deliv Rev，2018，1(123)：33-64.

[24] Li D，Lin S B，Cheng B. Complications and posttreatment care following invasive laser skin resurfacing：a review[J]. J Cosmet Laser Ther，2018，20(3)：168-178.

[25] McBurney E I. Side effects and complications of laser therapy[J]. Dermatol Clin，2002，20(1)：165-176.

[26] Damiani E，Puglia C. Nanocarriers and microcarriers for enhancing the UV protection of sunscreens：an overview[J]. J Pharm Sci，2019，108(12)：3769-3780.

[27] Kaul S，Gulati N，Verma D，et. al. Role of nanotechnology in cosmeceuticals：a review of recent advances[J]. J Pharm (Cairo)，2018，2018：3420204.

[28] Lima E V A，Lima M M D A，Paixão M P，et al. Assessment of the effects of skin microneedling as adjuvant therapy for facial melasma：a pilot study [J]. BMC Dermatol，2017，17(1)：14.

[29] Wang X, Liu Z, Zhang T. Flexible sensing electronics for wearable/attachable health monitoring[J]. Small,2017,13(25):1602790.

[30] Guo Y, Guo Z, Zhong M, et al. A flexible wearable pressure sensor with bioinspired microcrack and interlocking for full-range human-machine interfacing[J]. Small,2018, 14(44):e1803018.

[31] Goodarzi P, Falahzadeh K, Nematizadeh M, et al. Tissue engineered skin substitutes [J]. Adv Exp Med Biol,2018,1107:143-188.

[32] Keen M A. Hyaluronic acid in dermatology[J]. Skinmed,2017,15(6):441-448.

[33] Garcês A, Amaral M H, Sousa Lobo J M, et al. Formulations based on solid lipid nanoparticles (SLN) and nanostructured lipid carriers (NLC) for cutaneous use: a review[J]. Eur J Pharm Sci,2018,112:159-167.

[34] Liang Z, Zhang J, Wu C, et al. Flexible and self-healing electrochemical hydrogel sensor with high efficiency toward glucose monitoring[J]. Biosens Bioelectron,2020,1 (155):112105.

[35] Panico A, Serio F, Bagordo F, et al. Skin safety and health prevention: an overview of chemicals in cosmetic products[J]. J Prev Med Hyg,2019,60(1):E50-E57.

[36] Gavazzoni Dias M F. Hair cosmetics: an overview[J]. Int J Trichology,2015,7(1): 2-15.

[37] Aziz Z A A, Mohd-Nasir H, Ahmad A, et al. Role of nanotechnology for design and development of cosmeceutical: application in makeup and skin care[J]. Front Chem, 2019,7:739.

[38] Bukhari S N A, Roswandi N L, Waqas M, et al. Hyaluronic acid, a promising skin rejuvenating biomedicine: a review of recent updates and pre-clinical and clinical investigations on cosmetic and nutricosmetic effects[J]. Int J Biol Macromol,2018,120 (Pt B):1682-1695.

[39] Gallardo A, Teixidó J, Miralles R, et al. Dose-dependent progressive sunscreens: a new strategy for photoprotection? [J]. Photochem Photobiol Sci,2010,9(4):530-534.

[40] Sherje A P, Jadhav M, Dravyaka B R, et al. Dendrimers: a versatile nanocarrier for drug delivery and targeting[J]. Int J Pharm,2018,548(1):707-720.

[41] Goleva E, Berdyshev E, Leung D Y, et al. Epithelial barrier repair and prevention of allergy[J]. J Clin Invest,2019,129(4):1463-1474.

[42] Kallis P J, Friedman A J, Lev-Tov H. A guide to tissue-engineered skin substitutes [J]. J Drugs Dermatol,2018,17(1):57-64.

[43] Witmanowski H, Błochowiak K. The whole truth about botulinum toxin—a review [J]. Dermatol Alergol,2020,37(6):853-861.

[44] Mitura S, Sionkowska A, Jaiswal A. Biopolymers for hydrogels in cosmetics: review [J]. J Mater Sci Mater Med,2020,31(6):50.

[45] Lee S H, Jun S H, Yeom J, et al. Optical clearing agent reduces scattering of light by the stratum corneum and modulates the physical properties of coenocytes via

hydration[J]. Skin Res Technol,2018,24(3):371-378.

[46] Stoica A E,Chircov C,Grumezescu A M. Nanomaterials for wound dressings:an up-to-date overview[J]. Molecule,202,25(11):2699.

[47] Obagi Z,Damiani G,Grada A,et al. Principles of wound dressings:a review[J]. Surg Technol Int,2019,10(35):50-57.

（李延）

Chapter 9
Applications of Biomedical Polymers in Cosmetic Dermatology

9.1   Overview of Cosmetic Dermatology

Cosmetic dermatology is a science that studies the anatomical structure and physiological function of human skin and implements the maintenance, improvement, repair and shaping of human skin health and beauty and regularity based on the theory of dermatology and the combination of medicine and aesthetics. It is a main clinical application discipline of aesthetic medicine. The main areas of cosmetic dermatology include skin beauty basic theory, skin health and beauty, hair health and beauty, laser and photon beauty treatment technology, beauty application technology, skin surgery, beauty Chinese medicine and treatment of skin diseases with lesions, et al.

According to the literature, cosmetic dermatology has a long history. In China, it is said to start from Dayu period (2277 BC to 2213 BC). According to the legend, when Dayu was at his 50th, wrinkles appeared in the corners of his eyes and forehead one after another. At that time, it was suggested to touch the face with wax grease to lighten the wrinkles. But the skin got hard after touching the wax. After many tests, someone suggested that the wheat flour and the dough should be applied to the face. This is the legend of the "Yu selects powder" in the ancient literature. In the Tang Dynasty, the great medical scientist Sun Simiao presented more than 80 skin beauty prescriptions in *Thousand Golden Preions*, which is the earliest known literature on beauty prescriptions in China. Li Shizhen's *Compendium of Materia Medica* in the Ming Dynasty also recorded more than 700 beauty prescriptions.

According to historical records, the ancient Egyptians had the earliest conscious of using cosmetics. The ancient Egyptians loved aromatic products. They kept collecting natural spices from India, Arabia and other places, and used them to make perfumes and cosmetics.

The ancient Egyptians attached great importance to the health and beauty of the skin. After bathing, they applied a lot of sesame oil, perfumes or ointment to moisturize the skin. In order to resist the hot and dry climate, they applied animal grease to the skin to prevent skin dryness.

In general, the development of modern cosmetic dermatology is mainly divided into five generations. The first generation: the age of ordinary oil and skin care. It is characterized by the use of pure physical properties of cosmetics (e. g. , animal oil) which taken from natural unprocessed oil (heating at most), mainly to achieve moisturization and prevent cracking. The second generation: oil-water mixture skin care era. It is the first generation of cosmetics produced by industrial integration. It also has the effect of moisturizing and preventing chapped, but it is more hygienic, convenient and pure than the first generation. The representative products of this generation include petroleum jelly. The third generation: the era of natural plant cosmetics. It is the first generation of cosmetics produced by high-tech plant purification technology. It is characterized by hygiene, convenience, beauty, high purity, certain effects, and complex raw materials. The representative products of this generation include the earlier cucumber facial cleanser. The fourth generation: the era of bio-hormone ecological cosmetics. It is the first generation of cosmetics produced by high-tech biological engineering technology. It is characterized by hygiene, convenience, beauty, high purity, strong efficacy, complex raw materials, easy absorption, and pure fragrance. The fifth generation: nanotechnology natural essence cosmetics era. It is the first generation of cosmetics dealt with molecular micro-processing technology, and it is also the application of the most advanced chemical technology in the field of cosmetics.

9.2 Applications of Biomedical Polymers in Skin Barrier Repair

The human skin barrier (Figure 9-1) is divided into anatomic barrier and functional barrier. The outermost structure of the skin is the stratum corneum of the epidermis, which forms a cuticle epidermal permeability barrier to prevent the loss of water and electrolytes. Other protective or barrier effect of epidermis include immune defense, UV protection and protection from oxidative damage. Many patients with inflammatory skin diseases have significant disorders of skin barrier structure and function. The stratum corneum moisture content of the cheek skin lesions decreases, the fat content decreases, and the percutaneous water loss increases. Repeated chronic inflammation leads to the destruction of the patient's skin barrier. Chronic photodamage is an important predisposing factor for aggravating the destruction of the skin barrier. When the skin barrier is damaged, erythema, edema, blisters and pigmention appear after a short period of ultraviolet radiation. Prolonged ultraviolet radiation causes skin thickening, elastic fiber damage, wrinkles and other capacious changes.

The skin barrier can be repaired with existing biomedical polymer materials.

9.2.1 Hyaluronic acid (HA)

HA is a linear non-sulfated glycosaminoglycan polymer, which is the main component of the extracellular matrix (ECM). ECM is a key regulator that affects the metabolism of cells. The molecular weight of HA is critical to its various functions. The high molecular weight HA fragments reflect intact tissue, anti-angiogenesis, and immunosuppressive states, while smaller HA fragments, which are usually inducers of inflammation and angiogenesis, are considered as pressure signals. Due to its super capacity to retain large amounts of water, HA is responsible for the skin's moisture content. In addition, HA is involved in wound healing and aging processes.

9.2.2 Antioxidants

Clinical commonly used antioxidants include fruit acid, salicylic acid and so on. Fruit acid was introduced into the field of skin treatment in 1974 for the treatment of ichthyosis. It refers to a class of alpha hydroxyacids, which is a family including glycolic acid, tartaric acid, citric acid, lactic acid, etc. Salicylic acid, as a chemical peeling agent for the skin, was originally extracted from willow bark. Topical treatment with salicylic acid or fruit acid can significantly improve erythema, inflammatory papules and pigmentation. The mechanism is that when the antioxidant is applied to the skin, fruit acid activates the cell ion channel TRPV3, and excessive calcium ions enter the cells to induce apoptosis, thus softening the stratum corneum and accelerating the exfoliation of the stratum corneum, so that the melanin in the keratinocytes is exfoliated together, and a lighter skin color reveals. Long-term use can stimulate the synthesis of collagen and mucopolysaccharide in the dermis, which will lighten the skin wrinkle, and it is better for the wrinkle caused by photoaging skin (due to the degeneration and reduction of collagen in the dermis). In addition, the use of antioxidants can soften keratin and promote drug penetration, thereby improving the efficacy of external medicine.

9.2.3 Botulinum toxin

Botulinum toxin consists of the Gram-positive-spore-forming anaerobic *Clostridium botulinum* and causes a chemical reaction to innervate the nerve by inhibiting the release of the neurotransmitter acetylcholine from the end of the peripheral axon. There are currently a botulinum neurotoxin A (BoNTA) and a botulinum neurotoxin B (BoNTB) toxin available in clinical practice. Botox® (Allergan Corporation, Irvine, California, USA) is a type A toxin and is currently approved by the US Food and Drug Administration (FDA) for a variety of indications (including blepharospasm and strabismus). Botulinum toxin has been approved for the use in cosmetics and for hyperhidrosis of the hands and feet. Botulinum toxin injection treatment can be used to improve resistant facial flush, and the wrinkles of the frontal face caused by skin barrier destruction and chronic light damage in patients with rosacea.

9.3 Applications of Biomedical Polymers in Skin Defect Repair

9.3.1 Skin substitutes materials

Skin is the largest organ of the human body and is more vulnerable than any other part of the body. Injuries of skin can range from small wounds that heal spontaneously within a few days, to even large third-degree burns that threaten the lives of patients. In acute large-area wounds and burns, elderly and diabetic patients, the normal wound healing response and the skin's inherent tissue regeneration ability are far from enough. This is a challenge for skin repair. Biomedical polymer materials are natural and synthetic polymer biomaterials with special functions produced by the organic combination of medicine and polymer science. They can have different physical and chemical properties through the control of the composition and structure to meet different needs. They also have some advantages that they are easy to process and easy to disinfect and sterilize, and have good biocompatibility. It has been applied throughout the entire medical field, and now the biomedical polymer materials related to alternative materials for skin defect repair are summarized as follows.

9.3.1.1 Natural biomedical polymer materials

The design of tissue engineering scaffolds is to simulate the function of living extracellular matrix in tissues. Therefore, researchers have explored the use of extracellular matrix proteins as materials for tissue engineering scaffolds, such as collagen, gelatin (i. e. , hydrolyzed form of collagen), elasticity protein and HA. These materials as scaffold materials for skin tissue engineering can combine other natural polymer fibrin (e. g. , hemagglutinin) and pullulan (i. e. , natural biopolymer produced by fungi) to play a synergistic role.

9.3.1.2 Synthetic biomedical polymer materials

Synthetic polymers are produced from hydrocarbons in the laboratory, such as poly(lactic acid) (PLA), poly(lactic-co-glycolic acid) (PLGA), and polyurethane (PU). Although they may lack the inherent cell interaction mechanisms in natural biomedical polymer materials, their precise controllability in terms of composition and repeatability, and their ability to combine with natural biomedical polymer materials make them ideal for skin regeneration applications.

生物医用高分子在皮肤疾病诊疗和健康中的应用(双语版) ■ · 402 ·

9.3.1.3　Natural and synthetic composite scaffolds

Using a unique combination of natural and synthetic materials to make tissue engineering scaffolds has been explored by many researchers, as a method of utilizing the inherent biocompatibility of natural materials while making up for its lack of sufficient mechanical strength. Natural biomedical polymer materials have the disadvantages of low mechanical properties and fast degradation, which hinders its clinical application. In contrast, most synthetic biomedical polymer materials have good mechanical and physical properties, which can be controlled during the production process. The combination of different synthetic and natural ingredients makes the composite scaffold exhibits better controllable degradation rate and chemical properties. To further solve the above problems, skin cell biology and *in-situ* manufacturing technologies are needed, including 3D printing and other technologies. Interdisciplinary communication is essential for tissue regeneration, and skin repair and regeneration are no exception.

9.3.2　Skin graft materials

For patients who are unable to repair the skin injury without the skin tissue donor area, or are unwilling to accept the skin tissue donor area injury, allogeneic tissue or tissue substitutes should be used for repair. Allograft and xenografts are still the main methods to solve the problem of insufficient sources of autologous skin or no conditions for autologous skin transplantation. They can not only prevent the loss of electrolytes, proteins and other body components, but also reduce the contamination of wound pathogenic microorganisms, reduce the pain of the wound, improve the patient's compliance with other treatments, and also improve the survival rate of autologous skin transplantation. However, allogeneic and heterogeneous tissues often have problems such as immune rejection, absorption, deformation, and non-suitable bovine mechanical properties. Therefore, biomedical polymer materials made according to different needs have been playing an important role in clinical application as skin tissue graft materials.

9.3.2.1　Temporary skin graft materials

Among biomedical polymer materials, collagen-based materials are currently the focus of research. Transparent polymer films, polymeric foam films, hydrocolloids, diaphragm hydrogels, amorphous hydrogels, sponge foams and other materials have been developed. Collagen reconstructed by polymerization and cross-linking can form structural materials with certain strength and stability. It has high hydrophilicity, non-toxicity, biocompatibility *in vivo*, good biodegradability and other biological characteristics. Using collagen as the main material, one has developed artificial skin graft materials characterized by histological engineering technology, such as Biobrane® and Dermagraft®.

9.3.2.2　Semi-permanent skin graft materials

There are Integra® and other materials that have been studied more deeply. It is a collagen scaffold composed of bovine collagen and shark chondroitin sulfate, with a layer of silicone membrane attached to the surface. It can be transplanted on wounds with rich blood supply and no infection, and provides a role similar to dermal substitutes. With the establishment of blood flow from 10 days to 3 weeks or so, the silicone membrane can be removed and another layer of autologous epidermis thinner than 0.020 cm (0.080 inch) can be transplanted. This composite method of forming dermis on synthetic materials and then autologous epidermal transplantation is different from temporary skin graft materials. Here, the research on temporary skin graft materials and permanent skin graft materials are integrated.

9.3.2.3　Permanent skin graft material

The permanent skin graft material is Epicel®, and it is also known as "test tube skin". In 1975, Rhinewald and Green invented an alternative epidermal material for artificial epidermal cell culture *in vitro*. Due to the lack of dermal components, the wound surface after transplantation has the disadvantages of easy infection, ulceration, and scar formation. However, Epicel® is transplanted on Integra® and Alloderm® artificial dermal substitute materials that have established blood supply, and has shown good results in long-term clinical observation.

With the rapid development of biology and bioengineering technology, in today's diversified skin substitute market, clinicians should choose the most suitable treatment and application according to the wound situation. Ideal skin substitutes should include the following attributes: enhance tissue regeneration, control pigmentation, barrier protection and anti-infection function, regenerate accessory structures (e.g., hair follicles and sweat glands), easy to handle and apply, and long shelf life. There is still a certain distance between the existing skin substitutes and people's expectations. How to make full use of the advantages of skin substitutes and overcome their shortcomings is the development trend of future research.

9.4　Applications of Biomedical Polymers in Anti-Aging

9.4.1　Rhytidectomy

Collagen fiber is the most abundant component of dermal connective tissue, and its main ingredient is collagen. Collagen in dermis is mainly composed of type I collagen (85%-90%), type II collagen (8%-11%) and type V collagen (2%-4%). Elastic fiber plays an important role in maintaining skin elasticity. Elastic fiber is composed of elastin and filiform protein. Elastic fibers and collagen fibers are tangled together to maintain the integrity, strength and elasticity of the skin. After being damaged by external environment and light aging, the structures of collagen and elastin are destroyed, resulting in the decrease of skin elasticity and the generation of wrinkles.

In order to prevent and eliminate wrinkles, there are many ways in the fields of medicine, chemistry and skin beauty, such as physical methods, including laser and bioelectricity. In this section, we will mainly discuss the chemical related anti-wrinkle methods.

9.4.1.1 Botulinum toxin

Botulinum toxin is safe and effective in the treatment of wrinkles in the upper, middle and lower parts. After 3-7 days of botulinum toxin treatment, muscle paralysis wrinkles will disappear. After 3-6 months, synaptic regeneration will reverse the paralysis (Figure 9-2). Botulinum toxin is a kind of drug with high safety, and its application in the cosmetic field is relatively safe. However, it needs to be used in accordance with the dose range in the area to optimize patient satisfaction and maintain the natural effect.

9.4.1.2 Hyaluronic acid

Hyaluronic acid (HA) is a non-sulfated glycosaminoglycan polymer with a linear conformation, which is the main component of extracellular matrix (ECM). The total amount of HA in the skin is more than 50%. Due to its strong water holding capacity, HA can increase the moisture content of the skin, which is inherently helpful to increase the skin luster visually. The content of HA in epidermis is decreased with the increase of age. UV also causes the loss of HA and water, resulting in wrinkles.

Evidence-based analysis revealed that the anti-wrinkle efficacy of HA is molecular weight dependent which is expected to be due to differences in percutaneous absorption of different molecular weights of HA across the stratum corneum. In a clinical trial involving 76 female aged between 30 and 60 having periocular wrinkles, these patients were applied with 0.1% cream formulation containing different molecular weights of HA (50, 130, 300, 800, and 2000) twice daily for a period of 60 days. The greater improvements were observed in the skin hydration level, skin elasticity, and reduction in peri-ocular wrinkles in women applied with cream formulation containing low molecular weight HA. In view of molecular weight dependent percutaneous absorption, the swift anti-wrinkle and skin rejuvenating effects of nano-HA containing topical formulations were expected to be due to superior percutaneous absorption of ultra-small HA molecules.

HA can also be used for soft tissue filling. After 2007, HA soft tissue filling has become one of the popular non-surgical cosmetic methods, second only to Botox skin filling treatment. The mechanism of dermal filling is shown in Figure 9-3. HA filling in dermis is rarely allergic, relatively painless and has little side effects; Yet, it can not maintain the effect for a long time, with the need of repeat filling. HA soft tissue filling may cause inflammation, swelling, ecchymosis and asymmetry, which may depend on the injection technology. It is usually necessary to inject different doses of HA into different parts of the face and massage to prevent facial unevenness. HA filling has become the main method for the treatment of wrinkles. After filling, collagen synthesis can be optimized for several months or even for a long time.

9.4.1.3 Poly(lactic acid) (PLA)

PLA is a volume stimulant, instead of a direct filler. Unlike HA, one of the advantages of PLA is to stimulate the production of collagen to maintain the anti-wrinkle effect for a long time. However, the injection of PLA may produce subcutaneous papules, which requires a small amount of multiple injections. The frequently injected area is the cheek, chin, temple, etc. and fan-shaped injection is conducted in this area. Yet, it is impossible to predict the possible effect since it is not a filling material, so the amount of injection needs to be controlled.

9.4.2 Wearable polymer

With the increasing demand for wearable devices (e. g. , sports bracelets), more and more polymers combined with flexible electronic technology are applied to wearable portable devices for life health monitoring, including the detection of heart rate, pulse, body temperature, blood pressure and biological indicators in sweat (Figure 9-4). The requirements of wearable polymer are as follows: ① It is a functional material that can realize the integration of different functional devices; ② It can meet the requirements of mechanical stability and skin affinity of flexible electronic devices at the same time.

At present, flexible electronic devices can be installed on wearable polymers (e. g. , polydimethylsiloxane (PDMS)) and other film patches to achieve the detection of daily physiological indicators, such as daily monitoring of skin temperature, skin pH and calcium level. Such flexible electronic devices can be connected to wireless devices through bluetooth, and are sensitivity and repeatability. The layered network made of carbon nanotubes and gold nanotubes can produce a good linear response to the urea level in body fluids, and can be used as a sensor for various biomedical detection. Poly (ethylene terephthalate) (PET) film loaded with hollow spherical nanoparticles (NPs) containing glucose oxidase, can detect glucose.

There are also films made of other wearable polymers that can be applied to the skin for drug delivery and disease treatment. Polyimide (PI) film and poly(*p*-xylene) film are also used to carry flexible electronic devices such as LED lights and microarray syringes that can be implanted subcutaneously to monitor blood pressure and drug injection. Agarose hydrogel, which is loaded with NPs and heatable flexible electronic devices, can build effective platform for temperature control. It can be used in chronic wounds and burns of skin, which can maintain slobber's moisture, prevent pathogen damage and promote transdermal delivery of drugs and growth factors.

9. 5　Applications of Biomedical Polymers in Hair Cosmetics

9.5.1　Hair care products

The biomedical polymer materials in hair care products are mainly found in the conditioning agent, which are designed to provide one or more of the following functions: increase the convenience of wet and dry combing; smooth, seal and realign damaged areas of the hair shaft; reduce porosity; impart shiny and a silky feel to hair; provide some protection against thermal and mechanical damage; moisturize; increase volume and body; eliminate static electricity. Accordingly, some of the common biomedical polymer materials as follows are added to hair care products to meet the above requirements(Table 9-1).

Table 9-1　The categories and functions of biomedical polymer materials in hair care products

Categories	Functions
Silicones (e. g. , dimethicone, dimethiconol)	Imbue softness to hair, improve dry combing capability and increase shine
Cationic polymers（e. g. , polyquaternium-10, cationic guar derivatives)	Make hair softer, smoother, easier to comb, and less static; and also act as surfactant agents for hair cleaning
Hydroxyethylcellulose	Improve the dispersion of materials and foam stability, viscosity and fluidity
PEG -2M	Help a variety of conditioning components such as cations and oils absorb on hair or skin and form a film, making hair smooth enough to comb easily
Chitosan	Improve hair combing and make hair elastic and shiny
Xanthan gum	Stabilize emulsions and foams, and help remove dirt

9.5.2　Hair growth products

Common polymers in traditional hair growth formulations include algae polysaccharides, mucopolysaccharides, dextran-40 and so on, generally acting as nutrients to assist hair growth. In recent years, attempts have been made to load some drugs, such as 5α reductase inhibitors, and even traditional Chinese medicine into nanocapsules, targeting hair follicles, for example, the natural polymer chitosan coated dutasteride nanocapsules.

9.6 Applications of Biomedical Polymers in Functional Skin Care Products

9.6.1 Moisturizing products

The categories and functions of biomedical polymer meterials in moisturizing products are shown in Table 9-2.

Table 9-2 The categories and functions of biomedical polymer materials in moisturizing products

Categories	Functions
Ceramide liposome	Ceramide can limit the water loss from the skin to the environment, reduce transepidermal water loss (TEWL), and thus increasing the water content of the stratum corneum
Hyaluronic acid	HA can draw water from the stratum basale, atmosphere, and from the underlying epidermis to increase skin hydration
Collagen	Natural moisturizing factors such as glycine, hydroxyproline, and hydroxylysine containing in collagen molecule maintain skin moisture. Hydrophilic groups such as hydroxyl and carboxyl groups on the outside of the collagen molecule make it easy to form hydrogen bonds with water, improving the water storage capacity of skin
Beta-glucan	Beta-glucan can form a film on the skin to fully lock in moisture and prevent moisture loss
Poly(glutamic acid)	Poly(glutamic acid) has a strong water absorption. Additionally, it can inhibit the hyaluronidase activity, thus having a strong moisturizing ability
Silicones(e. g. , dimethicone,caprylyl methicone)	Silicones help form a protective moisture barrier, healing and protecting dry skin areas
Chitin	Chitin interacts with proteins and lipids ,forming a protective film attached to keratin and lipids, and plays a role in maintaining skin moisture
Others (pullulan polysaccharide, tremella fuciformis polysaccharide, sour bean polysaccharide, sclerotinia gum, etc.)	Film-forming moisturizing

9.6.2　Skin whitening products

The categories and functions of biomedical polymer materials in skin whitening products are shown in Table 9-3.

Table 9-3　The categories and functions of biomedical polymer materials in skin whitening products

Categories	Functions
Collagen	Tyrosine residues in collagen compete with tyrosine in the skin to combine with the active center of tyrosinase, inhibiting tyrosinase to catalyze conversion of tyrosine to dopa in the skin, thus preventing melanin production in the skin to achieve whitening effect
Poly(glutamic acid)	Poly(glutamic acid) can significantly inhibit tyrosinase activity, thereby inhibiting skin melanin production
Silk fibroin	Silk fibroin can block ultraviolet rays

9.6.3　Sunscreen products

UV absorbents are active ingredients in sunscreen products that prevent harmful UVB (290-320 nm) and UVA(320-400 nm) from reaching the active layer beneath the skin's surface. To enhance efficiency, UV absorbents must be retained on the uppermost surface of the skin as a protective film and should also remain photostable throughout the entire UV exposure period. Skin penetration and photolysis of UV absorbents are undesirable since skin penetration decreases expected UV protection while photolysis leads to changes in color and appearance, and increases phototoxicity of the sunblock. And decomposed products of UV absorbents may leads to allergies.

The most popular UV absorbents are lipophilic molecules with relatively low molecular weight. Although measures are taken to promote photostability, such as addition of photostabilizers and use of high molecular weight UV absorbents to minimize skin absorption, they still are capable of penetrating skin and being systemically absorbed. Thus, developing innovative formulations of non-penetrating UV absorbents is still necessary.

Under the circumstances, encapsulating UV absorbents in different structured materials is a useful strategy to prevent skin penetration and enhance the photoprotective potential of sunscreen actives. Encapsulation encompasses many supramolecular systems, such as solid lipid NPs, nanostructured lipid carriers, nanoemulsions, polymer NPs, silica NPs, and dendrimers. This section provides a brief description of the novel nanocarriers which are being used for sunscreen products.

9.6.3.1　Solid lipid NPs (SLNs)

SLNs are the first lipid NPs developed from substituting the liquid lipid (oil) of an oil/water nanoemulsion with physiologically, well tolerated and biodegradable melt-emulsified lipids which are solid at room and body temperature. They consist of a hydrophilic shell and a hydrophobic core which allows the encapsulation of hydrophobic compounds. Their mean particle size ranges from 40 nm to 1000 nm.

SLNs have UV resistant properties and act as physical sunscreens on their own. SLNs as carrier for 3,4,5-trimethoxybenzoylchitin and vitamin E sunscreen are developed to enhance UV protection. However, they have some drawbacks: ① little stable, since they are prone to drug expulsion phenomena during storage or usage because of the complexity of the physical state of the lipid, and to the simultaneous presence of alternative colloidal structures; ② insufficient drug loading due to the limited solubility of drugs in the solid lipid matrix; ③ not suitable for oil-based formulations as they will dissolve.

9.6.3.2 Nanostructured lipid carriers (NLCs)

NLCs are considered as the second generation of the lipid nanoparticles. NLCs have been developed so that the drawbacks associated with SLNs can be overcome. Based on SLNs, NLCs replace solid oil with a mixture of solid oil and liquid oil, which makes them have a more irregular defect structure, thus generating more space to accommodate more active substances, effectively improving its coating rate and the stability of active substances in the long-term storage process. Compared with SLNs, NLCs are more convenient for the coating of active ingredients because of its incomplete crystallization and amorphous state. At present, there are three main structures of NLCs coating active ingredients: amorphous type, imperfect type and multiple type.

Compared to SLNs, NLCs show higher drug-loading capacity for entrapped bioactive compound because of the distorted structure which helps in creating more space. Other limitations of SLNs (e.g., reduced particle concentration and expulsion of drug during storage) are solved by manipulating the formulation of NLCs. They are formulated by biodegradable and physiological lipids that show very low toxicity. NLCs have modulated drug delivery profile by a biphasic drug release pattern. In this case, the drug is released initially with a burst release, followed by a sustained release at a constant rate. They possess numerous advantageous features, including increased skin hydration due to occlusive properties, and the small size ensures close contact to the stratum corneum leading to the increased amount of drug penetration into the skin. There are stable drug incorporation during storage and enhanced UV protection system with reduced side effects. Using NLCs loaded sunscreen can greatly improve the sunscreen effect of the system, reduce its irritation to the skin, reduce the dosage of chemical sunscreen, and improve the compatibility and stability of the sunscreen system.

9.6.3.3 Nanoemulsions

Nanoemulsions are a combination of a surfactant with an oil or water phase. Depending on the composition, nanoemulsions have different types, such as oil in water, water in oil, and bicontinuous nanoemulsions. They exhibit various sizes ranging from 50 nm to 200 nm. They have very low oil/water interfacial tension and a lipophilic core, which is surrounded by a monomolecular layer of phospholipids. These properties make it more suitable for the delivery of lipophilic compounds. Nanoemulsions show several advantages, including low viscosity, high kinetic stability, high interfacial area, and high solubilization capacity. In cosmetics formulation, nanoemulsions provide rapid penetration and active transport of active ingredients and hydration to the skin.

9.6.3.4　Polymer nanoparticles (PNs)

PNs are colloidal carrier systems composed of a polymer core with a diameter of submicron level. According to their structural organization, composition and distribution of the active compound, they can be classified into nanocapsules (NCs) and nanospheres (NSs). In the former one, the active compounds are entrapped inside, whereas in the latter, they are adsorbed on the surface. The polymer lipid walls of NCs are ideal for sustained release of lipophilic compounds and protect them from photodegradation phenomena. The properties of PNs depend on the polymer composition, organic solvent and surfactant dosage, which can affect the particle size, surface properties and release rate of UV active.

The main advantages of PNs are that they can provide controlled/sustained release of the UV absorbents, hence prolonging their residence time on the skin, improving photostability of the sunscreen agents and preventing skin absorption.

9.6.3.5　Silica NPs (SNs)

SNs could confine UV absorbents within a hollow silica matrix or precursors of UV filters to a silica matrix for chemically binding with UV absorbents. Their particle sizes vary from 10 nm to 10 μm. There is a new generation of UV absorbents based on the photochemical transformation of suitable precursors upon exposure to sunlight. The UV absorbents are generated from their precursors on demand, affording protection at the time, place and degree required, increasing their UV blocking ability as UV exposure is increased. The protective ability of these UV absorbents was shown to be further enhanced by encapsulation in SNs (average particle size was 100-1000 nm) as demonstrated for a silyl precursor of BP-3 that was copolymerized with alkoxysilane using sol-gel technology. The encapsulation improved the yield of transformation of the BP-3 precursor by increasing the absorbance of the final product 3-fold compared to non-encapsulated BP-3. From the chemical point of view, encapsulation in a rigid matrix is expected to improve the light conversion efficiency by restricting the mobility of the radicals formed in the initial steps of the reaction. Furthermore, chemical incompatibilities of the UV filter with other components of the sunscreen formulation are prevented by the physical barrier between them. From a biological point of view, confinement in the silica matrix should lead to a reduction in the toxicologic and allergenic potential of the UV filters as well. Finally, as silica is a natural and chemically inert material, a reduction of the environmental impact of such supramolecular sunscreens relative to molecular filters can also be expected, as long as the UV filter is not released.

9. 6. 3. 6　Dendrimers

Dendrimers are highly branched, unimolecular, globular, micellar nanostructure, and multivalent NPs. Their diameters range from 2 nm to 20 nm. A dendrimer is typically built from a core on which series of branches are engrafted in an arborescent way and often adopts a spherical three-dimensional morphology. Its properties (e. g., monodispersity, polyvalence, and stability) make it an ideal carrier with precision and selectivity. Dendrimers provide controlled release from the inner core and drugs are incorporated in interior as well as being attached on the surface.

Due to the definite 3D structure and several surface functional groups, dendrimers can act by encapsulation of drugs within the dendritic structure or by forming electrostatic/covalent bonds between drugs with terminal functional groups of dendrimers. Two mechanisms of the drug delivery from drug-dendrimer conjugate have been reported in the literature. The first mechanism is owed to *in vivo* cleavage of covalent bonds between drug and dendrimer in existence of enzymes or an environment required for bond breaking. The second mode of drug release is the alteration in physical conditions, temperature and pH which are not dependent on external factors.

9.7　Applications of Biomedical Polymers in Laser Cosmetology

After years of development, laser cosmetology has been widely used in clinical practice. Skin has a high scattering characteristic, which is determined by its refractive index mismatch of different tissue structures. In laser surgery, part of the incident laser beam can reflect from the surface. When photons penetrating the surface, reflection, refraction, scattering, and absorption can occur in the tissue. When the scattered light overlaps with the incident light, the light energy of the subcutaneous tissue is superimposed, and the light is absorbed by the target tissue, causing damage to the target tissue. However, the high scattering characteristics of the skin reduce the penetration depth of the light in the tissue, the light reaching the target tissue in the skin is less than the incident light, and the target tissue absorbs less energy. Increasing the energy density of the laser increases the energy absorption of the target chromophores, but it also increases the risk of skin damage such as blister, pigmentation, and scarring. Some recent studies have shown that optical clearing agents(OCAs) can reduce the scattering of light in tissues and enhance the penetration depth of laser (Figure 9-5). Therefore, they have a certain prospect in the field of skin laser beauty. They can enhance the therapeutic effect of deep skin diseases, reduce the energy required to clear target tissues, and thus reducing the skin damage caused by laser. In addition, laser operation often causes a few skin injury, such as erythema and edema, and medical dressings can be used to promote skin healing at this moment. In laser surgery, it is very important to reduce skin scattering and prevent skin injury, which can produce good effects. In this section, we mainly introduce the application of OCAs and medical dressings in laser surgery.

9.7.1 Applications of optical clearing agents(OCAs)

9.7.1.1 Mechanisms of optical clearing and types of OCAs

OCAs are a kind of chemical reagents with high refractive index, high permeability and good biocompatibility. The effect of these agents on the tissue are reversible. Currently, there are three main proposed mechanisms of optical clearing (OC). (ⅰ) Refractive matching:OCAs penetrate into the tissue, improve the refractive index of the interstitial fluid, make the refractive index of each tissue components match, reduce the scattering of light in the tissue, and enhance the penetration depth of light. (ⅱ) Dehydration: the entry of the hyperosmolar OCAs into the tissue results in the loss of moisture and the decrease of the refractive index mismatch. (ⅲ) Reversible dissociation of collagen fibers: some OCAs are capable of destabilizing the collagen structure, and reducing light scattering of collagen tissue. Collagen fiber is the main scattering source of dermis.

OCAs are mainly classified as follows: (ⅰ) Alcohols: e. g. , glycerol, poly(ethylene glycol) (PEG), poly(propylene glycol), mannitol, sorbitol and xylitol. (ⅱ) Sugars: e. g. , glucose, dextrose, fructose, ribose and sucrose. (ⅲ) Organic acids: e. g. , oleic and linoleic acids. (ⅳ) Other organic solvents: e. g. , dimethyl sulphoxide (DMSO) or thiazone. (ⅴ) X-ray contrast agents: e. g. , Omnipaque™.

Although these OCAs are considered non-toxic, long-term use in the body may results in tissue edema and irritation, local hemostasis, shrinkage and even tissue necrosis. In this case, injection of OCAs into the skin may cause necrosis. The penetration of OCAs depends on a number of factors, including the type, refractive index, concentration and tissue exposure time of OCAs, as well as the original turbidity of the biological tissue and permeability to a particular OCA.

9.7.1.2 Manners to promote the penetration of OCAs

The barrier function in the stratum corneum prevents the penetration of OCAs, which requires a longer time for skin OC. However, the long-term application of hyperosmolar OCAs may cause skin damage. Some methods to accelerate the penetration of OCAs are as follows: (ⅰ) Chemical enhancers: azone, oleic acid, dimethyl sulfoxide (DMSO), propylene glycol and thiazone can enhance the permeability of OCAs. At present, these chemical enhancers are seldom used *in vivo*, and their safety and penetration effect need to be further studied. (ⅱ) Physical methods to remove the stratum corneum surface layers: e. g. , adhesive tape, and microdermabrasion. (ⅲ) Other factors: e. g. , photothermal, laser, electrophoresis, and ultrasound. Although these methods can improve the effect of OCAs and reduce the action time of OCAs, they may have other side effects. For example, some chemical enhancers can be toxic to the human body, and physical methods can also cause skin damage.

9.7.1.3 The applications of OCAs *in vivo* and *in vitro*, and the prospect of OCAs in laser cosmetology

Currently, OCAs have not been used in clinic, but they have broad prospects for improving laser therapy. Studies on light transparency of skin tissues are mainly *in vitro* experiments, and few *in vivo* experiments (animal experiments). Due to the safety and biocompatibility of OCAs and the different drug metabolism between *in vitro* and *in vivo* tissues, their application in the human body is limited. *In vitro* experiments, the method of administration is usually *in vitro* tissue immersion, while *in vivo* experiments, the methods of administration are usually surface painting and subcutaneous injection. The solution of glycerin, sugar, polyethylene glycol, propylene glycol or acetic acid has a reversible clearing effect on tissues and can be used *in vivo*. However, the concentration should not be too high to avoid tissue damage and necrosis. Glycerin is often used *in vivo* experiments. When its concentration is more than 30%, it can cause skin edema and other adverse reactions. The effect of thiazone and Omnipaque™ *in vivo* was better without obvious side effect. Many studies have shown that the application of OCAs can improve the OC effect of skin *in vivo* and *in vitro*, increasing the detection depth of molecular optical imaging. There have been few studies on the combine application of OCAs and lasers; however, it has been reported that the combination of OCA (a mixture of polypropylene glycol and polyethylene glycol) and lasers is more effective and less damaging in the treatment of human skin tattoos than in the control group. Yet, the case number is small and further study is needed. There are many challenges in the application of OCAs in the human body. Development of a kind of OCAs with low toxicity, good biocompatibility, direct applying to the skin and rapid metabolism, is of great significance for laser cosmetology.

9.7.2 Applications of medical dressings in postoperative laser repair

9.7.2.1 Definition and classification of medical dressings

Medical dressing is a kind of biomedical material that can stick to the wound, control the infection, promote the repair of the skin injury and avoid the formation of the scar. Biomedical dressings can be divided into passive dressings, interactive dressings and bioactive dressings. The different materials, physical forms, architecture of theses dressings leading to functions and applicable wound types are also different.

(ⅰ) Passive dressings, such as gauze and tulle dressings, are used to cover the wound and restore the structural function.

(ⅱ) Interactive dressings, such as foams, hydrogels and hydrocolloids, are used to prevent the penetration of bacteria in the wound.

(ⅲ) Bioactive dressings, such as collagen, hyaluronic acid, chitosan (CS), alginate and elastin, are biocompatible, biodegradable and non-toxic. They can be used separately and in combination. Interactive dressings and bioactive dressings belong to modern dressings that can prevent wound dehydration and promote healing. Hydrogel dressing is considered ideal for wound dressings. Nanotechnology is also being used in medical dressings, organic and non-organic NPs (e. g., polymeric NPs and silver NPs, respectively) can carry growth factors, antimicrobials and drugs to stimulate wound healing. A variety of biomedical dressings have been reported for skin burns: such as Ag^+ sulfadiazine-containing nanosheet-based ultra-thin films, NO-releasing polymer films, and tyrothricin (cyclic polypeptide antibiotic)-containing CS-based film-forming gel layers. These dressings are non-toxic, which can inhibit inflammation, reduce scarring, and promote epithelialization and granulation tissue formation.

9.7.2.2 Postoperative complications of laser and early application of medical dressings

During laser surgery, laser device, treatment style, preoperative evaluation, parameter setting and operation, medical history of patients (e. g., abnormal scarring, excessive sun exposure) or history of medication (e. g., aspirin, nonsteroidal anti-inflammatory drugs) may affect the risk of laser complications. These complications include early complications of skin (e. g., erythema, edema, infection), mid-term complications (e. g., hyperpigmentation, hypopigmentation), late complications (e. g., scarring). The early use of medical dressings after laser surgery can release early complications and reduce the risk of mid-term and late complications. The first two weeks after surgery is regarded as the key period of wound care. Medical dressings used for laser postoperative skin repair include the followings: (ⅰ) Open dressings: ointment or cream can be directly applied on the skin surface, which can promote wound healing and care easily, such as aquaphor. But this method may increase the risk of acne, milia and infection. (ⅱ) Closed dressings: This method can provide a moist wound healing environment, and has good effects. The disadvantages of closed dressings include high cost, long time of use, adhere to skin uneasily, and no absorption layer. Dressings commonly used in facial care after laser surgery include composite foam (Flexzan and Revitaderm), hydrogel (2ⁿᵈ Skin), polymer film (Silon-TSR), and polymer mesh (N-terface and Mepitel). It is recommended to use closed dressings for at least 24 h after laser surgery, no more than 4 days, and convert to open dressings on the 5th day to help reducing the infection rate. The purpose of wound care in the first week after laser surgery is to prevent skin infection, avoid environmental irritation, and achieve reepithelialization.

In summary, the modern biomedical dressings have a broad prospect in laser cosmetology, and they need to be further improved in terms of drug penetration and activity, water retention, air permeability, skin adhesion and so on.

9.8 Challenges and Perspectives

With the development of modern science and technology, especially the major breakthrough of biotechnology, the application of biomedical polymer materials in the field of beauty will be more extensive, and the demand is also increasing. New biomedical polymer materials have the advantages of good biocompatibility, better biological activity and non-toxic side effects, etc. New materials are constantly appearing, bringing more new choices for cosmetic dermatology. The research on biomedical polymer materials by many research teams at home and abroad provides more reference data for its application in skin repair, functional cosmetics, skin fillers, auxiliary laser therapy and other aspects. The safety, histocompatibility and interaction mechanism of biomedical polymer materials in human skin and tissues need to be further studied. In addition, the commercial application of biomedical polymer materials still needs to be further explored. It is believed that with the development of more related studies, the application of biomedical polymer materials in cosmetic dermatology will have a wider prospect. We believe that biomedical polymer materials can be developed more rapidly, thus promoting the development of beauty industry.

Questions

1. What characteristics should biomedical polymer substitute materials have?
2. How to use biomedical polymer materials to repair the skin barrier?
3. What effects can biomedical polymer materials have in laser cosmetology?
4. Which functional skin care products can biomedical polymer materials be used in?
5. What roles are the nanostructured lipid carriers play in sunscreen products?

Extended Reading

[1] Draelos Z D. Cosmetic dermatology: products and procedures[M]. Hoboken N J: Blackwell Publishing Ltd.,2010.

[2] Baran R,Maibach H I. Textbook of cosmetic dermatology[M]. 4th ed. London:Informa Healthcare,2010.

[3] Sarbana K. Lasers in dermatological practice [M]. New York: Mcgraw-hill Education,2014.

[4] 赵长生,孙树东.生物医用高分子材料[M].2版.北京:化学工业出版社,2016.

[5] Carruthers J,Carruthers A. 软组织填充剂与医学美容——美容皮肤科实用技术[M].刘秉慈,译.北京:人民军医出版社,2007.

(Li Yan)

第十章
可穿戴电子皮肤器件

第一节　电子皮肤概述

皮肤是人体最大的器官,是人体的物理屏障,也是人体感知环境的重要器官,具有优异的自愈合能力及感觉(如温度、痛觉、压力等)传感性能。皮肤中包含多种感觉受体,可将皮肤与环境的物理接触转变为电信号,进而传输到中枢神经系统,最终由大脑的躯体感觉皮层做出判断,实现对外界环境的感知。

当皮肤受损时,特别是较大面积的损伤或缺失时,皮肤难以自愈,导致物理屏障作用减弱。此时,皮肤中的感觉受体受到破坏,导致人体对外界环境的触觉感受减弱甚至丧失。目前,植皮是治疗大面积皮肤损伤的主要手段,但仍存在皮肤来源有限及皮肤功能重建难度高等问题。此外,由于机器人与人工智能的快速发展,人们期望赋予机器人更多的功能,例如与人类相似的皮肤传感性能。具有皮肤传感性能的机器人在病患看护、疾病诊断与监测方面具有重要的应用,可实现较为复杂的交互任务。上述需求推动了电子皮肤的快速发展。

所谓电子皮肤(e-skin),就是模拟人体真实皮肤功能的人造皮肤器件(图 10-1),也被称为智能皮肤(smart skin)。电子皮肤器件不仅具有皮肤的感觉传递功能,还可以被赋予更多的功

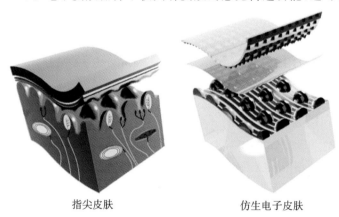

指尖皮肤　　　　　　　　仿生电子皮肤

图 10-1　人类指尖皮肤剖面图与电子皮肤示意图

Figure 10-1　Cross-sectional view of human fingertip skin and schematic diagram of e-skin

能。例如,可将化学或生物传感器集成于电子皮肤中,实现对环境或人体的气体或液体物质的检测,从而对环境变化或人体生理状态变化进行监测。电子皮肤有望作为假体移植到人体,替代缺失或病变的皮肤。此外,电子皮肤在软体机器人方面有非常广阔的应用前景,有望赋予机器人更多的功能,通过模拟皮肤的传感作用来完成交互式任务。

电子皮肤器件的发展经历了单一功能器件到多功能集成器件的过程。根据不同的需求和应用场景,人们可对电子皮肤器件的结构和功能进行设计,体现出非常强的灵活性。本章将介绍电子皮肤器件的设计要素、种类及应用。

第二节 电子皮肤器件设计要素

电子皮肤器件是对人体真实皮肤的模拟,不仅要有与皮肤相似的力学性能,而且要实现皮肤的部分功能。因此,电子皮肤器件要满足三个要求:①具有与真实皮肤类似的力学性质,如低模量、可拉伸性、柔性等;②可实现真实皮肤的功能,如对压力、应变、剪切、温度等刺激的传感;③可集成真实皮肤不具有的功能,如对生理电信号、化学物质等信号的传感,实现对人体健康的监测。为了满足以上要求,在设计电子皮肤器件时,需要针对不同的功能和用途,从材料和器件结构等角度综合考虑,以获得性能优异的器件。

一、材料的选择

电子皮肤与真实皮肤具有相似的力学性质,因此制备电子皮肤的材料需要具有优异的柔性、可拉伸性、生物相容性及自修复性等,以保证其生物安全性和使用寿命。材料的选择和制备策略在模拟真实皮肤的力学性质方面起到关键作用。此外,为了实现电子皮肤的传感功能,需要使用具有优异电学性能(包括导电与介电性能)的材料。下面对电子皮肤的基底材料、介电材料、导电材料的选择进行简要介绍。

(一)基底材料

为模拟皮肤优异的柔性及可拉伸性,柔性较好的高分子材料常用作电子皮肤的基底材料(见扩展阅读1),目前使用最多的是聚二甲基硅氧烷(PDMS,通常称为硅胶)。这种材料不仅具有非常好的柔性、可拉伸性及生物相容性,还具有优异的化学稳定性和高透明度等。通过紫外线照射后,PDMS还可具有较强的表面黏附力,一方面可与皮肤良好贴合,另一方面,对器件中的电极材料具有较好的结合力,避免器件在人体运动过程中脱落或器件结构发生变化。此外,聚氨酯具有非常好的弹性,也可作为基底材料制备可拉伸的印刷电路,在电子皮肤领域也具有重要的应用价值。其他材料如传统的电纺丝纤维膜、纺织品等也可作为电子皮肤的基底材料,但由于可拉伸性和透明性较差,其应用受到一定的限制。

(二)介电材料

在基于晶体管和电容器的电子皮肤器件中,需要使用聚合物介电材料作为绝缘层,要求其具有较高的介电常数和较低的漏电流。上面介绍的PDMS本身也是一种常用的聚合物介电材料。在介电聚合物的发展过程中,人们发现,化学结构的设计(例如在聚合物链上修饰氰基、氟原子等极性基团),添加高介电常数的纳米粒子(如二氧化钛、钛酸钡等纳米粒子)等方法可提高聚合物材料的介电常数。在提高介电性能的同时,需要保证材料的生物相容性、柔性及可拉伸性。由于电子皮肤器件处于反复拉伸、弯曲等动态过程中,介电材料的耐久性、自修复性等因素也会显著影响器件的稳定性,在制备器件时需要注意。

（三）导电材料

导电材料是电子皮肤中的关键材料。目前,人们已经将多种导电材料应用于电子皮肤中。例如碳纳米管、石墨烯等碳材料具有优异的电学、力学性能及高化学稳定性,已被广泛用于电子皮肤的制备。近年来,半导体纳米线(如硅、砷化镓、硒化镉纳米线等)及金属纳米线(如金、银、铜纳米线等)也被用于电子皮肤的制备。但由于纳米线的制备方法通常较为复杂、成本较高,其应用受到一定的限制。近年来,人们将有机聚合物导体材料应用于电子皮肤的制备。常见的聚合物导体材料包括聚 3-己基噻吩、聚苯胺、聚吡咯、聚(3,4-乙撑二氧噻吩)/聚苯乙烯磺酸复合物(PEDOT:PSS)等。有机半导体材料通常加工性能好,力学性能更接近人体皮肤。因此,相对于碳纳米管、石墨烯、金属(金、银、铜等)纳米线等材料,有机半导体材料更适合用于制备大面积柔性电子皮肤器件。

二、器件可拉伸性的实现

人体皮肤具有优异的可拉伸性,因此电子皮肤需要有与人体皮肤相似的可拉伸性,这样在使用过程中才能保持与皮肤良好的贴合性,并且延长工作寿命。为了获得电子皮肤优异的可拉伸性,一方面需要开发具有优异弹性的材料,另一方面需要对材料在器件中的排列结构进行设计,从而获得具有优异可拉伸性的电子皮肤器件。前文"材料的选择"主要介绍了柔性、可拉伸性材料的选择,主要是从材料的固有可拉伸性出发,选择具有适当可拉伸性的材料,增强器件的可拉伸性。下面将主要从材料在器件中的集成结构出发,介绍增强器件可拉伸性的方法。

传统的无机半导体/导体材料通常模量高、脆性高、可拉伸性差,在柔性器件应用方面受到诸多限制。为解决这些问题,研究人员从材料的几何构型出发,发展了一系列制备具有优异可拉伸性材料的方法。

第一种方法是通过拉伸使连续薄膜产生裂隙。首先将刚性的连续导体/半导体薄膜置于弹性基底上,然后对基底进行单向或双向拉伸。由于薄膜具有脆性,在拉伸基底的过程中,薄膜断裂形成裂隙。随着拉伸程度的增大,裂隙变宽或裂隙数量变多,材料获得良好的可拉伸性。通过控制拉伸程度,薄膜在产生裂隙的同时可维持导电通路(图 10-2(a))。Graz 等人通过该策略将金膜复合于弹性基底上,其拉伸程度达到 100% 时仍能保持良好的导电性。

第二种方法是使一维纤维状材料在基底铺展。由于一维材料的随机取向,基底可形成导电网络通路。在基底拉伸时,材料仍能与基底直接接触,导电网络可随着基底的拉伸发生形变。即使在形变量较大时,导电网络也不会被破坏(图 10-2(b))。例如 Lee 和 Ko 团队利用银纳米线作为导电材料制作了具有高拉伸性和高导电性的电极材料,其形变量可达 460%,并且在拉伸时其薄膜电阻仍然较低。

第三种方法是利用微加工法对导电材料进行图案化(图 10-2(c)),形成弯曲或螺旋结构,然后将其与弹性基底复合。具有螺旋结构的导电材料可随基底的拉伸发生较大形变,类似于弹簧在拉力作用下发生可逆形变,从而赋予复合材料良好的可拉伸性。Gonzalez 等人对导电材料的多种图案化结构对器件可拉伸性的影响进行了研究,他们发现当导电材料以蛇形或马蹄形置于基底中时,材料的可拉伸性最好,在形变量达 100% 时仍能保持良好的导电性。多层蛇形结构叠加的方式可进一步提升其可拉伸性。

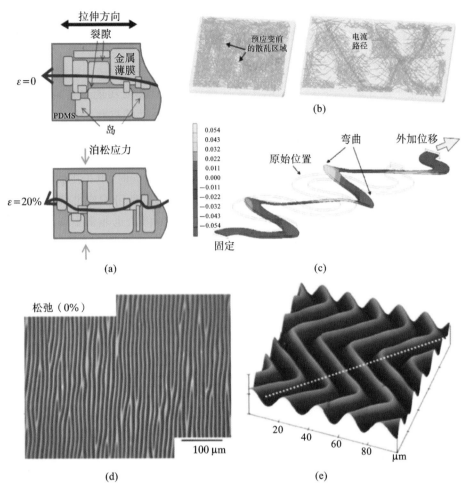

图 10-2　几种提升器件可拉伸性的方法

(a)拉伸弹性基底,使刚性导体/半导体薄膜产生裂隙,同时保持导电通路;(b)利用一维纤维状材料构建网络结构,拉伸变形时,仍保持导电通路;(c)将导电材料以蛇形或马蹄形置于基底中,提升可拉伸性;(d)单向预拉伸可制备线性褶皱;(e)双向拉伸可制备人字形褶皱

Figure 10-2　Several methods to improve the stretchability of the device

(a)Stretching the elastic substrate to create cracks in the rigid conductor/semiconductor film;(b)Using one-dimensional fibrous materials to build a deformable network structure;(c)The conductive materials are placed in the substrate in a serpentine or horseshoe shape to improve the stretchability;(d)Unidirectional pre-stretching can produce linear folds;(e)Bidirectional stretching can produce herringbone folds

　　第四种方法是将高模量的导体材料复合于预拉伸的弹性基底上。在基底收缩时,导体材料出现褶皱。单向预拉伸可制备线性褶皱(图 10-2(d)),双向拉伸可制备人字形褶皱(图 10-2(e))。此外,还可通过微加工方法预先在弹性基底表面构筑褶皱结构,然后将导电材料复合于褶皱的表面。通过该方法制备的褶皱结构也具有良好的可拉伸性。褶皱策略适用于多种材料,包括无机半导体、金属、复合材料、石墨烯、碳纳米管等。由于褶皱的存在,柔性器件在被拉伸时,其中的导体材料的形变主要源自其几何结构的变化,材料本身不会产生大形变。利用褶皱策略不仅可赋予器件良好的可拉伸性,还可避免材料本身的反复变形,有利于延长器件的使用寿命。

第三节　电子皮肤器件种类及其应用

　　皮肤的功能非常复杂,与之对应的电子皮肤器件所需具备的功能也非常多(见扩展阅读2)。首先,电子皮肤器件需要对皮肤的触觉传感进行模拟,从而使皮肤受损或肢体缺失的患者重建皮肤对外界环境的触感,也可赋予机器人更加丰富和精确的触觉响应性,完成更为复杂的人机交互任务。其次,电子皮肤器件作为一种可穿戴器件,也可被赋予化学传感性能,包括对体液及气体化学成分的传感,从而实现对人体健康进行监测。同时,电子皮肤器件还可被赋予疾病治疗的功能。当监测到人体健康发生变化时,电子皮肤器件可响应性释放其负载的特定药物,进而对疾病进行治疗。另外,对于可穿戴设备,其能源供给也非常重要。通过材料及器件结构设计,可赋予电子皮肤器件储能及供能的功能。此外,将多种功能集成,可制备多功能电子皮肤器件,从而在一定程度上实现电子皮肤的智能化,可用于监测血压、呼吸频率、身体运动、体温变化等。本节将对具有不同功能的电子皮肤器件进行简要介绍。

一、力学刺激传感器件

　　人体皮肤能感觉到复杂的外部力学刺激,包括压力、拉伸、剪切、弯曲、振动、滑动等。对电子皮肤器件来说,从材料和器件结构上进行设计来实现对力学刺激的传感,就显得尤为重要。

　　皮肤与外界环境接触时产生压力与应变。根据压力与应变的不同,人体可判断接触的物质的基本性质。压力与应变的识别与传递是皮肤的重要功能之一,因此也是电子皮肤模拟的重要功能之一。在电子皮肤器件中,主要通过器件的电阻、电容、摩擦电效应等对外界作用力的响应性实现压力和应变的传感。其中,基于电容和电阻变化的电子皮肤不仅结构简单,而且能够探测动态和静态的刺激信号,因而得到最广泛和深入的研究。

　　基于电阻变化的电子皮肤可通过三种途径实现压力或应变的传感:①聚合物基复合材料中导电逾渗网络的变化;②导电材料与电极之间接触电阻的变化;③导电材料本身电阻的变化。电子皮肤器件将作用力变化转变为器件电阻的变化,是一种非常简单、常用的策略。

　　例如,将单壁碳纳米管在弹性基底(如 PDMS)上进行排列形成薄膜,可制备应变传感器。当拉伸弹性基底时,碳纳米管薄膜发生断裂,从而在膜中形成缝隙,导致薄膜的电阻增加。形变程度越大,膜中产生的缝隙越大,电阻也越大。因此,可通过测量电阻变化来实现应变的传感。该器件可被集成到衣物、创可贴、手套等表面,从而达到对人体不同运动(如呼吸、说话、行走、手势等)的传感(图 10-3),有望实现电子皮肤在健康监测、虚拟现实、机器人等领域的广泛应用。此外,金属纳米线也可作为导电材料构建应力传感器。压力导致纳米线与电极之间的接触程度发生变化,进而使器件的电阻发生变化。通过固定电压,测量器件电流随应力的变化,从而实现应力的传感。

　　基于电容变化的电子皮肤主要通过压力或应变改变器件电极之间的距离、面积、介电层的介电常数实现压力或应变的传感。例如,利用微结构化的 PDMS 薄膜作为介电层,可制备基于电容器原理的压力传感器。如图 10-4 所示,器件中 PDMS 薄膜表面具有金字塔形的微结构阵列。当受到外界压力时,该薄膜依然能保持良好的弹性形变能力,从而赋予 PDMS 薄膜灵敏的响应性。外界压力导致介电层厚度发生改变,进而使电容器的电容发生改变,也可使场效

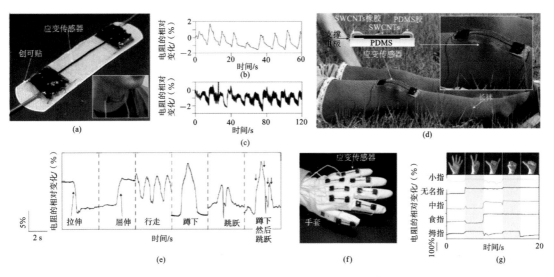

图 10-3 利用碳纳米管制备的应变传感器用于探测不同类型的人体运动

（a）集成于创可贴上的器件；（b、c）呼吸和说话产生的运动导致器件电阻的变化；（d）集成于丝袜上的器件；（e）不同类型的运动导致不同的电阻变化模式；（f）集成于手套上的器件；（g）通过电阻的变化对手势进行识别

Figure 10-3 Strain sensor device made of carbon nanotubes are used to detect different types of human movements

（a）Devices integrated in band-aids；（b and c）Breath and speech motions cause changes in device resistance；（d）Devices integrated on stockings；（e）Different types of motions lead to different resistance change patterns；（f）A device integrated on a glove；（g）Recognition of gestures through changes in resistance

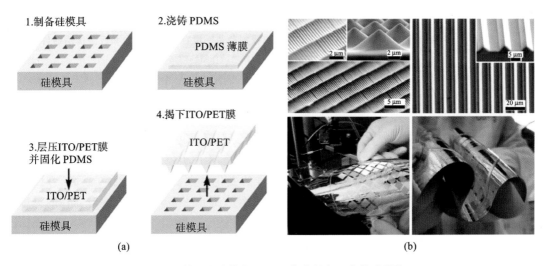

图 10-4 基于微结构化 PDMS 薄膜制备压力传感器件

（a）利用微结构化的 PDMS 薄膜作为介电层制备基于电容器原理的压力传感器；（b）该器件中微结构的扫描电镜图及器件的实物图

Figure 10-4 Pressure sensor device made of microstructured PDMS film

（a）Using a microstructured PDMS film as a dielectric layer to fabricate a pressure sensor device based on the principle of capacitance；（b）SEM images of the microstructure in the device and the photos of the device

应晶体管的输出电流发生改变,由此实现压力的传感。此外,在 PDMS 基底中引入单壁碳纳米管,在拉伸和松弛基底后,纳米管发生弯曲,基于此可构建基于平行板电容器的压力和应变传感器(图 10-5)。该器件具有对压力非常灵敏的传感性能及非常迅速的响应速度,对压力和应变的传感具有空间分辨能力,这进一步扩展了该器件在电子皮肤方面的应用。

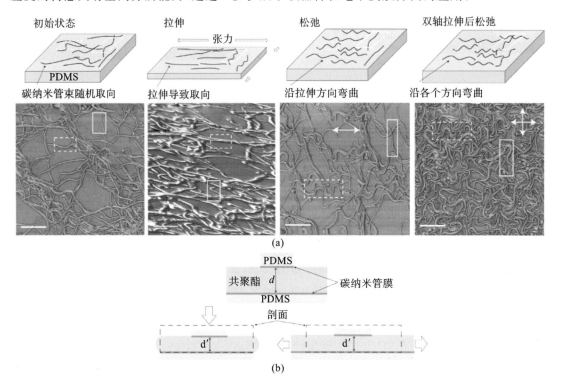

图 10-5 利用表面含碳纳米管阵列的 PDMS 薄膜制备基于电容原理的压力和应变传感器件
(a)对基底的双向拉伸使碳纳米管弯曲;(b)该器件的结构示意图

Figure 10-5 The use of PDMS films containing carbon nanotube arrays on the surface to fabricate pressure and strain sensor devices based on the change in capacitance

(a)Bending the carbon nanotubes by biaxial stretching of the substrate;(b)Schematic diagram of the structure of the device

灵敏度是压力传感器较为重要的性能参数之一。灵敏度可以被定义为电信号(如电容、电阻、电流、电压等)随外界压力变化曲线的斜率。通常情况下,压力传感器的灵敏度与传感材料的压缩模量有关:给定压力时,应变越高则电信号的变化越大,器件的灵敏度越高。对于前面介绍的基于电容和压阻变化的压力传感器,目前已经发展出了多种方法来提升器件的灵敏度。

对于电容型器件,介电层的微结构化可提升其灵敏度。例如,上述在 PDMS 表面制备金字塔形的阵列,在施加压力时,金字塔尖端很大的压强使 PDMS 产生很大的形变,导致电容变化增大,达到提升灵敏度的目的。多孔结构也可用于提升压力传感器的灵敏度。孔结构可将应力集中在孔之间的框架结构上,当施加差别很小的压力时,器件的导电性发生显著的改变,可实现灵敏度的提升。

对于压阻型器件,改变导电材料之间的接触点或接触面积的方式可改变接触电阻,从而提升器件灵敏度。例如,可将碳材料(碳纳米管、石墨烯等)与交叉电极阵列集成,在外力作用下,器件内部电极与导电材料的接触点或接触面积的变化程度大,可显著提升器件的灵敏度,可用于血压及手腕脉搏等较小压力的连续测量。

灵敏度的提升通常也会导致器件可测量范围的缩小,灵敏度高的传感器在压力增加时,其灵敏度降低。欲实现电子皮肤对人体皮肤的真实模拟,就需要在提升灵敏度的同时增大其传感范围。Cho 等人在器件中功能层表面制备半球形阵列,制备了压阻型的压力传感器,其在工作范围(0～12 kPa)内的灵敏度达到了 8.5 kPa^{-1}。此外,还可利用具有表面褶皱的电极制备电容型的压力传感器,通过压力改变电极面积来实现灵敏度和传感范围的增加。

人体皮肤除了能够感知应力应变以外,还对外力方向、滑动等不同的刺激具有精确的感知能力,例如皮肤能够区分作用力的方向,还能感知物体在皮肤表面的滑动。对电子皮肤器件来说,只有实现其对不同力学刺激的精确感知能力,才能在假体、机器人等方面获得广泛应用。从器件角度上讲,对滑动及力方向的传感需要器件对动态的力学刺激进行探测,因此主要利用压电和摩擦电原理来设计电子皮肤器件。聚偏氟乙烯是典型的压电材料,可在其表面制备不同的突起,利用不同的材料在这些突起表面滑动时产生的振动来探测材料在器件表面的滑动状态,进而对材料的表面粗糙度进行感知(图 10-6(a))。基于摩擦电原理的纳米发电机也可用于探测器件表面的滑动状态。通过在器件中置入碳纳米管/PDMS 复合电极,当表面有物体滑动时,这些电极对移动物体做出响应,从而探测物体在器件表面的移动方向。

通过器件结构设计,同一个器件上可实现多种电信号(如电阻、电容、电流、电压等)的测量,由此可实现法向和切向作用力的区分。图 10-6(b)所示的力学传感器由一个顶电极和四个底电极组成,顶电极和底电极之间由介电材料分隔,由此形成四个电容器。通过检测四个电容器电容的变化,可实现法向和切向作用力的区分。Bergbreiter 等人将三块导电材料置于一块导电材料周围,设计了一种力学传感装置。当不同方向上的力作用于器件上时,中间区域与周围导电材料之间的相对距离和接触面积发生变化,导致器件的电阻和电容发生改变,通过分析输出信号,该器件可识别作用力的大小和方向。可同时实现力的大小和方向探测的器件可集成到机械臂上,实时探测机械臂在抓取、移动物体时所受到的压力和剪切力。

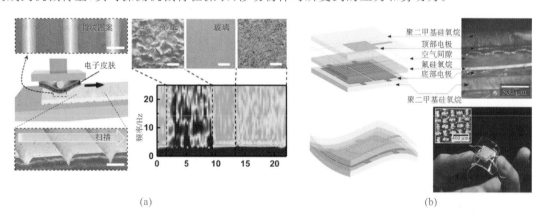

(a)　　　　　　　　　　　　　　　　　　　　(b)

图 10-6　对不同力学刺激具有精确感知能力的器件

(a)基于压电效应的器件用于材料表面粗糙度的传感;(b)利用多个电容变化实现法向和切向作用力的区分

Figure 10-6　Devices that have the ability to accurately detect different mechanical stimuli

(a)A device based on the piezoelectric effect is used to sense the surface roughness of a material;(b)The use of multiple capacitance changes to realize the distinction between normal phase and tangential force

二、温度传感器件

人体皮肤不仅能感知力学刺激,还能通过温度感受器感知人体和外界环境温度的变化。

人体温度的异常变化通常意味着健康状况的变化。因此,设计具有温度传感功能的电子皮肤器件对探测人体中暑、感染等导致的体温异常具有重要的应用价值。

目前,商业化的温度传感器主要基于金属基或陶瓷基半导体材料的热阻效应。这些材料由于具有一定的刚性,难以在柔性电子皮肤领域得到广泛的应用。因此,需要对这些材料进行结构设计,使其具有更好的可拉伸性。例如,可将金属热阻材料设计为蛇形弯曲结构或网状结构,使其具有很好的可拉伸性,可用于柔性电子皮肤的设计与制备。此外,非金属热阻材料(如碳纳米管、石墨烯、聚合物半导体等材料)也可用作电子皮肤的温度传感材料。根据材料电阻率随温度的变化趋势,其可分为两类:第一类热阻材料的电阻率随温度升高而增大,第二类热阻材料的电阻率随温度升高而降低。两类材料均可用于温度传感电子皮肤的设计。例如Wang 等人利用铜纳米线(第一类热阻材料)形成的网状结构制备了温度传感器,该器件在 25～48 ℃之间的灵敏度为 $0.7\ \Omega\cdot℃^{-1}$,在体温区(37 ℃)附近具有较高的灵敏度。Cho 等人利用还原氧化石墨烯(第二类热阻材料)制备了温度传感器,通过调控石墨烯的还原程度,获得了更高的灵敏度和更宽的温度探测区间。

除了热阻效应,热电效应及热释电效应也可用于设计温度传感电子皮肤。与基于热阻效应的温度传感器不同,基于这两种原理的器件无须供能即可工作,在电子皮肤器件方面具有一定的优势。具有热电效应的材料可在温差下产生电流(即塞贝克效应),通过检测电流从而探测温度。例如,Zhu 等人利用多孔聚氨酯和热电效应材料 PEDOT:PSS 制备了温度传感器,其温度探测精度小于 0.1 ℃。将这种器件集成为阵列后,可用于探测人手部温度的分布。具有热释电效应的材料在温度改变时会由于电极化而产生瞬时电压,通过检测电压的变化即可探测温度。例如,Ko 等人利用还原氧化石墨烯与聚偏氟乙烯的复合材料制备了温度传感器,获得了较高的灵敏度(每摄氏度变化 2.93%)与较宽的温度探测区间(0～100 ℃)。

三、生理电信号传感器件

人体内器官、组织、神经等的活动均会产生生理电信号,这些生理电活动与心律不齐、心肌梗死、神经肌肉病变、癫痫发作等疾病紧密相关。因此,对生理电信号进行监测,可进一步获得人体生命体征信号。例如心电图可记录心脏活动,肌电图可显示肌肉组织的活动状态,脑电图可记录大脑的运行状态等。

目前常用的生理电信号传感设备(如心电图仪、脑电图仪等)可精确地监测人体的生理电信号。然而,由于设备体积大、便携性差等缺点,患者难以长期实时监测生理电信号的变化。针对这个问题,研究人员开发了一种柔性、超薄、超轻、生物相容的表皮生理电信号传感器件。他们将蛇形的金属线集成到弹性体材料上,通过调节材料的组成使其与皮肤的力学性质相匹配,从而制备了具有生理电信号传感功能的电子皮肤。该器件不仅可记录心电图和肌电图,而且可与其他传感器(如应变传感器、无线充电单元、LED 显示器等)进行集成,从而得到多功能的电子皮肤器件(图 10-7(a))。

生理电信号需要经过医生的复杂分析才能得出结论,这限制了患者的使用。针对此问题,研究人员开发了一种可显示不同颜色的心电图监测器件(图 10-7(c))。他们将晶体管放大器与颜色可调的有机发光二极管集成到心电图监测器件中。当器件显示为红色时,心电图为正常状态;当器件显示蓝色时,表明心脏活动异常。该器件为心脏病患者提供了可视化监测心脏活动的方案,更适合患者长期实时监测心脏活动。

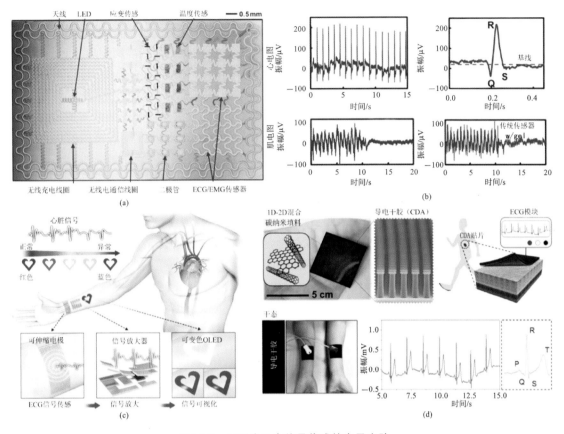

图 10-7 用于生理电信号传感的电子皮肤

(a)可测量心电图、肌电图的多功能电子皮肤器件,此器件还集成了温度、形变传感器及无线通信单元;(b)利用该器件测量得到的心电图和肌电图;(c)可随心电图信号异常发生颜色改变的电子皮肤器件示意图;(d)仿壁虎脚部结构制备的可监测心电图的电子皮肤器件

Figure 10-7 E-skins for electrophysiological signal sensing

(a)A multifunctional e-skin device that can measure ECG and EMG. This device also integrates temperature and strain sensors and wireless communication units;(b)ECG and EMG measured with this device;(c)A schematic diagram of an e-skin device that can change color with abnormal ECG signals;(d)An e-skin device that can monitor ECG made by imitating the structure of gecko's foot

为了更加精确地获得生理电信号,器件的电极需要与皮肤紧密接触。传统心电图仪的电极通过在电极与皮肤之间涂抹凝胶来实现紧密接触;而在柔性电子皮肤器件中,可通过对器件材料的设计实现与皮肤的紧密贴合。例如,Jeon 等人通过仿壁虎脚部结构的方法制备了可监测心电图的电子皮肤器件。该器件的电极可与皮肤之间通过静电吸引和物理接触的方式形成紧密贴合。即使在人体正常运动时,该器件的电极也不会与皮肤发生脱离,依然能够准确地测量心电图(图 10-7(d))。

器件的可拉伸性也是确保其可以与皮肤保持紧密贴合的重要条件。特别是在人体不规则、常运动的部位(如关节处),器件的可拉伸性可使电极在重复拉伸、扭曲的过程中仍然与皮肤保持良好的贴合性。银纳米线通常作为可拉伸电极材料,它具有优异的导电性与可加工性。但其生物相容性较差,并且容易氧化导致导电性变差。针对这个问题,可利用银-金核壳纳米线制备可拉伸性优异的电极,其生物相容性更好,耐氧化性更强,同时保持高导电性。该器件在生理电信号监测方面表现出优异的性能,不仅可以应用于人体皮肤表面,而且可应用于动物心脏表面。

尽管电子皮肤器件在生理电信号传感领域取得了快速发展,但是其离实际应用还较远(见扩展阅读3)。目前在该领域还存在一些问题,例如对电信号的分析还有赖于人工,而将处理器集成于电子皮肤还存在较大挑战;电子皮肤器件中电极和弹性体材料的化学稳定性和生物相容性还需提高。在人体日常活动中,长时间、不规则的运动导致器件与皮肤之间的贴合稳定性较差,影响生理电信号的精确传感和稳定性。这些问题的解决有赖于器件结构的优化及材料性能的提升。

四、化学传感器件

人体体液中含有水、电解质、代谢产物、激素等成分,这些成分的组成和含量与人体健康状况息息相关。因此,通过在电子皮肤中集成化学传感器,对体液的化学成分进行分析,可在分子水平上采集人体的生理健康信息,这对疾病的早期诊断和预防有重要的作用。

化学传感电子皮肤器件从原理上主要可分为电化学传感器、化学阻抗传感器、晶体管传感器等。当器件与目标化合物接触时,化学传感器的电势、电流、电阻等随着目标化合物的种类和浓度发生改变,由此获得目标化合物的信息。例如在电化学传感器中,可设计制备具有离子选择性的电极,当其与目标离子化合物接触时,可通过测量器件电势改变实现化学物质的识别(电势测定法);也可在电极上固定氧化还原酶,当电极上固定的酶与催化目标化合物发生氧化还原反应时,通过器件的电流变化可对目标化合物进行检测(电流测定法)。化学阻抗传感器通常是将传感元件置于两个电极之间,当传感元件与目标化合物接触或发生反应时,其电阻发生改变,由此实现化学物质的传感。而晶体管传感器主要由半导体层、介电层和三个电极(源电极、漏电极和栅电极)组成,可视为在化学阻抗传感器中增加了一层介电层和一个栅电极,可实现对化学传感信号的放大,进一步提升器件的灵敏度。

在体液传感中,对水含量的监测与分析是非常重要的,特别是对电子皮肤器件来说,检测皮肤中水含量的高低可辅助诊断皮肤疾病,如皮炎、银屑病、湿疹、瘙痒等。皮肤水含量可通过测量皮肤的阻抗、热导率、光谱性质等方法得到。相对于传统手段,通过电子皮肤器件测量皮肤水含量更具有优势。图10-8(a)所示的是基于阻抗变化原理设计的测量皮肤水含量的电子皮肤器件。该器件由一个采样系统和两个电极组成,其中采样系统提供不同频率的交流电。皮肤的阻抗随水含量发生变化,导致输出电流的振幅和相位发生改变,测量输出电流振幅和相位的变化,可测得皮肤的水含量。

在实际应用中,人体体液中的电解质、代谢产物、激素等成分较为复杂,浓度非常低,因此电子皮肤中的化学传感器需要具有对不同组分的高度选择性,以及非常低的检测限和高灵敏度。此外,体液中的化学物质体现了人体的健康水平,因此器件需要具有较高的稳定性以及很好的重复性,其得到的检测数据才能作为疾病早期诊断的依据。

近年来,研究人员在分析汗液成分的可穿戴化学传感电子皮肤器件方面取得了显著进展。该类器件主要由电化学电极组成,通过电势测量法或电流测量法分析汗液中的葡萄糖、乳酸、乙醇、酸碱度、电解质等成分。

在制备基于电流测量的传感器时,人们首先在电极上固定葡萄糖氧化酶、乳酸氧化酶、乙醇氧化酶等,这些酶将选择性地使目标化合物发生氧化还原反应。器件中电流的大小与待测

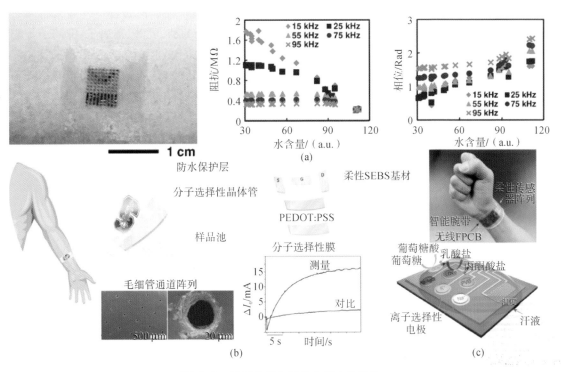

图 10-8 用于化学传感的电子皮肤器件

(a)测量皮肤水含量的电子皮肤器件,皮肤阻抗和输出电流相位随水含量发生改变;(b)检测汗液中的皮质醇的电子皮肤器件示意图;(c)同时检测汗液中的葡萄糖、乳酸、钠离子、钾离子等成分的皮肤器件示意图

Figure 10-8 E-skin devices for chemical sensing

(a) An e-skin device that measures skin water content; (b) A schematic diagram of an e-skin device that detects cortisol in sweat; (c) Schematic diagram of the e-skin device for detecting glucose, lactic acid, sodium ion, and potassium ion in sweat

物的浓度呈线性关系,因此通过测量电流的变化即可测得目标化合物的浓度。例如,Mercier 等人利用此方法制备得到可穿戴的电子皮肤传感器,利用电极上的乳酸氧化酶与汗液中乳酸发生氧化还原反应,通过测量器件电流的变化可测得汗液中乳酸的浓度。

在基于电势测量的传感器中,具有离子选择性的电极的电势依赖于目标物的浓度,通过测量电势的变化可对汗液中的带电物质如铵根离子、钾离子、钠离子等进行测量。例如,Davis 等人开发了一种可同时提取汗液并实时检测汗液中葡萄糖、钠离子、氯离子等的可穿戴器件。Takei 等人在此基础上发展了一种电荷耦合器件,用于汗液酸碱度的测量,进一步提高了器件的灵敏度。

电子皮肤化学传感器也可用于监测汗液中的激素成分。然而,汗液中激素的浓度非常低,因此对传感器的要求非常高。Salleo 等人基于有机电化学晶体管开发了一种检测汗液中的皮质醇的电子皮肤器件(图 10-8(b))。该器件含有分子印迹层,可选择性地与皮质醇分子结合,从而限制了器件中离子的运动。进而,通过测量晶体管中电流的变化,皮质醇的浓度可被计算出来。他们将该器件用于人体手臂,实时检测汗液中的皮质醇含量,取得了良好的效果。

尽管具有单一检测功能的化学传感器可反映人体汗液中的化学组成,但由于不同的生理变化可导致汗液中含有相同的化学物质,因此单一化学传感器难以准确地检测人体的健康状况。为避免这一问题,研究人员将多种传感器集成到同一平台上,同时检测汗液中的多种化学成分、人体温度、脉搏等数据,从而更加准确地判断人体的健康状况。例如,Javey等人将多种传感器集成到可穿戴电子皮肤器件,用于同时检测汗液中的葡萄糖、乳酸、钠离子、钾离子等成分(图10-8(c))。更为重要的是,检测得到的信息可直接无线传输到移动设备或者云服务器中,达到实时监测人体健康的目的。Kim等人将温度、湿度、葡萄糖、酸碱度传感器等集成到一个电子皮肤器件中,同时检测人体温度、汗液中的葡萄糖含量及汗液的酸碱度。

在组织液提取与检测方面,电子皮肤也表现出巨大的潜力。Wang等人设计了一种葡萄糖传感器,通过非侵入性的方式提取组织液,并检测其中的葡萄糖浓度。此外,组织液传感器还可以与汗液传感器进行集成,同时检测组织液和汗液中的葡萄糖水平,能够更为准确地体现人体的血糖水平。

五、皮肤给药器件

与传统药物治疗相比,针对患者不同的病理状况进行个性化治疗更具优势。个性化治疗要求在治疗过程中对患者的各项生理指标进行实时监测,跟踪患者的恢复情况,从而调整治疗方案,如药物的选择及剂量等。针对此需求,研究人员将生理电信号传感器、化学传感器等与药物控释器件集成到柔性电子皮肤中,通过生理电信号和体液化学组成的变化,实时监测人体健康状况的变化,由此反馈给药物控释器件,按实际需求控制药物的释放速度与释放量,从而更加及时、高效、个性化地对患者进行治疗。药物控释器件可与多种器件进行集成,按患者治疗需求进行设计。目前,该方法已成为新一代的经皮给药技术,具有非常好的应用前景。

例如,Kim等人设计了一种集形变传感、信息存储和药物控释于一体的电子皮肤器件(图10-9)。他们利用硅膜制备的形变传感器,可检测人体由于帕金森病导致的运动障碍,收集到的信息可存储于器件中的存储模块。通过分析人体的生命体征信息,在发现异常后,将信息反馈到药物控释模块。当药物控释模块接收到药物释放的信号时,加热部件开始工作,促进药物释放,增强药物的扩散能力及透皮能力。

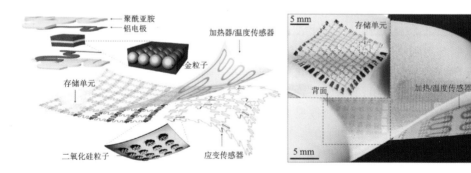

图10-9　集形变传感、信息存储和药物控释于一体的电子皮肤器件
Figure 10-9　A multifunctional e-skin device fabricated by integrating strain sensor, information storage unit, and controlled drug release unit

此外,还可将生理电信号传感器与药物控释模块进行集成,形成多功能的电子皮肤器件。当检测到生理电信号出现异常时,药物控释模块开始工作,实现透皮给药。还可在器件中集成离子电渗电极,通过离子电渗方法促进药物的穿透性,使药物能更高效地渗透到皮肤深层,从而达到更高的药物利用率和更好的治疗效果。

通过电子皮肤中的化学传感器来检测人体体液的化学组成,可对人体健康状况进行监测。

研究人员将化学传感器与药物控释器件相结合,可实现疾病的诊断与治疗一体化。如图10-10所示,将葡萄糖传感器、温度/湿度传感器、酸碱度传感器集成到一体,可通过检测汗液中的葡萄糖水平获得人体的血糖水平。进而,将加热模块和负载了二甲双胍药物的微针贴片与上述传感器件集成。其中的微针贴片用温度响应性材料制备,在低温时,微针保持完整状态,可避免其中的药物变性;在高温时,微针快速溶解在体液中,释放其中的药物。此外,微针还可穿透真皮层,提升药物的透皮吸收率。当葡萄糖传感器检测到人体血糖水平超过正常值时,加热模块对微针贴片进行加热,使二甲双胍从微针中释放,经皮肤吸收进入循环系统,从而达到控制血糖水平的目的。

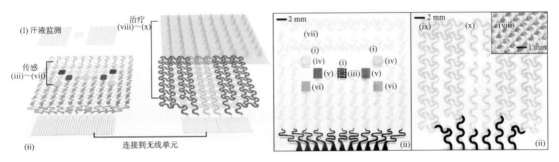

图 10-10　将葡萄糖传感器与药物控释微针贴片结合制备的诊疗一体化器件
Figure 10-10　An integrated diagnosis and treatment device prepared by combining a glucose sensor with a drug controlled release microneedle patch

经皮给药电子皮肤器件的出现解决了经皮给药中存在的穿透性差、效率低等难题,并且实现了患者健康状况的实时监测、药物释放的智能控制,极大地促进了经皮给药技术的发展(见扩展阅读4)。然而,该领域还存在一些困难与挑战,例如:经皮给药电子皮肤器件的稳定性和可靠性还需要进一步提高;目前通过经皮给药电子皮肤器件可检测和治疗的疾病还有限;一些大分子药物(如多肽、核酸、蛋白质等),还难以通过电子皮肤器件实现经皮给药。上述问题的解决有赖于器件结构、材料、药物等方面的深入发展,使器件的各个模块之间形成协同效应,提升其传感精度及药物递送效率,进一步扩大经皮给药器件的应用范围,实现患者的个性化治疗。

六、电子皮肤能源器件

随着电子皮肤器件的发展,它将越来越多地被用于人体健康的长期监测。大部分器件在工作的过程中需要消耗能量,以实现生理信号的识别与记录、物理与化学刺激的传感、药物的控制释放等功能。这就要求实现器件的不间断供能。为达到这一目的,研究人员将可拉伸的能源存储器件(如超级电容器、锂离子电池等)或能源转换器件(如太阳能电池、纳米发电机等)集成到电子皮肤中,进一步拓展了电子皮肤器件的应用范围。

超级电容器是一种通过电极与电解质之间形成的界面双层来存储能量的新型元器件,具有充放电速度快、功率密度高、工作寿命长等优势,受到人们的广泛关注。通常,超级电容器由三个部分组成:电极、电解质及阻隔层,其中材料结构与材料的电化学性质显著影响超级电容器的性能。目前,已有多种具有可拉伸性的材料被用于制备超级电容器,如碳纳米管、碳纤维、石墨烯、金属纳米线等。根据应用需求,可将超级电容器设计为一维、二维、三维结构。例如

Peng 等人设计制备了一维纤维状的超级电容器,他们首先将一层碳纳米管组装到弹性纤维表面,然后组装一层凝胶电解质;最后在最外层覆盖一层碳纳米管,由此形成同轴纤维状超级电容器,可用于编织智能织物及电子皮肤器件。Wei 等人利用碳纳米管薄膜作为电极,电纺丝聚氨酯纤维膜作为阻隔层,以 PDMS 作为弹性基底,构建了二维超级电容器。该器件在反复拉伸和充、放电过程中表现出非常好的稳定性,可用在电子皮肤器件中,即使人体在长时间运动中,也可稳定地为其他传感器件提供能源。Niu 等人在 2016 年报道了一例基于聚苯胺、碳纳米管和海绵电极的三维固态超级电容器。他们通过重复蘸涂-干燥的方法将碳纳米管负载到电极的海绵式骨架上,然后在其表面聚合苯胺,获得了具有可逆压缩-回复性能的超级电容器。当其形变量超过 60% 时,该器件仍能保持几乎不变的电容量。

除了超级电容器外,还可将柔性电池直接集成到电子皮肤器件中,为其提供能源。相对于超级电容器,电池具有更高的能量,更加适合于需要长期工作的电子皮肤器件。锂离子电池由于具有轻便、能量高等优势,已得到非常广泛的应用。为了满足电子皮肤应用的需求,柔性锂离子电池获得了快速发展。目前,研究热点集中在将电解质材料(如 $LiCoO_2$,$LiMn_2O_4$,$Li_4Ti_5O_{12}$ 等)和电极材料进行柔性化设计。类似于超级电容器,可将锂离子电池设计为一维纤维状、二维片状以及三维多孔状等,并且在结构上采取褶皱、弯曲、蛇形等设计,使锂离子电池具有较好的可拉伸性。Huang 和 Rogers 团队报道了柔性锂离子电池的设计方法,该电池以柔性硅橡胶作为基底,在双向拉伸量达 300% 时,其电量密度仍能达到 $1.1\ mA \cdot h \cdot cm^{-2}$。更为重要的是,该柔性锂离子电池中还可集成柔性的无线充电系统,为电池的长期使用提供保障,从而为电子皮肤器件及其他可移植器件提供稳定的能源。

随着电池领域的快速发展,研究人员已开发出多种便携电池,例如锌-空气电池、铝-空气电池等。从理论上讲,这些金属-空气电池比锂离子电池具有更高的能量密度,更加适合为电子皮肤器件提供能源。例如,Peng 等人利用碳纳米管制备了弹簧状的阴极,构建了纤维状的柔性锌-空气电池。该电池在高电流密度下表现出优异的充、放电性能,非常适合为小型设备供能。该纤维状的电池可用于纺织成织物,用于电子皮肤、智能手表等。

此外,太阳能电池的快速发展为电子皮肤器件的供能也提供了更多的选择。然而,太阳能电池在电子皮肤方面的应用也受到一些限制,例如当电子皮肤应用到人体时,光源的可获得性和光源的强度受到限制。此外,太阳能电池材料主要是刚性材料,可用于柔性太阳能电池的材料还较少。目前,基于有机光伏材料,研究人员已开发出多种柔性太阳能电池。例如,利用聚噻吩类材料与富勒烯衍生物进行复合,可获得柔性非常好的太阳能电池。该类电池可与皮肤保持紧密贴合,重复充、放电 1000 次后仍能保持稳定的能源供给。类似于金属-空气电池,太阳能电池也可设计为一维纤维状,由此获得更好的拉伸性,并且可通过纺织来制备多种形式的织物,大大促进了电子皮肤、可穿戴器件的发展。

近年来,研究人员发展了多种纳米发电机,从人体运动(如心跳、血流、行走、呼吸、肌肉伸缩等)中获取机械能并将其转变为电能,从而为可穿戴器件提供能源。目前,柔性纳米发电器件主要有两种:纳米压电器件和纳米摩擦电器件。

对于压电器件,其中的压电材料在外力作用下发生形变时,内部会产生极化现象,同时在它的两个相对表面出现正负相反的电荷。基于该原理,Baik 等人在柔性 PDMS 基底上集成了压电单元(图 10-11(a)),制备了柔性压电器件。他们首先将聚苯乙烯小球沉积在二氧化硅基底上作为模板,然后将压电材料(如氧化锌、锆钛酸铅等)沉积到小球表面,在灼烧除去聚苯乙烯小球模板后,得到空心半球状的压电材料阵列;然后将其包埋进 PDMS 基底中,形成可拉伸的压电薄膜。该器件的输出电压可达到 4 V,电流密度达到 $0.13\ \mu A \cdot cm^{-2}$。通过多层压电材料的堆叠还可进一步提高输出电压和电流密度。

摩擦电器件基于摩擦起电和静电感应现象的耦合,两种材料之间发生摩擦时产生电荷,通过外力使电荷分离,由此形成电势差,经由外部电路即可形成电流。例如 Bao 和 Kim 团队利用 PDMS 和单壁碳纳米管制备了摩擦电器件,如图 10-11(b)所示,该器件由多层结构组成,可在多种力学刺激(如压力、拉伸、弯曲、振动等)下产生电能。此外,该器件还可同时输出电阻和电容变化信号,实现对上述力学刺激的传感。这种同时具有供能和传感性能的器件可用于自供能电子皮肤器件,可长期监测人体温度、生理电信号、血压等生理指标的变化,在人体健康监测设备方面具有重要的应用价值。

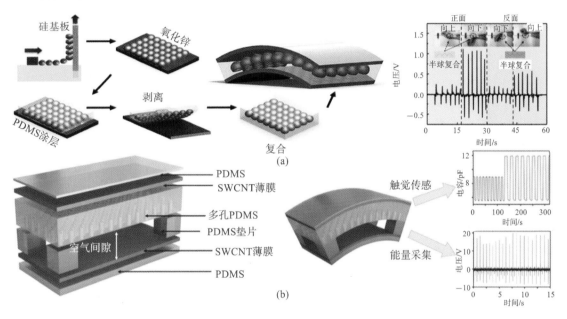

图 10-11 压电和摩擦电器件

(a)基于空心半球状的压电材料阵列的柔性压电器件,可将手腕的弯曲运动转变为电能;(b)基于单壁碳纳米管的柔性摩擦电器件,可在弯曲时产生电能

Figure 10-11 Piezoelectric device and triboelectric device

(a)A flexible piezoelectric device based on a hollow hemispherical piezoelectric material array can convert the bending motion of the wrist into electrical energy;(b)A flexible triboelectric device based on single-walled carbon nanotubes can generate electricity when it is bent

第四节 挑战与展望

本章主要介绍了电子皮肤的发展近况,包括电子皮肤器件的材料选择、结构设计与优化、种类与应用等。电子皮肤不仅可模拟人体皮肤的基本功能,实现压力、应变、摩擦等力学刺激的传感,还可用于化学、电学等方面的传感。通过多功能集成,电子皮肤可实现对人体健康的监测、疾病的诊断等功能,还可应用于假体皮肤、机器人等领域(见扩展阅读 5)。

尽管近年来电子皮肤器件领域取得了很大进展,但该领域还存在一些难题与挑战。例如在材料方面,电子皮肤器件中的导体、半导体、介电材料、基底材料等具有良好的可拉伸性、生物相容性、自愈合性等性能。然而,材料之间的界面还存在接触电阻大、容易脱落等问题,需要在材料界面的性质方面进一步优化,提升器件性能。在传感性能方面,电子皮肤器件存在测量稳定性及传感滞后现象,这严重影响了器件质量的稳定性和测量的灵敏度。因此,需要从材料性质和器件结构设计方面进一步改进。另外,目前大面积皮肤器件的制备工艺和多功能集成工艺还不成熟,存在器件阻抗大、信噪比低等缺点,需要进一步在器件设计制备工艺方面深入发展。此外,电子皮肤器件的监测数据存储、无线信号传输、稳定自供能等方面的发展还处于初级阶段,还难以实现信号分析、存储、传输等过程的稳定,需要在材料、器件结构、多器件集成等方面系统考虑,以实现智能电子皮肤的应用。

思 考 题

　　1. 请查阅文献,说出目前已开发出的模拟皮肤功能的柔性电子器件。它们的工作原理是什么?

　　2. 人体皮肤对多种刺激信号具有非常灵敏的感知能力,而电子皮肤在检测复杂信号时,灵敏度和准确性大大下降。为解决这一问题,你认为应该如何选择器件材料和设计器件结构?

　　3. 为更好地模拟皮肤功能,需要实现皮肤对痛觉、痒觉等刺激的传感。通过查阅资料,你认为如何设计电子皮肤器件才能满足上述要求?

　　4. 电子皮肤在反复运动过程中容易造成器件的损伤和失效。人体皮肤的损伤可通过自修复功能进行修复,而电子皮肤器件如何才能实现自修复功能?

　　5. 人体皮肤受伤后可逐渐恢复,但也可能留下瘢痕。通过查阅文献,你认为应该如何通过器件结构设计及功能集成,利用电子皮肤辅助修复伤口及淡化瘢痕?

扩 展 阅 读

[1]　Benight S J,Wang C,Tok J B H,et al. Stretchable and self-healing polymers and devices for electronic skin[J]. Prog Polym Sci,2013,38(12):1961-1977.

[2]　Hammock M L,Chortos A,Tee B C,et al. The evolution of electronic skin (e-skin):a brief history,design considerations,and recent progress[J]. Adv Materi,2013,25(42):5997-6038.

[3]　Yang J C,Mun J,Kwon S Y,et al. Electronic skin:recent progress and future prospects for skin-attachable devices for health monitoring,robotics,and prosthetics[J]. Adv Mater,2019,31(48):e1904765.

[4]　Lee H,Song C,Baik S,et al. Device-assisted transdermal drug delivery[J]. Adv Drug Deliv Rev,2018,127:35-45.

[5]　Bauer S,Bauer-Gogonea S,Graz I,et al. 25th anniversary article:a soft future:from robots and sensor skin to energy harvesters[J]. Adv Mater,2014,26(1):149-161.

参 考 文 献

[1]　Boutry C M,Negre M,Jorda M,et al. A hierarchically patterned,bioinspired e-skin able

to detect the direction of applied pressure for robotics[J]. Sci Robot,2018,3(24):
eaau6914.

[2] Mao H Y,Laurent S,Chen W,et al. Graphene:promises,facts,opportunities,and
challenges in nanomedicine[J]. Chem Rev,2013,113(5):3407-3424.

[3] Takei K,Takahashi T,Ho J C,et al. Nanowire active-matrix circuitry for low-voltage
macroscale artificial skin[J]. Nat Mater,2010,9(10):821-826.

[4] Arias A C,MacKenzie J D,McCulloch I,et al. Materials and applications for large area
electronics:solution-based approaches[J]. Chem Rev,2010,110(1):3-24.

[5] Graz I M,Cotton D P,Lacour S P. Extended cyclic uniaxial loading of stretchable gold
thin-films on elastomeric substrates[J]. App Phys Lett,2009,94(7):071902.

[6] Lee P,Lee J,Lee H,et al. Highly stretchable and highly conductive metal electrode by
very long metal nanowire percolation network[J]. Adv Mater,2012,24(25):3326-3332.

[7] Gonzalez M,Axisa F,Bulcke M V,et al. Design of metal interconnects for stretchable
electronic circuits[J]. Microelectron Reliab,2008,48(6):825-832.

[8] Lipomi D J,Tee B C K,Vosgueritchian M,et al. Stretchable organic solar cells[J]. Adv
Mater,2011,23(15):1771-1775.

[9] Choi W M, Song J, Khang D Y, et al. Biaxially stretchable "wavy" silicon
nanomembranes[J]. Nano Lett,2007,7(6):1655-1663.

[10] Ha M, Lim S, Ko H. Wearable and flexible sensors for user-interactive health-
monitoring devices[J]. J Mater Chem B,2018,6(24):4043-4064.

[11] Yang J C, Mun J, Kwon S Y, et al. Electronic skin:recent progress and future
prospects for skin-attachable devices for health monitoring,robotics,and prosthetics
[J]. Adv Mater,2019,31(48):e1904765.

[12] Yamada T,Hayamizu Y,Yamamoto Y,et al. A stretchable carbon nanotube strain
sensor for human-motion detection[J]. Nat Nanotechnol,2011,6(5):296-301.

[13] Mannsfeld S C B,Tee B C K,Stoltenberg R M,et al. Highly sensitive flexible pressure
sensors with microstructured rubber dielectric layers[J]. Nat Mater,2010,9(10):
859-864.

[14] Lipomi D J,Vosgueritchian M,Tee B C K,et al. Skin-like pressure and strain sensors
based on transparent elastic films of carbon nanotubes[J]. Nat Nanotechnol,2011,6
(12):788-792.

[15] Pang Y,Zhang K,Yang Z,et al. Epidermis microstructure inspired graphene pressure
sensor with random distributed spinosum for high sensitivity and large linearity[J].
ACS Nano,2018,12(3):2346-2354.

[16] Bae G Y,Pak S W,Kim D,et al. Linearly and highly pressure-sensitive electronic skin
based on a bioinspired hierarchical structural array[J]. Adv Mater,2016,28(26):5300-
5306.

[17] Park J,Kim M,Lee Y,et al. Fingertip skin-inspired microstructured ferroelectric skins
discriminate static/dynamic pressure and temperature stimuli[J]. Sci Adv,2015,1(9):

e1500661.

[18] Charalambides A, Bergbreiter S. Rapid manufacturing of mechanoreceptive skins for slip detection in robotic grasping[J]. Adv Mater Technol, 2017, 2(1): 1600188.

[19] Viry L, Levi A, Totaro M, et al. Flexible three-axial force sensor for soft and highly sensitive artificial touch[J]. Adv Mater, 2014, 26(17): 2659-2664.

[20] Han S, Kim M K, Wang B, et al. Mechanically reinforced skin-electronics with networked nanocomposite elastomer[J]. Adv Mater, 2016, 28(46): 10257-10265.

[21] Bae G Y, Han J T, Lee G, et al. Pressure/temperature sensing bimodal electronic skin with stimulus discriminability and linear sensitivity [J]. Adv Mater, 2018, 30 (43): e1803388.

[22] Zhang F, Zang Y, Huang D, et al. Flexible and self-powered temperature-pressure dual-parameter sensors using microstructure-frame-supported organic thermoelectric materials[J]. Nat Commun, 2015, 6: 8356.

[23] Kim D H, Lu N S, Ma R, et al. Epidermal electronics[J]. Science, 2011, 333(6044): 838-843.

[24] Koo J H, Jeong S, Shim H J, et al. Wearable electrocardiogram monitor using carbon nanotube electronics and color-tunable organic light-emitting diodes[J]. ACS Nano, 2017, 11(10): 10032-10041.

[25] Kim T, Park J, Sohn J, et al. Bioinspired, highly stretchable, and conductive dry adhesives based on 1D-2D hybrid carbon nanocomposites for all-in-one ECG electrodes [J]. ACS Nano, 2016, 10(4): 4770-4778.

[26] Huang X, Yeo W H, Liu Y, et al. Epidermal differential impedance sensor for conformal skin hydration monitoring[J]. Biointerphases, 2012, 7(1-4): 52.

[27] Parlak O, Keene S T, Marais A, et al. Molecularly selective nanoporous membrane-based wearable organic electrochemical device for noninvasive cortisol sensing[J]. Sci Adv, 2018, 4(7): eaar2904.

[28] Gao W, Emaminejad S, Nyein H Y Y, et al. Fully integrated wearable sensor arrays for multiplexed *in situ* perspiration analysis[J]. Nature, 2016, 529(7587): 509-514.

[29] Imani S, Bandodkar A J, Mohan A V, et al. A wearable chemical-electrophysiological hybrid biosensing system for real-time health and fitness monitoring [J]. Nat Commun, 2016, 7: 11650.

[30] Emaminejad S, Gao W, Wu E, et al. Autonomous sweat extraction and analysis applied to cystic fibrosis and glucose monitoring using a fully integrated wearable platform [J]. Proc Natl Acad Sci U S A, 2017, 114(18): 4625-4630.

[31] Nakata S, Shiomi M, Fujita Y, et al. A wearable pH sensor with high sensitivity based on a flexible charge-coupled device[J]. Nat Electron, 2018, 1: 596-603.

[32] Lee H, Song C, Hong Y S, et al. Wearable/disposable sweat-based glucose monitoring device with multistage transdermal drug delivery module [J]. Sci Adv, 2017, 3 (3): e1601314.

[33] Lee H，Choi T K，Lee Y B，et al. A graphene-based electrochemical device with thermoresponsive microneedles for diabetes monitoring and therapy［J］. Nat Nanotechnol，2016，11(6)：566-572.

[34] Chen Y，Lu S，Zhang S，et al. Skin-like biosensor system via electrochemical channels for noninvasive blood glucose monitoring［J］. Sci Adv，2017，3(12)：e1701629.

[35] Lee H，Song C，Baik S，et al. Device-assisted transdermal drug delivery［J］. Adv Drug Deliv Rev，2018，127：35-45.

[36] Son D，Lee J，Qiao S，et al. Multifunctional wearable devices for diagnosis and therapy of movement disorders［J］. Nat Nanotechnol，2014，9(5)：397-404.

[37] Yang Z，Deng J，Chen X，et al. A highly stretchable，fiber-shaped supercapacitor［J］. Angew Chem Int Ed Engl，2013，52(50)：13453-13457.

[38] Li X，Gu T，Wei B. Dynamic and galvanic stability of stretchable supercapacitors［J］. Nano Lett，2012，12(12)：6366-6371.

[39] Niu Z，Zhou W，Chen X，et al. Highly compressible and all-solid-state supercapacitors based on nanostructured composite sponge［J］. Adv Mater，2015，27(39)：6002-6008.

[40] Xu S，Zhang Y，Cho J，et al. Stretchable batteries with self-similar serpentine interconnects and integrated wireless recharging systems［J］. Nat Commun，2013，4：1543.

[41] Xu Y，Zhang Y，Guo Z，et al. Flexible，stretchable，and rechargeable fiber-shaped zinc-air battery based on cross-stacked carbon nanotube sheets［J］. Angew Chem Int Ed Engl，2015，54(51)：15390-15394.

[42] Chun J，Kang N R，Kim J Y，et al. Highly anisotropic power generation in piezoelectric hemispheres composed stretchable composite film for self-powered motion sensor［J］. Nano Energy，2015，11：1-10.

[43] Park S，Kim H，Vosgueritchian M，et al. Stretchable energy-harvesting tactile electronic skin capable of differentiating multiple mechanical stimuli modes［J］. Adv Mater，2014，26(43)：7324-7332.

（许江平）

Chapter 10
Wearable Electronic Skin Devices

10.1   Overview of Electronic Skin

Skin is the largest organ in human body and a physical barrier between human body and the environment. Skin is also the most important organ for sensing, with very excellent properties, including self-healing ability, tactile sensing capability (e. g. , temperature, pain and pressure), and others. The skin involves a variety of specific sensory receptors, which can convert physical contact into electric signals. Then, the electric signals are transmitted to the central nervous system and ultimately processed by the brain's somatosensory cortex.

When the skin is damaged in a large area, it is difficult for the skin to self-heal, resulting in the loss of physical barrier, the destruction of the sensory receptors in the skin, and even the loss of tactile sense. At present, dermatoplasty is the main method for treating large areas of skin damage. However, there are still problems, such as limited skin sources and high difficulty in skin function reconstruction. In addition, due to the rapid development of robots and artificial intelligence, people expect to give robots more functions, such as skin sensing performance similar to humans. Robots with skin sensing capabilities have important applications in patient care, disease diagnosis and monitoring, and can achieve more complex interactive tasks. The above-mentioned demands have promoted the rapid development of electronic skin (e-skin).

The so-called e-skin, also known as smart skin, refers to an artificial skin device that simulates the functions of the real human skin (Figure 10-1). The e-skin devices can not only have the sensory function of the skin, but also can integrate more functions that the real skin doesn't have. For example, chemical or biological sensors can be integrated into the e-skin to detect gas and liquid substances in the environment and the human body, so as to monitor environmental changes or changes in the physiological state of the human body. E-skin is expected to be transplanted to the human body as a prosthesis to replace missing or diseased skin. In addition, e-skin has very broad application prospects in soft robots. It is expected to give robots more functions to complete interactive tasks through simulating the sensing function of skin.

The development of e-skin devices has gone through a process from single functional devices to multifunctional integrated devices. According to different demands and application scenarios, people can design the structures and functions of the e-skin devices. This chapter will introduce the design principles, types and applications of e-skin devices.

10.2 Design Principles of E-Skin Devices

The e-skin device is a simulation of the real skin of the human body. It must not only have mechanical properties similar to skin, but also have the functions of skin. Therefore, the e-skin device must meet three requirements: ① It has mechanical properties similar to real skin, such as low modulus, high stretchability, and high flexibility; ② It can realize the functions of real skin, such as sensing of pressure, strain, shear and temperature; ③ It can integrate functions that real skin does not have, such as the sensing of physiological electric signals and chemical substances, to realize the monitoring of human health. To meet the above requirements, it is necessary to comprehensively consider materials and device structures for different functions and uses.

10.2.1 Materials

E-skin has similar mechanical properties to real skin. Therefore, materials for preparing e-skin should have excellent flexibility, stretchability, biocompatibility, and self-healing ability, to ensure its biological safety and service life. Material selection and preparation strategies play a key role in simulating the mechanical properties of real skin. In addition, in order to realize the sensing function of the e-skin, it is necessary to use materials with excellent electrical properties (including conductive and dielectric properties). This section will briefly introduce the selection of substrate materials, dielectric materials, and conductive materials for e-skin.

10.2.1.1 Substrate materials

The most widely used substrate material is polymer materials (see extended reading 1), such as polydimethylsiloxane (PDMS, usually called silica gel). This material not only has very good flexibility, stretchability and biocompatibility, but also has excellent chemical stability and high transparency. In addition, PDMS have strong surface adhesion after UV irradiation, enabling it to fit well with the skin and strongly bind to the electrodes in the device, which prevents the device from falling off from the skin. In addition, polyurethane, which has very good elasticity, can also be used as a substrate material to prepare stretchable printed circuits. Therefore, polyurethane also has important applications in e-skin. Other materials, such as traditional electrospun fiber membranes and textiles, can also be used as the substrate material of e-skin, but their stretchability and transparency are poor. As a result, their applications are subject to certain restrictions.

10.2.1.2　Dielectric materials

In e-skin devices which are based on transistors and capacitors, polymer dielectric materials are used as insulating layers, which require higher dielectric constant and lower leakage current. The PDMS described above is a commonly used polymer dielectric material. In the development of dielectric polymers, it was discovered that through the design of chemical structures (for example, the modification of polar groups such as cyano groups and fluorine atoms on the polymer chain), the addition of high-permittivity nanoparticles (e.g., titanium dioxide, barium titanate) can increase the dielectric constant of polymer materials. While improving the dielectric properties, it is necessary to ensure the biocompatibility, flexibility and stretchability of the material. As the e-skin devices are usually in repeated stretching and bending, the durability and self-healing properties of dielectric materials are also important, which need to be paid attention during the device preparation.

10.2.1.3　Conductive materials

Conductive materials are the key materials in e-skin. At present, people have applied a variety of conductive materials to e-skin. As the carbon materials, such as carbon nanotubes and graphene have excellent electrical and mechanical properties and high chemical stability, they are widely used in the preparation of e-skin. In recent years, semiconductor nanowires (e.g., silicon, gallium arsenide, and cadmium selenide nanowires) and metal nanowires (e.g., gold, silver, and copper nanowires) have also been used in the preparation of e-skin. However, because the preparation methods of nanowires are usually more complicated and costly, their applications are subject to certain restrictions. In recent years, organic polymer conductor materials have been applied to the preparation of e-skin. Common materials include poly-3-hexylthiophene, polyaniline, polypyrrole, poly(3,4-ethylenedioxythiophene)/polystyrene sulfonic acid (PEDOT:PSS), etc. Organic semiconductor materials generally have good processing properties, and their mechanical properties are closer to those of human skin. Therefore, compared with materials such as carbon nanotubes, graphene, and metal nanowires, organic semiconductor materials are more suitable for preparing large-area flexible e-skin devices.

10.2.2　Realization of device stretchability

Human skin has excellent stretchability. Therefore, e-skin needs to have stretchability similar to that of human skin in order to maintain a good fit with the skin during use. In order to achieve excellent stretchability, on the one hand, it is necessary to develop materials with excellent elasticity. On the other hand, it is necessary to design the alignment structure of the materials in the devices. The previous section mainly introduced the selection of flexible and stretchable materials, mainly focused on the inherent stretchability of the materials. This section will focus on the integrated structure of the materials in the devices, and introduce methods for enhancing the stretchability of the devices.

Traditional inorganic semiconductor/conductor materials usually have high modulus, high brittleness, and poor stretchability. They are subject to many restrictions in the application of flexible devices. In order to solve these problems, researchers have developed a series of methods for preparing materials with excellent stretchability by designing the geometric configuration of the materials.

The first method is to create cracks in the continuous film by stretching. Firstly, a rigid continuous conductor/semiconductor film is placed on an elastic substrate, and then the substrate is unidirectionally or bidirectionally stretched. As the film is brittle, it breaks to form cracks when the substrate is stretched. As the degree of stretching increases, the cracks become wider and the number of cracks increases. Consequently, the material obtains good stretchability. By controlling the degree of stretching, the film can be cracked while maintaining a conductive path (Figure 10-2(a)). For example, Graz et al. used this strategy to integrate a gold film on an elastic substrate, which can still maintain good conductivity when the strain reaches 100%.

The second method is to spread the one-dimensional fibrous material on the substrate. Due to the random orientation of the one-dimensional material, a conductive network path can be formed on the substrate. When the substrate is stretched, the material can still maintain direct contact with the substrate, and the conductive network can deform. Even when the deformation is large, the conductive network will not be destroyed (Figure 10-2(b)). For example, Lee and Ko's team used silver nanowire as conductive material to make electrode material with high stretchability and high conductivity. The strain of the electrode could reach 460%, and the resistance was still low when stretched.

The third method is to use micro-fabrication technique to pattern the conductive materials (Figure 10-2(c)) into a curved or spiral structure, and then put the conductive materials on an elastic substrate. The conductive materials with a spiral structure can undergo very large deformation with the stretching of the substrate, thereby giving the composite materials good stretchability. Gonzalez et al. studied the effect of various patterned structures of conductive materials on the stretchability of the device. They found that when the conductive materials were placed in the substrate in a serpentine structure or a horseshoe shape, the stretchability of the materials was the best, which could still maintain good conductivity when the strain reaches 100%. The stretchability could be further improved by stacking multiple serpentine structures.

The fourth method is to composite a high modulus conductive material with a pre-stretched elastic substrate. When the substrate shrinks, wrinkles on the conductive material appear. Unidirectional pre-stretching can produce linear folds (Figure 10-2(d)), and bidirectional stretching can produce herringbone folds (Figure 10-2(e)). In addition, it is also possible to construct a wrinkle structure on the surface of the elastic substrate in advance by a micro-fabrication method, and then put the conductive material on the surface of wrinkle. The pleated structure prepared by this method also has good deformability. This strategy is applicable to a variety of materials, including inorganic semiconductors, metals, composite materials, graphene, carbon nanotubes, etc. Due to the existence of wrinkles, when the flexible device is stretched, the deformation of the conductive materials therein is mainly derived from the change of its geometric structure, and the material itself does not produce large deformation. The use of the wrinkle strategy can not only give the device good stretchability, but also avoid the repeated deformation of the material itself, which is beneficial for prolonging the service time of the device.

10.3　Types of E-Skin Devices and Their Applications

The function of skin is very complicated. Therefore, the corresponding e-skin devices should be multifunctional (see extended reading 2). First of all, the e-skin devices need to simulate the tactile sensing of the skin, so that patients with damaged skin or missing limbs can reconstruct the skin's tactile sensing to the external environment. It can also give the robot more precise tactile responsiveness, to complete more complicated human-computer interaction tasks. Secondly, as a wearable device, the e-skin devices can also be endowed with chemical sensing properties, including sensing the chemical components of body fluids and gases, so as to realize the function of human health monitoring. In addition, the e-skin devices can also be integrated with disease treatment functions. When a change in human health is monitored, the e-skin devices can responsively release its loaded specific drug to treat the disease. In addition, for wearable devices, its energy supply is also very important. Through the material and device structure design, the e-skin devices can be used for energy storage and energy supply. In addition, by integrating multiple functions, multifunctional e-skin devices can be prepared, thereby realizing the intelligence of the e-skin, which can be used to monitor blood pressure, respiratory rate, body movement, body temperature changes, etc. In this section, the e-skin devices with different functions will be briefly introduced.

10.3.1　Mechanical sensor devices

Human skin can feel complex external mechanical stimuli, including pressure, stretching, shearing, bending, vibration, sliding, and others. For e-skin devices, it is particularly important to design the materials and device structures to realize the sensing of mechanical stimuli.

When the skin is in contact with the external environment, pressure and strain are generated. According to the difference in pressure and strain, the human body can judge the basic properties of the environment. The sensing of pressure and strain is important for the e-skin. In e-skin devices, the sensing of pressure and strain is mainly realized through the changes of the device's resistance, capacitance, and triboelectric effect responding to the external forces. Among them, the e-skin devices based on the principle of capacitance and resistance change are not only simple in structure design, but also able to detect dynamic and static stimulus signals. Therefore, they have received the most extensive and in-depth research.

The e-skin devices based on the resistance change can realize the sensing of pressure or strain through three ways: ① the change of the conductive percolation network in the polymer composite material; ② the change of the contact resistance between the conductive material and the electrode; ③ the conductivity changes in the resistance of the materials. This kind of e-skin device transforms the applied force into the change of the device resistance, which is a very simple and commonly used strategy.

For example, by arranging single-walled carbon nanotubes on an elastic substrate (e.g., PDMS) to form film, a strain sensor could be prepared. When the elastic substrate was stretched, the carbon nanotube film was broken. Therefore, gaps formed in the film, resulting in an increase in the resistance. The greater the degree of deformation, the greater the gap produced in the film and the greater the resistance. Therefore, strain sensing can be achieved by measuring resistance changes. The device could be integrated into the surface of clothing, band-aids, gloves, etc., to achieve the sensing of different human movements, such as breathing, speaking, walking, and gestures (Figure 10-3). This kind of e-skin device is expected to be widely used in health monitoring, virtual reality, robots and other fields. In addition, metal nanowires can also be used as conductive materials to construct stress sensors. The pressure causes a different degree of contact between the nanowire and the electrode, which further changes the resistance of the device. By fixing the voltage, the change of current with the stress is measured to realize the stress sensing.

E-skin devices based on changes in capacitance mainly realize pressure or strain sensing by changing the distance, area, and dielectric constant of the dielectric layer between the device electrodes. For example, by using a microstructured PDMS film as a dielectric layer, a pressure sensor based on capacitor can be prepared. As shown in Figure 10-4, the surface of the PDMS film in the device has an array of pyramid-shaped microstructure. When exposed to external pressure, the film can still maintain good elastic deformation ability, giving the PDMS film sensitive responsiveness. The external pressure causes the change of thickness of the dielectric layer, which further changes the capacitance of the capacitor and the output current of the field effect transistor, thereby realizing pressure sensing. In addition, single-walled carbon nanotubes are introduced into the PDMS substrate. After the substrate is stretched and relaxed, the nanotubes are bent, and the pressure and strain sensors based on parallel plate capacitors can be constructed (Figure 10-5). The device has very sensitive pressure sensing performance and fast response speed, and has spatial resolution for the sensing of pressure and strain, which further improves the applicability of the device in e-skin.

Sensitivity is an important performance parameter of pressure sensors. Sensitivity can be defined as the slope of the curve of electrical signals (such as capacitance, resistance, current, and voltage) with external pressure. Generally, the sensitivity of a pressure sensor is related to the modulus of compression of the material. At a given pressure, the greater the change in the electrical signal, the higher the sensitivity of the device. For the aforementioned pressure sensors based on changes in capacitance and piezoresistance, a variety of methods have been developed to improve the sensitivity of the device.

For the e-skin devices based on capacitor, the microstructure of the dielectric layer can improve the sensitivity. For example, the above-mentioned pyramid-shaped array is prepared on the surface of the PDMS. The pressure at the tip of the pyramid is very large, which causes a large deformation of the PDMS, leading to an increase in capacitance change. As a result, the sensitivity is significantly enhanced. The porous structure can also be used to increase the sensitivity of the pressure sensor. The holes can concentrate stress on the frame structure. When a small pressure is applied, the conductivity of the device changes significantly, and the sensitivity can be improved.

For piezoresistive devices, the contact resistance can be changed by changing the contact point or contact area between conductive materials, thereby improving the sensitivity of the device. For example, carbon materials (carbon nanotubes, graphene, etc.) can be integrated with cross-electrode arrays. Under the action of external force, the contact points or contact areas between the internal electrodes of the device and the conductive materials vary greatly. The sensitivity of the device is significantly improved, which can be used in the measurements of small pressures such as blood pressure and wrist pulse.

The increase in sensitivity usually results in a decrease in the measurable range of the device. The sensitivity of a sensor with high sensitivity will be decreased when the pressure increases. Thus, it is necessary to increase its sensing range while increasing the sensitivity. Cho et al. prepared a hemispherical array on the surface of the functional layer in the device, and prepared a piezoresistive pressure sensor with a sensitivity of 8.5 kPa^{-1} in the working range of 0-12 kPa. In addition, a capacitive pressure sensor can be prepared with electrodes with wrinkles on the surface, and the electrode area can be changed by pressure to achieve an increase in sensitivity and sensing range.

In addition to sensing stress and strain, human skin also has precise sensing capabilities for detecting the direction of force. For example, the skin can distinguish the direction of force, and it can also sense the sliding of objects on the surface of the skin. For e-skin devices, only by achieving their precise perception of different mechanical stimuli, can they be widely used in prostheses, robots, and others. From the perspective of devices, the sensing of sliding and force directions requires the devices to detect dynamic mechanical stimuli. Therefore, e-skin devices are mainly designed based on piezoelectric and triboelectric materials. Poly(vinylidene fluoride) is a typical piezoelectric material. Different protrusions can be prepared on its surface. The vibration caused by the sliding of different materials on the surface of these protrusions is used to detect the sliding state of the material on the surface of the device and the surface roughness of the material (Figure 10-6(a)). The nano-generator based on triboelectricity can also be used to detect the sliding state of the surface of the device. By inserting carbon nanotube/PDMS composite electrodes in the device, these electrodes can respond to the moving objects and detect the moving directions of the objects on the surface of the device.

Through the device structure design, a variety of electrical signals (e. g. , resistance, capacitance, current, and voltage) can be measured on the same device, so that the normal and tangential forces can be distinguished. The mechanical sensor shown in Figure 10-6(b) is composed of a top electrode and four bottom electrodes, which are separated by a dielectric material, forming four capacitors. By detecting the changes of the four capacitances, the normal and tangential forces can be distinguished. Bergbreiter et al. put three pieces of conductive material around one piece of conductive material and designed a mechanical sensing device. When forces in different directions act on the device, the relative distance and contact area between the middle area and the surrounding conductive materials change, triggering the changes in resistance and capacitance of the device. By analyzing the output signal, the device can identify the force size and direction. Devices that can simultaneously detect the magnitude and direction of the force can be integrated into the robotic arm, to detect the pressure and shear force on the robotic arm when grasping and moving objects.

10. 3. 2 Temperature sensor devices

Human skin can not only sense mechanical stimuli, but also perceive changes in the temperature of human body and the external environment. Abnormal changes in human body temperature usually mean changes in health. Therefore, designing a e-skin device with temperature sensing function has important application for detecting abnormal body temperature caused by heatstroke and infection.

At present, the commercial temperature sensors are mainly based on the thermal resistance effect of metal-based or ceramic-based semiconductor materials. These materials are difficult to be widely used in the field of flexible e-skin due to their rigidity. Therefore, it is necessary to design the structure of these materials to make them have better stretchability. For example, metal thermal resistance materials can be designed as a serpentine curved structure or a mesh structure, so that it has good stretchability and can be used in the design and preparation of flexible e-skins. In addition, non-metal thermal resistance materials, such as carbon nanotubes, graphene, and polymer semiconductor materials, can also be used as temperature sensing materials for e-skin. According to the changing trend of resistivity with temperature, the materials can be divided into two categories: the first type of thermal resistance material has an increase in resistivity with increasing temperature, and the second type of thermal resistance material has a decrease in resistivity with increasing temperature. Both types of material can be used in the design of temperature-sensing e-skin. For example, Wang et al. prepared a temperature sensor using a network structure formed by copper nanowires (the first type of thermal resistance material). The sensitivity of the device in the range of 25 ℃ to 48 ℃ is 0. 7 $\Omega \cdot ℃^{-1}$. Cho et al. used reduced graphene oxide (the second type of thermal resistance material) to prepare a temperature sensor. By adjusting the degree of reduction of graphene, temperature-sensing devices having higher sensitivity and a wider temperature detection range were obtained.

In addition to the thermal resistance effect, the thermoelectric effect and the pyroelectric effect can also be used to design temperature-sensing e-skins. Different from temperature sensors based on the thermal resistance effect, devices based on these two principles can work without power supply. The materials having thermoelectric effect can generate electric current under the temperature difference (Seebeck effect), and detect the temperature by detecting the current. For example, Zhu et al. used porous polyurethane and PEDOT:PSS to prepare a temperature sensor with detection accuracy of less than 0. 1 ℃. This device can be used to detect the temperature distribution of hand. The materials with pyroelectric effect will generate instantaneous voltage due to electrical polarization when the temperature changes. Therefore, the temperature can be detected by detecting the change in voltage. For example, Ko et al. prepared a temperature sensor using a composite material of reduced graphene oxide and poly(vinylidene fluoride), and obtained a higher sensitivity (changes 2. 93% per degree Celsius) and a wider temperature detection window (0-100 ℃).

10. 3. 3　Electrophysiological sensor devices

The activities of human organs, tissues, and nerves will produce electrophysiological signals. These electrophysiological activities are closely related to diseases such as arrhythmia, myocardial infarction, neuromuscular disease, and epileptic seizures. Therefore, through the monitoring of electrophysiological signals, human vital signs can be further obtained. For example, an electrocardiogram can record heart activity, an electromyography can show the activity state of muscle, and electroencephalogram can record the activity of brain.

Commonly used electrophysiological signal sensing equipment (e. g. , electrocardiograph, electroencephalogram meter) can accurately monitor the electrophysiological signals of the human body. However, due to their large size and poor portability, it is difficult for patients to long-term monitor changes of electrophysiological signals. To overcome these shortcomings, researchers have developed a flexible, ultra-thin, ultra-light, and biocompatible sensing devices for detecting epidermal electrophysiological signals. They integrated the snake-shaped metal wires into the elastomer material, and adjusted the composition of the material to match the mechanical properties of the skin, thereby preparing an e-skin with electrophysiological signal sensing function. The devices can not only record ECG and EMG, but also can be integrated with other sensors (e. g. , strain sensors, wireless charging units, and LED displays) to obtain a multifunctional e-skin device (Figure 10-7 (a)).

Since the electrophysiological signals need to be analyzed by the doctor, it is not convenient for the patients to use the devices. Therefore, researchers have developed an ECG monitoring device that can display different colors (Figure 10-7 (b)). They integrated transistor amplifiers and color-adjustable organic light-emitting diodes into the ECG monitoring device. When the device displays red, the ECG is normal; when the device displays blue, it indicates abnormal cardiac activity. The device provides a visualized monitoring of cardiac activity for patients with heart disease, and is more suitable for long-term real-time monitoring of cardiac activity for patients.

To obtain electrophysiological signals more accurately, the electrodes of the device need to be in close contact with the skin. The electrodes of the traditional electrocardiograph are in close contact by applying gel between the electrodes and the skin, while in flexible e-skin devices, the device materials can be designed to achieve close contact with the skin. For example, Jeon et al. prepared an e-skin device that can monitor an electrocardiogram by mimicking the structure of gecko foot. The electrode of the device can form a close fit with the skin through electrostatic attraction and physical contact. Even when the human body is moving normally, the electrode of the device will not detach from the skin, and it can still accurately measure the electrocardiogram (Figure 10-7(c)).

The stretchability of the device is also an important condition to ensure that it can maintain a close fit with the skin. Especially in irregular and frequently moving parts of the human body (e. g. , joints), the stretchability of the device allows the electrode to maintain a good fit with the skin during the repeated stretching and twisting process. Silver nanowires are generally used as stretchable electrode materials and have excellent electrical conductivity and processability. However, its biocompatibility is poor, and it is easy to oxidize and lead to poor conductivity. To solve this problem, silver-gold core-shell nanowires can be used to prepare electrodes with excellent stretchability, which have better biocompatibility and stronger oxidation resistance, and can maintain high electrical conductivity. The device exhibits excellent performance in monitoring electrophysiological signals, and can be applied not only to the surface of human skin, but also to the surface of animal heart.

Although e-skin devices have achieved rapid development in the field of electrophysiological signal sensing, they are still far from practical applications (see extended reading 3). At present, there are still some problems in this field. For example, the analysis of signals still depends on human, and there are still big challenges in integrating the processor into the e-skin. The chemical stability and biocompatibility of electrodes and elastomer materials in e-skin devices still need to be improved. The movement of human leads to poor adhesion stability between the device and the skin, which affects the accurate sensing and stability of electrophysiological signals. The solution of these problems depends on the optimization of the device structure and the improvement of material properties.

10. 3. 4　Chemical sensor devices

There are water, electrolytes, metabolites, hormones and other components in body fluid. The composition and content of these components can reflect the health of the human body. Therefore, by integrating chemical sensors in the e-skin to analyze the chemical components in body fluid, the health information can be detected at the molecular level, which plays an important role in the early diagnosis of diseases.

Chemical sensing e-skin devices can be divided into electrochemical sensors, chemical impedance sensors, and transistor sensors. When the device contacts the target compound, the potential, current, and resistance of the chemical sensor will change. By analyzing the signal change, the information about the target compound can be obtained. For example, in an electrochemical sensor, an ion-selective electrode can be designed and prepared. When it contacts the target ionic compound, measuring the potential changes can realize the identification of the chemical substance (potentiometry). The electrode can also be fixed with oxidoreductases, when the enzymes immobilized on the electrode and the catalytic target compounds undergo an oxidation-reduction reaction, measuring the current changes through the device can detect the target compounds (amperometric method). For chemical impedance sensors, the sensing element is usually placed between two electrodes. When the target compounds contact or react with the electrodes, its resistance changes, thus realizing chemical substance sensing. The transistor sensors are mainly composed of a semiconductor layer, a dielectric layer and three electrodes (e. g. , source, drain, and gate), which can be regarded as adding a dielectric layer and a gate electrode to the chemical impedance sensor. This kind of devices can realize the amplification of chemical sensing signals, further enhancing the sensitivity of the device.

In body fluid sensing, the monitoring and analysis of water content are very important, especially for e-skin devices, detecting the level of water content in the skin can be used to assist in the diagnosis of skin diseases, such as dermatitis, psoriasis, eczema, and itching. The skin water content can be obtained by measuring the impedance, thermal conductivity, and spectral properties of the skin. Compared with traditional methods, measuring skin water content through e-skin devices has more advantages. Figure 10-8(a) shows an e-skin device designed for measuring skin water content. The device consists of a sampling system and two electrodes. The sampling system provides alternating currents of different frequencies. The impedance of the skin changes with the water content, which causes the changes in amplitude and phase of the output current. By measuring the changes in amplitude and phase of the output current, the water content of the skin can be measured.

In practical applications, the electrolytes, metabolites, hormones and other components in human body fluid are relatively complex and have very low concentrations. Therefore, chemical sensors in e-skin need to have high selectivity to different components, as well as very low detection limits and high sensitivity. In addition, the chemical substances in body fluid reflect the health level of the human body. Therefore, the device needs to have high stability and good repeatability, thus the detection data obtained can be used for early diagnosis of diseases.

Recently, researchers have made significant progress in wearable chemical sensor devices that analyze the composition of sweat. This type of devices is mainly composed of electrochemical electrodes, and the components such as glucose, lactic acid, ethanol, pH, and electrolyte in sweat are analyzed by potentiometric method or amperometric method.

When preparing a sensor based on current measurement, people first immobilize glucose oxidase, lactate oxidase, alcohol oxidase, and other enzymes, on the electrode. These enzymes will selectively cause a redox reaction of the target chemicals. Since the current in the device has a linear relationship with the concentration of the analyte, the concentration of the target chemicals can be obtained by measuring the change in the current. For example, Mercier et al. used this method to prepare a wearable e-skin sensor. The redox reaction between lactate oxidase on the electrode and lactic acid in sweat can induce the change in current, which can be used to measure the concentration of lactic acid.

In sensors based on potential measurement, the potential of the ion-selective electrode depends on the concentration of the target. By measuring the change in potential, the charged substances in sweat can be measured, such as ammonium ions, potassium ions, and sodium ions. For example, Davis et al. developed a wearable device that can simultaneously extract sweat and then detect glucose, sodium ions, and chloride ions in the sweat. Takei et al. developed a charge-coupled device for the measurement of sweat pH, which further improved the sensitivity of the device.

E-skin chemical sensors can also be used to monitor the hormone components in sweat. However, due to the very low concentration of hormones in sweat, the sensitivities of the sensors should be very high. Salleo et al. developed a method for detecting cortisol in sweat based on organic electrochemical transistors (Figure 10-8(b)). The device contained a molecularly imprinted layer, which could selectively combine with cortisol molecules, thereby limiting the movement of ions in the device. Furthermore, by measuring the change in current in the transistor, the concentration of cortisol could be calculated. They used the device on the human arm to detect the cortisol content in sweat.

Although a chemical sensor with a single detection function can detect the chemical composition of human sweat, it is difficult for a single chemical sensor to accurately detect the health of the human body. To overcome this drawback, researchers integrated multiple sensors on the same platform to detect various chemical components in sweat, human body temperature, pulse and other data at the same time. Therefore, it is more accurate to judge the health of the human body through this way. For example, Javey et al. integrated multiple sensors into wearable devices that can be used to simultaneously detect glucose, lactic acid, sodium ions, potassium ions and other components in sweat (Figure 10-8(c)). More importantly, the detected information can be directly wirelessly transmitted to mobile devices or cloud servers to achieve real-time monitoring of human health. Kim et al. integrated temperature, humidity, glucose, and pH sensors into an e-skin device to detect human body temperature, glucose content in sweat, and sweat pH.

In tissue fluid extraction and detection, e-skin device also shows very strong potential. Recently, Wang et al. designed a glucose sensor that can non-invasively extract tissue fluid and detect the glucose concentration in it. In addition, the tissue fluid sensor can also be integrated with a sweat sensor to detect the glucose level in the tissue fluid and sweat at the same time, which can more accurately reflect the level of the human blood sugar.

10.3.5 Drug delivery skin device

Compared with traditional drug treatment, personalized treatment for different patients has more advantages. Personalized treatment requires of monitoring the patient's various physiological indicators during the treatment process and tracking the patient's recovery. With these information, doctors can adjust the treatment plan, such as the choice and dosage of drugs. Recently, researchers integrated electrophysiological signal sensors, chemical sensors, and drug controlled release devices into the flexible e-skin. Through the changes in electrophysiological signals and the chemical composition of body fluid, the device can feed back to the drug controlled release device, to control the release speed and the amount of the drug. The drug controlled release device can be integrated with a variety of devices according to the patient's treatment needs. At present, this method has become a new generation of transdermal drug delivery technology with very good application prospects.

For example, Kim et al. designed an e-skin device that integrated strain sensing, information storage, and controlled drug release (Figure 10-9). They used a silicon film to prepare a strain sensor that could detect movement disorders caused by Parkinson's disease. The collected information could be stored in the device. By analyzing the vital signs information of the human body, the information was sent to the drug controlled release module. When the drug controlled release module received the drug release signal, the heating component started to work to promote the release of the drug, and enhanced the diffusion and transdermal abilities of the drug.

In addition, the electrophysiological signal sensors can be integrated with the drug controlled release module to form a multifunctional e-skin device. When an abnormal electrophysiological signal is detected, the drug controlled release module starts to work to achieve transdermal drug delivery. Iontophoresis electrodes can also be integrated in the device to promote the penetration of drugs through iontophoresis, so that the drugs can penetrate deeper into the skin more efficiently, thereby achieving higher drug utilization and better therapeutic effects.

The e-skin can detect the chemical composition of human body fluid through chemical sensors to monitor the health of the human body. Researchers combine chemical sensors with drug controlled release devices to integrate the diagnosis and treatment of diseases. As shown in Figure 10-10, the glucose sensor, temperature sensor, humidity sensor, and pH sensor are integrated. Then the human blood sugar level can be obtained by detecting the glucose level in sweat. Furthermore, the heating module and the microneedle patch loaded with the metformin are integrated with the above-mentioned sensor device. The microneedle patch is made of temperature-responsive materials. At low temperatures, the microneedles remain intact, which can avoid the denaturation of the drugs in them; at high temperatures, the microneedles quickly dissolve in body fluid and release the drugs. In addition, the microneedles can penetrate the dermis to increase the transdermal absorption rate of the drugs. When the glucose sensor detects that the human blood glucose level exceeds the normal value, the heating module heats the microneedle patch, so that metformin is released from the microneedles and absorbed through the skin into the circulatory system, thereby achieving the control of blood glucose levels.

The emergence of transdermal drug delivery e-skin devices overcomes the problems of poor penetration and low efficiency in skin drug delivery, and realizes real-time monitoring of patient health status and intelligent control of drug release, which greatly promotes transdermal drug delivery technology (see extended reading 4). However, there are still some difficulties and challenges in this field. For example, the stability and reliability of transdermal drug delivery e-skin devices need to be further improved. At present, the diseases that can be detected and treated by transdermal drug delivery e-skin devices are still limited. Some macromolecular drugs (e. g. , peptides, nucleic acids, and proteins) are still difficult to achieve transdermal drug delivery through e-skin devices. The solution to the above problems depends on the in-depth development of device structures, materials, drugs, etc. , so that the various modules of the device can have a synergistic effect, improving its sensing accuracy and drug delivery efficiency.

10. 3. 6 Electronic skin for energy supply

With the development of e-skin devices, it will be increasingly used for long-term monitoring of human health. For most devices, they consume energy during work to realize functions such as identification and recording of physiological signals, sensing of physical and chemical stimuli, and controlled release of drugs. This requires the realization of uninterrupted energy supply of devices. To achieve this goal, researchers developed stretchable energy storage devices (e. g. , supercapacitors, lithium-ion batteries) or energy conversion devices (e. g. , solar cells, nanogenerators) which were integrated into the e-skin, further expanding the application range of e-skin devices.

Supercapacitor is a new type of component that stores energy through the double layer of the interface formed between the electrode and the electrolyte. It has the advantages of fast charging and discharging, high power density, and long working life, and has attracted widespread attention. Generally, a supercapacitor is composed of three parts: electrode, electrolyte and dielectric layer. The structure of the material and the electrochemical properties of the material significantly affect the performance of the supercapacitor. At present, a variety of stretchable materials have been used to prepare supercapacitors, including carbon nanotubes, carbon fibers, graphene, and metal nanowires. The supercapacitors can be designed in one-dimensional, two-dimensional, and three-dimensional structures. For example, Peng et al. designed and prepared one-dimensional fibrous supercapacitors. They first assembled a layer of carbon nanotubes on the surface of elastic fibers, and then assembled a layer of gel electrolyte, and finally covered a layer of carbon nanotubes on the outermost layer, to formed a coaxial fibrous supercapacitor which could be used for weaving smart fabrics and e-skin devices. Wei et al. constructed a two-dimensional supercapacitor using carbon nanotube film as electrodes, electrospun polyurethane fiber film as a dielectric layer, and PDMS as an elastic substrate. The device exhibits very good stability during repeated stretching and charging and discharging, and can be used in e-skin devices, for stably providing energy for other sensor devices. Niu et al. reported a case of three-dimensional solid-state supercapacitor based on polyaniline, carbon nanotubes and sponge electrodes in 2016. They loaded the carbon nanotubes on the sponge-like skeleton of the electrode through repeated dip-coating-drying methods, and then polymerized aniline on the surface to obtain a supercapacitor with reversible compression-recovery properties. When its strain exceeds 60%, the device can still maintain almost constant capacitance.

In addition to supercapacitors, flexible batteries can also be directly integrated into e-skin devices to provide energy for them. Compared with supercapacitors, batteries have higher energy and are more suitable for e-skin devices that require long-term work. Lithium-ion batteries have been widely used due to their advantages of portability and high energy. In order to meet the needs of e-skin applications, flexible lithium-ion batteries developed rapidly. At present, research focuses on the flexible design of electrolyte materials (e. g., $LiCoO_2$, $LiMn_2O_4$, $Li_4Ti_5O_{12}$) and electrode materials. Similar to supercapacitors, lithium-ion batteries can be designed in one-dimensional, two-dimensional, and three-dimensional structures. The team of Huang and Rogers reported the design method of a flexible lithium-ion battery. The battery uses flexible silicone rubber as a substrate. When the biaxial stretching reaches 300%, its power density can still reach $1.1\ mA \cdot h \cdot cm^{-2}$. More importantly, a flexible wireless charging system can also be integrated into the flexible lithium-ion battery, which can guarantee the long-term use of the battery, thereby providing stable energy for e-skin devices and other implantable devices.

With the rapid development of batteries, researchers have developed a variety of portable batteries, such as zinc-air batteries and aluminum-air batteries. In theory, these metal-air batteries have a higher energy density than lithium-ion batteries and are more suitable for providing energy for e-skin devices. For example, Peng et al. used carbon nanotubes to prepare a spring-like cathode and constructed a fibrous flexible zinc-air battery. The battery exhibits excellent charge and discharge performance under high current density, and is very suitable for powering small devices. The fibrous battery can be woven into fabrics, used in e-skin, smart watches, and others.

In addition, the rapid development of solar cells also provides more options for the energy supply of e-skin devices. However, the application of solar cells in e-skin is also subject to some restrictions. For example, when the e-skin is applied to the human body, the availability of light sources and the intensity of the light sources are limited. In addition, solar cell materials are mainly rigid materials, and there are a few materials that can be used for flexible solar cells. At present, using organic photovoltaic materials, researchers have developed a variety of flexible solar cells. For example, using polythiophene materials and fullerene derivatives can fabricate flexible solar cells. This type of batteries can maintain a close fit with the skin, and can still maintain a stable energy supply after repeated charging and discharging 1000 times. Similar to metal-air batteries, solar cells can also be designed in a one-dimensional fiber structure, thereby obtaining better stretchability, and various forms of fabrics can be fabricated by spinning, which greatly promotes the development of e-skin and wearable devices.

In recent years, researchers have developed a variety of nano-generators to convert mechanical energy obtained from human movements (such as heartbeat, blood flow, walking, breathing, and muscle contraction) into electrical energy for wearable devices. At present, there are two main types of flexible nano-generator devices: piezoelectric nano-generator and triboelectric nano-generator.

For piezoelectric devices, when the piezoelectric material is deformed, polarization will occur. At the same time, positive and negative charges will appear on the opposite surfaces. Baik et al. integrated a piezoelectric unit (Figure 10-11(a)) on a flexible PDMS substrate to prepare a flexible piezoelectric device. They first deposited polystyrene beads on a silica substrate as a template, and then deposited piezoelectric materials (e. g. , zinc oxide, lead zirconate titanate) on the surface of the beads, and then burned to remove the polystyrene beads template. Afterwards, a hollow hemispherical piezoelectric material array is obtained, which is then embedded in the PDMS substrate to form a stretchable piezoelectric film. The output voltage of the device can reach 4 V, and the current density can reach 0. 13 $\mu A \cdot$ cm^{-2}. The output voltage and current density can be further improved by stacking multiple layers of piezoelectric materials.

Triboelectric devices are based on the coupling of triboelectricity and electrostatic induction. When friction occurs between two materials, charges are generated, which are separated by external force, thereby forming a potential difference. For example, Bao and Kim's team used PDMS and single-walled carbon nanotubes to prepare a triboelectric device, as shown in Figure 10-11(b). The device can detect resistance and capacitance change signals at the same time, to realize the sensing of the above-mentioned mechanical stimuli. This device with both energy supply and sensing performance can be used for self-powered e-skin devices, which can be used in long-term monitoring of changes in human body temperature, physiological electrical signals, and blood pressure.

10.4　Challenges and Perspectives

This chapter mainly introduces the recent development of e-skin, including material selection, structural design and optimization, types and applications of e-skin devices, etc. E-skin can not only simulate the basic functions of human skin, and realize the sensing of mechanical stimuli such as pressure, strain, and friction, but also can be used for chemical and electrical sensing. Through multi-functional integration, the e-skin can realize functions such as human health monitoring and disease diagnosis, and can be applied to prosthetic skin, robots and other fields (see extended reading 5).

Although great progress has been made in the field of e-skin devices in recent years, there are still some problems and challenges in this field. For example, the conductors, semiconductors, dielectric materials, and base materials in e-skin devices have good stretchability, biocompatibility, and self-healing properties. However, the interface between the materials still has problems such as high contact resistance. It is necessary to further optimize the properties of the material interface to improve the performance of the device. In addition, the e-skin devices still have low measurement stability and high sensing hysteresis, which seriously affects the stability of the devices quality and measurement sensitivity. Therefore, further improvements are needed in terms of material properties and device structure design. Moreover, the current preparation process and multifunctional integration process of large-area skin devices are not yet mature. There are disadvantages such as large device impedance and low signal-to-noise ratio. Further development in device design and preparation processes is required. Also, the development of monitoring data storage, wireless signal transmission, and stable self-supply of e-skin devices is still in its infancy. It is difficult to achieve the stability of signal analysis, storage, transmission and other processes. Systematic consideration of device integration and other aspects may realize the application of smart e-skin.

Questions

1. Which kinds of flexible electronic devices have been developed to simulate the skin functions? How do they work?

2. Human skin has a very sensitive ability to perceive a variety of signals, while the sensitivity and accuracy of e-skin are greatly reduced when detecting complex signals. To solve this problem, how do you think the device materials and device structures should be selected?

3. To better simulate the skin functions, it is necessary to realize the skin's sensing of pain, itching and other stimuli. How do you think the e-skin device should be designed to meet the above requirements?

4. The e-skin devices will be damaged during repeated movement. While the human skin damage can be repaired through the self-healing ability, how can the self-healing function be realized in the e-skin devices?

5. The human skin has a self-healing ability, which can gradually recover after injury, but it may also leave scars. How do you think the e-skin can assist wounds repair and scars fade?

Extended Reading

[1] Benight S J, Wang C, Tok J B H, et al. Stretchable and self-healing polymers and devices for electronic skin[J]. Prog Polym Sci,2013,38(12):1961-1977.

[2] Hammock M L,Chortos A,Tee B C,et al. The evolution of electronic skin (e-skin):a brief history,design considerations,and recent progress[J]. Adv Materi,2013,25(42): 5997-6038.

[3] Yang J C,Mun J,Kwon S Y,et al. Electronic skin:recent progress and future prospects for skin-attachable devices for health monitoring, robotics, and prosthetics[J]. Adv Mater,2019,31(48):e1904765.

[4] Lee H,Song C,Baik S,et al. Device-assisted transdermal drug delivery[J]. Adv Drug Deliv Rev,2018,127:35-45.

[5] Bauer S,Bauer-Gogonea S,Graz I, et al. 25th anniversary article: a soft future: from robots and sensor skin to energy harvesters[J]. Adv Mater,2014,26(1):149-161.

(Xu Jiangping)

第十一章
生物医用高分子在皮肤伤口修复中的应用

第一节 皮肤伤口概述

一、伤口的产生和愈合

皮肤是人体最大的器官,它与周围环境直接接触,是人体的第一道屏障,具有防止体液丢失、调节体表温度等重要功能(相关内容见本教材第一章)。在某些情况(如外伤、手术等)下,正常皮肤的解剖结构与生理功能会遭到破坏而产生创伤,皮肤伤口按修复过程可以分为急性伤口和慢性伤口。急性伤口可来源于浅表擦伤至深部损伤,一般可在 3 周内愈合。而 2 个月未能愈合的急性伤口则发展为慢性伤口,如动、静脉溃疡或糖尿病伤口。皮肤伤口一般按照特定的顺序愈合,经过多个精细调控的过程。皮肤伤口愈合一般有完整的止血和炎症机制,而且内皮细胞、成纤维细胞等必须迁移到受伤区域并在损伤部位增殖。伤口愈合过程中会生成新的组织及结构。如图 11-1 所示,这些过程一般分为四大阶段,即止血期、炎症期、增生期和重构/成熟期(见扩展阅读 1、2)。

皮肤伤口的愈合过程开始于止血期。当血管破损时,血管收缩,血小板被激活并出现聚集,成为血小板凝块,起到初级止血作用。接着血小板又经过复杂的变化产生凝血酶,使邻近血浆中的纤维蛋白原变为纤维蛋白,相互交织的纤维蛋白使血小板凝块与血细胞缠结成血凝块。同时,血小板的突起伸入纤维蛋白网内。随着血小板微丝(肌动蛋白)和肌球蛋白的收缩,血凝块进一步收缩并变得更坚实,从而有效地发挥止血作用。另外,纤维蛋白溶解系统的激活会导致纤维蛋白降解。在这一过程中,肽类的释放则激发趋化性并增加毛细血管的通透性。由巨噬细胞和成纤维细胞以及角质形成细胞产生的细胞因子还可引发炎症反应,起到对损坏或坏死组织、微生物等的清除作用。随后是增生期肉芽组织形成、再上皮化以及结缔组织基质形成。肉芽组织由密集的巨噬细胞、成纤维细胞、毛细血管网、纤维连接蛋白、透明质酸及内皮细胞组成。在肉芽组织的形成过程中,巨噬细胞、成纤维细胞和内皮细胞相互依存。在重构/成熟期,组织强度更高的 Ⅰ 型胶原逐渐代替 Ⅲ 型胶原,皮肤变厚变韧。

缺氧是伤口愈合早期触发新生血管形成的重要因素。基底膜形成前伤口会持续渗液。同

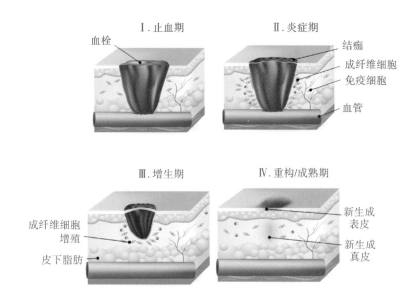

图 11-1　皮肤伤口愈合过程示意图
Figure 11-1　Schematic diagram of healing process of skin wounds

时,成纤维细胞从伤口边缘聚集,循环纤维细胞及间充质干细胞迁移到不成熟的结缔组织基质。再上皮化从伤口边缘开始。其中,上皮细胞失去半桥粒连接,通过纤维连接蛋白矩阵的迁移,再通过伤口,直至遇到相同的细胞。定向迁移和增殖需要一个有效、平衡以及酶支持的"剪切和粘贴"程序。经过这一过程,伤口边缘的上皮细胞直接接触,此为一级愈合。另外,迁移细胞连接一定时间后发生二级愈合。由于上皮的封闭延迟和肉芽组织的形成率较高,开放性伤口的愈合过程较慢。伤口愈合过程的最后阶段称为收缩阶段,开始于粒状组织内大量胶原的形成。在收缩阶段,伤口边缘之间的距离缩小直至紧密闭合伤口。这一过程的发生是由于成纤维细胞的分化以及祖细胞向肌成纤维细胞的分化,富含肌动蛋白骨架基质的肌成纤维细胞使基质收缩。伤口收缩后进入重塑过程,在此过程中基质的产生停止,成纤维细胞和肌成纤维细胞凋亡、退化。伤口愈合的最终结果可能是临床愈合后完全无瘢痕,也可能由于纤维化而留下明显瘢痕。

二、伤口敷料

伤口敷料是包扎伤口的材料,用以覆盖疮、伤口或其他暴露的损害。伤口敷料包括与伤口基底直接接触的初级敷料及覆盖在初级敷料之上起辅助作用的次级敷料。初级敷料根据创面的需要直接覆盖在创面上,起到治疗和保护创面的作用。次级敷料可以起到巩固初级敷料的作用,从而更加充分地满足伤口愈合的需要。

早期的伤口敷料产品包括纱布、胶布、天然或合成的绷带以及脱脂棉。纱布敷料由编织和非织造纤维棉、人造丝和涤纶制成。纱布敷料价格低廉,用于帮助很多伤口引流。但由于其干燥的性质,它们会黏附在伤口处,在移除过程中引起疼痛。纱布敷料可以为伤口提供一定的保护,但需经常更换以防止邻近健康组织浸渍其中,因此可能导致成本增加并造成重复性组织损伤。为此,在使用纱布作为敷料时,可将其浸渍到石蜡、碘或凡士林中以避免干燥并提供非黏附性的覆盖面。1971 年,Winter 博士首次提出了"湿性伤口愈合"的概念。他们研究发现,完整水疱的愈合速度比将水疱挑破后快两倍,并指出上皮细胞无法游移穿过干燥结痂的细胞层,因此需要花时间向痂皮下的湿润床游移,使得上皮细胞愈合的时间延长。而湿润环境则可以促进上皮细胞爬行,减少瘢痕形成。这一结论为现代湿性伤口愈合理论奠定了基础,同时也促进了新型湿性伤口愈合敷料的快速发展。相比于早期的传统敷料(如纱布、油纱等),新型敷料可以对伤口愈合产生积极作用,促进伤口止血和快速愈合。新型敷料主要包括水凝胶敷料、纤维敷料等,这些功能型敷料主要通过高分子材料加工制得。因此,以下部分将着重介绍高分子材料在新型伤口愈合敷料以及复合功能敷料方面的研究进展。

第二节　高分子水凝胶伤口敷料

一、水凝胶材料简介

大部分生物由柔软且含水的凝胶组成,它们能够感知外界环境的刺激并做出实时、快速的响应。在所有的人造材料中,水凝胶是与生物组织最相似的材料,它们通常是由亲水性高分子经轻度交联而形成的高分子网络,其网络间隙存在着可以在网络中流动的水分子;同时一些小分子也可以在高分子网络中移动,进行信息和物质的传递。水凝胶能够提供模拟细胞外基质的微环境,可以对细胞行为和组织功能进行调控。近年来,基于合成或天然高分子的水凝胶在生物医用领域得到了广泛关注。例如,由聚甲基丙烯酸羟乙酯制备的隐形眼镜,由重组蛋白或白蛋白形成的用于外科手术黏合的生物黏合剂,由藻酸盐多糖制备的伤口敷料,由透明质酸形成的用于填充修复的水凝胶等,这些材料均被广泛应用于临床。水凝胶具有良好的生物相容性、易成型加工、形状大小可控等特点,在三维组织工程基质、药物载体、生物复合材料等生物医学工程领域具有广泛的应用前景。

根据水凝胶的来源,其可以分为天然高分子水凝胶及合成型高分子水凝胶两类。天然高分子水凝胶主要由天然高分子材料形成,包括胶原、明胶、纤维蛋白、壳聚糖、海藻酸钠、透明质酸、硫酸软骨素、琼脂糖等。这类水凝胶的组成与结构类似于天然细胞外基质,具有良好的生物相容性、生物可降解性等;但是其力学性能普遍较低,难以满足承受组织修复的力学要求。合成型高分子水凝胶主要由合成高分子材料交联形成,如聚乙二醇、聚乙烯醇、聚甲基丙烯酸羟乙酯、聚丙烯酰胺、聚丙烯酸及其衍生物。合成型高分子水凝胶通常具有较高的力学性能,且结构和性能可控,重复性好,但由于缺乏生物学功能,其生物相容性相对较差,因此其应用也受到一定的限制。

根据水凝胶的交联方式,水凝胶可以分为物理交联型水凝胶和化学交联型水凝胶两类。物理交联型水凝胶由高分子链通过物理相互作用(如链缠绕)或超分子弱相互作用(如静电作用、氢键等)形成。形成物理交联型水凝胶的反应条件温和、无需化学交联剂。然而,该种水凝胶中的交联是非永久性的,因此当外界环境(如 pH、温度、离子浓度等)变化时,水凝胶可能会发生解离。化学交联型水凝胶通过自由基聚合反应、辐射、紫外线照射、化学引发与酶交联等方式使高分子链之间形成稳定的共价键来构建水凝胶网络。相比于物理交联型水凝胶,共价键交联使化学交联型水凝胶力学性能明显提高。然而,共价交联过程中残留的化学交联剂、有机溶剂、引发剂等可能会引起细胞毒性,因此化学交联型水凝胶的后处理显得尤为重要(见扩展阅读3）。

（一）仿生黏附水凝胶

受生物的启发或模仿生物的结构特征、作用方式或作用机制，设计合成的仿生水凝胶，在生物医用领域具有广阔的应用前景。其中，受天然贻贝、藤壶、管虫等海洋生物良好的水下附着力的启发，仿生黏附水凝胶近年来得到了越来越多的关注（见扩展阅读4）。仿生黏附水凝胶是指具有高黏附力和一定生物相容性的水凝胶，可替代传统的缝合手术伤口的闭合器械，并具有促进伤口愈合的功效。其黏附力来源于原位水凝胶形成的过程中，高分子中活性基团与生物组织中活性基团的相互作用或与被黏物表面间的多重超分子相互作用。例如，一些带有醛基的水凝胶可以与生物组织中的氨基共价结合，从而显示出对活组织的高黏附力。长春工业大学段莉洁教授等通过羧甲基壳聚糖的氨基和氧化右旋糖酐的醛基原位发生席夫碱反应，制备了原位可注射黏附水凝胶。在大鼠烧伤创面原位注入该水凝胶，发现该水凝胶可促进细胞黏附，并可促使上皮细胞迁移到伤口区域，从而促进皮肤再生。

贻贝分泌的足丝蛋白可在水中快速交联固化，具有较高的防水黏附能力，使其成为极具优势和潜力的生物黏合剂。贻贝的足丝蛋白中含有丰富的邻苯二酚结构，可通过多重相互作用与基底产生黏附，在湿态黏附中起到关键性作用。受贻贝超强的水下黏附能力的启发，研究者们开发出了多种多样的仿贻贝黏附水凝胶。华中科技大学张连斌等利用聚多巴胺（PDA）、还原性氧化石墨烯（rGO）、聚乙烯亚胺（PEI）、聚丙烯酰胺（PAM）制备了一种高黏附的水凝胶膜，可在太阳光的照射下加速伤口愈合。该水凝胶膜充分利用了聚多巴胺（PDA）的良好黏附性和还原性氧化石墨烯（rGO）的光热转换能力，在伤口上附着以后，该水凝胶膜将太阳能转化为热能，并局部加热伤口。局部温度的升高可抑制炎症反应，促进再上皮化、血管生成和胶原沉积，从而显著促进伤口愈合。天津大学刘文广教授等利用 PDA、聚乙二醇双丙烯酸酯（PEGDA700）和季戊四醇三丙烯酸酯（PETA）之间的 Michael 加成反应，合成了一种超支化聚合物 HB-PBAE。他们将 HB-PBAE、聚乙烯基咪唑（PVI）和明胶溶液混合，并加入 Fe^{3+} 得到了仿生黏附水凝胶。Fe^{3+} 可与邻苯二酚基团间形成配位键，从而稳定水凝胶。当需要更换敷料时，只需要在敷料上喷涂 Zn^{2+} 水溶液，水凝胶的黏附能力就会显著下降。同时，PVI 与 Zn^{2+} 形成了稳定的配位键，进一步增强了水凝胶的强度，从而能够方便、无损地更换敷料，并且在伤口处基本不会有明显的敷料残留，对伤口愈合有很好的促进作用（图11-2）。这种含金属离子的可逆黏附伤口敷料为新型伤口敷料的设计提供了一个新的思路。

（二）可注射水凝胶

可注射水凝胶是指注射前为流动的液体，通过注射器注入皮下组织或肌肉组织后，在注射部位可原位凝胶化的水凝胶。其形成机制是利用高分子材料对外界刺激的响应，使聚合物在生理条件下发生状态或构象的变化，完成由溶液向凝胶的转变。目前研究的可注射水凝胶主要包括普通水凝胶和智能刺激响应水凝胶（如温度响应性、pH 响应性、酶响应性水凝胶等）。可注射水凝胶能快速封闭任意形状的伤口，与伤口轮廓黏合形成物理屏障，还可维持皮肤的湿润环境，并且让伤口快速止血，同时预防伤口感染，因此在医用敷料方面具有重要的应用价值。

福建农林大学张敏等利用动态亚胺键设计开发了一种由胶原（COL）、壳聚糖（CS）和二苯甲醛修饰的 PEG2000 可注射水凝胶伤口敷料。COL/CS 水凝胶具有良好的热稳定性、可注射性、pH 敏感性和抗菌能力。COL/CS 水凝胶可以很好地黏附在组织表面，其作用于湿润的创面后，能促进伤口快速止血并有效地促进伤口愈合。上海大学尹静波教授等将多巴胺（DA）修

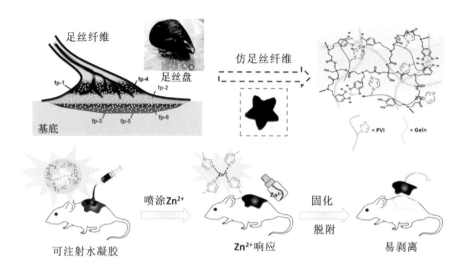

图 11-2　基于金属配位的仿生高黏附水凝胶及其促进伤口愈合的性能

Figure 11-2　Bioinspired adhesive hydrogels based on metal coordination for accelerating skin wound healing

饰到醛改性的海藻酸盐(ALG)骨架中以形成双功能化的海藻酸盐,通过酰肼改性聚(L-谷氨酸)和双功能化海藻酸盐的席夫碱反应,制备了可注射生物黏合水凝胶(PGA/ALG-CHO 水凝胶)。PGA/ALG-CHO 水凝胶可快速凝胶化,邻苯二酚基团与组织之间的氢键和 π-π 堆积等多种相互作用形成水凝胶的网络屏障,使其具有优越的止血性能。上海交通大学医学院附属瑞金医院、上海市伤骨科研究所的刘志宏等利用牛血清白蛋白(BSA)类细胞外基质的特性来模拟细胞外基质,通过巯基化的牛血清蛋白、KK 多肽和 Ag^+ 的协同交联,成功构建了具有促进血管生成和抗菌能力的可注射多肽蛋白水凝胶,用于促进感染伤口的愈合。在该蛋白水凝胶体系中,Ag^+ 作为交联剂不仅能提供抗菌性能,还能引入 $K_2(SL)_6K_2(KK)$ 多肽,使水凝胶具有促进血管生成的能力。体内动物实验结果表明,多肽蛋白水凝胶在伤口愈合早期具有可观的胶原沉积和血管形成能力,可使新生组织迅速再生,并出现新的毛囊(图 11-3)。

二、止血水凝胶敷料

皮肤创伤的一个直接结果是出血。过度失血是引起伤员死亡的主要原因。使用适当的止血器材进行急救处理,可以有效地减少伤亡。止血带是常用的止血器材,但其在除四肢外的人体其他部位的应用往往受限。因此,快速止血材料以及敷料一直是急救领域研究的热点。目前,常见的止血敷料主要包括橡胶敷料、泡沫敷料、静电纺丝纤维敷料、膜敷料、水凝胶敷料等。在这些敷料中,水凝胶因具有特定的网状交联结构,具有半通透性,可阻隔细菌侵入、防止创面感染、允许氧气和水通过等,在止血敷料临床应用中具有重要价值。

止血水凝胶敷料可通过在凝胶中引入止血因子(如止血多肽、止血药等)或赋予凝胶物理阻隔作用得到。维也纳科技大学 Paul Slezak 教授等利用点击化学的方法,将凝血酶受体激活肽 6(thrombin receptor agonist peptide-6,TRAP-6)接枝到聚乙烯醇(PVA)凝胶表面,得到止血多肽修饰的 PVA-TRAP-6 水凝胶。由于 TRAP-6 多肽具有激活血小板的重要功能,该止血水凝胶不仅表现出良好的生物相容性,而且能够显著缩短凝血时间,可作为止血敷料应用于组织与器官的创面出血(图 11-4)。浙江大学欧阳宏伟等模仿细胞外基质(ECM)的组成设计

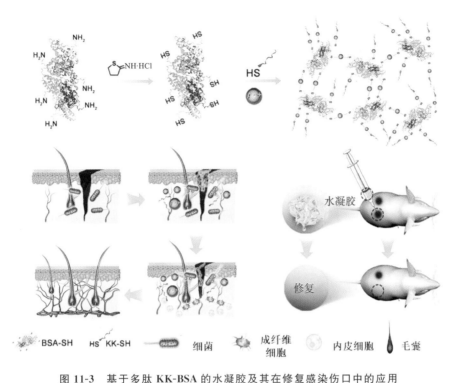

图 11-3　基于多肽 KK-BSA 的水凝胶及其在修复感染伤口中的应用

Figure 11-3　Hydrogels based on polypeptide KK-BSA for infected wound treatments

了一种光反应胶黏剂。这种生物大分子基质水凝胶可在紫外线照射后快速凝胶化和固定,黏附和封闭动脉以及心肌壁的出血点。该凝胶可以承受高达 290 mmHg 的血压,明显高于大多数临床环境下的血压。他们的研究结果表明,这种水凝胶可以阻止 4~5 mm 长的猪颈动脉切口和直径为 6 mm 的猪心脏穿透孔的高压出血。该类水凝胶具有良好的耐受性,并且作为创伤性伤口密封胶具有显著的临床优势。

此外,将具有止血功能的无机纳米颗粒(如二氧化硅、硅藻土等)引入水凝胶中也可得到能高效止血的水凝胶敷料。带电荷的硅酸盐能够有效地凝聚血液中的凝血因子,胶原蛋白的快速吸水功能则能够有效浓缩血液组分。将两者的优势有效结合,可获得具有多种功能的新型止血材料。基于这一设计理念,莱斯大学 Hartgerink 等以硅酸盐纳米片与胶原蛋白作为基质材料,将这两种材料按照适当的比例复合,通过交联得到了纳米复合型水凝胶。由于硅酸盐与胶原蛋白的协同作用,这种纳米复合型水凝胶具有高效富集凝血因子和快速浓缩血液成分的多种功效,能够起到快速止血的效果。

三、抗菌敷料

在水凝胶敷料的使用过程中,水凝胶敷料直接与组织表面接触,可以减少体液的流失。同时,该过程也需要防止伤口的二次感染。因此,水凝胶敷料应具有较好的抗菌性能,这样其在使用过程中才能抑制伤口表面细菌的生长。为了满足应用的需求,抗菌性水凝胶敷料应运而生。根据抗菌剂引入方式的不同,抗菌性水凝胶可分为负载抗菌剂水凝胶和本征型抗菌水凝胶。

负载抗菌剂水凝胶直接将抗菌剂负载到水凝胶内部。根据抗菌剂种类的不同,负载抗菌

生物医用高分子在皮肤疾病诊疗和健康中的应用(双语版) ∙∙∙∙∙∙∙∙∙∙∙∙∙∙∙∙∙∙ ▪ ∙460∙

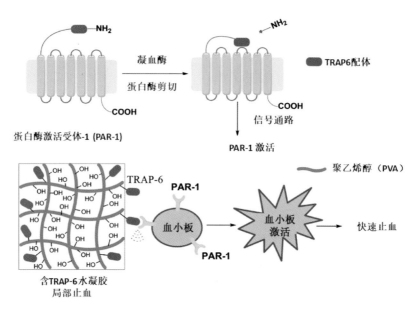

Figure 11-4　Schematic diagram of platelet activated hydrogel matrix synthesis

剂水凝胶大致可分为负载金属离子或金属纳米颗粒(比如 Ag^+、Fe^{3+}、Ag 纳米颗粒)、抗生素和非抗生素类抗菌药物三种类型的水凝胶。西安交通大学陈鑫等将乙二胺四乙酸铁(EDTA-Fe^{3+})与透明质酸(HA)进行物理交联,得到一种可由感染部位的细菌触发抗菌性并且能够快速自愈合的水凝胶。EDTA-Fe^{3+} 与透明质酸之间的动态离子键可以在数分钟内快速重建,赋予水凝胶良好的自愈合性能。当应用于创口处时,HA 可以在感染部位发生降解,水凝胶能够局部释放出 Fe^{3+} 络合物。这些 Fe^{3+} 络合物可被周围细菌迅速吸附并还原为 Fe^{2+},Fe^{2+} 与细菌和炎性细胞产生的过氧化氢(H_2O_2)通过 Fenton 反应形成羟基自由基来破坏细菌结构,从而达到杀菌的目的(图 11-5)。

　　与负载抗菌剂水凝胶不同,形成本征型抗菌水凝胶的聚合物网络具有抗菌功能。常见的本征型抗菌水凝胶可分为两类:阳离子聚合物水凝胶和抗菌肽水凝胶。本征型抗菌水凝胶主要通过与带负电荷的细菌细胞膜相互作用,使得细胞膜的结构被破坏,细胞间质流出,从而杀死细菌。西安交通大学雷波等基于单分散的 PDA 官能化的生物活性玻璃纳米颗粒和抗菌性多肽 F127-ε-聚-L-赖氨酸制备了一种抗菌水凝胶。该纳米复合物水凝胶对具有多重耐药性的细菌表现出高效抗菌性,且能够有效促进胶原组织的形成和血管再生。

四、热刺激伤口敷料

　　热刺激是一种古老而有效的促进伤口愈合的方法。在伤口周围施加局部热量可增加血流量、刺激成纤维细胞增殖并减少炎症。该方法对加强伤口周围的新陈代谢、促进伤口愈合具有重要意义。近年来,很多研究证实,采用光热疗法(PTT)可促进伤口组织再生,且该疗法作为辅助疗法已在临床中被广泛使用。目前,PTT 多使用面积小、能量高的激光器作为光源,这种光源显示出极好的组织穿透能力,对周围组织的损害极小,并且已经成功地与纳米药物结合,主要用于治疗与肿瘤或细菌感染相关的伤口。

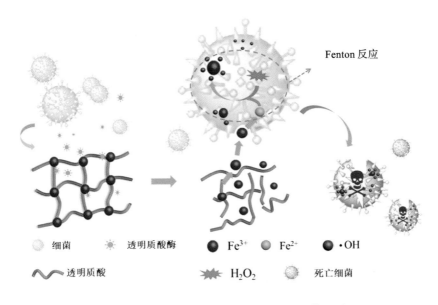

Fenton 反应

细菌   透明质酸酶 Fe^{3+} Fe^{2+} ·OH

透明质酸 H_2O_2 死亡细菌

图 11-5   EDTA-Fe^{3+}-HA 水凝胶的制备与抗菌机制

Figure 11-5   Preparation and antibacterial mechanism of EDTA-Fe^{3+}-HA hydrogels

将光热材料复合到水凝胶或者其他支架材料中是构建热刺激伤口敷料的重要途径。华中科技大学杨操等制备了一种含有纳米羟基磷灰石/氧化石墨烯（nHA/GO）复合颗粒的新型多功能支架。在波长为 808 nm 的近红外光（NIR）照射下，该支架可通过热消融促进肿瘤细胞死亡并促进成骨作用。进一步的研究表明，这种新型的光热支架不仅可以杀死人体的骨肉瘤细胞，还可以促进组织再生，在治疗骨肉瘤切除组织损伤中具有重要应用前景。另外，光热抗菌水凝胶也是治疗细菌性伤口感染的一种重要策略。如图 11-6 所示，西北农林科技大学王丽等将具有光热性能的锑烯纳米片（AM NSs）掺入壳聚糖（CS）的网络结构，构建了具有优异抗菌能力的复合水凝胶（CS/AM NSs 水凝胶）。与细菌一起培养时，CS/AM NSs 水凝胶可通过 CS 与细菌细胞膜的相互作用将细菌聚集在其表面。随后，CS 固有的杀菌特性可将细菌杀死。引入近红外光后，AM NSs 可以有效地将光能转换为热能，以消除残留细菌。由于 CS 的捕获作用与 AM NSs 的光热作用之间的协同作用，CS/AM NSs 水凝胶对大肠杆菌和金黄色葡萄球菌具有良好的抗菌性能。该复合凝胶在感染的全层缺损伤口愈合试验中也显示出良好的生物相容性和抗菌性能。

随着抗生素的滥用，对耐药菌感染伤口进行快速有效的灭菌成为伤口修复领域的严峻挑战。中国科学院上海硅酸盐研究所常江等制备了以聚多巴胺（PDA）和铜掺杂硅酸钙陶瓷（Cu-CS）为主要成分的多功能复合水凝胶（PDA/Cu-CS 水凝胶）。该复合水凝胶中的 PDA/Cu 络合物具有光热性能和抗菌活性。通过复合水凝胶的光热作用及铜离子独特的"热离子效应"，该水凝胶显示出对耐甲氧西林金黄色葡萄球菌和大肠杆菌的高效、快速和长期抑制作用。另外，该水凝胶具有显著的生物活性，能够有效地去除伤口中的感染区域，并在感染性皮肤伤口愈合过程中促进血管的生成和胶原蛋白的沉积。此外，西安交通大学郭保林等开发了一种具有自愈合和光热抗菌活性的可注射物理双网（DN）水凝胶黏合剂。该水凝胶可用于治疗多药耐药细菌感染（如耐甲氧西林金黄色葡萄球菌感染），并促进伤口愈合。

尽管在促进伤口愈合方面有很好的效果，但 PTT 疗法通常需要使用激光器，这在一定

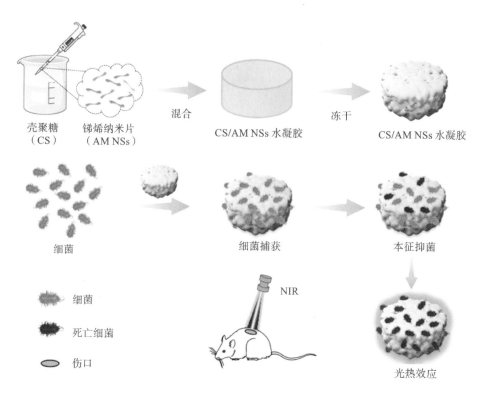

图 11-6　CS/AM NSs 水凝胶的制备及其在治疗细菌性感染伤口中的应用

Figure 11-6　Preparation of chitosan-based hydrogels incorporated with antimonene nanosheets for rapid capture and elimination of bacteria

程度上限制了其应用。使用更为便捷的太阳光来局部加热伤口以促进伤口愈合具有更为重要的实际应用价值。华中科技大学张连斌等提出利用太阳光照射光热水凝胶薄膜来加速伤口愈合的策略(图 11-7)。该聚丙烯酰胺水凝胶含有聚多巴胺(PDA)和还原氧化石墨烯(rGO),可黏附在伤口表面并将太阳能转化为热能,从而实现局部加热伤口。局部温度的升高抑制了炎症反应,并增强了上皮再生、血管生成和胶原沉积。

五、电刺激伤口敷料

生物体内存在跨上皮/内皮电势。当组织损伤时,跨上皮/内皮电势会发生改变,从而产生一种稳定且大小恒定的直流电场,即内源性电场。研究发现,伤口边缘处的电流明显大于伤口中心,且该电流会随着伤口的愈合而变化。该电场产生的内源性电信号在皮肤的自我修复过程中起着重要的作用。因此,通过在伤口局部施加外部电场就有可能修饰、增强内源生物电信号,并引导和调控成纤维细胞、神经元细胞、内皮细胞的分布、迁移、增殖、分化等,从而加速皮肤组织的定向修复。经过多年的探索,伤口部位的电刺激疗法已作为一种重要的临床策略被用于组织修复领域,其具体的作用体现在减轻伤口水肿、炎症反应,增加血液微循环,加速伤口闭合等方面。

伤口修复和组织再生是涉及许多生理信号的复杂过程。因此,采用具有生物活性和生理信号响应能力的新型伤口敷料来加速伤口愈合是一种非常具有前景的策略。目前,电刺激水凝胶伤口敷料的相关研究主要集中在导电水凝胶电极的制备及其在伤口修复相关领域的应用

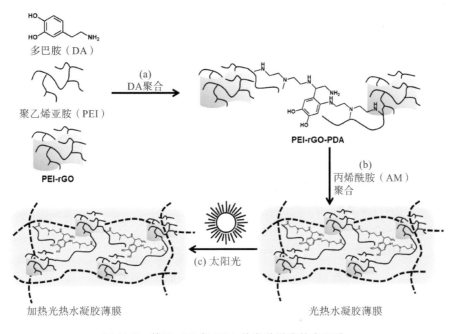

图 11-7 基于 rGO 与 PDA 的自黏附光热水凝胶

Figure 11-7 Self-adhesive photothermal hydrogel based on rGO and PDA

上。例如,西南交通大学鲁雄等受贻贝的启发,制备了聚多巴胺(PDA)还原的氧化石墨烯(pGO)结合壳聚糖(CS)和丝素蛋白(SF)的水凝胶(pGO-CS/SF 水凝胶)。该材料具有良好的力学强度、电活性和抗氧化性能,可用作电刺激伤口敷料。体外研究表明,电活性 pGO-CS/SF 水凝胶可以响应电信号并促进细胞行为,还可以通过去除过量的 ROS 来减少细胞氧化。在体内全层皮肤缺损模型中的研究表明,该类水凝胶敷料可有效地促进伤口愈合。

四川大学王云兵等开发了一种导电水凝胶敷料,通过将甲基丙烯酸-3-磺丙基酯共价掺入聚甲基丙烯酸-2-羟乙酯(polyHEMA)水凝胶网络中,以原位掺杂聚吡咯(PPY),在弱碱性生理条件下保持水凝胶的高电导率(图 11-8)。该水凝胶在防止细菌黏附和蛋白质吸收方面优于商业化的 Hydrosorb® 敷料,这有助于降低更换敷料时感染和继发性损害的可能性。使用糖尿病大鼠的体内实验表明,当使用这种 polyHEMA/PPY 水凝胶进行电刺激时,其愈合速度快于普通电极。因此,这种 polyHEMA/PPY 水凝胶有望用于慢性伤口的电刺激治疗。

此外,导电水凝胶的抗菌性能和力学性质也是其应用于伤口修复的重要因素。华中科技大学杨光等针对身体可拉伸部位(包括肘部、膝盖、腕部和项枕等)的皮肤伤口通常会因频繁运动而愈合延迟的问题,利用聚(3,4-乙撑二氧噻吩)、聚(苯乙烯磺酸盐)、瓜尔胶泥制备了一种可注射、生物相容性好、可自愈的导电凝胶材料(PPGS),并用于治疗各种伤口。吉林大学林权等将聚多巴胺修饰的银纳米颗粒(PDA@AgNPs)、聚苯胺和聚乙烯醇通过超分子组装得到柔软的导电水凝胶。该水凝胶对革兰阴性菌和革兰阳性菌表现出广泛的抗菌活性,并可以实时监测人体的运动。另外,PDA@AgNPs/CPHs 也可通过促进血管生成,加速胶原蛋白沉积,抑制细菌生长和控制伤口感染,对糖尿病伤口起到显著治疗作用。

另外,在临床操作中,电刺激疗法常常需要使用较大的设备,难以实现实时治疗。因此,亟须开发能够在伤口部位产生电场以用于皮肤伤口愈合的可穿戴和即时护理的设备。由于体积小巧,酶生物燃料电池(EBFC)和纳米发电机等自供电器件引起了研究者们的关注。日本东

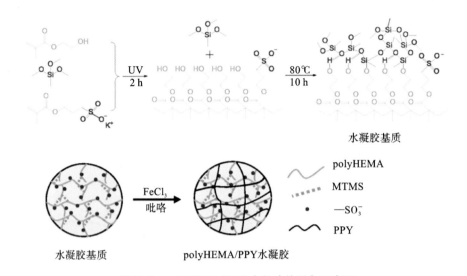

图 11-8 polyHEMA/PPY 水凝胶的制备示意图

Figure 11-8 Schematic diagram of preparation of polyHEMA/PPY hydrogel

北大学 Nishizawa 等使用柔性酶电极和可拉伸水凝胶制备了内置酶生物燃料电池(EBFC)的可拉伸生物电膏,该生物燃料电池通过酶电化学反应可在皮肤表面产生超过 12 h 的离子电流。动物实验结果表明,该电膏的离子流可促使伤口愈合更快、更顺畅。此外,华中科技大学张连斌等开发了一种由自黏附水凝胶和压电纳米发电机构成的混合皮肤贴片(HPSP,图 11-9),它由仿贻贝黏附的水凝胶基质和基于取向 PVDF 纳米纤维的压电纳米发电机组成。该压电纳米发电机具有与皮肤相近的杨氏模量,可以自黏附在伤口部位,并在局部产生由运动引起的电压。作为一种可穿戴的实时电刺激设备,该贴片大大加快了伤口愈合过程,与常规纱布敷料相比,利用该器件可使全层皮肤缺损的闭合时间缩短约 1/3。

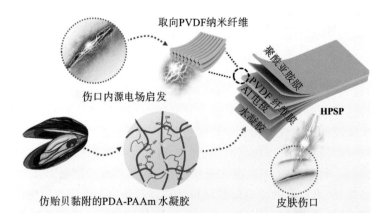

图 11-9 具有自黏附性能的水凝胶和压电纳米发电机的复合皮肤贴片

Figure 11-9 Bioinspired hybrid patches with self-adhesive hydrogel and piezoelectric nanogenerator

六、可控释放活性组分(生长因子、气体)的伤口敷料

临床上,有时需要补充适当的活性成分(如生长因子或某些气体)来促进慢性伤口的愈合。

因此,开发含有可控释放活性组分的伤口敷料用于治疗慢性伤口具有重要意义。生长因子(growth factors)是一类多肽类物质,它通过与特异的、高亲和的细胞膜受体结合来调节细胞生长和其他细胞功能,其在信号转导、调控细胞的增殖和分化、维持组织以及细胞有序的生长发育等方面具有重要的意义。重组人表皮生长因子(rhEGF)在临床上已经广泛用作治疗伤口的一种生物制剂,可有效地促进细胞再生和组织修复;但在直接使用时,其也面临着不易储存和蛋白变性等挑战。为解决这些问题,西南交通大学韩璐等将多巴胺插入黏土纳米片中,并在两层之间进行有限的氧化,然后添加丙烯酰胺单体并原位聚合得到水凝胶基体。该水凝胶具有优异的黏附性能,并可负载 rhEGF。负载有 rhEGF 的水凝胶在大鼠全层皮肤缺损实验中表现出优异的促伤口愈合性能。

尽管生长因子疗法效果好,但其费用目前偏高。因此,开发新型高效、低成本的促伤口愈合敷料具有重要的临床价值。O_2、NO、H_2S 等气体疗法已被证明具有促进伤口愈合的潜力,具有疗效佳、生物相容性好等优势。研究表明,充足的氧气供应是伤口组织生长和重塑的前提。然而,伤口处的微循环不足会导致缺氧,不利于伤口的愈合。因此,增加伤口周围的氧气含量是促进伤口愈合的重要策略之一,当前的氧气疗法(如高压氧和局部气态氧)主要采用气态氧输送,其在穿透皮肤方面的效果不佳,这限制了氧气疗法在促进伤口愈合方面的广泛应用。南京大学吴锦慧等开发了一种包覆有微藻的水凝胶贴片,通过微藻的光合作用产生溶解氧,该贴片可以促进体外细胞增殖、迁移和血管的形成,并能促进糖尿病小鼠慢性伤口的愈合(图 11-10)。

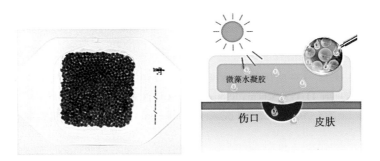

图 11-10 包覆微藻的水凝胶贴片及其促进慢性伤口愈合示意图

Figure 11-10 Schematic diagram of microalgae hydrogel patch and its promotion of chronic wound healing

此外,根据波尔效应,还可使用 CO_2 代替直接使用的 O_2 来进行皮肤伤口治疗,以促进伤口愈合。当 CO_2 溶解在伤口周围的组织中时,pH 的降低将触发血红蛋白在该部位释放更多的 O_2,从而有效地促进伤口愈合。与直接使用 O_2 相比,CO_2 在体液中的溶解度高,因此它在伤口上的作用更为便利。更重要的是,按需在伤口上精确释放 CO_2 气体的策略已引起越来越多的关注。

台湾成功大学 Yeh 等设计了一种金属离子-配体配位的纳米粒子,在近红外光(NIR)照射下,该纳米粒子结合的碳酸氢根分解生成 CO_2,用于伤口愈合。考虑到纳米粒子本身在使用过程中可能产生的毒性和迁移问题,华中科技大学张连斌等制备了含有温度响应 Pluronic F127 嵌段共聚物(BCP)和表面带有氨基的碳纳米颗粒(CNP)复合水凝胶。带有氨基的 CNP 可负载碳酸氢根;在光照下,CNP 可将光能转化为热能来触发碳酸氢盐分解。因此,该光热水凝胶可在伤口部位局部释放 CO_2,进而改善局部微循环,增加组织氧浓度,加速伤口愈合。此外,除单独的气体递送外,还可将气体递送与光热疗法结合起来加速伤口愈合。南方医科大学顺德医院邓凯贤等报道了一种由甲基丙烯酸酯修饰的明胶(GelMA)、NO 供体 BNN6、β-环糊精修饰的氧化石墨烯、多巴胺接枝的透明质酸复合而成的水凝胶(图 11-11)。在近红外光的照射下,复合水凝胶可释放 NO 气体,并局部产生热量。光热疗法和气体疗法的协同作用可以提高抗菌效率并降低耐药性,可在全层皮肤修复小鼠模型中改善胶原蛋白的沉积和血管的生成,促进细菌感染伤口皮肤的再生。

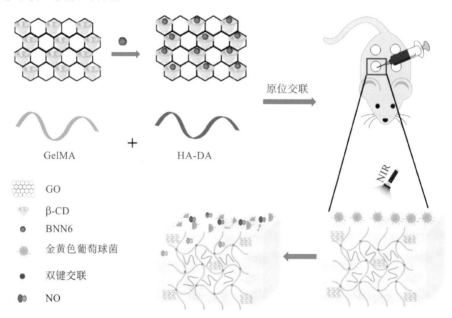

图 11-11　GO-βCD-BNN6 水凝胶释放 NO 与抗菌促愈合作用示意图
Figure 11-11　Schematic diagram of GO-βCD-BNN6 hydrogels for
NO release and promoting infected wound healing

第三节　功能性聚合物纤维敷料

聚合物纤维也是一类重要的伤口敷料。用于人体内的医用纤维材料必须具有良好的生物相容性。按材料种类,聚合物纤维可分为天然高分子纤维和合成高分子纤维,目前对功能性聚合物纤维敷料的研究具有重要意义,功能性聚合物纤维敷料具有广阔的开发前景。

一、纤维敷料制备技术

理想的伤口敷料应该无毒、不致敏,且能保持伤口环境湿润,允许气体交换,可以吸收伤口渗出物,形成利于伤口愈合的微环境并抑制细菌生长。将常用的纤维敷料(如棉纱布)覆盖在破损皮肤上即可用于伤口的临床护理和治疗。但是,纱布极易造成伤口与敷料间的粘连,容易导致二次创伤及细菌滋生等后果。近些年,纤维敷料制备技术蓬勃发展,具有高比表面积、高孔隙率的微米-纳米结构的纤维膜(微纳纤维膜)已成为一种新型的伤口修复敷料。相比于其他敷料,微纳纤维膜更为轻薄、透气且功能多样,越来越受到人们的重视。制备微纳纤维膜的技术有多种,包括拉伸法、模板合成、相分离、自组装和静电纺丝技术等。

静电纺丝技术是目前研究最广泛的纤维制备技术。该技术以高压静电为驱动力,将聚合物溶液(或熔体)液滴在静电场力的作用下拉伸变形,随着溶剂的挥发或熔体的冷却形成纤维。静电纺丝具有工艺简单、选材广泛(几乎包含从天然高分子,如海藻酸钠、明胶、壳聚糖、纤维素、丝素蛋白、透明质酸及明胶等,到化学合成的各种物质,如聚己内酯、聚乙烯醇、聚乳酸、聚偏氟乙烯等的所有高分子)、成本低、纺丝方式多样等特点,此外,纤维取向、直径、形貌、厚度以及纤维的内外结构便于调控(见扩展阅读 5)。

静电纺丝纤维用作医用敷料具有诸多优势:①纤维尺寸、结构可调。静电纺丝所得的纤维直径分布在几纳米到几微米之间,具有较好的机械强度,其多级的几何尺寸与细胞外基质(ECM)的微观结构和生物功能相似。目前,静电纺丝膜已被用作支架材料应用于组织工程,为细胞的增殖和迁移、活性物质的传递等提供了支持和引导的场所,有利于表皮迁移、血管生成和组织重塑;②静电纺丝膜具有高渗透性和高孔隙率,能够快速吸收伤口处出现的组织液,有利于伤口透气并能够阻止细菌进入,防止感染;③静电纺丝膜还可通过优化纤维材料等产生优异的止血效果及伤口贴合性;④静电纺丝膜可作为载药平台(如可负载抗炎药、生长因子、抗生素等),按需调整药物递送速度,促进伤口愈合。图 11-12 展示了常用的直接制备负载药物的静电纺丝纤维敷料的方法,包含共混、同轴和乳液静电纺丝三种。共混静电纺丝通常得到活性成分分散在整个纤维中的纤维,而同轴静电纺丝和乳液静电纺丝可以很好地合成核/壳形态纤维,以适应不同的释药需求。

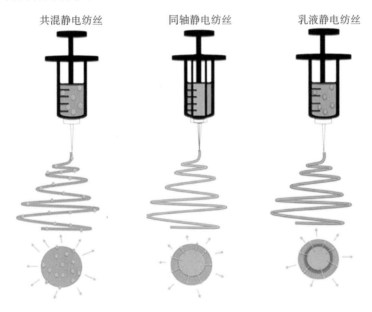

图 11-12　负载药物的静电纺丝纤维敷料的制备示意图

Figure 11-12　Schematic diagram of preparation of drug-loaded electrospun fiber dressings

此外,对静电纺丝纤维进行后处理也可提高伤口愈合效率。一般来说,静电纺丝纤维的表面可能缺少一些特定的生物活性。然而,静电吸附、物理浸涂、层层组装或表面化学反应等方法可赋予纤维所需的功能。例如,有研究者将聚乙烯醇(PVA)静电纺丝膜浸入壳聚糖溶液中,使壳聚糖的功能转移到 PVA 膜上,就可以提供给 PVA 膜即时的止血活性。还有研究者将表皮生长因子(EGF)通过化学键固定在表面氨基化的 PCL 和 PCL-PEG 嵌段共聚物的共混纤维表面,用以治疗糖尿病溃疡。研究表明,负载 EGF 的纤维敷料可增加角质形成细胞特异性基因,从而加速伤口愈合。

二、表面浸润性

一些严重的皮肤伤口如烫伤、溃疡等,会造成伤口组织液过度渗出,形成难以愈合的高渗出性伤口。其 24 h 内的渗出液量可超过 10 mL,敷料浸润率在 75% 以上,极易造成伤口和敷料的粘连,更换敷料时会给患者造成巨大的痛苦和不便。因此,高渗出性伤口对敷料的表面浸润性能有更高的要求。用于高渗出性伤口的敷料需要吸收和排出渗出液,还必须保持伤口的湿润度以促进愈合。常用的纱布不能保持湿润,这将延迟伤口愈合。目前,湿式敷料(如海藻酸盐凝胶、亲水纤维、泡沫敷料和银离子敷料)可吸收伤口组织液并保持伤口湿润,促进肉芽组织生长并抵抗细菌感染,是高渗出性伤口的首选。然而,当伤口组织液过多时,伤口过度水化将带来严重问题。传统的湿式亲水敷料可以吸收伤口部分组织液,但由于其固有的亲水性,不可避免地会在伤口和敷料之间的界面处留下伤口组织液。残留的伤口组织液会持续使伤口水化,并使愈合过程复杂化,增加感染风险。生物界面在伤口组织液与生物材料之间的相互作用中起着重要作用。伤口敷料的表面润湿性通常会影响伤口周围组织液的润湿行为。类似于大多数传统敷料,亲水材料很容易被伤口组织液润湿,从而使伤口过度水化,并导致周围正常组织的浸渍。相反,作为敷料的防水外层,疏水材料可防止外部液体与伤口的意外接触,但是它们不能促进伤口组织液的排出。最近,一些具有不对称(Janus 型)润湿性的膜材料由于其独特的水滴运输能力得到了广泛关注,如具有润湿性梯度的聚酯织物、聚氨酯(PU)/聚醋酸乙烯酯复合纤维膜、单面氟化棉织物膜(图 11-13)。控制表面润湿性为设计具有有效转移伤口组织液能力的伤口敷料提供了重要机遇。

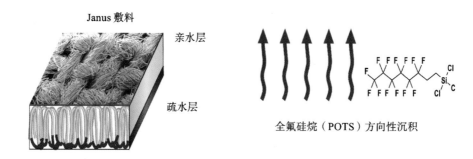

图 11-13　Janus-C 膜制备示意图
Figure 11-13　Schematic illustration for the preparation of the Janus-C membrane

中国科学院理化技术研究所王树涛等在亲水棉质医用纱布表面通过静电纺丝得到一层疏水的聚氨酯纳米纤维阵列薄层,形成能够主动将伤口处多余渗出液按单一方向"压"出伤口的敷料,保持伤口与敷料界面适度的干爽性,防止伤口部位过度水化,同时促进伤口愈合(图 11-14)。使用时,将敷料疏水一侧面向伤口组织,亲水棉质医用纱布提供的毛细作用将过多的渗出液通过疏水性纳米纤维泵送到亲水一侧,从而防止渗出液过度润湿伤口。但是在去除多余渗出液的过程中,仍会有一些细菌黏附在创面从而导致后期感染。因此,他们还在上述敷料的基础上引入银纳米粒子以使敷料具备一定的抗菌性能。

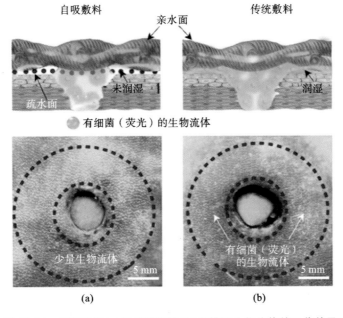

图 11-14　自吸敷料(a)和传统敷料(b)对模拟生物流体的吸收效果对比

Figure 11-14　Comparison between the treatment of simulated biofluid (a mixture of green fluorescence-labeled *S. aureus* and FBS) by (a) self-pumping dressing and (b) conventional dressing on the murine dorsum model

三、止血纤维敷料

传统止血材料(如止血纱布、绷带和止血海绵等)的止血效果一般较差,且不具备主动止血功能,只能满足一般或常规出血创面的止血需求。此外,这些材料一般不能在体内降解,难以被机体吸收,因此使用范围受到限制。近年来的研究发现,在纱布、海绵等表面修饰一层多孔、柔软且吸水后具有优异黏附性和凝血作用的纤维会大大提高其止血性能。美国麻省理工学院Hammond等将多肽(RADA16-I)纳米纤维通过层层组装技术负载到纱布或明胶海绵表面,得到具有主动凝血功能的快速止血纱布或海绵。RADA16-I自组装多肽纳米纤维能够有效地聚集并交联血液中的成分,可大大提高纱布或海绵的止血效果。复旦大学附属浦东医院禹宝庆等用介孔二氧化硅负载姜黄素与聚乙烯吡咯烷酮共混静电纺丝制备了纳米纤维贴片,用于伤口的快速止血和抗菌。研究发现,纳米纤维贴片具有良好的生物相容性,并且能够对金黄色葡萄球菌起抑制作用。此外,体内止血研究发现,混合纳米纤维贴片在与血液接触时可迅速转变为水凝胶,然后激活凝血系统以阻止伤口出血。

此外,在提高材料止血效果的基础上,如何进一步优化其制备过程也引起了科研工作者和产业界的广泛关注。青岛大学龙云泽等开发了一种户外使用的便携式静电纺丝装置(约150 g),该装置可在伤口处原位沉积负载有CuS的复合纳米纤维。复合纳米纤维敷料可实现快速止血并消灭超级细菌。这种原位生成的电纺丝纳米纤维可有效地贴附于创口的粗糙表面,其贴合性明显优于压在创面上的传统纳米纤维贴片。此外,该原位生成的纳米纤维敷料不仅可以加速止血(短于6 s),而且可以缩短超级细菌感染创面的愈合时间(18 天)。双功能纳米纤维与便携式静电纺丝设备结合,可在户外快速止血的同时消灭超级细菌,从而显著改善户外急救的效果(图 11-15)。

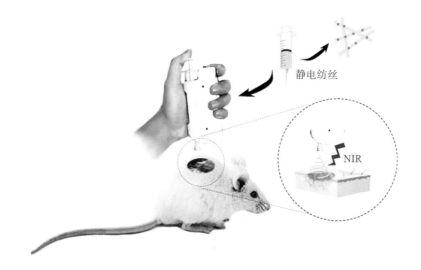

静电纺丝

NIR

图 11-15　便携式静电纺丝装置及其原位伤口敷料制备示意图
Figure 11-15　Portable electrospinning device for *in-situ* wound dressing preparation

四、抗菌性纤维敷料

细菌感染严重威胁着伤口愈合的进程。因此,预防细菌感染对完成伤口修复至关重要。向静电纺丝纤维中添加无机、有机或金属抗菌剂是赋予纤维敷料抗菌性的重要策略。

目前,临床操作中常通过口服或注射抗生素的方式来治疗细菌感染伤口。长期使用广谱抗生素会带来细菌耐药问题,若其释放浓度小于最小抑菌浓度则会加剧耐药的不良后果。因此,如何控制抗生素的释放浓度一直是抗菌纤维敷料的重要研究方向。He 等人将恩诺沙星负载到 PVDF 静电纺丝纳米纤维中,在 0~12 h 内,药物释放呈突释行为,累积释放量达到 60%,可以快速杀灭细菌。剩余药物可持续释放 3 天,可有效抑制细菌的增殖。

此外,将以纳米银、纳米锌以及碳基纳米材料为代表的无机抗菌剂负载到纤维中也是常用的抗菌策略,这些纤维敷料可以杀死细菌,降低炎症反应或促进上皮增殖、再生。有研究者使用 PVA 作为还原剂,制备了含纳米银颗粒的 PVA 静电纺丝纤维,该纤维对大肠杆菌和金黄色葡萄球菌均表现出抑制作用,抑菌效率也远高于负载硝酸银的伤口敷料。

中国科学院上海硅酸盐研究所常江等人通过溶胶-凝胶法合成了掺杂锌的介孔二氧化硅纳米球(HMZS),并将负载有盐酸环丙沙星(CiH)的含锌中孔二氧化硅纳米球(CiH-HMZS)掺入聚己内酯(PCL)静电纺丝纤维中,制备了新型伤口愈合敷料。如图 11-16 所示,该复合纤维敷料可以通过释放硅离子来促进血管生成和皮肤再生、释放锌离子来增强毛囊再生,同时抑制细菌的生长活性;并且盐酸环丙沙星与锌具有协同的抗菌作用,可用于抑制细菌感染伤口中的细菌生长并增强包括皮肤毛囊再生在内的皮肤伤口愈合。

虽然这些无机材料表现出优异的广谱抑菌性能,但其大量使用仍然存在一定的安全风险。此外,一些有机高分子(如高分子季铵盐、含胍基高分子等)或是由某些氨基酸组装而成的抗菌多肽也具有优异的抑菌性能。以它们为主体的静电纺丝纤维膜甚至可以克服多药耐药(MDR)细菌的感染。西安交通大学雷波等开发了一种由荧光和抗菌功能杂化的多肽纳米纤维的弹性体用于抑制 MDR 细菌感染和促进伤口愈合(图 11-17)。杂化纳米纤维基质由聚(柠檬酸盐)-ε-聚赖氨酸(PCE)和聚己内酯(PCL)组成。PCL-PCE 杂化纳米纤维基质表现出仿生

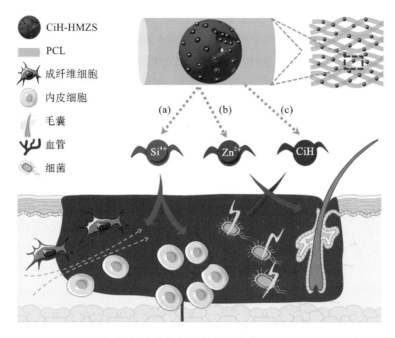

图 11-16　具有离子/药物释放特性的多功能静电纺丝纤维复合膜

Figure 11-16　Multifunctional electrospun fiber composite membrane with ion/drug release characteristics

的弹性行为,高抗菌活性(包括杀死 MDR 细菌的能力)和良好的生物相容性,并可以有效地预防 MDR 细菌引起的伤口感染,显著增强伤口愈合和皮肤再生能力。

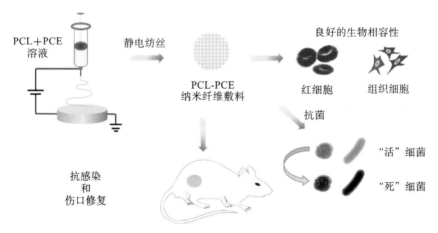

图 11-17　基于仿生弹性体多肽的纳米纤维基质用于多药耐药细菌治疗和伤口愈合/皮肤再生

Figure 11-17　Biomimetic elastomeric polypeptide-based nanofibrous matrix for overcoming multidrug-resistant bacteria and enhancing full-thickness wound healing/skin regeneration

第四节　挑战与展望

在本章中,我们介绍了新型高分子敷料在促进伤口愈合和止血方面的进展。通过采用水凝胶、功能性聚合物纤维等,结合化学组成、网络结构、表面浸润性等调控手段,有效实现自黏附、抗菌、渗液排出等独特功能,促进伤口修复。另外,利用水凝胶为载体,有效结合光热组分、纳米发电机以及功能性纳米载体,可实现对伤口的外界刺激,促进伤口愈合。相比于传统的敷料,新型敷料从伤口愈合的本质出发,针对伤口修复的机制、可能存在的感染等问题,通过激活自体因素促进伤口修复、抑制细菌感染,从而达到促进伤口愈合的目的,因而具有广阔的发展前景。然而,我们也注意到,对于一些慢性难愈合伤口以及存在耐药菌感染的伤口,实现其快速愈合仍然是该领域的重要挑战。现阶段的功能性敷料更多的是在小型动物模型上进行验证,其能否在大动物以及人体伤口愈合中发挥相同的作用仍需进一步测试,尤其是对于一些使用纳米粒子、纳米器件的功能性敷料,材料的生物安全性需要进一步验证,以确保其不会在大幅度运动过程中发生泄漏以及脱落。此外,发展更加便捷、低成本的制备手段,使新型功能性敷料从实验室走向产业化道路仍然需要材料科学、临床医学、相关企业的深度交叉与合作。随着不同学科间的相互融合,随着材料科学、界面科学、纳米器件等相关领域的快速发展,我们相信在不久的将来,新型高分子伤口敷料将会更多地出现并应用于临床治疗领域,造福广大患者。

思 考 题

1. 试述传统干性敷料和水凝胶伤口敷料各自的优势与不足。
2. 聚合物纤维敷料的制备方法有哪些?
3. 哪些外界环境因素有利于伤口愈合? 如何实现?
4. 水凝胶用于伤口敷料有哪些要求?
5. 如何提高伤口修复的效果?

扩 展 阅 读

[1] 丁炎明.伤口护理学[M].北京:人民卫生出版社,2017.

[2] 陈孝平.外科学[M].2 版.北京:人民卫生出版社,2010.

[3] 薛巍,张渊明.生物医用水凝胶[M].广州:暨南大学出版社,2012.

[4] Ye Q,Zhou F,Liu W M. Bioinspired catecholic chemistry for surface modification[J]. Chem Soc Rev,2011,40(7):4244-4258.

[5] Homaeigohar S,Boccaccini A R. Antibacterial biohybrid nanofibers for wound dressings [J]. Acta Biomater,2020,107:25-49.

参 考 文 献

[1] Gao Y,Du H,Xie Z,et al. Self-adhesive photothermal hydrogel films for solar-light assisted wound healing[J]. J Mater Chem B,2019,7(23):3644-3651.

[2] Xie T,Ding J,Han X,et al. Wound dressing change facilitated by spraying zinc ions [J]. Mater Horiz,2020,7(2):605-614.

[3] Ding C,Tian M,Feng R,et al. Novel self-healing hydrogel with injectable,pH-responsive,strain sensitive,promoting wound-healing,and hemostatic properties based on collagen and chitosan[J]. ACS Biomater Sci Eng,2020,6(7):3855-3867.

[4] Yan S,Wang W,Li X,et al. Preparation of mussel-inspired injectable hydrogels based

on dual-functionalized alginate with improved adhesive, self-healing, and mechanical properties[J]. J Mater Chem B, 2018, 6(40): 6377-6390.

[5] Cheng L, Cai Z, Ye T, et al. Injectable polypeptide-protein hydrogels for promoting infected wound healing[J]. Adv Funct Mater, 2020, 30(25): 2001196.

[6] Qin X, Labuda K, Chen J, et al. Development of synthetic platelet-activating hydrogel matrices to induce local hemostasis[J]. Adv Funct Mater, 2015, 25(42): 6606-6617.

[7] Hong Y, Zhou F, Hua J, et al. A strongly adhesive hemostatic hydrogel for the repair of arterial and heart bleeds[J]. Nat Commun, 2019, 10(1): 2060.

[8] Kumar V A, Taylor N L, Jalan A A, et al. A nanostructured synthetic collagen mimic for hemostasis[J]. Biomacromolecules, 2014, 15(4): 1484-1490.

[9] Tian R, Qiu X, Yuan P, et al. Fabrication of self-healing hydrogels with on-demand antimicrobial activity and sustained biomolecule release for infected skin regeneration [J]. ACS Appl Mater Interfaces, 2018, 10(20): 17018-17027.

[10] Zhou Y, Xi Y, Xue Y, et al. Injectable self-healing antibacterial bioactive polypeptide-based hybrid nanosystems for efficiently treating multidrug resistant infection, skin-tumor therapy, and enhancing wound healing[J]. Adv Funct Mater, 2019, 29(22): 1806883.

[11] Wang H, Li M, Hu J, et al. Multiple targeted drugs carrying biodegradable membrane barrier: anti-adhesion, hemostasis, and anti-infection[J]. Biomacromolecules, 2013, 14(4): 954-961.

[12] Li D, Nie W, Chen L, et al. Fabrication of curcumin-loaded mesoporous silica incorporated polyvinyl pyrrolidone nanofibers for rapid hemostasis and antibacterial treatment[J]. RSC Adv, 2017, 7(13): 7973-7982.

[13] Liu X, Zhang J, Liu J, et al. Bifunctional CuS composite nanofibers via *in situ* electrospinning for outdoor rapid hemostasis and simultaneous ablating superbug fabrication of curcumin loaded mesporous silica incorporated[J]. Chem Eng J, 2020, 401: 126096.

[14] Li Z, Milionis A, Zheng Y, et al. Superhydrophobic hemostatic nanofiber composites for fast clotting and minimal adhesion[J]. Nat Commun, 2019, 10: 5562.

[15] Hou S, Liu Y, Feng F, et al. Polysaccharide-peptide cryogels for multidrug-resistant-bacteria infected wound healing and hemostasis[J]. Adv Healthc Mater, 2019, 9(3): 1901041.

[16] Zhang X, Zhang C, Yang Y, et al. Light-assisted rapid sterilization by a hydrogel incorporated with Ag_3PO_4/MoS_2 composites for efficient wound disinfection[J]. Chem Eng J, 2019, 374: 596-604.

[17] Qiao Z, Lv X, He S, et al. A mussel-inspired supramolecular hydrogel with robust tissue anchor for rapid hemostasis of arterial and visceral bleedings[J]. Bioact Mater, 2021, 6(9): 2829-2840.

[18] Bu Y, Zhang L, Sun G, et al. Tetra-PEG based hydrogel sealants for *in vivo* visceral hemostasis[J]. Adv Mater, 2019, 31(28): e1901580.

[19] Wang L,Zhang X,Yang K,et al. A novel double-crosslinking-double-network design for injectable hydrogels with enhanced tissue adhesion and antibacterial capability for wound treatment[J]. Adv Funct Mater,2020,30(1):1904156.

[20] Zhao X,Liang Y,Guo B,et al. Injectable dry cryogels with excellent blood-sucking expansion and blood clotting to cease hemorrhage for lethal deep-wounds, coagulopathy and tissue regeneration[J]. Chem Eng J,2021,403:126329.

[21] Chen W,Wang R,Xu T,et al. A mussel-inspired poly(γ-glutamic acid) tissue adhesive with high wet strength for wound closure[J]. J Mater Chem B,2017,5(28): 5668-5678.

[22] Bai S,Zhang X,Cai P,et al. A silk-based sealant with tough adhesion for instant hemostasis of bleeding tissues[J]. Nanoscale Horiz,2019,4(6):1333-1341.

[23] Wang R,Li J,Chen W,et al. A biomimetic mussel-inspired ε-poly-L-lysine hydrogel with robust tissue-anchor and anti-infection capacity[J]. Adv Funct Mater,2017,27 (8):1604894.

[24] Shin M,Ryu J,Park J,et al. DNA/tannic acid hybrid gel exhibiting biodegradability, extensibility,tissue adhesiveness,and hemostatic ability[J]. Adv Funct Mater,2015, 25(8):1270-1278.

[25] Ma L,Feng X,Liang H,et al. A novel photothermally controlled multifunctional scaffold for clinical treatment of osteosarcoma and tissue regeneration[J]. Mater Today,2020,36:48-62.

[26] Liu Y,Xiao Y,Cao Y,et al. Construction of chitosan-based hydrogel incorporated with antimonene nanosheets for rapid capture and elimination of bacteria[J]. Adv Funct Mater,2020,30(35):2003196.

[27] Xu Q,Chang M,Zhang Y,et al. PDA/Cu bioactive hydrogel with "hot ions effect" for inhibition of drug-resistant bacteria and enhancement of infectious skin wound healing [J]. ACS Appl Mater Interfaces,2020,12(28):31255-31269.

[28] Zhao X,Liang Y,Huang Y,et al. Physical double-network hydrogel adhesives with rapid shape adaptability, fast self-healing, antioxidant and NIR/pH stimulus-responsiveness for multidrug-resistant bacterial infection and removable wound dressing[J]. Adv Funct Mater,2020,30(17):1910748.

[29] Duo S,Zhou N,Xie G,et al. Surface-engineered triboelectric nanogenerator patches with drug loading and electrical stimulation capabilities:toward promoting infected wounds healing[J]. Nano Energy,2021,85:106004.

[30] Zhao X,Liang Y,Huang Y,et al. Physical double-network hydrogel adhesives with rapid shape adaptability, fast self-healing, antioxidant and NIR/pH stimulus-responsiveness for multidrug-resistant bacterial infection and removable wound dressing[J]. Adv Funct Mater,2020,30(17):1910748.

[31] Lu Y,Wang Y,Zhang J,et al. *In-situ* doping of a conductive hydrogel with low protein absorption and bacterial adhesion for electrical stimulation of chronic wounds[J]. Acta

Biomaterialia,2019,7(89):217-226.

[32] Li S,Wang L,Zheng W,et al. Rapid fabrication of self-healing, conductive, and injectable gel as dressings for healing wounds in stretchable parts of the body[J]. Adv Funct Mater,2020,30(31):2002370.

[33] Zhao Y,Li Z,Song S,et al. Skin-inspired antibacterial conductive hydrogels for epidermal sensors and diabetic foot wound dressings[J]. Adv Funct Mater,2019,29 (31):1901474.

[34] Kai H,Yamauchi T,Ogawa Y,et al. Accelerated wound healing on skin by electrical stimulation with a bioelectric plaster[J]. Adv Health Mater,2017,6(22):1700465.

[35] Du S,Zhou N,Gao Y,et al. Bioinspired hybrid patches with self-adhesive hydrogel and piezoelectric nanogenerator for promoting skin wound healing[J]. Nano Res,2020,13 (9):2525-2533.

[36] Han L,Lu X,Liu K,et al. Mussel-inspired adhesive and tough hydrogel based on nanoclay confined dopamine polymerization[J]. ACS Nano,2017,11(3):2561-2574.

[37] Chen H,Cheng Y,Tian J,et al. Dissolved oxygen from microalgae-gel patch promotes chronic wound healing in diabetes[J]. Sci Adv,2020,6(20):eaba4311.

[38] Li W P,Su C H,Wang S J,et al. CO_2 delivery to accelerate incisional wound healing following single irradiation of near-infrared lamp on the coordinated colloids[J]. ACS Nano,2017,11(6):5826-5835.

[39] Xie G,Zhou N,Gao Y,et al. On-demand release of CO_2 from photothermal hydrogels for accelerating skin wound healing[J]. Chem Eng J,2021,403:126353.

[40] Huang S,Liu H,Liao K,et al. Functionalised GO nanovehicle with nitric oxide release and photothermal activity-based hydrogels for bacteria-infected wound healing[J]. ACS Appl Mater Interfaces,2020,12(26):28952-28964.

[41] Rieger K A,Birch N P,Schiffman J D. Designing electrospun nanofiber mats to promote wound healing—a review[J]. J Mater Chem B,2013,1(36):4531-4541.

[42] Tian X,Jin H,Sainio J,et al. Droplet and fluid gating by biomimetic janus membranes [J]. Adv Funct Mater,2014,24(38):6023-6028.

[43] Shi L,Liu X,Wang W,et al. A Self-pumping dressing for draining excessive biofluid around wounds[J]. Adv Mater,2019,31(5):e1804187.

[44] Zhang Y,Chang M,Bao F,et al. Multifunctional Zn doped hollow mesoporous silica/polycaprolactone electrospun membranes with enhanced hair follicle regeneration and antibacterial activity for wound healing[J]. Nanoscale,2019,11(13):6315-6333.

[45] Xi Y,Ge J,Guo Y,et al. Biomimetic elastomeric polypeptide-based nanofibrous matrix for overcoming multidrug-resistant bacteria and enhancing full-thickness wound healing/skin regeneration[J]. ACS Nano,2018,12(11):10772-10784.

（张连斌）

Chapter 11

Applications of Biomedical Polymers in Skin Wound Repair

11. 1   Overview of Skin Wounds

11. 1. 1   Production and healing of skin wounds

Skin is the largest organ of the human body, which is in direct contact with the surrounding environment and acts as a protective barrier at the interface between the human body and the surrounding environment. The skin has many important functions, including preventing the loss of body fluids and regulating body surface temperature. Due to certain factors, such as an injury and a surgery, the anatomical structure and physiological functions of normal skin can be destroyed and skin trauma occurs. Skin wounds can be classified into acute or chronic wounds depending on the healing process. Acute wounds originate from superficial abrasions to deep injuries, and they can usually heal within 3 weeks. Acute wounds that fail to heal within 2 months usually develop into chronic wounds, such as certain types of ulcers or diabetic wounds. Wound healing requires multiple processes to occur in a specific order. As shown in Figure 11-1, these processes are generally divided into four major stages, namely hemostasis, inflammation, migration, and remodeling/maturation.

The wound healing process begins with hemostasis, i. e. , blood clots form and the wounds close. At this stage, blood vessels constrict to stop bleeding, and platelets are activated. Platelets play several important roles in wound healing, including regulating hemostasis during the aggregation phase and secondary hemostasis during the coagulation phase. Platelets can also produce biologically vasoactive mediators and chemokines, such as proteases, cytokines, and growth factors. Cytokines send chemotactic signals to inflammatory cells and cell populations. Fibrin is formed during secondary hemostasis. The fibronectin clot acts as a temporary matrix, allowing epithelial cells and fibroblasts to migrate to the wound. A blood clot forms and thrombin is activated. Activation of the fibrinolytic system leads to fibrin degradation. In this process, peptides are released to stimulate chemotaxis and increase capillary permeability. Cytokines can also trigger an inflammatory response and play a role in removing debris, damaged or necrotic tissues, and microorganisms, which is followed by granulation tissue formation, re-epithelization, and connective tissue matrix formation. The granulation tissue is composed of dense macrophages, fibroblasts, capillary networks, fibronectin, hyaluronic acid, and endothelial cells. During the formation of granulation tissue, macrophages, fibroblasts, and endothelial cells are interdependent.

Hypoxia is an important factor that triggers the formation of new blood vessels at early stage of wound healing. Before the basement membrane is formed, the wound will continue to seep fluid. At the same time, fibroblasts gather from the edge of the wound, and circulating fibroblasts and mesenchymal stem cells migrate to the immature connective tissue matrix. Re-epithelialization begins at the edge of the wound, where epithelial cells lose hemidesmosome connections and migrate across the wound through a temporary fibrin—fibronectin matrix until they encounter the same cells. Directional migration and proliferation require an effective, balanced, and enzyme-supported "cut and paste" program. After this process, the epithelial cells on the edge of the wound are in direct contact, which is called primary healing. In addition, secondary healing occurs after the migrating cells connect for a certain period. Due to the delayed epithelial closure and the higher formation rate of granulation tissue, the healing process of open wounds is slower. The final stage of the wound healing process is called the contraction stage and begins with the formation of large amounts of collagen in the granular tissue. In the contraction phase, the distance between the edge of the wound is reduced until the wound is tightly closed. This process occurs due to the differentiation of fibroblasts and the differentiation of progenitor cells into myofibroblasts. Myofibroblasts rich in actin skeletal matrix cause the matrix to contract. After the wound shrinks, it enters the remodeling process, in which the production of the matrix is stopped, and fibroblasts and myofibroblasts undergo apoptosis and degeneration. The final result of wound healing may be completely scarless, or it may leave obvious scars due to fibrosis.

11.1.2 Wound dressings

Wound dressings are materials that wrap wounds to cover sores, wounds, or other damage. Wound dressings include primary dressings that are in direct contact with the wound bed and secondary dressings that play an auxiliary role on top of the covered primary dressings. The primary dressings directly cover the wound surface, to treat and protect the wound surface. The secondary dressings can play a role in consolidating the primary dressing, to more fully meet the needs of wound healing.

Early wound dressing products include gauze, tape, natural or synthetic bandages, and absorbent cotton. The gauze dressings are made of woven and non-woven fiber cotton, rayon, and polyester. Because they are cheap and easy to obtain, they are suitable for drainage of many wounds. While due to their dry nature, they can adhere to the wound and cause pain during removal. The gauze dressings can provide some protection to the wound, but it needs to be changed frequently to prevent the maceration of healthy adjacent tissues, which may increase costs and cause repetitive tissue damage. Therefore, when using gauze as a dressing, it can be impregnated with paraffin, iodine, or petroleum to avoid drying, providing a non-adhesive coverage. In 1971, Dr. Winter firstly proposed the concept of "wet wound healing". They found that the intact blister healed about 2 times quicker than the broken blister, and pointed out that because the epithelial cells could not migrate through the dry or crusted cell layer, they took time to migrate to the moist bed under the scab, allowing the epithelial cells heal longer. A moist environment could promote epithelial cells crawling and reduced scar formation. This conclusion laid the foundation for modern wet wound healing theory, and at the same time promoted the rapid development of new wet wound healing dressings. Compared with the early traditional dressings (e. g. , gauze, oily gauze), new dressings have a positive effect on the wound, promoting hemostasis and the rapid healing of the wound. New dressings mainly include hydrogel dressings and fiber dressings, and these functional dressings are mainly produced by polymer materials. Therefore, the following sections will focus on the research progress of polymer materials in new wound healing dressings and composite functional dressings.

11. 2   Polymer Hydrogel-Based Wound Dressings

11. 2. 1   Introduction of hydrogel materials

Most organisms are composed of soft and water-containing gels. They can sense external environmental stimuli and generate real-time and fast responses. Among all artificial materials, hydrogels are the most similar materials to biological tissues. They are polymer networks formed by light cross-linking of hydrophilic polymers. Water molecules and some small molecules can move in the polymer network. Hydrogels can provide a microenvironment that mimics extracellular mechanisms and can regulate cell behavior and tissue function. In recent years, hydrogels based on synthetic or natural polymers have received extensive attention in the biomedical field. For example, contact lenses made of poly (hydroxyethyl methacrylate), bioadhesives made of recombinant protein or albumin for surgical bonding, wound dressings made of alginate polysaccharides, and hydrogels made of hyaluronic acid are widely used in clinical practice. Hydrogels have good biocompatibility, easy molding and processing, and controllable shape and size, and have broad application prospects in biomedical engineering fields, including three-dimensional tissue engineering matrices, drug carriers, and biocomposites.

According to their source, hydrogels can be classified into two types: natural polymer hydrogels and synthetic polymer hydrogels. Natural polymer hydrogels are mainly formed by natural polymer materials, including collagen, gelatin, fibrin, chitosan, sodium alginate, hyaluronic acid, chondroitin sulfate, agarose, etc. The compositions and structures of the natural polymer hydrogels are similar to the natural extracellular matrix, and they have the advantages of good biocompatibility and biodegradability. However, its mechanical properties are generally low and cannot meet the mechanical requirements for the repair of load-bearing tissues. Synthetic polymer hydrogels are mainly formed by cross-linking synthetic polymer materials, such as poly(ethylene glycol), poly(vinyl alcohol), poly(hydroxyethyl methacrylate), polyacrylamide, poly(acrylic acid), or their derivatives. Generally, synthetic polymer hydrogels have high mechanical properties, controllable structure and performance, and good repeatability. Yet, the lack of biological functions and poor biocompatibility should be considered for synthetic polymer hydrogels.

According to the cross-linking method of hydrogels, they can be divided into physically crosslinked hydrogels and chemically crosslinked hydrogels. Physically crosslinked hydrogels refer to the formation of polymer chains through physical interactions (e. g., chain entanglement) or weak supramolecular interactions (e. g., ionic interactions, hydrogen bonds). The reaction conditions for the formation of the physically crosslinked hydrogel are mild and no chemical cross-linking agent is required. Since the physical cross-linking is nonpermanent, the hydrogel may dissociate when the external environment (e. g., pH, temperature, ion concentration) changes. The chemically crosslinked hydrogels are constructed using free radical polymerization, ultraviolet irradiation, and enzymatic cross-linking in which a stable covalent bond between polymer chains is generated to construct a hydrogel network. Compared with physically crosslinked hydrogels, their mechanical properties can be significantly improved, but residual chemical cross-linking agents, organic solvents, initiators, etc. may cause potential cytotoxicity. Therefore, the post-treatment for the materials is particularly important.

11. 2. 1. 1 Bioinspired adhesive hydrogels

Inspired by the fascinating biological structure and functions, bioinspired hydrogels have a broad application prospect in the biomedical field. Among them, taking inspiration from the underwater adhesion of natural mussels, barnacles, and other marine organisms, bioinspired adhesive hydrogels have received more and more attention in recent years. Bioinspired adhesive hydrogels refer to hydrogels with high adhesion and biocompatibility, which can replace traditional surgical suture wound closure devices and have the effect of promoting wound healing. The adhesion mainly comes from the interaction between the active groups in the polymer and the active groups in the biological tissue or the multiple supramolecular interactions with the surface. For example, some hydrogels with aldehyde groups can covalently bond with amino groups in biological tissues, thereby exhibiting high adhesion strength to living tissues. Duan et al. prepared an *in-situ* injectable viscous hydrogel by Schiff base reaction between the amino group of carboxymethyl chitosan and the aldehyde group of oxydextran. Injecting the hydrogel on the burn wound in rats can promote cell adhesion and make epithelial cells migrate to the wound area to promote skin regeneration.

The adhesive protein secreted by mussels has a fast curing speed, high waterproof adhesion ability, and excellent adhesion diversity in water, making it a biological adhesive with great advantages and potential. The catechol group, which is rich in mussel's adhesive protein, plays key roles in wet adhesion and adhesion diversification. Inspired by the strong underwater adhesion ability of mussels, a variety of mussel-like adhesion hydrogels have been developed. For example, Zhang et al. used polydopamine (PDA), reduced graphene oxide (rGO), branched polyethyleneimine (PEI), and polyacrylamide (PAM) to prepare a highly adhesive hydrogel film. After being attached to the wound, the hydrogel converted solar energy into heat energy and heated the wound locally. An increase of the local temperature at the wound site could reduce inflammation and promoted re-epithelialization, angiogenesis, and collagen deposition, thereby significantly promoting wound healing. Liu et al. synthesized a hyperbranched polymer HB-PBAE by the Michael addition reaction between polydopamine (PDA), poly(ethylene glycol diacrylate) (PEGDA700), and pentaerythritol triacrylate (PETA). Then, HB-PBAE, poly(1-vinyl imidazole) (PVI), and gelatin solution were mixed, and Fe^{3+} was added to prepare a bioinspired adhesive hydrogel. Fe^{3+} can form coordination bonds with catechol group to stabilize the hydrogel. When the dressing needs to be changed, Zn^{2+} aqueous solution can be sprayed on the dressing and the adhesive ability of the hydrogel is significantly reduced. At the same time, PVI and Zn^{2+} form a stable coordination bond, which further enhances the strength of the hydrogel. It can be easily and non-destructively replaced, and there is no obvious dressing residue on the wound, which promotes wound healing (Figure 11-2). This kind of dressing change promoted by metal ions may provide a new idea for the design of wound dressings.

11.2.1.2　Injectable hydrogels

Injectable hydrogels refer to hydrogels that were fluid before injection, and after injecting into the subcutaneous tissue or muscle tissue through a syringe, they form gel *in-situ* at the wound sites. The formation mechanism is based on the polymer material's response to external stimuli to change the state or conformation of the polymer under physiological conditions and complete the conversion process from solution to gel. The injectable hydrogels usually respond to external stimuli (e. g. , temperature, pH, enzyme). Because these hydrogels have excellent biocompatibility and mechanical properties, they can quickly close wounds of any shape, bond with the contour of the wound to provide a physical barrier, also maintain the moist environment of the skin, and quickly stop bleeding and prevent wounds infection. These hydrogels are potentially useful in medical dressing.

Zhang et al. designed and developed a PEG2000-based injectable hydrogel by collagen

(COL), chitosan (CS), and dibenzaldehyde through dynamic imine bond. COL/CS hydrogel has good thermal stability, injectability, pH sensitivity, and antibacterial capability. COL/CS hydrogel can adhere well to the tissue surface. After the COL/CS hydrogel acts on the moist wound surface, it can effectively promote wound healing and rapid wound hemostasis. Yin et al. introduced dopamine (DA) to aldehyde-modified alginate (ALG) skeleton to form bifunctional ALG and obtained injectable bioadhesive hydrogel (PGA/ALG-CHO hydrogel) with hydrazide-modified poly(L-glutamic acid). The injectable bioadhesive hydrogel (PGA/ALG-CHO hydrogel) possessed various interactions (e. g. , hydrogen bond and π-π stacking between catechol groups and tissues), endowing it with superior hemostatic capability. Liu et al. mimicked the characteristics of the extracellular matrix by using sulfhydryl bovine serum protein, KK polypeptide, and Ag^+ to build a protein-based injectable hydrogel that can promote the healing of infected wounds. In this protein-based hydrogel, Ag^+, as a cross-linking agent, can not only provide a sterile microenvironment and strong antibacterial ability but also introduce $K_2(SL)_6K_2$ (KK) peptides to generate blood vessels. In addition, the results of *in vivo* experiments also showed that the protein-based hydrogel has considerable collagen deposition and vascularization ability in the early stage of wound healing so that new tissues are rapidly regenerated and new hair follicles appear (Figure 11-3).

11.2.2 Hemostatic hydrogel dressings

A direct result of skin trauma is the occurrence of bleeding. Excessive blood loss is the main cause of death. The use of appropriate hemostatic equipment for first aid treatment can effectively reduce casualties. Since the application of tourniquets in parts of the human body other than the limbs is often limited, rapid hemostatic materials have always been a hot topic in the field of first aid. Currently, the common types of hemostatic dressings mainly include rubber dressings, foam dressings, electrospun fiber dressings, membrane dressings, hydrogel dressings, etc. Among these dressings, hydrogels are of great importance in the application of hemostatic dressings due to their specific crosslinked network structure, semi-permeable, bacterial invasion blockage, wound infection prevention, and allow for the passage of oxygen and water.

Hemostatic hydrogel dressings can be obtained by introducing hemostatic factors (e. g. , hemostatic polypeptides, hemostatic drugs) into the gel or via a strong physical barrier. For example, Paul Slezak et al. used click chemistry to graft thrombin receptor agonist peptide-6 (TRAP-6) onto poly(vinyl alcohol) (PVA) to obtain a hemostatic polypeptide modified PVA-TRAP-6 hydrogel. Since TRAP-6 has a significant function of activating platelets, the hemostatic hydrogel not only exhibits a good biocompatibility, but also significantly shortens the clotting time, and can be used as a hemostatic dressing for wounds and bleeding in tissues and organs (Figure 11-4). Ouyang et al. designed a light-responsive adhesive that mimicked the composition of the extracellular matrix (ECM), which could quickly gel and fix after ultraviolet irradiation, and adhered and sealed the bleeding artery and myocardial wall. The adhered hydrogel could withstand blood pressure up to 290 mmHg, which is significantly higher than the blood pressure in most clinical settings. This hydrogel can prevent 4-5 mm porcine carotid artery incisions and 6 mm diameter heart penetration holes in the porcine heart. The treated pigs survived after using this hydrogel for hemostatic treatment, which is well tolerated and has significant clinical advantages as a wound sealant.

In addition, the introduction of inorganic nanoparticles (NPs) (e. g. , silica, clays) with hemostatic function into hydrogels is also an effective manner to obtain hemostatic hydrogel dressings. The negatively charged silicate can effectively condense the coagulation factors in the blood, and the fast water absorption of inorganic nanoparticles can effectively concentrate blood components. Hartgerink et al. prepared a nanocomposite hydrogel and the result showed that through the synergistic effect of silicate and collagen, the nanocomposite hydrogel has multiple functions of efficiently enriching coagulation factors and rapidly concentrating blood components, and can achieve rapid hemostasis.

11.2.3　Antibacterial dressings

During the use of the hydrogel wound dressings, the hydrogel dressings directly contact the surface of the tissue, which can reduce the loss of body fluids, and it is also necessary to prevent secondary infection of the wound. Therefore, hydrogel dressings should have good antibacterial properties, which can inhibit the growth of bacteria on the wound surface during use, and at the same time prevent the infection of microorganisms outside the body. In order to meet this requirement, antibacterial hydrogel dressings have emerged, which can be obtained by loading antibacterial agents or modifying hydrogel with the antibacterial motif.

The antibacterial agents loaded hydrogels refer to the hydrogels that directly load the antibacterial agent into the hydrogels. According to different types of antibacterial agents, hydrogels loaded with antibacterial agents can be roughly divided into three types. They are hydrogels loaded with metal ions or metal NPs (such as Ag^+, Fe^{3+}, Ag NPs), antibiotics, and non-antibiotics antibacterial drugs. For example, Chen et al. used ferric ethylenediaminetetraacetate (EDTA-Fe^{3+}) to crosslink hyaluronic acid (HA) to obtain antibacterial hydrogels. When being applied to wounds, HA can be degraded at the site of infection, and the hydrogels can locally release Fe^{3+} complexes. These Fe^{3+} complexes can be rapidly absorbed by surrounding bacteria and reduced to Fe^{2+}. Fe^{2+} reacts with hydrogen peroxide (H_2O_2) produced by bacteria and inflammatory cells to form hydroxyl radicals through Fenton reaction to destroy the bacterial structure, thereby achieving sterilization (Figure 11-5).

Unlike hydrogels loaded with antibacterial agents, inherent antibacterial hydrogels refer to hydrogels with inherent antibacterial properties prepared by introducing components with antibacterial functional groups. Inherent antibacterial hydrogels can be divided into cationic polymer hydrogels and antimicrobial peptide-based hydrogels. The inherent antibacterial hydrogels mainly kill the bacteria by interacting with the negatively charged bacterial cell membrane, and the cell membrane structure is destroyed and the intercellular substance flows out. Lei et al. prepared an antibacterial hydrogel based on monodisperse PDA-functionalized bioactive glass NPs and antibacterial polypeptide F127-ε-poly-L-lysine. The nanocomposite hydrogel exhibited highly effective antibacterial properties against bacteria with multidrug resistance and effectively promoted the formation of collagen tissue and the regeneration of blood vessels.

11.2.4　Thermal stimulation wound dressings

As an ancient yet effective method, the application of local heat around the wound can increase blood flow, stimulate the proliferation of fibroblasts, and reduce inflammation. The local heating method can strengthen the metabolism around the wound and promote wound healing. In recent years, many scientific studies have confirmed that the use of photothermal therapy (PTT) can promote wound tissue regeneration, and this therapy has been widely used clinically as adjuvant therapy. Currently, PTT mostly uses lasers with a small area and high energy as the light source, showing excellent tissue penetration ability and minimal damage to surrounding tissues and has been successfully combined with nano-drugs for the treatment of tumor-related or bacterial wounds.

Combining photothermal materials into hydrogels or other scaffold materials is an important way to achieve thermal stimulation wound dressings. For example, Yang et al. developed a multifunctional scaffold containing nano-hydroxyapatite/graphene oxide (nHA/GO) composite particles. Under the NIR irradiation, the scaffold can effectively kill human osteosarcoma cells and also promote tissue regeneration, providing a promising clinical tool for treating osteosarcoma resection tissue damage. In addition, the use of photothermal antibacterial hydrogels are also an important strategy for the treatment of bacterial wound infections. As shown in Figure 11-6, Wang et al. constructed a composite hydrogel (CS/AM NSs hydrogel) with outstanding antibacterial ability by incorporating antimonene nanosheets (AM NSs) with extraordinary photothermal properties into the network structure of chitosan (CS). When being cultured with bacteria, CS/AM NSs hydrogel could aggregate on the surface of the bacteria through the interaction of CS and bacterial cell membrane. Subsequently, the inherent bactericidal properties of CS would kill certain bacteria. Under the NIR, AM NSs could effectively convert light energy into heat energy to eliminate residual bacteria. Due to the synergy between the capture effect of CS and the photothermal effect of AM NSs, CS/AM NSs hydrogel showed good antibacterial properties against *Escherichia coli* (*E. coli*) and *Staphylococcus aureus* (*S. aureus*).

With the abuse of antibiotics, rapid and effective sterilization of wounds infected by drug-resistant bacteria inevitably becomes a serious challenge in the field of wound healing. Chang et al. prepared a multifunctional composite (PDA/Cu-CS) hydrogel mainly composed of polydopamine (PDA) and copper-doped calcium silicate ceramic (Cu-CS). The PDA/Cu complex in the composite hydrogel played a key role in enhancing photothermal performance and antibacterial activity. The unique "hot ions effect" produced by heating copper ions through the photothermal effect of the composite hydrogel showed high-efficiency, rapid, and long-term inhibition of methicillin-resistant *S. aureus* and *E. coli*. The composite hydrogel showed significant biological activity and could effectively remove existing infections in the wound area, and significantly promoted angiogenesis and collagen deposition during the healing process of infectious skin wounds. In addition, Guo et al. developed an injectable double network hydrogel adhesive with high self-healing efficiency and photothermal antibacterial activity to treat multidrug-resistant bacterial infections (MRSA) in the wound. The hydrogel exhibited good tissue adhesion, degradability, photothermal antibacterial activity.

Usually, laser-based PTT still has limitations. Since the penetration depth of NIR is usually less than 1 cm, long-distance light irradiation cannot be achieved, which will hinder its practical application in wound healing. By using appropriate photothermal materials, solar energy can be effectively converted into heat energy. Therefore, it is expected to use sunlight to locally heat the wound to promote wound healing. Zhang et al. proposed a strategy of using self-adhesive photothermal hydrogel films to accelerate wound healing under sunlight (Figure 11-7). The polyacrylamide hydrogel contains PDA and rGO, which can adhere to the wound and convert solar energy into heat energy, thereby locally heating the wound. The increase of local temperature reduces inflammation and enhances epithelial regeneration, angiogenesis, and collagen deposition.

11.2.5　Electrical stimulation wound dressings

As known, a transepithelial/endothelial potential exists in the organism. When the tissue is damaged, the potential will change, thereby generating a stable and constant direct-current (DC) electric field, i.e., the endogenous electric field. Studies have found that the current at the edge of the wound is significantly greater than that at the center of the wound, and the current changes as the wound heals. The internal electrical signal generated by the electric field plays an important role in the healing process of the skin wound. Therefore, by applying an external electric field locally to the wound, it is possible to modify and enhance endogenous bioelectric signals and guide and regulate the distribution, migration, proliferation, and differentiation of fibroblasts, neuronal cells, and endothelial cells, thereby accelerating the orientation of skin tissue repair. Recently, electrical stimulation (ES) therapy at the wound site has been used as an important clinical strategy in the field of tissue repair by reducing wound edema and inflammation, increasing blood microcirculation, and accelerating wound closure.

Wound repair and tissue regeneration are complex processes involving many physiological signals. Therefore, it is possible to use new types of wound dressings with effective biological activity and physiological signal response to accelerating wound healing.

At present, researches about ES hydrogel wound dressings are mainly focused on the preparation of conductive hydrogel electrodes and their applications in wound healing. For example, Lu et al. prepared a rGO-CS/SF hydrogel based on PDA, rGO, chitosan (CS), and silk fibroin (SF). The obtained hydrogel showed good mechanical strength, electrical activity, and anti-oxidizing capability. The composite hydrogels were used as an ES wound dressing. *In vitro* studies have shown that the electroactive rGO-CS/SF hydrogel can respond to electrical signals and promote cell behavior, and it can also reduce cell oxidation by removing excess reactive oxygen species (ROS). Studies in the full-thickness skin defect model *in vivo* showed that it could effectively promote wound healing.

Similarly, Wang et al. prepared a conductive polyHEMA/polypyrrole (PPY) composite hydrogel (Figure 11-8). When this polyHEMA/PPY hydrogel was used to electrically stimulate diabetic rats, the wound healing was much faster than that achieved by the ES strategy based on commercially available electrodes.

In addition, antibacterial properties and mechanical properties should also be considered when designing a conductive hydrogel. Yang et al. developed injectable, biocompatible, self-healing, and conductive hydrogels (PPGS) based on poly(3,4-ethylenedioxythiophene), poly (styrene sulfonate), and guar cement for various wounds. The results showed that PPGS had great potential in the fields of tissue engineering and biomedicine. Lin et al. obtained conductive hydrogels (i. e. , PDA@AgNPs/CPHs) by using PDA-modified silver NPs (PDA @AgNPs), polyaniline, and poly(vinyl alcohol), which exhibited extensive antibacterial activity against gram-negative bacteria and gram-positive bacteria and could monitor the large-scale movement of the human body in real-time. In addition, PDA@AgNPs/CPHs have a significant therapeutic effect on diabetic foot wounds by promoting angiogenesis, accelerating collagen deposition, inhibiting bacterial growth, and controlling wound infections.

In addition, the use of ES therapy in clinical operations is often restricted by bulky equipment, and it is difficult to achieve real-time treatment. There is an urgent need for wearable and point-of-care equipment that can generate an electric field at the wound site for skin wound healing. Therefore, self-powered devices such as enzyme biofuel cells and nanogenerators have also attracted growing attention, which is small in size and can produce ES without the need for a commercial power source. For example, Nishizawa et al. used flexible enzyme electrodes and stretchable hydrogels to prepare a stretchable bio-electric paste with a built-in enzyme biofuel cell, which generated ionic current on the skin surface through an enzyme electrochemical reaction. Animal experiment results showed that the ion current of electrospun fibers can promote wounds to heal faster and smoother. Zhang et al. developed a hybrid skin patch with a self-adhesive hydrogel and piezoelectric nanogenerator (HPSP, Figure 11-9), which consists of a mussel-like adhered hydrogel matrix and oriented PVDF nanofibers as piezoelectric nanogenerators. The HPSP has Young's modulus similar to that of the skin. It can self-adhere to the wound site, and locally generate a voltage caused by motions. As a wearable real-time ES device, the patch greatly accelerates the healing process and shortens the closure time of full-thickness skin defects by about 1/3.

11.2.6 Wound dressings for controlled active ingredients release

The treatment of chronic wounds sometimes requires appropriate supplementation of active ingredients, such as growth factors or certain gas stimulation to facilitate wound healing. Therefore, the development of wound dressings containing the controlled release of active ingredients will play an increasingly important role in the treatment of chronic wounds. The growth factor is a kind of polypeptide substance that regulates cell growth and other cell functions by binding to specific, high-affinity cell membrane receptors. It is used in signal transduction, regulation of cell proliferation and differentiation, and tissue maintenance. Recombinant human epidermal growth factor (rhEGF) is widely used clinically in wound treatment as a biological agent that strongly promotes cell regeneration and tissue repair, but its direct use faces the challenge of requiring long-term low-temperature storage. To this end, Han et al. inserted dopamine into clay nanosheets with partial oxidation and incorporated the nanocomposites into polyacrylamide hydrogels. The hydrogels exhibited repeatable and long-lasting adhesion. In addition, the rhEGF could be loaded into the hydrogels, and the rat full-thickness skin defect experiment showed that the hydrogels can be excellent dressings for accelerating wound healing.

The development of effective yet economical methods to improve wound healing is always highly desirable. Due to the advantages of high treatment efficiency and good biocompatibility, gas therapy by using O_2, NO, H_2S, and others have been proved to have the potential to promote wound healing. Studies have shown that adequate oxygen supply is a prerequisite for wound tissue growth and remodeling. However, insufficient microcirculation at the wound can lead to hypoxia, which is not beneficial for the healing of skin wounds. Therefore, increasing the oxygen content around the wound is one of the most important strategies to promote wound healing. Current oxygen therapies, including hyperbaric oxygen (HBO) and local gaseous oxygen (TGO), mainly use gaseous oxygen delivery, which is not effective in penetrating the skin. Wu et al. developed an oxygen-generating patch made of living microalgae hydrogel, which could generate dissolved oxygen (Figure 11-10). The transport performance of the dissolved oxygen generated by the patch is more than 100 times than TGO. The patch could promote cell proliferation and migration, and tube formation *in vitro*, and improve chronic wound healing and skin graft survival in diabetic mice.

In addition, according to the principle of the Bohr effect, CO_2 can be used instead of direct use of O_2 for skin wound treatment to promote healing. When CO_2 dissolves in the tissue surrounding the wound, the decrease in pH will trigger the hemoglobin to release more O_2 locally at the site, thereby effectively promoting the healing of the wound. Compared with the direct use of O_2, CO_2 has a high solubility in body fluids, thus it is more convenient for controlled delivery. In particular, the strategy of accurately releasing CO_2 gas on the wound on demand has attracted more and more attention.

Yeh et al. designed a metal ion-ligand coordination NP and used NIR to trigger CO_2 release for wound healing. Zhang et al. developed a photothermal hydrogel for on-demand and local delivery of CO_2 by combining thermally responsive block copolymer (BCP) of Pluronic F127 and carbon NP (CNP) with amino groups to accelerate the healing of skin wounds. When the hybrid hydrogel was irradiated with light, CNP can convert light energy into heat energy, triggering the decomposition of bicarbonate and local release CO_2 at the wound site, which speeded up wound healing by improving local microcirculation and increasing tissue oxygen concentration. In addition, gas delivery can also be combined with photothermal therapy (Figure 11-11).

11.3 Functionalized Polymer Fiber Dressings

Polymer fibers are also important dressing materials used in skin wound treatment. Medical fiber materials used in the human body must have good biocompatibility. Therefore, the current research on functionalized polymer fiber dressings has important significance and broad development prospects.

11.3.1 Preparation of polymer fibers

Ideal wound dressings should be non-toxic, non-sensitizing, and they can allow gas exchange, absorb wound exudate to protect the wound, form a microenvironment conducive to wound healing, and inhibit bacterial growth. Commonly used fiber dressings, such as cotton gauze, were used for clinical wound care and treatment by covering the damaged skin. However, gauze is prone to cause adhesion between the wound and the dressing, which causes secondary trauma and bacterial growth. In recent years, the preparation technology of fiber dressings has developed vigorously. The micro-nano structured fiber membrane with high specific surface area and high porosity is a new type of wound dressing. Compared with other dressings, it is lighter, thinner, more breathable, and has various functional directions. There are many technologies for preparing micro-nano structured fiber membranes, such as stretching method, template synthesis, phase separation, self-assembly, and electrospinning technology.

Among the preparative technologies of fiber dressings, electrospinning technology is currently the most widely studied technology. Electrospinning technology is a fiber production method that uses electric force to draw charged threads of polymer solutions or polymer melts up to fiber diameters in the order of some hundred nanometers. The electrospinning process is simple, low cost, with wide selection of materials.

Compared with other forms of fiber materials, electrospun fibers show many advantages in medical dressings. Firstly, they have structural advantages. The diameter of the fibers obtained by electrospinning technology ranged from a few nanometers to a few microns, and it has good mechanical strength. Its multi-level geometric size is similar to the microstructure and biological function of the extracellular matrix (ECM). At present, the electrospun fiber membrane is often used as a scaffold material for tissue engineering. It provides support and guidance for the proliferation and migration of cells and the transfer of active substances, which is conducive to angiogenesis and tissue remodeling. Secondly, electrospun fiber membrane usually has high permeability and porosity, which can quickly absorb the tissue fluid that appears in the wound, facilitating the ventilation of the wound and preventing bacterial infection. Thirdly, the electrospun fiber membrane can also achieve an excellent hemostatic effect by optimizing the fiber material and the electrospun fiber membrane can be used as a drug loading platform to enhance its drug delivery efficacy. For example, it can be loaded with anti-inflammatory drugs, growth factors, antibiotics, etc., and the drug delivery speed can be adjusted as needed to promote wound healing. Figure 11-12 shows the commonly used strategies for directly preparing drug-loaded electrospun fiber dressings, including blending, coaxial, and emulsion electrospinning. Blended electrospinning usually produces fibers containing active agents dispersed throughout the fiber, while coaxial electrospinning and emulsion electrospinning synthesize core/shell morphologies well to meet different drug loading requirements.

In addition, post-treatment of electrospun fibers can also improve wound healing properties. Generally, the surface of electrospun fibers may lack the properties required for specific biological applications. The property can be imparted by electrostatic adhesion, dip coating, layer-by-layer assembly, or surface chemical reaction. For example, PVA electrospun membranes can be coated with chitosan by simply immersing the PVA membrane in a chitosan solution, which can provide instant hemostatic activity. Epidermal growth factor (EGF) can also be fixed on the surface of the fibers through a facile grafting strategy. *In vivo* wound studies have shown that EGF conjugated fibers can increase keratinocyte-specific genes. Therefore, the incorporation of growth factors can promote gene expression, thereby accelerating wound healing.

11.3.2 Surface wettability

Some serious skin wounds (e. g. , scalds, ulcers) can cause excessive exudation of wound tissue fluid, forming highly exudative wounds that are difficult to heal. The amount of exudation in 24 h can exceed 10 mL, and the dressing infiltration rate is more than 75%. It is also easy to cause adhesion of the wound and dressing, and will cause great pain and inconvenience to the patients. Therefore, high-exudation wounds have higher requirements for the surface infiltration performance of dressing materials. Dressings for high-exudation wounds need to absorb and drain exudate, while they must also maintain the moistness of the wound to promote healing. The commonly used gauze cannot keep moist, which would delay wound healing. At present, wet dressings (e. g. , alginate gels, hydrophilic fibers, foams, and silver ion dressings) can absorb wound tissue fluid and keep the wound moist, promote granulation growth and resist bacterial infections, and are the first choice for high-exudation wounds. Excessive wound tissue fluid caused excessive wound hydration is a serious problem. Generally, traditional wet hydrophilic dressings can absorb part of the wound tissue fluid, but due to its inherent hydrophilicity, it is inevitably to produce wound tissue fluid at the interface between the wound and the dressing. Residual wound tissue fluid will continue to hydrate the wound and complicate the healing process. The biological interface plays an important role in the interaction between wound tissue fluid and biological materials. The surface wettability of the wound dressings usually affects the wetting behavior of the tissue fluid around the wound. Like most traditional dressings, hydrophilic materials are easily wetted by wound tissue fluid, which can over-hydrate the wound. On the contrary, as a waterproof outer layer of the dressing, hydrophobic materials can prevent accidental contact of external liquid with the wound, but they cannot promote the removal of wound tissue fluid. Recently, several asymmetrically (Janus type) wetting materials have shown unique ability to transfer fluid, such as polyester fabrics with wettability gradients, polyurethane (PU)/poly (vinyl acetate) composite fiber membranes, and single-sided fluorinated cotton fabric membrane (Figure 11-13). Therefore, manipulation of surface wettability may provide opportunities for designing wound dressings with effective wound tissue fluid capabilities.

Wang et al. prepared electrospun hydrophobic polyurethane (PU) nanofiber membranes onto a hydrophilic ultrafine fiber network and constructed a self-absorbent dressing as a biological fluid pump (Figure 11-14). The network provided drainage force to pump excess biological fluid through the hydrophobic nanofiber membrane to discharge the fluid unidirectionally from the hydrophobic side to the hydrophilic side, thereby preventing the biological fluid from wetting the wound. In the infected wound model, they showed that this self-pumping dressing can heal wounds faster than conventional dressings. This study provided new clues to manage excess biological fluid around wounds to promote faster wound healing and the self-pumping dressing has great potential as the next generation dressing for clinical wound healing.

11.3.3 Hemostatic fiber dressings

Traditional hemostatic materials and products are mainly hemostatic gauze, bandages, and hemostatic sponges. Clinical applications have found that these products have poor hemostatic effects and do not have the ability to actively stop bleeding. They can only meet the hemostatic needs of general or conventional bleeding wounds, and they are not degradable in the body. It is difficult to be absorbed by the body, therefore their applications are quite limited. In recent years, scientists have discovered that the surface modification of gauze, sponge, etc. , with a layer of porous, soft, and water-absorbing fibers with excellent adhesion and blood coagulation will greatly improve their hemostatic properties. For example, Hammond et al. loaded RADA16-I self-assembled polypeptide nanofibers on the surface of gauze or gelatin sponge through layer-by-layer assembly technology to obtain a fast hemostatic gauze or sponge with active coagulation function. Since RADA16-I self-assembled polypeptide nanofibers can effectively aggregate and cross-linking components in the blood, the hemostatic effect of gauze or sponge is greatly improved. Yu et al. prepared hybrid electrospun poly(vinyl pyrrolidone) fibers with curcumin-loaded mesoporous silica for rapid hemostasis and antibacterial wound dressings. It is found that the nanofiber mat has no obvious toxic effect on cell growth, and can enhance the antibacterial effect on *S. aureus in vitro*. In addition, the hybrid nanofiber mat could quickly turn into hydrogel when in contact with blood and then activated the coagulation system to prevent bleeding from the wound.

In addition, based on improving the hemostatic effect of the materials, further optimization of the preparation process has also aroused the widespread interest of scientific researchers. Long et al. developed a portable electrospun device (about 150 grams) for outdoor use, which can realize the green synthesis of CuS composite nanofibers. These composite nanofibers can be deposited on the wound *in-situ* while achieving rapid hemostasis and elimination of super bacteria outdoors without the use of other materials or equipments. The compactness of this *in-situ* electrospun nanofiber on the rough surface of the wound is better than that of the traditional nanofiber pad pressed on the wound. Therefore, nanofibers can not only accelerate hemostasis (< 6 s), but also shorten the healing time of superbacterial infection wounds (18 days). These dual-function nanofibers combined with portable electrospun equipment can be used for outdoor rapid hemostasis and simultaneous ablation of super bacteria, which can significantly improve outdoor first aid (Figure 11-15).

11.3.4 Antibacterial fiber dressings

Bacterial infections seriously threaten the wound healing process, and preventing bacterial infections is essential to complete wound healing. The addition of inorganic, organic, or metal antibacterial agents to electrospun fibers has always been an important strategy for obtaining antibacterial fiber dressings.

At present, in clinical operations, systemic antibiotics are often used to treat wound infections. The long-term use of antibiotics with strong potency and rapid sterilization will bring bacterial resistance. If the release concentration is less than the minimum inhibitory concentration, the adverse consequences of resistance will be aggravated. Therefore, controlling a reasonable antibiotic release concentration has always been an important aspect of antibacterial fiber dressings. He et al. loaded enrofloxacin antibiotics into PVDF electrospun nanofibers. Within 0-12 h, the drug release showed a burst behavior, and the cumulative release reached 60%, which can quickly kill bacteria, and then the residual drug continued to release up to 3 days. The sustainable release of the loaded drugs can effectively inhibit the proliferation of bacteria.

In addition, many studies have shown that loading inorganic antibacterial agents including Ag, Zn, and carbon-based nanomaterials, into fibers can kill bacteria, reduce inflammation, or promote epithelial proliferation and regeneration. Some researchers used PVA as a reducing agent to prepare Ag-NPs loaded PVA electrospun fibers. The fibers showed inhibitory effects on *E. coli* and *S. aureus*, and the antibacterial efficiency was much higher than that of wound dressings loaded with silver nitrate.

Chang et al. synthesized zinc-doped hollow mesoporous silica nanospheres (HMZS) by the sol-gel method and loaded them into polycaprolactone (PCL) electrospun fiber to prepare a new type of wound healing dressing. As shown in Figure 11-16, the composite electrospun fiber dressing can promote angiogenesis and skin regeneration by releasing Si ions, and enhance hair follicle regeneration and inhibit bacterial growth by releasing zinc ions.

Besides these inorganic materials, some organic polymers, such as quaternary ammonium salts, guanidine group-containing polymers, or antibacterial peptides, also have excellent antibacterial properties. Loading these motifs into the electrospun fiber membranes can even overcome multidrug resistance (MDR) bacterial infections. Recently, Lei et al. developed an elastic, photoluminescence, and antibacterial hybrid polypeptide-based nanofiber matrix as a multifunctional platform for inhibiting MDR bacteria and enhancing wound healing (Figure 11-17). The hybrid nanofiber matrix is composed of poly(citrate)-ε-polylysine (PCE) and polycaprolactone (PCL). The PCL-PCE hybrid nanofiber matrix exhibits biomimetic elastic behavior, strong antibacterial activity (including the ability to kill MDR bacteria) and excellent biocompatibility, and can effectively prevent wound infections caused by MDR bacteria and enhance wound healing and skin regeneration.

11.4   Challenges and Perspectives

In this chapter, we have reviewed the recent progress of functionalized polymer dressings in promoting wound healing and hemostasis. By using hydrogels, functionalized polymer fibers, etc., and tuning their chemical composition, network structure, surface wettability, and other features, they can effectively achieve unique functions such as self-adhesion, antibacterial, and exudate removal, thereby promoting wound healing. In addition, the hydrogels can be used as a carrier to effectively combine the photothermal components, nanogenerators, and functional nanocarriers to achieve external stimulation to the wound and promote wound repair. Compared with traditional dressings, functionalized polymer dressings are aimed at the mechanism of wound repair, possible infections and other issues, by activating autologous factors to promote wound repair and inhibit bacterial infections, so as to achieve the purpose of promoting wound healing, which is of great importance as the next-generation dressings. However, we have also noticed that for some chronic hard-to-heal wounds and wounds with drug-resistant bacteria infection, achieving rapid healing is still an important challenge in this field. Moreover, these functionalized polymer dressings are still in their infancy and are more verified in small animal models. It remains challenging to verify their functions in wound healing in large animals and humans. Especially for some functionalized dressings that use nanoparticles and nanodevices, the biological safety of these materials needs to be further verified to ensure that they will not be greatly affected because of leakage and shedding issues. In addition, the development of more convenient and low-cost preparative methods for these functionalized polymer dressings to come true still requires the in-depth crossover and cooperation of scientists and engineers from materials science, clinical medicine, and related industries. With the integration of different disciplines and the rapid development of materials science, interface science, nanodevices, and other related fields, we believe that in the near future, more functionalized polymer dressings will appear and be used in clinical treatment, and ultimately benefiting the patients.

Questions

1. Describe the advantages and disadvantages of traditional dry and hydrogel-based wound dressings.

2. What are the preparative methods of polymer fiber dressings?

3. What external environmental factors are conducive to wound healing? How to achieve?

4. What are the requirements for using hydrogels as wound dressings?

5. How to improve the effect of wound repair?

Extended Reading

[1] 丁炎明. 伤口护理学[M]. 北京:人民卫生出版社,2017.

[2] 陈孝平. 外科学[M]. 2 版. 北京:人民卫生出版社,2010.

[3] 薛巍,张渊明. 生物医用水凝胶[M]. 广州:暨南大学出版社,2012.

[4] Ye Q,Zhou F,Liu W M. Bioinspired catecholic chemistry for surface modification[J]. Chem Soc Rev,2011,40(7):4244-4258.

[5] Homaeigohar S,Boccaccini A R. Antibacterial biohybrid nanofibers for wound dressings [J]. Acta Biomater,2020,107:25-49.

(Zhang Lianbin)